Essentials of Cardiac Imaging

2nd Edition

Foreword

James T. T. Chen has been repeatedly and appropriately characterized by medical students and residents as a real "national treasure." The depth and breadth of his experience in cardiac imaging, coupled with his extraordinary ability to communicate complex concepts in an easily understood fashion, have made him a favorite of generations of physicians. Having had the opportunity to work closely with Dr. Chen for nearly twenty years, I can personally attest to his outstanding abilities as both a diagnostician and teacher. We were delighted when, in 1987, Dr. Chen published the first edition of *Essentials of Cardiac Roentgenology*. It was widely predicted at that time that the book would become a classic, and indeed it has emerged as a favorite text for residents, medical students, and faculty interested in this fascinating field.

Since publication of that edition, there have been important advances in cardiac imaging. In this new edition, Dr. Chen, with the help of well-recognized experts, has updated the book to include comprehensive discussions of such technologies as computed tomography, magnetic resonance imaging, nuclear cardiology, and echocardiography. In keeping with the tenets of modern medicine and, more importantly, with his own personal philosophy, Dr. Chen stresses that one must always choose the least invasive, least expensive, and most effective method for establishing a diagnosis. He routinely emphasizes evaluation beginning with the simplest, least expensive procedures and moving toward more sophisticated and expensive procedures only as required to establish specific diagnoses. While he reviews multiple ways to establish a diagnosis, he continually indicates to the physician the least invasive, most cost-effective manner to arrive at the correct one.

Dr. Chen has incorporated clinical information as it relates to cardiac imaging in order to stress that it is the whole patient who must be evaluated, not simply the images. As a result, while clearly directed toward radiologists, *Essentials of Cardiac Imaging*, 2nd edition, will also prove extremely useful for cardiologists, thoracic surgeons, and their trainees.

The first edition of *Essentials of Cardiac Roentgenology*, quickly became a classic in its field. The second edition provides further enhancements and refinements to an already-outstanding text while preserving the practicality, depth, and breadth of experience Dr. Chen has conveyed to legions of physicians during a career spanning more than thirty years. The text is a fitting reflection of Dr. Chen's excellence and strongly reflects his commitment to his field and his students. Those who have not had the opportunity to work directly with him will profit immensely from the wisdom shared through *Essentials of Cardiac Imaging*, 2nd edition.

Carl E. Ravin, M.D.
Professor and Chairman
Department of Radiology
Duke University
Durham, North Carolina

Essentials of Cardiac Imaging

2nd Edition

James T. T. Chen, M.D.
Professor of Radiology
Duke University School of Medicine
Durham, North Carolina

With contributions by

R. Edward Coleman
Donald P. Frush
Michael W. Hanson
Robert J. Optican
Edward F. Patz, Jr.
H. Dirk Sostman
William Stanford
Jean-Paul Vallée

FOREWORD BY CARL E. RAVIN, M.D.
Professor and Chairman
Department of Radiology
Duke University School of Medicine
Durham, North Carolina

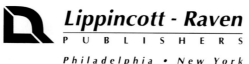

Lippincott - Raven
P U B L I S H E R S
Philadelphia • New York

Acquisitions Editor: James Ryan
Developmental Editor: Brian Brown
Manufacturing Manager: Dennis Teston
Production Manager: Maxine Langweil
Production Editor: Jonathan Geffner
Cover Designer: Joseph DePinho
Indexer: Mary Kidd
Compositor: Maryland Composition
Printer: Courier Westford

Library of Congress Cataloging-in-Publication Data
Chen, James T. T.
      Essentials of cardiac imaging / James T. T. Chen, with contributions by
R. Edward Coleman . . .   [et al.]; foreword by Carl E. Ravin—2nd ed.
        p. cm.
      Rev. ed. of: Essentials of cardiac roentgenology / James T. T.
Chen. c1987.
      Includes bibliographical references and index.
      ISBN 0-316-13784-7
      1. Heart—Imaging. 2. Heart—Diseases—Diagnosis. I. Chen,
James T. T. Essentials of cardiac roentgenology.
      [DNLM: 1. Heart Diseases—diagnosis. 2. Diagnostic Imaging—
methods.   WG 141 C518e   1997]
      RC683.5.I42C47   1998
      616.1′20754vdc21
      DNLM/DLC
      for Library of Congress   97-19921
                                                              CIP

To my wife, Alice

Contents

Contributors

R. Edward Coleman, M.D. *Professor and Director, Division of Nuclear Medicine, Department of Radiology, Duke University Medical Center, P.O. Box 3949, Durham, North Carolina 27710*

Donald P. Frush, M.D. *Assistant Professor, Division of Pediatric Radiology, Department of Radiology, Duke University Medical Center, Erwin Road, Durham, North Carolina 27710*

Michael W. Hanson, M.D. *Assistant Professor of Radiology and Internal Medicine, Chief of Nuclear Cardiology, Division of Nuclear Medicine, Department of Radiology, Duke University Medical Center, P.O. Box 3949, Durham, North Carolina 27710*

Robert J. Optican, M.D. *Department of Diagnostic Radiology, Baptist Memorial Hospital, 899 Madison, Memphis, Tennessee 38103*

Edward F. Patz, M.D. *Associate Professor, Department of Radiology, Duke University Medical Center, P.O. Box 3808, Durham, North Carolina 27710*

H. Dirk Sostman, M.D. *Professor and Chairman, Department of Radiology, New York Hospital–Cornell Medical Center, 525 East 68th Street, New York, New York 10021*

William Stanford, M.D. *Professor, Department of Radiology, The University of Iowa College of Medicine, 200 Hawkins Drive, Iowa City, Iowa 52242*

Jean-Paul Vallée, M.D. *Research Fellow, Center of Advanced Resonance Magnetic Imaging, Department of Radiology, Duke University Medical Center, Durham, North Carolina 27710; University Hospital of Geneva, Division of Radiodiagnostic, 24, Micheli-du-Crest, 1211 Geneva 14, Switzerland*

Preface to First Edition

The purpose of *Essentials of Cardiac Roentgenology* is to provide a practical approach to cardiac roentgenology in light of pathophysiology and clinical information. Such basic skill, once acquired, is equally effective in the interpretation of images obtained by other cardiac diagnostic procedures.

There are seventeen chapters. The first five provide background information crucial to the understanding of the following twelve, which deal with the full spectrum of cardiac problems. An attempt is made to strike a balance between congenital and acquired diseases. In order to define the role of cardiac roentgenology in the age of high technology, other imaging modalities such as angiocardiography, echocardiography, scintigraphy, computed tomography, magnetic resonance imaging, and digital subtraction angiocardiography are briefly introduced. The chapters on pulmonary vascularity, cardiovascular calcifications, and cardiac fluoroscopy are particularly comprehensive because of their paramount importance in the practice of cardiac radiology.

Emphasis has been placed on diagnostic signs of common diseases. For example, any fluoroscopically detected coronary calcification in the presence of anginal chest pain is diagnostic of occlusive coronary artery disease 94% of the time.

Statistical guidance to the interpretation of roentgen signs is also stressed because of its high predictive value. A right-sided aortic arch with mirror-image branching, for example, is associated with serious intracardiac defects in 98% of cases; of these, over 90% will turn out to be tetralogy of Fallot.

By deriving full diagnostic information from the chest roentgenogram and by learning the potential of other imaging techniques, the reader should be in a position to decide whether, and what, additional diagnostic procedures are needed, as well as to plan the strategy for catheterization or surgery.

Although primarily intended for radiologists, cardiologists, and thoracic surgeons, this text should also prove valuable to the medical students, residents, and fellows who need to master the subject of cardiac imaging.

J. T. T. C.

Preface

Since the publication of the first edition of this book, under the title *Essentials of the Cardiac Roentgenology*, the improvements in cardiac imaging have been swift and abundant. This makes the task of choosing and sequencing a wide variety of modalities in the diagnosis of a given disease more challenging than ever. With the help of experts both at Duke and other medical centers, I have tried to provide a concise state-of-the-art book encompassing all major areas of cardiac imaging with special emphasis on the role of each technique in patient management. Although such discussions thread through each of the 20 chapters, they are the theme of Chapter 1, entitled ''Cardiac Imaging Systems.''

Chapters 2 to 6 focus in detail on radiography, computed tomography, magnetic resonance imaging, nuclear cardiology, and echocardiography, respectively, addressing the advantages and limitations of each and their usefulness relative to each other. The interpretation of data obtained from cardiac catheterization is the theme of Chapter 7, entitled ''Cardiovascular Hemodynamics.'' The next three chapters are also fundamental to the diagosis of heart disease. These are: Chapter 8, entitled ''Pulmonary Vascularity;'' Chapter 9, entitled ''Radiographic Anatomy;'' and Chapter 10, entitled ''Cardiovascular Calcifications.'' The basics of cardiac imaging have thus been presented in the first ten chapters. Such background information is crucial to the understanding of clinical applications of each modality discussed in the second ten chapters.

Efforts have also been made to incorporate clinical information to the discussion of cardiac imaging so that the whole patient, not just his or her cardiac images, can be seen in better perspective. Although primarily intended for radiologists, this work should prove useful also for cardiologists, thoracic surgeons, and their trainees. Some senior medical students may also find the materials relevant to their basic needs.

Acknowledgements

I am grateful to Charles E. Putman and Carl E. Ravin for their continued support and encouragement, to the contributors of new chapters, and to my colleagues at Duke in radiology and in cardiology, thoracic surgery and pediatric and adult catherization laboratories. Many of the best illustrations are angiocardiograms from the Pediatric Catheterization Laboratory, reflecting the excellent work being done there.

My best ideas came from the daily contact with my residents, fellows, colleagues, and students throughout my years of teaching. Their intellectual curiosity and questioning minds make teaching a learning experience. Their feedback after going out into the real world continues to be my inspiration for continual improvement.

My thanks to Louis Humphrey and his staff for a smoothly running computer, to Duke Medical Photography, to Keith A. Tarpley in the Radiology Photo Lab, and to Vera Mills for getting materials ready at all times.

I would also like to extend a word of appreciation for the cordial cooperation and valuable suggestions from Nancy E. Chorpenning, Tammerly Booth, and Richard Wilcox. Special thanks to James Ryan, Acquisitions Editor; Brian Brown, Developmental Editor; and Jonathan Geffner, Senior Production Editor at Lippincott–Raven Publishers.

Essentials of Cardiac Imaging

2nd Edition

Essentials of Cardiac Imaging,
James T. T. Chen,
Lippincott–Raven Publishers, Philadelphia © 1998.

CHAPTER 1

Cardiac Imaging Systems

James T. T. Chen

The heart can be imaged in a number of ways, from the simple and economical to the sophisticated and expensive. The former category is exemplified by radiography and the latter by magnetic resonance imaging (MRI), but they range over the spectrum to include echocardiography, angiocardiography, nuclear imaging, and computed tomography (CT). In terms of cost-effectiveness, we should always choose the less invasive, the less expensive, and the more effective method for our patients. Such important decisions should be made on two bases: a thorough understanding of the heart in health and disease and complete familiarity with the advantages and limitations of each imaging method.

RADIOGRAPHY AND FLUOROSCOPY

Despite the advent of newer and more sophisticated techniques, radiography aided by fluoroscopy remains the mainstay of cardiac imaging because of its ready availability (usually it is the first examination), its familiar presentation format, and its established value in most areas of cardiology. One certainly should try to derive full diagnostic information from the first examination before considering additional tests (1). More sophisticated, invasive, and expensive methods should be considered when the risk assumed (as for selective angiocardiography) is less than the potential achievable benefit.

In certain cases, a good deal of information can first be extracted from chest radiographs, thus making additional studies almost unnecessary. In congenital valvular aortic stenosis in patients older than 40 years, the combination of a mildly prominent left ventricle and clear lungs speaks for the absence of heart failure (Fig. 1-1). The isolated ascending aortic dilatation suggests chronic disease and therefore the likelihood of a congenital etiology (Fig. 1-1). The severity of the stenosis is evidenced by a large area of valvular calcifi-

cation (Fig. 1-2). The pattern of calcification (Fig. 1-2; see also **Fig. 10-8D,E**) is also suggestive of a bicuspid valve (see **Chapter 11** and **Table 10-1**). The doming of the thickened aortic valve is more easily visible on angiocardiography (Fig. 1-3), echocardiography (Fig. 1-4), and electron beam CT than other modalities.

One can also see the striking poststenotic dilatation of the aorta on angiocardiography (Fig. 1-3) and spin-echo MRI (Fig. 1-5). To show the interior changes of a severely hypertrophied left ventricle, MR images are the best (Fig. 1-5). Calcified aortic valves can also be depicted with gradient-echo MRI (Fig. 1-6), but the best technique for this purpose is electron beam CT (Fig. 1-7) (2). For practical purposes, in addition to chest radiographs, the only other preoperative assessment that may be needed is transthoracic echocardiography. This test serves to rule out other cardiovascular abnormalities, to estimate the systolic gradient across the valve, and to assess left ventricular function (see **Chapter 6**).

In a symptomatic population, any fluoroscopically detected coronary calcification (Fig. 1-8) is diagnostic of major atherosclerotic coronary artery stenosis 94 percent of the time (3). The sensitivity of this test is, however, rather low at 40%. Radiography has even poorer sensitivity, but grossly calcified vessels are clearly visible on film (Fig. 1-9). Electron beam CT is the most sensitive tool in the detection of coronary calcification (Fig. 1-10) and, therefore, also in the identification of early coronary atherosclerosis in asymptomatic individuals with known risk factors. Aggressive therapeutic intervention in these people may lessen their risk of future coronary events (see **Chapter 3**).

Cardiac fluoroscopy can also help determine whether and what additional imaging procedures are needed for those with fluoroscopically detected coronary calcification. In the presence of diffuse and severe left ventricular asynergy (indicative of significant myocardial ischemia and dysfunction), for example, the next test should probably be PET (positron emission tomography) to assess myocardial viability before echocardiography, exercise or pharmacologic

Department of Radiology, Duke University School of Medicine, Durham, North Carolina 27710, U.S.A.

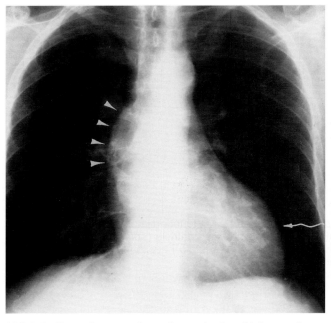

FIG 1-1. Posterior–anterior radiograph of a middle-aged man with congenital valvular aortic stenosis (AS) (same patient as shown in **Fig. 11-1A**). There is only mild cardiomegaly with increased convexity of the hypertrophied left ventricle (*arrow*). The ascending aorta is markedly dilated (*arrow-heads*).

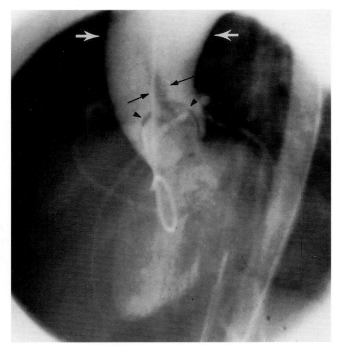

FIG 1-3. Aortogram of patient with valvular AS (same patient as shown in **Fig. 11-6A**) shows late opacification of the left ventricle due to changing catheter position during the injection of contrast medium. Note the negative jet (*small opposing arrows*), doming of the thickened aortic valve (*arrowheads*), and marked poststenotic dilatation of the ascending aorta (*large opposing arrows*).

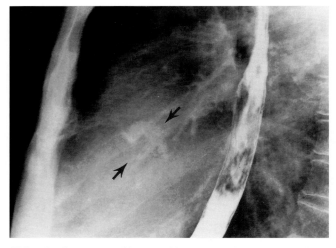

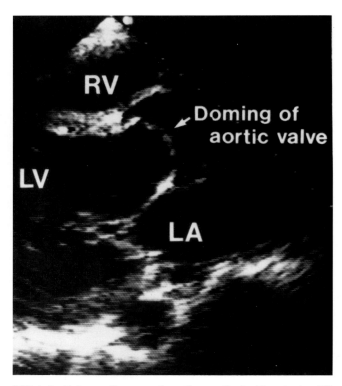

FIG 1-2. A 55-year-old man with exertional dyspnea and angina pectoris. The lateral radiograph shows a heavily calcified aortic valve (*arrow*) indicative of severe aortic stenosis. Moreover, the shape of the calcium deposit is suggestive of one of the patterns of a bicuspid valve (the "mushroom" type) (compare with **Fig. 10-8D,E**).

FIG 1-4. Echocardiogram of another patient with valvular AS shows a similar updoming of the stenotic aortic valve (*arrow*). RV, right ventricle; LV, left ventricle; LA, left atrium.

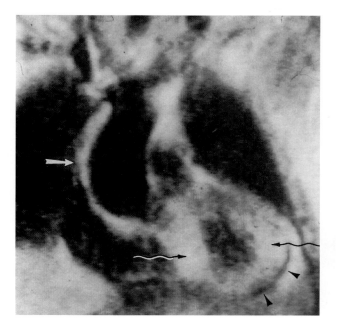

FIG 1-5. Coronal spin-echo MR image of a patient with valvular AS shows considerable poststenotic dilatation of the aorta (*arrow*), markedly hypertrophied left ventricle (*spiral arrows*), and normal pericardium (*arrowheads*). Also note that the volume in the left ventricle is actually smaller than normal. (Reproduced with permission from Lieberman JM, Alfidi RJ, Nelson AD, et al. Gated magnetic resonance imaging of the normal and diseased heart. *Radiology* 1984;152:465–470.)

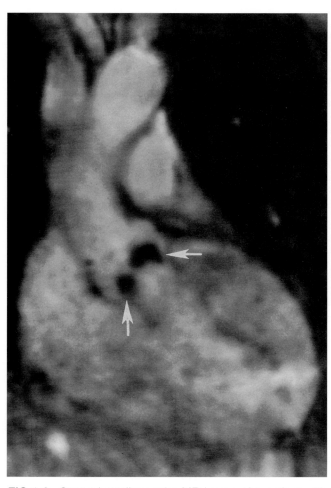

FIG 1-6. Coronal gradient-echo MR image of a patient with valvular AS shows signal-void areas (*arrows*) representing the calcified valve.

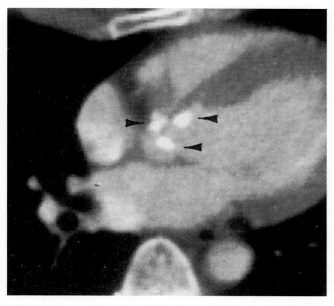

FIG 1-7. Long-axis view of the heart obtained with electron beam CT demonstrates discrete calcification of all three aortic cusps (*arrowheads*). (Reproduced with permission from Stanford W, Rumberger JA. *Ultrafast computed tomography in cardiac imaging: principles and practice.* Mt. Kisco, N.Y.: Futura, 1992.)

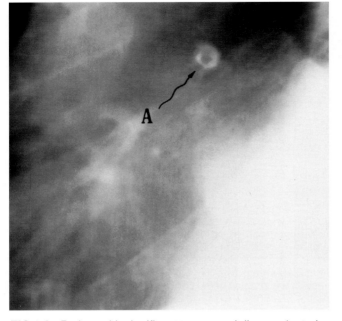

FIG 1-8. Patient with significant two-vessel disease (anterior descending and right coronary artery). The only calcified coronary artery visible (*arrow*) on fluoroscopy (as a ring-like density) is the origin of the anterior descending artery in the left anterior oblique (LAO) view. A, anterior descending artery.

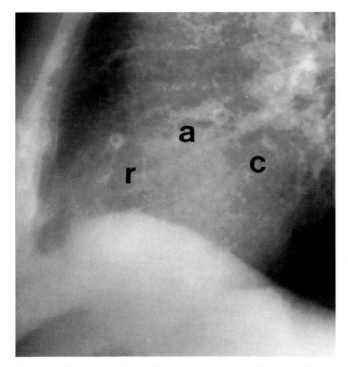

FIG 1-9. Patient with significant three-vessel disease. On the lateral chest radiograph there is heavy calcification of all three major coronary arteries. a, anterior descending; c, circumflex; r, right.

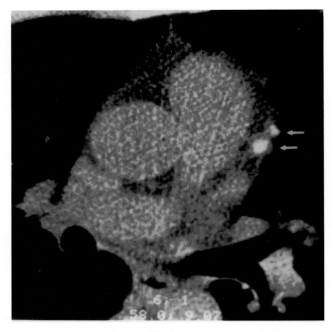

FIG 1-10. Electron beam CT shows discrete calcific plaques (*arrows*) in the anterior descending coronary artery.

stress testing, and cardiac catheterization. Although it is more expensive, PET has proved superior in assessing the viability of the myocardium in the context of severe ischemia and asynergy (4) (see **Chapter 5**). If the myocardium is viable, these patients may recover their contractile function after revascularization in 75% to 85% of the segment. If not, the only surgery to be considered is cardiac transplantation. In the long run, PET may prove to be more cost-effective. If asynergy is confined to one segment of the heart—even with accompanying congestive heart failure—cardiac catheterization, left ventriculography, and selective coronary arteriography should probably be done in preparation for coronary artery bypass procedures, aneurysmectomy, or mitral valve repair.

For the diagnosis of pericardial effusion, almost all imaging methods are applicable (5). However, for practical purposes, only echocardiography (Fig. 1-11) is needed if radiographs have not already provided the definitive diagnosis (Fig. 1-12). If echocardiography proves to be technically difficult to perform because of obstructive emphysema, extreme obesity, marked chest deformity, or poor cooperation on the part of the patient, CT should be the next choice (Fig. 1-13) (see **Chapter 3**). Cardiac fluoroscopy is a valuable adjunct to chest radiography for its ability to image the highly mobile subepicardial fat stripes. Once the fat stripe is found, the pericardium will be easily identified as a linear or bandlike density immediately in front of the lucent fat (Fig. 1-5; see also **Chapter 2**). The efficacy of MRI for evaluating the pericardium has been proved (Figs. 1-5 and 1-14; see also **Chapter 4**), but it should not be the first choice when simpler techniques can provide a quick and

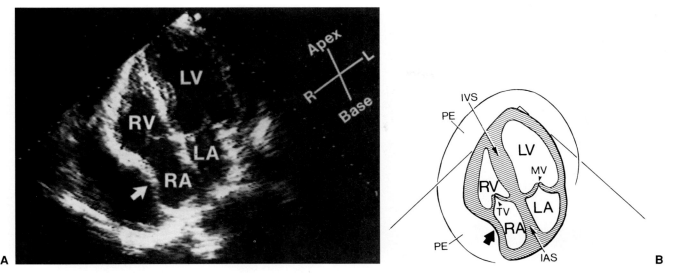

FIG 1-11. Transthoracic echocardiogram (**A**) and diagram (**B**) show systolic compression of the right atrium (RA) by the pericardial effusion (PE), suggesting the presence of cardiac tamponade. The same patient is shown in **Fig. 14-21**. LA, left atrium; LV, left ventricle; RV, right ventricle; RA, right atrium; IVS, interventricular septum; IAS, interatrial septum.

reliable diagnosis. Pericardiocentesis coupled with pneumopericardium is excellent for making visible the two layers of the pericardium (see **Fig. 14-14**), but it should be undertaken only for treating cardiac tamponade because of its invasive nature.

ECHOCARDIOGRAPHY

Echocardiography uses reflected, pulsed ultrasound to make visible cardiac structures. The ultrasound waves are generated when an appropriate piezoelectric crystal is struck by alternating electric current. The sound waves so produced have high frequencies that are far beyond the audible range.

The piezoelectric crystal can also convert mechanical energy into electrical energy. Therefore, the transducer used in echocardiography is both a transmitter and a receiver of ultrasound pulses. Unlike x-rays, ultrasound waves require matter to propagate, and they may be viewed as compression and relaxation of the propagating medium in the direction of the beam. At any interface between tissues of different density and elasticity (different acoustic impedances), the ultrasound waves are reflected back to the transducer. The returned echo is represented on the oscilloscope as target spikes in the amplitude modulation (A-mode), dots in the brightness modulation (B-mode), or lines in the time motion modulation (M-mode) (6) (see **Fig. 6-1**). Since blood has

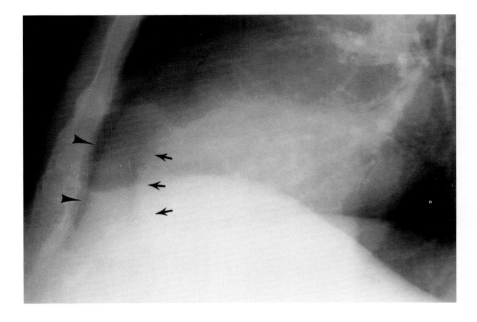

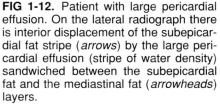

FIG 1-12. Patient with large pericardial effusion. On the lateral radiograph there is interior displacement of the subepicardial fat stripe (*arrows*) by the large pericardial effusion (stripe of water density) sandwiched between the subepicardial fat and the mediastinal fat (*arrowheads*) layers.

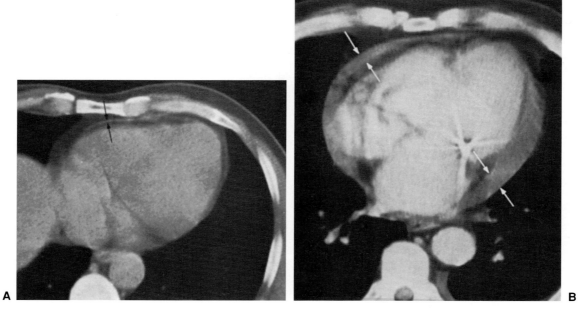

FIG 1-13. Conventional CT slices show normal pericardium (**A**) and large pericardial effusion (**B**).

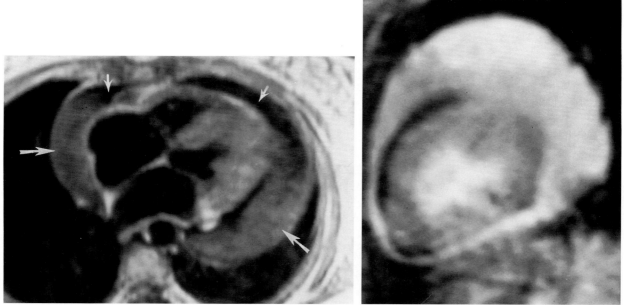

FIG 1-14. A 41-year-old woman with diffuse connective tissue disease. Her spin-echo MR image (**A**) shows a large pericardial effusion (*arrows*). The usual low-intensity pericardial effusion (*small arrows*) is seen superiorly and anteriorly. The protein elements within the effusion (*large arrows*) have gravitated to the inferior and posterior compartments of the pericardium. Her gradient-echo sagittal MR image (**B**) shows a large effusion distributed mainly in the superior and posterior portions of the pericardial cavity.

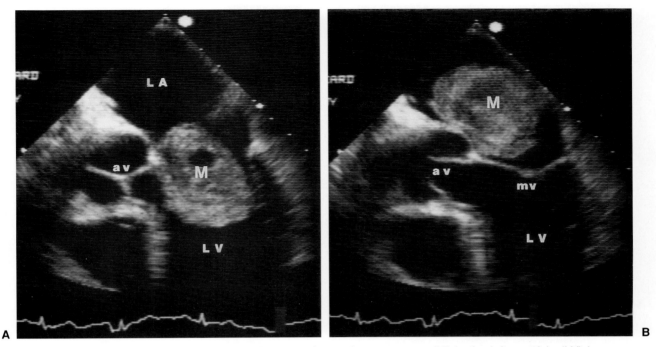

FIG 1-15. Transesophageal echocardiograms show a large myxoma (M) in the left ventricle (LV) in diastole (**A**). The M returns to the left atrium in systole (**B**). av, aortic valve; mv, mitral valve.

a different acoustic impedance from that of the soft-tissue structures within the heart (e.g., cardiac valves), these structures can be readily imaged with ultrasound (Fig. 1-15).

When normal saline is injected intravenously, tiny air bubbles (microcavitations) are produced in the bloodstream. The microcavitations reflect the ultrasound waves and are visualized as a swiftly moving cloud of signals on echocardiography. This technique is termed contrast ultrasonography (7). As the microcavitations pass through the right atrium, both right-to-left and left-to-right shunting across the atrial septum can be outlined. In the presence of tricuspid insufficiency, the echo-loaded blood is seen to oscillate widely between the right atrium and ventricle. In systole, the cloud of echoes may flow rapidly from the right ventricle through the right atrium all the way to the inferior vena cava and hepatic veins.

There are two image presentation formats, the time-motion mode (M-mode) and two-dimensional real-time (2D-RT) echocardiography. M-mode examinations are accomplished by moving photographic paper across the B-mode display to record the movement of cardiac structures (**Fig. 6-1**). In this format, the depth of an echo is shown along the vertical axis, and time is measured along the horizontal axis. M-mode echocardiography shows the motion of a certain point of the heart instead of the familiar anatomic structures, and therefore it may be difficult for the inexperienced observer to understand the data so obtained. Alternatively, cardiac structures can be imaged in real time in two dimensions by the 2D-RT echocardiographic technique (see **Chapter 6**). This method provides a fan-shaped field of vision, con-

forming more closely to the actual anatomic structure of the heart. M-mode scanning is limited by a small imaging area. The heart is adequately imaged only through the fourth or fifth left intercostal space. Real-time echocardiography is more versatile than M-mode scanning and can approach the heart from several acoustic windows (**Fig. 6-2**) other than the parasternal portal. They are the subxiphoid, apical (**Fig. 6-4**), and suprasternal approaches (8).

The best feature of echocardiography is its noninvasive nature. For diagnostic purposes, the ultrasound waves are of high frequencies and low intensities. No definite adverse biologic effects from pulsed diagnostic ultrasound waves have been found since clinical and epidemiologic investigations began 35 years ago (8). Two-dimensional echocardiography has become the standard cardiac ultrasound imaging method, providing anatomic and some functional information of the pericardium, the myocardium, the cardiac valves, and the great vessels. It is also frequently used for the purpose of detecting intracardiac masses and congenital heart diseases. Currently, M-mode echocardiography is not performed routinely, but occasionally it is used as an adjunct to the 2D-RT study (see **Chapter 6**).

Doppler ultrasound and transesophageal echocardiography have now become popular. The former technique provides direct hemodynamic information not available with 2D studies (see **Fig. 6-8**). And with the latter method, one can obtain better cardiac images from within the thorax (Fig. 1-15; see also **Fig. 6-14**), not obstructed by the overlying soft tissues, bones, and lungs that ultrasound waves must

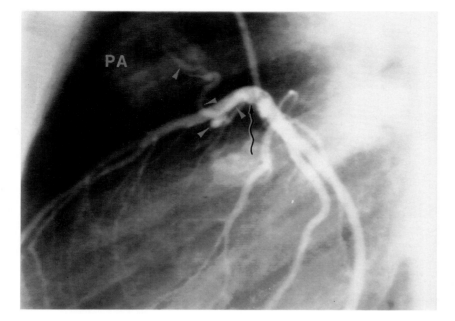

FIG 1-16. Selective left coronary arteriogram shows a fistula from the left main coronary artery to the pulmonary artery (PA). The origin of the fistula is marked by a long arrow; the course of the fistula is followed by arrowheads.

traverse with the transthoracic 2D approach (see **Chapter 6**).

SELECTIVE ANGIOCARDIOGRAPHY

Selective angiocardiography using radiopaque contrast media is commonly performed as a part of the cardiac catheterization procedure (9). It is the most informative in vivo imaging technique of the heart. When coupled with the hemodynamic data already obtained with catheterization, a complete evaluation of the cardiovascular status is usually achieved. In a predetermined site of the heart, a single bolus of contrast medium is delivered rapidly under low pressure through a large-caliber catheter. As the lumens of the cardiovascular structures are sequentially opacified, films are taken with either a rapid film changer or a 35-mm camera. The film changer provides films at a programed rate of up to 12 per second and has the advantage of showing excellent anatomic detail. The movie camera operates at the speed of 60 frames per second and is better suited to the evaluation of dynamic alterations (e.g., a narrow jet across a small ventricular septal defect or through a coronary artery fistula) (Fig. 1-16). Angled views have also been used to eliminate the superimposition of certain intracardiac structures in con-

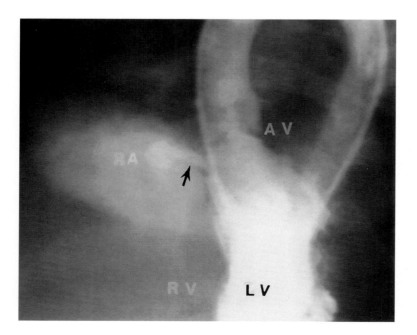

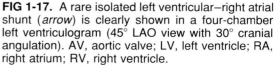

FIG 1-17. A rare isolated left ventricular–right atrial shunt (*arrow*) is clearly shown in a four-chamber left ventriculogram (45° LAO view with 30° cranial angulation). AV, aortic valve; LV, left ventricle; RA, right atrium; RV, right ventricle.

ventional angiographic projections (10,11). The new technique is extremely important in the diagnosis of complex congenital anomalies (Fig. 1-17), hidden coronary artery stenoses, and abnormalities of the main pulmonary artery and its bifurcation.

Unfortunately, a small but definite risk is involved in receiving intravascular contrast media, and this risk frequently cannot be predicted or prevented. Up to 15 percent of patients experience minor reactions to these media, such as nausea, vomiting, and hives. Major reactions include bronchospasm and anaphylactic shock. Deaths occur in 0.1% to 0.2% of patients receiving conventional, ionic, high-osmolality intravascular contrast agents (12,13). The death rate

in patients receiving a low-osmolality, nonionic medium is approximately five times lower (12).

NUCLEAR CARDIAC IMAGING

Some of the most exciting developments in cardiology are radionuclide studies of the heart and vessels (see **Chapter 5**). These studies provide a noninvasive in vivo evaluation of myocardial perfusion, cellular viability, and ventricular function. The perfused, viable myocardium can be studied with either of two radioactive tracers: thallium 201 (Tl-201), which is a cyclotron-produced radionuclide with a half-life

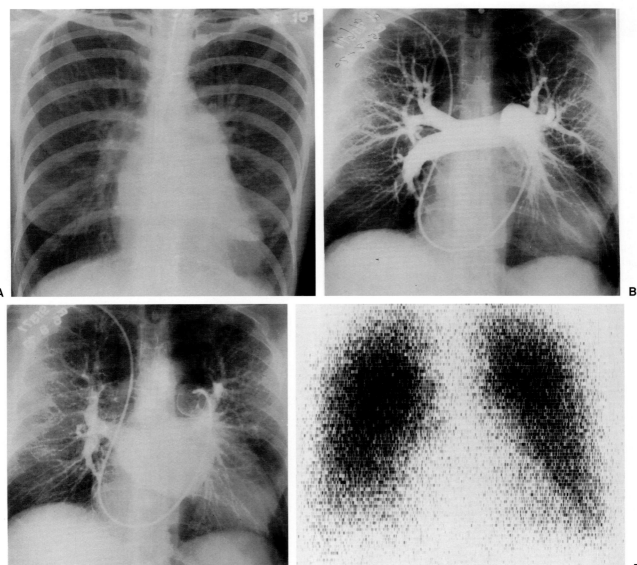

FIG 1-18. Patients with critical mitral valve stenosis showing striking cephalization of pulmonary blood flow. **A:** PA radiograph; **B:** pulmonary arteriogram; **C:** venous phase of B; **D:** pulmonary perfusion scan.

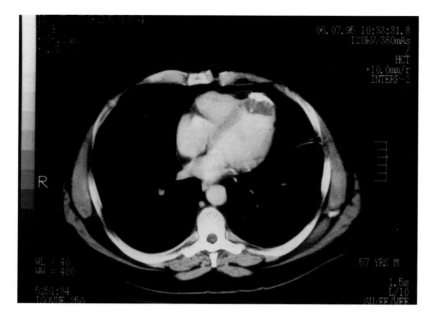

FIG 1-19. Helical CT shows apical left ventricular aneurysm with calcification and mural thrombus. This is the same patient as shown in **Fig. 3-10.**

of 73 hours, or technetium 99m Sestamibi (^{99m}Tc Cardiolite), with a half life of 6 hours, which can be prepared on site from a commercial kit. A defect on the exercise image that fills in on the redistribution image suggests ischemia. If the defect does not fill in on the redistribution image, the pattern would be most suggestive of previous myocardial infarction (see **Fig. 2**).

The most commonly used methods for assessing blood flow and ventricular function are the first-pass technique and the gated-equilibrium (MUGA) technique (see **Fig. 5-3**). These studies are suited to the evaluation of ischemic, valvular, congenital, and pulmonary heart diseases. Positron emission tomography has been used as an alternative but superior method to the Tl-201 or ^{99m}Tc Sestamibi studies to assess myocardial perfusion and viability. It is the only method currently available for evaluating in vivo myocardial metabolism. Myocardial perfusion can be evaluated with either nitrogen-13-labeled ammonia or rubidium 82. Metabolism in corresponding areas of myocardium can be evaluated with F-18 fluoro-2-deoxyglucose, the uptake of which requires viable myocardial cells. Thus, one of the indications of this study is for identification of viable myocardium. Normally, the heart does not metabolize glucose for its energy needs. However, when a myocardial segment is ischemic, it will preferentially shift to the anaerobic metabolism of glucose, which is a second indication for this study, that is, the identification of ischemic but viable myocardium (see **Chapter 5**). Despite the presence of severe asynergy, the underlying myocardium may frequently be viable and can benefit from revascularization. This occurred in 82% of patients in one study (see **Chapter 5**).

Pulmonary perfusion imaging with ^{99m}Tc macroaggregates of albumin (MAA) helps confirm the pulmonary blood flow pattern seen on chest radiographs and angiograms, for example, cephalization in severe mitral valve stenosis (Fig. 1-18) and left lateralization seen in valvular pulmonary stenosis (see **Fig. 8-17**). Changing body posture from upright to supine does not by itself alter the fixed abnormal pulmonary blood flow pattern (see **Chapter 8**).

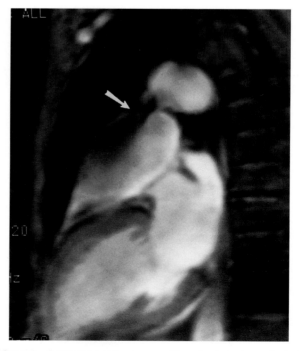

FIG 1-20. A 62-year-old woman with patent ductus arteriosis (PDA) has a turbulent jet (*arrow*) from the aorta to the pulmonary trunk visible in an oblique cine MR image. This is the same as shown in **Fig. 4–24B.**

COMPUTED TOMOGRAPHY

Conventional CT, helical (spiral) CT, and electron beam CT (EBCT) all have applications in cardiac imaging (Fig. 1-19). Because of its much shorter (50- to 100-msecond) scan times, which help minimize cardiac and respiratory lack of sharpness, EBCT is superior (Fig. 1-10) to conventional and helical CT in the evaluation of the heart and great vessels (see **Chapter 3**).

MAGNETIC RESONANCE IMAGING

Magnetic resonance imaging is a noninvasive, multiplanar imaging technique capable of accurately assessing both the anatomy and the function of the heart and great vessels (Fig. 1-20) (see **Chapter 4**).

REFERENCES

1. Elkin M. Issues in radiology related to the new technologies. *Radiology* 1982;143:1–6.
2. Stanford W, Rumberger JA. *Ultrafast computed tomography in cardiac imaging: principles and practice.* Mt. Kisco, N.Y.: Futura, 199;2552.
3. Margolis JR, Chen JTT, Kong Y, et al. The diagnostic and prognostic significance of coronary calcification: a report of 800 patients. *Radiology* 1980;137:609–616.
4. Di Carli M, Sherman T, Khanna S, et al. Myocardial viability in asynergic regions subtended by occluded coronary arteries: relation to the status of collateral flow in patients with chronic coronary artery disease. *J Am Coll Cardiol* 1994;23:860–868.
5. Shabetai R. Diseases of the pericardium. In: Schlant RC, Alexander RW, eds. *The heart*, 8th ed. New York: McGraw–Hill, 1994:1647–1674.
6. Johnson ML, Kisslo JA. Basic diagnostic echocardiography. *Disease-A-Month* 1976;23:3–58.
7. Gramiak R, Shah PM, Kramer DH. Ultrasound cardiography: contrast studies in anatomy and function. *Radiology* 1969;92:939–948.
8. Fleischer AC, James AE. *Introduction to diagnostic sonography.* New York: Wiley, 1980.
9. Franch RH, King SB, Douglas JS. Techniques of cardiac catheterization including coronary arteriography. In: Schlant RC, Alexander RW, eds. *The heart*, 8th ed. New York: McGraw–Hill, 1994:2381–2452.
10. Elliott LP, Bargeron LM, Soto B, et al. Axial cineangiography in congenital heart disease. *Radiol Clin North Am* 1980;18:515–546.
11. Burrows PE, Smallhorn JF, Moes CAF. Congenital cardiovascular disease. In: Putman CE, Ravin CE, eds. *Textbook of diagnostic imaging*, 2nd ed. Philadelphia: Saunders, 1994:1739–1780.
12. McClennan BL. Adverse reactions to iodinated contrast media: recognition and response. *Invest Radiol* 1994;29(suppl. 1):S41–S50.
13. Hudson ER, Smith TP, McDermott VG, et al. Pulmonary angiography performed with iopamidol: complications in 1,434 patients. *Radiology* 1996;198:61–65.

Essentials of Cardiac Imaging,
James T. T. Chen,
Lippincott–Raven Publishers, Philadelphia © 1998.

CHAPTER 2

Radiography and Fluoroscopy

James T. T. Chen

Radiologic analysis of the heart must be performed in an orderly, systematic fashion based on a firm understanding of normal and abnormal anatomy and physiology. The examination can be divided into four essential steps: radiographic examination, fluoroscopic examination, statistical guidance, and clinical correlation.

RADIOGRAPHIC EXAMINATION

Cardiac Series

Although four-view cardiac series had been used for decades as the initial radiologic examination of the heart, this procedure has now been simplified to two-view radiography. However, it is still useful to gain familiarity with the two oblique views that are frequently used in other cardiac imaging techniques, particularly in nuclear cardiology, conventional angiocardiography, echocardiography, cine computed tomography (CT), and cine magnetic resonance imaging (MRI). The conventional four-view cardiac series are used to register all aspects of the cardiovascular silhouette: the posteroanterior (PA) view with barium, the left-lateral (lateral) view with barium, a 45° right-anterior oblique (RAO) view with barium, and a 60° left-anterior oblique (LAO) view without barium (Fig. 2-1).

Objective Observation

To avoid biased preconception, it is desirable to first interpret the radiograph without prior knowledge of the patient's case. The clinical and other laboratory data should eventually be correlated with the radiographic findings at the conclusion of the radiographic analysis.

Department of Radiology, Duke University School of Medicine, Durham, North Carolina 27710, U.S.A.

Sequential Radiographic Analysis

An Overview

The first step is to survey the radiograph, thus obtaining an overview of the entire situation. At this time, it is wise to search briefly for abnormalities not directly related to the cardiovascular system that may reflect heart disease. For instance, bilateral rib notching is an important manifestation of coarctation of the aorta (1) (Fig. 2-2). A small and subluxed arm in a patient with an atrial septal defect suggests the diagnosis of Holt–Oram syndrome (2) (Fig. 2-3). A narrowed anteroposterior diameter of the thorax may be the cause of an innocent murmur (3). The combination of a right-sided stomach, a dilated azygos vein, and an absent image of the inferior vena cava strongly suggests the presence of congenital interruption of the inferior vena cava (4,5) (Fig. 2-4). When clinical information is lacking, changes in the bones and soft tissues of the thorax may provide a clue to the type and purpose of previous surgery performed on the patient (5) (Fig. 2-5).

Pulmonary Vasculature

The lung reflects the underlying pathophysiology of the heart. Therefore, a careful evaluation of the pulmonary vasculature will narrow the differential diagnoses considerably. For example, right-sided ventricular failure is manifested by scanty flow, small vessels, and unusually radiolucent lungs (Fig. 2-6). Left-sided ventricular failure is characterized by pulmonary edema and a cephalic flow pattern (Fig. 2-7) (see **Chapter 8**).

Cardiac Size

Radiographic mensuration of cardiac size is crucial in the diagnosis of heart disease. All enlarged hearts are abnormal hearts, but all normal-sized hearts are not necessarily normal.

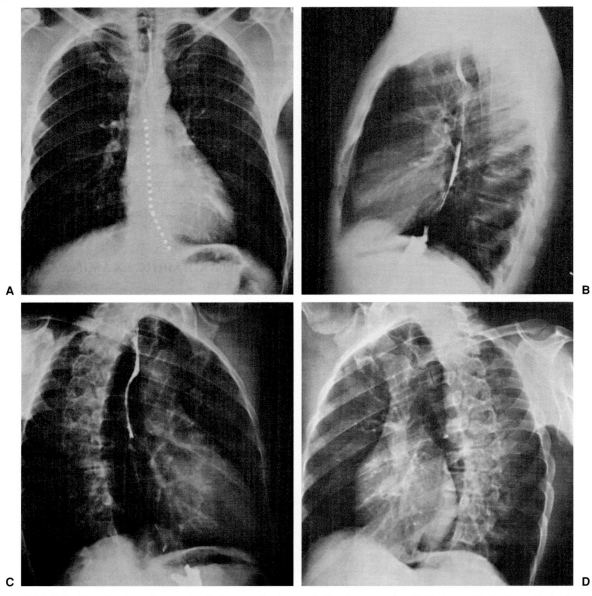

FIG 2-1. Standard cardiac series in four projections. **A:** Posteroanterior (PA) view with barium. Dotted line marks the lower course of the esophagus. **B:** Left lateral (Lateral) view with barium. **C:** Right anterior oblique (RAO) view at 45° with barium. **D:** Left anterior oblique (LAO) view at 60° without barium.

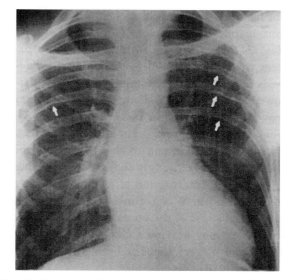

FIG 2-2. PA view of a patient with coarctation of the aorta showing notching of the ribs bilaterally (*arrows*). The coarctation is located in the lower thoracic aorta. The 3 sign is absent in the region of the aortic arch.

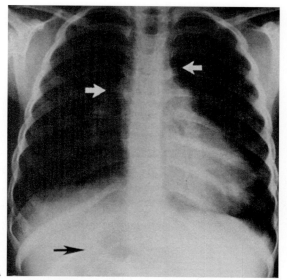

A

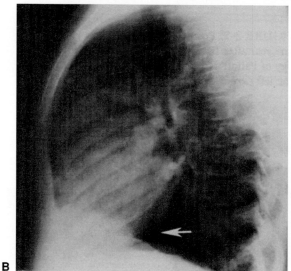

B

FIG 2-4. Patient with levocardia, right-sided stomach, a small ventricular septal defect, and interruption of the inferior vena cava. **A:** PA view shows the gastric air bubble (*black arrow*) to be on the right side. The azygos vein (*white arrow on right*) is dilated. The aortic arch is normal (*white arrow on left*). Pulmonary vascularity is slightly increased bilaterally. **B:** Lateral view shows an absence of image of the inferior vena cava (*arrow*).

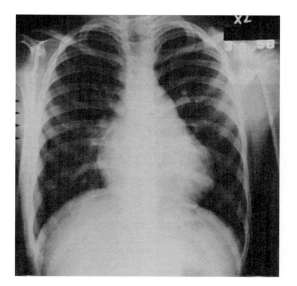

FIG 2-3. PA radiograph of a boy with subluxation of the atrophic right arm (*arrows*) and evidence of an atrial septal defect.

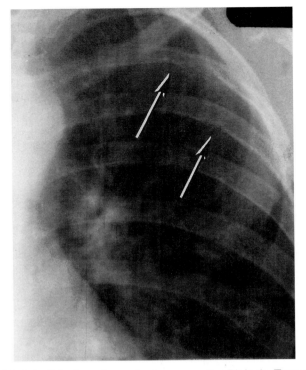

FIG 2-5. PA view of a patient 1 year after Blalock–Taussig operation for tetralogy of Fallot. Note multiple notched upper ribs on the left (*arrows*).

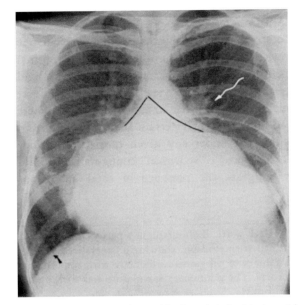

FIG 2-7. PA view of a patient with chronic left-sided ventricular failure from rheumatic mitral, aortic, and tricuspid insufficiency. Note gross cardiomegaly, striking cephalization of pulmonary vascularity, and interstitial pulmonary edema. The *black arrow* points to well-defined septal lines. the *white arrow* points to peribronchial cuffing of edema fluid. Black lines mark the widened subcarinal angle by the huge left atrium.

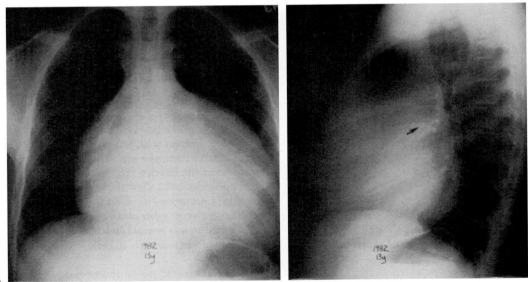

FIG 2-6. Radiographs of a 13-year-old patient with Ebstein's anomaly. He was in profound right-sided ventricular failure. The tricuspid valve was insufficient, and there was a right-to-left shunt at the atrial level. **A:** PA view shows gross cardiomegaly with decreased pulmonary vascularity and hyperlucent lungs. **B:** Lateral view shows striking right-sided cardiomegaly and small hila (*arrow*).

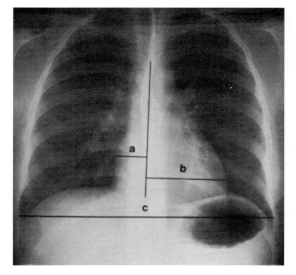

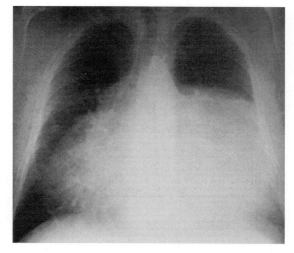

FIG 2-8. PA view of a normal person, showing the method of determining the cardiothoracic ratio. First a midline is drawn. Second, the maximum distances from this line to the right (a) and to the left (b) cardiac borders are measured. Third, the maximum internal diameter of the chest (c) is measured. The transverse diameter of the heart = a + b. The cardiothoracic ratio = (a + b)/c.

FIG 2-10. Radiograph of a patient with pericarditis with effusion, showing a generalized enlargement of the cardiac silhouette with smooth borders. The pulmonary vasculature was within normal limits.

The diagnosis of microcardia (as seen in Addison's disease) often requires retrospective assessment after the heart has regained its normal capacity with therapy. The cardiothoracic ratio on the PA chest radiograph remains the most simple yardstick for measuring cardiac size (Fig. 2-8). The average ratio in normal adults is 0.45.

Gross cardiomegaly before the development of congestive heart failure primarily reflects volume overload. The differential diagnosis includes valvular insufficiency (Fig. 2-9A), hyperkinetic state, left-to-right shunt, and severe bradycardia. Pericardial effusion is a well-known imitator of genuine cardiomegaly (Fig. 2-10). Mild cardiomegaly often results from pressure overload alone, as in valvular aortic stenosis (Fig. 2-11A), systemic hypertension, and pulmonary arterial hypertension. Significant cardiomegaly (with a cardiothoracic ratio >0.5) in patients with pressure overload strongly

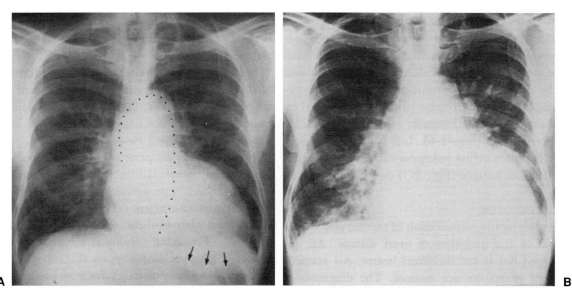

A   B

FIG 2-9. A: PA view of a patient with aortic insufficiency. The left ventricle enlarges leftward and downward (arrows). The stomach air bubble is depressed by the dilated left ventricle. The dotted line marks the dilated thoracic aorta in its entirety. B: Six months later the patient suffered congestive heart failure. Note increased cardiomegaly with pulmonary edema.

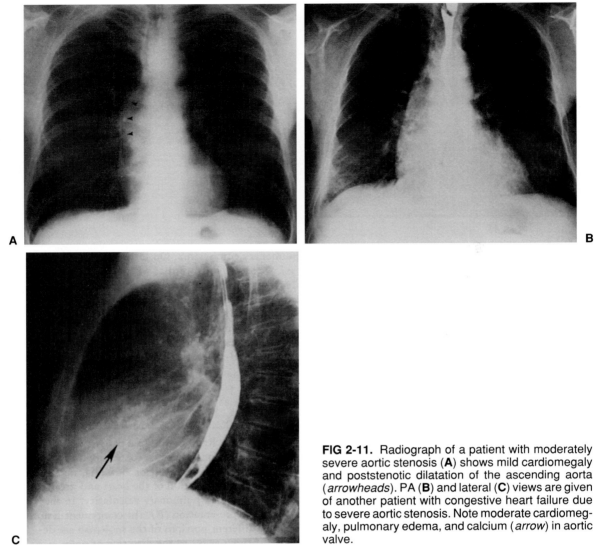

FIG 2-11. Radiograph of a patient with moderately severe aortic stenosis (**A**) shows mild cardiomegaly and poststenotic dilatation of the ascending aorta (*arrowheads*). PA (**B**) and lateral (**C**) views are given of another patient with congestive heart failure due to severe aortic stenosis. Note moderate cardiomegaly, pulmonary edema, and calcium (*arrow*) in aortic valve.

suggests the onset of congestive heart failure (Fig. 2-11B). Microcardia results primarily from depletion of the circulating blood volume, as in Addison's disease, starvation, anorexia nervosa, and obstructive emphysema (Fig. 2-12).

Cardiac Contour

To appreciate an abnormal cardiac contour, one must first become familiar with the normal radiographic appearance of the heart and great vessels in each view (see **Chapter 9**). Next, one must know what to expect as well as where and how frequently certain anatomic alterations will occur in a given cardiac condition. For instance, a ''snowman'' configuration suggests the presence of total anomalous pulmonary venous connection to the left vertical vein (Fig. 2-13).

A bulge along the left-lower cardiac border on the PA view has many causes, namely, loculated pericardial effusion, congenitally corrected transposition of the great arteries, idiopathic hypertrophic subaortic stenosis, and left ventricular aneurysm. However, only the last entity is associated with a sharply demarcated double density in the retrosternal area on the lateral view (1) (Fig. 2-14). Coeur en sabot, or boot-shaped heart, is typically noted in patients with tetralogy of Fallot (1) (Fig. 2-15).

Abnormal Density

The double density cast by an enlarged left atrium on the PA projection is well known (Fig. 2-16). However, if the left atrium is enormous, it may actually form the right cardiac border beyond the normal-sized or less dilated right atrium. Consequently, it is the right atrium that casts a double density on the PA view (Fig. 2-7). A pretracheal density is the hallmark of total anomalous pulmonary venous connection to the left vertical vein (Fig. 2-13C), even in neonates long

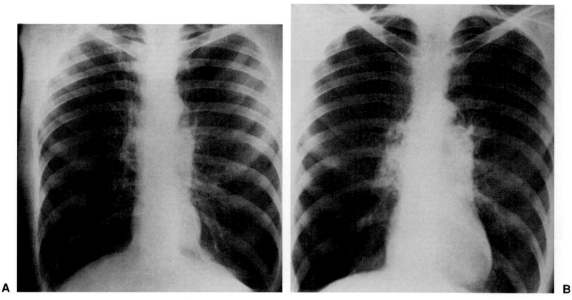

A   B

FIG 2-12. Radiographs of a patient with severe pulmonary emphysema. On initial examination (**A**), there was microcardia, which resulted primarily from decreased cardiac output and secondarily from overinflated lungs. On reexamination 3 years later (**B**), the size of the heart had increased considerably despite worsening of emphysema. These changes were highly suggestive of, and eventually proved to represent, severe right-sided heart failure.

before a snowman configuration is noticeable on the PA view.

One should also search diligently for intracardiac calcifications, which frequently have profound clinical implications. Any radiographic evidence of cardiac valve calcification is diagnostic of stenosis of that valve with or without associated insufficiency. The heavier the calcification, the worse the valve stenosis, regardless of other radiographic signs (6,7) (see **Chapter 10**).

Abnormal Lucency

Distinct radiographic lucencies in and about the heart are usually abnormal. The tracheobronchial tree may be displaced by enlarged cardiovascular structures and thus become conspicuous. For example, a right-sided aortic arch with an aberrant left-sided subclavian artery may show marked leftward and anterior displacement of the trachea (see **Figs. 16-72 and 16-73**). A huge left atrium almost always displaces the major bronchi (Fig. 2-17). The presence of pericardial effusion, thickening, or both usually provides a background of water density for the subepicardial fat stripe to be seen more clearly (8) (Fig. 2-18).

Cardiac Position

When dextrocardia is present, there is usually a mirror image of both the heart and the abdominal viscera. The incidence of associated intracardiac defects in this circumstance is only slightly increased (from 0.7% to 5.0%). When dextro-

cardia is associated with situs solitus (both the aortic arch and the stomach are left-sided) there would be a high incidence (98%) of congenital cardiac anomalies (Fig. 2-19) (4) (see also **Chapter 16**).

Great Arteries

Evaluation of the great arteries is an integral part of radiographic diagnosis of heart disease. Dilatation of the entire aorta is typical of severe aortic insufficiency (Fig. 2-9), whereas selective dilatation of the ascending aorta is characteristic of valvular aortic stenosis (Fig. 2-11). The position and number of the aortic arch may strongly suggest or, conversely, militate against congenital cardiac defects. For example, a very high incidence of congenital heart disease is associated with the avian type of right-sided aortic arch (9), but there is is no such association with double aortic arch (see discussion on aortic arch anomalies in **Chapter 16**). In the presence of double aortic arch, the heart is usually normal.

The descending aorta is closely applied to the lateral margin of the left atrium. In the presence of left atrial enlargement, the descending aorta may be displaced to the left side, providing a useful clue to this condition (Fig. 2-20). The combination of a small aorta and a large pulmonary trunk on the PA view often results from leftward rotation of the heart along its long axis. As the great arteries necessarily rotate laterad with a shifting heart, the aortic arch folds in on itself, becoming hidden in the mediastinum; the pulmonary

Text continues on page 23.

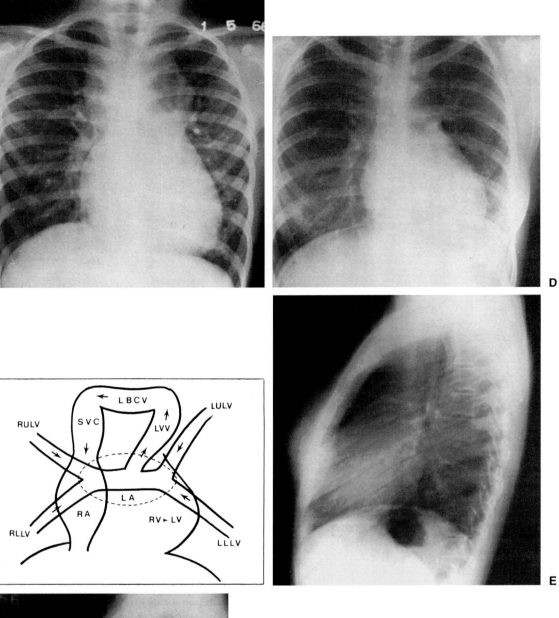

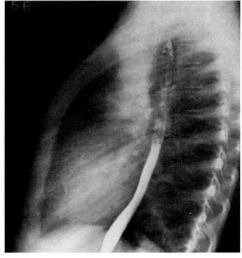

FIG 2-13. Radiographs of a patient with total anomalous pulmonary venous connection to the left vertical vein. In PA view (**A**), note the "snowman" configuration of the heart and great vessels with increased pulmonary vascularity. In the schematic representation (**B**), the component lesions forming different portions of the snowman are depicted. Arrows point to the direction of pulmonary venous blood flow. LA, left atrium; LBCV, left brachiocephalic vein; LLLV, left-lower-lobe vein; LULV, left-upper-lobe vein; LVV, left vertical vein; RA, right atrium; RLLV, right-lower-lobe vein; RULV, right-upper-lobe vein; RV → LV, convex left cardiac border formed by the left ventricle, which has been displaced by the enlarged right ventricle; SVC, superior vena cava. In the lateral view (**C**), there is a pretracheal density, representing superimposition of LVV on SVC. Postoperative PA (**D**) and lateral (**E**) views show considerable improvement.

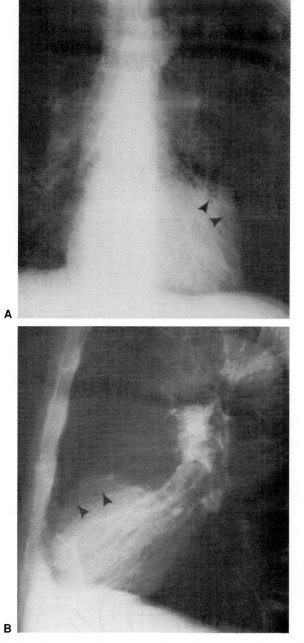

A

B

FIG 2-14. PA (**A**) and lateral (**B**) views of an anterolateral wall aneurysm (*arrows*) protruding leftward and anteriorly from the left ventricle. Note the sharply demarcated double density on the lateral view, representing superimposition of the aneurysm on the normal right ventricle.

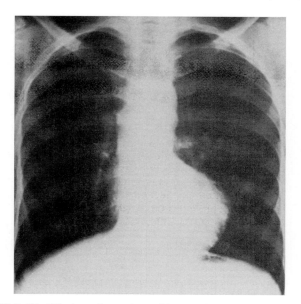

FIG 2-15. PA view of a patient with pseudotruncus arteriosus (severe tetralogy of Fallot with pulmonary atresia and ventricular septal defect). A classic coeur en sabot configuration is present. Note that the pulmonary vascularity is markedly diminished. The aorta is dilated, reflecting a large right-to-left shunt across the ventricular septal defect. The pulmonary trunk is concave from infundibular pulmonary stenosis and hypoplasia of the pulmonary trunk. The cardiac apex is upturned, reflecting an enlarged right ventricle displacing the left ventricular apex leftward, posteriorly, and upward.

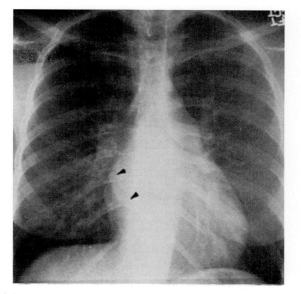

FIG 2-16. PA view of a patient with mitral stenosis and insufficiency. A double density (*arrows*) is clearly visible, representing severe left-sided atrial enlargement.

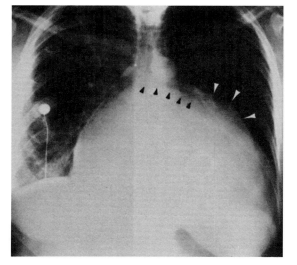

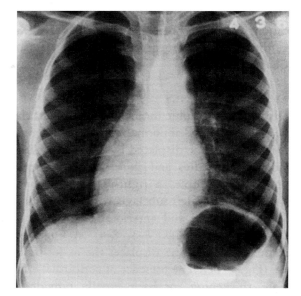

FIG 2-17. Radiograph of a patient with severe rheumatic mitral insufficiency. A disk valve is seen in the mitral position. The left atrium is enormous, displacing and compressing the left mainstem bronchus (*black arrowheads*). The subcarinal angle is markedly widened. *White arrowheads* point to the enlarged left atrial appendage.

FIG 2-19. PA view of a patient with dextrocardia with situs solitus, L-loop transposition of the great arteries, ventricular septal defect, and pulmonary stenosis. The apex of the ventricles points to the right side, whereas the stomach and the aorta remain on the left.

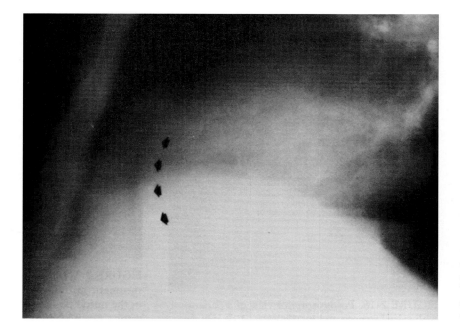

FIG 2-18. Radiograph of a patient with pericardial effusion showing a distinct radiolucent line (*arrows*) in the retrosternal area. This line represents the displaced subepicardial fat stripe between the water density of pericardial fluid and that of myocardium.

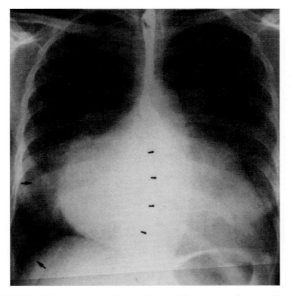

FIG 2-20. Radiograph of a patient with severe rheumatic mitral insufficiency, whose lighter PA view is shown in Fig. 2-7. Barium is now present in the esophagus, which outlines the anteromedial border of the descending aorta. Note that both the esophagus and aorta are displaced to the left by the enlarged left atrium (*small arrows*). *Horizontal arrow* on right points to the double density, and horizontal arrow on left points to the enlarged left atrial appendage. Kerley's lines (*oblique arrow*) are poorly distinguished.

trunk moves into the left lung, thus appearing larger than it actually is.

The mechanism of leftward rotation of the heart is two-fold. First, there is the intrinsic torque from an enlarging right ventricle in the presence of a normal left ventricle (e.g., in atrial septal defect, mitral stenosis, and precapillary pulmonary hypertension). Second, there is extrinsic torque from a flat bony thorax that compresses the heart anteroposteriorly and rotates it to the left (e.g., in straight back syndrome (3), pectus excavatum, and scoliosis). Therefore, in the presence of a left-to-right shunt, the combination of an inconspicuous aorta and a huge pulmonary trunk on the PA view is highly suggestive of an atrial septal defect (Fig. 2-3).

Pleura

A right-sided pleural effusion is typical of left-sided heart failure. Bilateral effusions suggest bilateral cardiac decompensation or a noncardiac condition. A pseudotumor or vanishing tumor (Fig. 2-21) may accompany congestive heart failure (10).

Esophagus

The esophagus is in close contact with a number of important cardiovascular structures. Any deviation or compression of the barium-filled esophagus may provide a clue to the underlying cardiac disorder. With left atrial enlargement, the esophagus is typically deviated posteriorly and to the right (Fig. 2-22). However, no esophagus is long enough to maintain the usual pattern of displacement when it is stretched against a giant left atrium. Instead, the esophagus simply flops to the left side, lining up with the similarly deviated descending aorta. This deviation is termed esophageal escape. Esophageal escape in the face of a gigantic left atrium is most commonly seen in long-standing, severe rheumatic mitral insufficiency (Fig. 2-20).

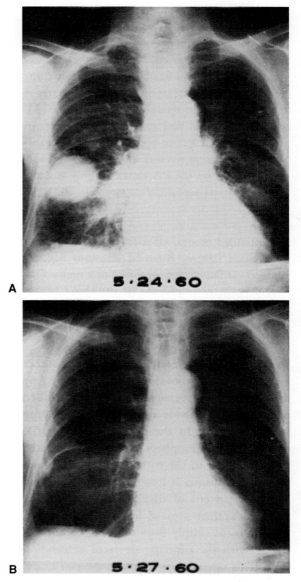

FIG 2-21. Radiographs of a patient with left-sided congestive heart failure. PA view (**A**) shows cardiomegaly, pulmonary edema, and a rounded opacity in the right midlung. PA view taken 3 days later (**B**), after the patient responded to anticongestive therapy, shows almost complete disappearance of the rounded opacity, which represented an interlobar pleural effusion in the minor fissure, a so-called pseudotumor.

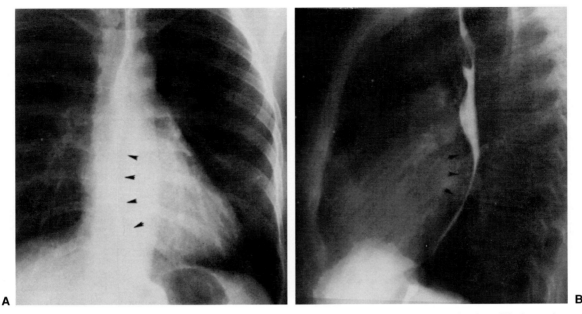

FIG 2-22. Radiographs of a patient with mitral valve stenosis shows deviation of the barium-filled esophagus to the right side (*arrows*) on the PA view (**A**) and posteriorly (*arrows*) on the lateral view (**B**).

The esophagus also reflects dynamic changes of the heart and aorta, thereby portraying certain hemodynamic disturbances (see discussion on cardiac fluoroscopy). In the evaluation of the aorta, it is advantageous to opacify the esophagus with a barium paste. The barium column outlines the anteromedial wall of the descending aorta, providing a useful landmark. An inserted nasogastric tube serves the same function.

Other Radiologic Techniques

At times, the diagnosis may escape the routine radiographic examination just described. In this situation, a number of other radiologic techniques may be considered. For example, conventional tomography is helpful in registering valvular calcifications in large patients (see **Fig. 10-6C,D**); CT scanning may be used as a noninvasive method to confirm or refute the diagnosis of a pulmonary arteriovenous fistula or a pulmonary vein varix (Fig. 8–22D,E,F).

With a large pleural effusion, the obscured cardiac borders can be brought into relief by changing the patient's body posture from erect to supine or lateral decubitus. Likewise, a hidden pulmonary infarct can be made visible by the same maneuver. Occasionally, a supine cross-table lateral view may be used to show the heart falling away from the sternum in patients with congenital absence of the left pericardium (see **Fig. 14-9C**).

Thoroughness and Comparison

Thoroughness of each examination and comparison with serial radiographs fill in unexpected or unexplained gaps.

Generalized massive edema including the chest wall along with mild cardiomegaly suggests cardiopulmonary alterations of renal origin (Fig. 2-23). Evaluating cardiac size over time is always important (Fig. 2-12).

FLUOROSCOPIC EXAMINATION

Fluoroscopy provides direct dynamic information (11,12) not obtainable on a radiograph. For example, a young person with aortic insufficiency may show left ventricular enlargement without dilatation of the aorta on a radiograph taken largely in diastole (Fig. 2-24). Under the fluoroscope, however, the dilated and hyperpulsatile aorta and left ventricle are virtually diagnostic of the disease (Fig. 2-25). A detailed discussion of cardiac fluoroscopy follows.

STATISTICAL GUIDANCE

Judicious use of statistics (1,9) more frequently than not leads us to the correct diagnosis. However, the final conclusion should be based only on radiologic manifestations. If the statistical suggestion fits the radiographic findings, the diagnosis is certain. If not, other differential diagnoses should then be considered.

CLINICAL CORRELATION

The radiologist is in a unique position as a consultant to the clinician. His or her responsibilities include suggesting the best possible diagnosis, assessing prognostic features revealed by the radiologic examination, and, at times, consulting about therapy. From time to time, both the clinical and

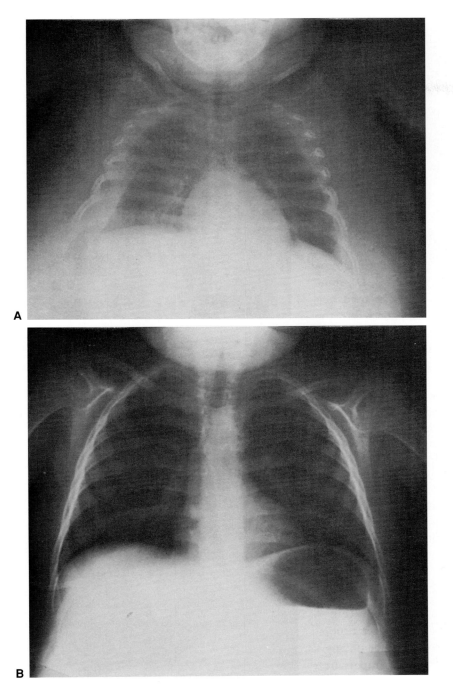

FIG 2-23. PA view (**A**) of a child with nephrotic syndrome and anasarca shows striking edema of the soft tissues of the thorax, pulmonary edema, pleural effusion, and mild cardiomegaly. Same view 2 weeks later (**B**) shows a dramatic improvement.

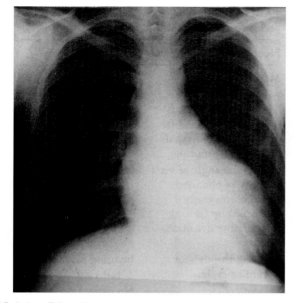

FIG 2-24. PA radiograph of a young adult with severe aortic insufficiency shows a large left ventricle, normal pulmonary vascularity, and a normal aorta.

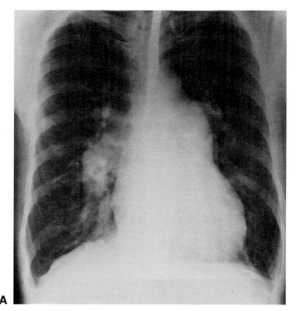

A

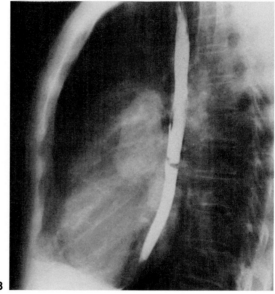

B

FIG 2-26. PA (A) and lateral (B) views of a patient with 2° atrial septal defect and a 3:1 left-to-right shunt, which was misinterpreted as mitral valve stenosis because of similar auscultatory findings. Radiologically, however, both views show a uniform increase in pulmonary vasculature and pure right-sided cardiomegaly. There is neither cephalization of the pulmonary vascularity nor left atrial enlargement to suggest mitral stenosis.

the radiologic diagnoses may be correct but not consistent. For example, the clinical manifestations of a ventricular septal defect may be convincing [e.g., a grade 5 holosystolic murmur caused by a high-velocity flow across a small ventricular septal defect (VSD)], while the radiographic signs are entirely within normal limits. The radiologist must be aware that a left-to-right shunt smaller than 2:1 in adults is extremely difficult, if not impossible, to detect. On the other hand, our colleagues might occasionally mistake a 2° atrial septal defect for mitral stenosis because of similar physical

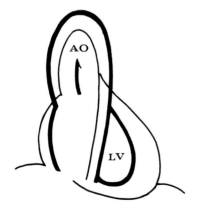

FIG 2-25. A schematic drawing of the radiograph of the same patient as in Fig. 2-24 depicts the fluoroscopic findings. The thin lines outline the diastolic phase of the heart and aorta; the thick lines outline the systolic phase of the heart and aorta. Note the normal aorta (AO) and dilated left ventricle (LV) in diastole and the dilated aorta and smaller left ventricle in systole.

findings; the radiographic features of each, however, are characteristic (Fig. 2-26).

Both the radiologist and the cardiologist must understand that no pressure gradient is detectable across a mildly stenotic vessel or cardiac valve (e.g., <50% reduction in diameter or <75% reduction in cross-sectional area of a valve or a vessel), even though the radiographic evidence of such a lesion is convincing and the angiocardiographic findings of the stenosis are unequivocal. After reviewing all clinical and laboratory information, reexamination of the films or the patient or both may become necessary. Following detailed radiologic analysis of some finer points, a correct diagnosis may be strengthened or a wrong impression corrected.

CARDIAC FLUOROSCOPY

There are two basic radiologic approaches to heart disease, namely, radiography and fluoroscopy. The former deals with anatomic details by filming at short exposure times that stop the motion; the latter explores the dynamic features that are discernible only in motion. Fluoroscopy was born with the discovery of x-rays in 1895, when Roentgen first saw his own hand on a fluorescent screen (13). For decades thereafter, fluoroscopy played a greater role than radiography in the field of radiographic diagnosis. The early radiographic technique was rather primitive and time consuming and yielded poor results. Compared with radiography, fluoroscopy was more versatile and often provided a clearer image and a more timely diagnosis (14). During the early part of this century the value of cardiac fluoroscopy became well recognized. With the improvement of radiographic technique after World War I, the use of fluoroscopy gradually declined. Other factors that contributed to its decline included the fear of radiation, the desire to save time, and the clumsiness of the conventional fluoroscope.

Following the advent of image intensification, enthusiasm for cardiac fluoroscopy has been rekindled. The modern image intensifier, using cesium iodide phosphors and televised viewing, can brighten the fluoroscopic image at least 10,000 times. The image intensifier permits cone vision under dim light, which allows for better perception of details. The use of videotape for instant replay and review has eliminated the need for reexamination of the patient. Experience with the image intensifier (15–17) has not only confirmed the previously proclaimed value of cardiac fluoroscopy but also established new roles for the procedure. Most notable among its new applications is the detection of coronary artery disease in both symptomatic (15,18) and asymptomatic (19,20) patients. With the advance of newer and more sophisticated cardiac imaging techniques, this simple and effective tool has been underused in most cases.

Technique

With the image intensifier, the procedure of cardiac fluoroscopy is markedly simplified. However, several important aspects need to be emphasized to ensure a safe and successful operation.

Radiation Protection

Although the advent of image intensification has eliminated most of the disadvantages of the conventional fluoro-

scope, the basic rules of radiation protection should still be strictly observed. The fluoroscope must meet the minimum specifications outlined in Handbook No. 60 of the National Bureau of Standards. The output of the fluoroscope at the tabletop should be limited to 0.5 rad per minute for children. For adults, the routine settings are 1.8 mA, 101 kV, and 3-mm aluminum filtration, with a focal spot tabletop distance of 18 inches (21).

Fluoroscopy should be used selectively, only after studying the pertinent radiographs, and with a definite goal. The approach should be systematic and well organized so that the task can be accomplished expeditiously within 2 to 3 minutes. The examining field should be the minimum, confined only to the point of interest. Unnecessary radiation to the patient or the examiner should be avoided. In this connection, adequate training of our residents in diagnostic imaging cannot be overemphasized.

Rapport with the Patient

During or before the time of fluoroscopy, the operator is able to talk to and establish a good rapport with the patient. A well-informed patient is usually relaxed and cooperative. Another advantage of fluoroscopy is that the physician can gain additional valuable information that is affordable only through contact with the patient. By conversing with and examining the patient, new light may be shed on the problems. For instance, finding a protuberant and firm abdomen should suggest the possibility of right-sided heart failure with tricuspid insufficiency.

Suspension of Respiration

Breath holding during cardiac fluoroscopy is desirable. It should be done with ease. Suspension of respiration after taking a small breath is ideal. Holding too big a breath for too long and too frequently tends to encourage an involuntary Valsalva maneuver. The end results of that are false-positive asynergy of the left ventricle and fainting spells. On the other hand, short and easy suspension of respiration helps eliminate all motions except for the rhythmic excursions of cardiovascular origin. If the patient simply cannot cooperate, a slow, quiet breathing pattern should be encouraged.

Positions

The examination is usually performed with the patient erect. The four views taken are the PA, the left lateral (lateral), the RAO, and the LAO. Depending on which structures are to be looked at, the degree of rotation for oblique views varies from 20° to 70°. For instance, if the left coronary arteries are the point of interest, a shallow LAO view at 25 to 35° is preferred to a steeper oblique view. Alternatively, if the purpose of the examination is to visualize aortic valve calcification, a >60° LAO view is usually required.

In conditions of extreme obesity, equivocal cardiac asynergy, and very small calcification, the recumbent position is preferred. The fluoroscopic image of an obese patient improves dramatically when he or she is lying down, since the thick layers of soft tissue are compressed and pushed aside from the examining field. Other favorable adjustments are also triggered by changing the body posture from upright to recumbent. For example, the heart is less affected by gravity when a patient is supine and therefore more relaxed. Physiologically, the cardiac output increases and the heart rate decreases. These adjustments bring about a truer picture of cardiac contractility and facilitate the detection of small cardiac calcifications.

X-ray Exposure

The x-ray exposure should be adjusted for each view, according to the body thickness to be penetrated. Obviously, more radiation is needed in the lateral than in the PA projection. The proper exposures for the oblique views fall somewhere between. As a rule, the kilovoltage ranges from 75 to 120, and the milliamperage between 1.5 and 3.5. Too much milliamperage blurs off the heart-lung interface as well as the small calcifications and delicate fat stripes. Too much kilovoltage reduces the contrast of the picture. Again, for the purpose of radiation protection, the x-ray beam should be collimated to the smallest possible size and the fluoroscopic time should be limited to <5 minutes.

Practical Applications

Cardiac fluoroscopy is indicated for the following purposes:

1. To complement radiography
2. To evaluate cardiovascular dynamics
3. To detect small cardiovascular calcifications
4. To visualize subepicardial fat stripes and other important cardiovascular landmarks
5. To differentiate cardiac from noncardiac diseases
6. To evaluate cardiac pacemakers, valve prostheses, and radiopaque foreign bodies
7. To study juxtaposed noncardiac structures
8. To assist cardiac catheterization and angiocardiography

Complementing Radiography

Radiography and fluoroscopy are complementary diagnostic techniques. Fluoroscopy should be used in every diagnostic dilemma, for there is no real substitute. For instance, the initial radiographs of a child or young adult with severe aortic insufficiency may show nothing more than a large left ventricle that by itself is nonspecific (Fig. 2-24). On

fluoroscopy, however, the telltale sign of a hyperpulsatile aorta immediately comes to view (Fig. 2-25). Judicious use of fluoroscopy as an adjunct to radiography is based on a firm understanding of the advantages and disadvantages of each method.

Evaluating Cardiovascular Dynamics

Fluoroscopy provides uninterrupted vision of the moving heart throughout the cardiac cycle. The behavior of the heart and vessels in systole, as portrayed under the fluoroscope, is of special importance when evaluating a number of heart diseases. This information, however, is not available on the radiograph, which is usually exposed during diastole. For instance, the systolic expansion of the aorta in aortic insufficiency (see Fig. 2-24) and the systolic expansion of the left atrium in mitral insufficiency (22) (Fig. 2-27) are seldom recorded on the radiograph, but can be readily appreciated fluoroscopically. The view of systolic expansion can be strengthened by the aid of barium; barium outlines the esophagus, which is displaced by the enlarging left atrium in systole. Similarly, a broad-based left ventricular aneurysm may evidence nothing abnormal radiographically. Under the fluoroscope, however, the vigorous systolic expansion of a thin-walled aneurysm is unmistakable (Fig. 2-28).

Although the poststenotic dilatation of the ascending aorta in valvular aortic stenosis can be seen on the film, the "snapping" pulsation of the ascending aorta in systole (Fig. 2-29), as revealed on the image intensifier, gives one added confidence in the diagnosis. In a patient with severe mitral stenosis, the rapid expansion of the right atrium and venae cavae in systole vividly portrays the presence of functional tricuspid insufficiency (Fig. 2-30). To appreciate the dynamic deviations from normal, Figs. 2-25, 2-28, 2-29, and 2-30 should be compared with Fig. 2-31, which depicts the dynamic characteristics of a normal heart.

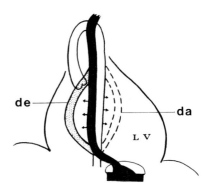

FIG 2-27. Schematic drawing of the posterior wedging sign of mitral insufficiency. The aorta in white and the esophagus in black are together in diastole. They are splayed apart by the enlarging left atrium in systole. da, laterally displaced aorta; de, laterally displaced esophagus; LV, left ventricle. Arrows point to the direction of displacement of the respective organs.

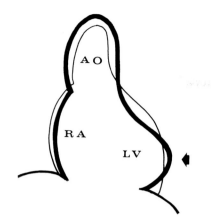

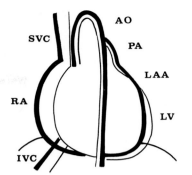

FIG 2-30. A schematic drawing of the rapid systolic expansion of the dilated right atrium (RA), superior vena cava (SVC), and inferior vena cava (IVC) as a result of tricuspid insufficiency in long-standing severe mitral stenosis. AO, aorta; LAA, left atrial appendage; LV, left ventricle; PA, pulmonary artery.

FIG 2-28. A schematic drawing of the fluoroscopic findings of a broad-based left ventricular aneurysm. In ventricular diastole (image outlined by thin lines), the left ventricle shows a smooth border without evidence of an aneurysm. In ventricular systole (image outlined by thick lines), however, the aneurysm bulges outward (*arrow*) in a direction opposite to the rest of the left ventricular wall. AO, aorta; LV, left ventricle; RA, right atrium.

In pericardial effusion, the damping of aortic pulsations is highly suggestive of cardiac tamponade. The rationale behind such a relationship is simple. The aortic arch is outside the pericardium, and its pulsation is not affected by the pericardial effusion under low pressure. As the intrapericardial pressure rises, however, the heart is compressed from all sides. In turn, cardiac function is progressively compromised with smaller stroke volumes ejected from the left ventricle, leading to more feeble pulsation of the aorta.

Uneven distribution of pulmonary blood flow is a common phenomenon of valvular pulmonary stenosis with an intact ventricular septum. More blood is channeled into the left lung at the expense of the right (23). The dynamic aspect of this pathophysiology is a remarkable increase in the pulsation of the dilated pulmonary trunk and its left branch; at

the same time, the pulsation of the shrunken right pulmonary artery is markedly decreased.

A uniform increase in pulmonary blood flow is the hallmark of a large left-to-right shunt. The caliber and length of all pulmonary vessels are strikingly increased in both lungs. The dynamic expression of these alterations is a remarkable amplification in pulsation of all the vessels. Under such circumstances, the body's natural defense is to develop a mechanism by which the excessive flow through the lung can be reduced. Fluoroscopically, such a mechanism is manifested by a progressive discrepancy in size and pulsation between the central and peripheral vessels, transforming shunt vascularity into the centralized flow pattern of Eisenmenger syndrome (see **Chapter 8**).

Detecting Cardiovascular Calcifications

Detection and localization of cardiovascular calcifications are of major clinical importance (7,15,17–20) (see **Chapter**

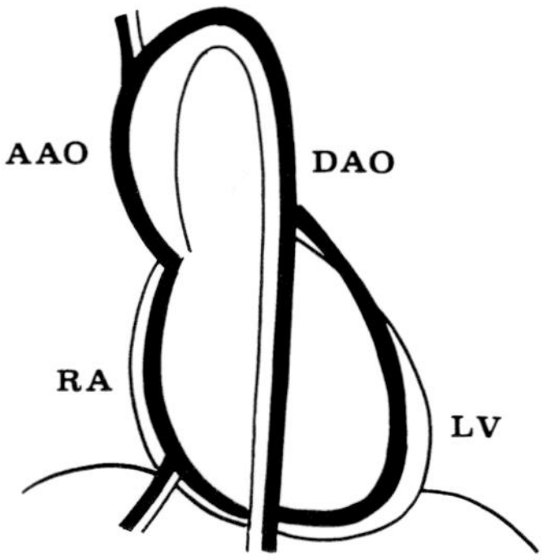

FIG 2-29. A schematic drawing of the snapping type of systolic expansion of the ascending aorta (AAO) in valvular aortic stenosis compared with the normal pulsation of the aortic arch and descending aorta (DAO). LV, left ventricle; RA, right atrium.

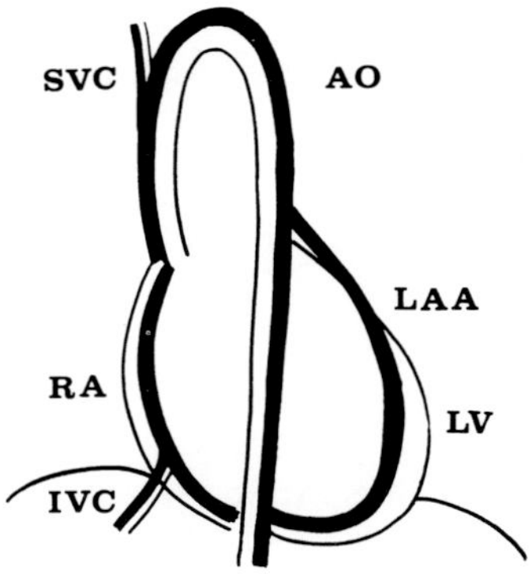

FIG 2-31. A schematic drawing of the dynamic characteristics of a normal heart. AO, aorta; IVC, inferior vena cava; LAA, left atrial appendage; LV, left ventricle; RA, right atrium; SVC, superior vena cava.

10). Although large cardiovascular calcifications (17) can be seen on the radiograph, confirmation frequently requires a fluoroscopic examination. Small calcifications, however, are fuzzed out by motion in the radiograph. Their detection relies entirely on a dynamic study under the image intensifier. By virtue of their vigorous rhythmic movements, even tiny flecks of calcium in the walls of the coronary arteries can be clearly seen fluoroscopically. A coronary artery always moves in a direction perpendicular to its long axis. The excursions of the right and circumflex coronary arteries are more vigorous than those of the anterior and posterior descending branches. Electron beam CT has become the most sensitive tool in the detection of coronary or other small cardiac calcifications (see **Chapters 3 and 10**).

Detecting Subepicardial Fat Stripes

The subepicardial fat stripes are important landmarks in the radiographic diagnosis of heart disease. They are cushion-like structures situated between the myocardium and the pericardium. Being small, delicate, and highly mobile, they usually are not visible on radiography except in the lateral view behind the sternum. Fluoroscopically, however, the fat stripes are easily seen as pulsating linear lucencies against the water density of myocardium.

Because the coronary arteries are embedded in the subepicardial fat stripes, the arteries can be identified by locating the fat stripes. For instance, if the calcified coronary artery (dark line under the fluoroscope) coincides with the fat stripe (bright line) within the left atrioventricular groove, it can be identified as the circumflex. The anterior descending artery moves synchronously with the fat stripe in the anterior interventricular groove. The right coronary artery travels along with the fat stripe in the right atrioventricular groove, as does the posterior descending artery with that in the posterior interventricular groove (Fig. 2-32). In a similar fashion, a radiopaque foreign body can be localized and a calcified valve identified in the heart by their relationships to the cardiac grooves marked by the subepicardial fat.

In the diagnosis of pericardial disease, the subepicardial fat stripes serve as a watershed between the myocardium

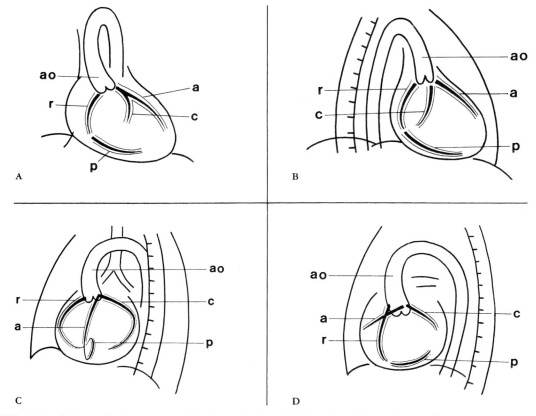

FIG 2-32. Schematic drawings depict the subepicardial fat stripes in relation to the coronary arteries in four views. **A:** Posteroanterior view. **B:** Right anterior oblique view. **C:** Left anterior oblique view. **D:** Left lateral view. a, anterior descending coronary artery, which is embedded in the anterior interventricular groove; ao, aorta; c, circumflex coronary artery, which is embedded in the left atrioventricular groove; p, posterior descending coronary artery, which is embedded in the posterior interventricular groove; r, right coronary artery, which is embedded in the right atrioventricular groove. The white halo surrounding each coronary artery in black represents the subepicardial fat stripes in the groove of the heart between chambers.

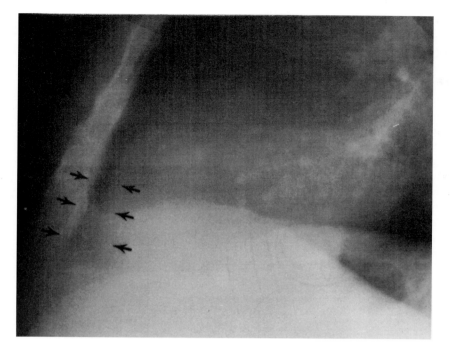

FIG 2-33. Normal hairline density of the pericardium sandwiched between the mediastinal fat (*anterior arrows*) and the subepicardial fat (*posterior arrows*), visible retrosternally in the lateral view.

and the pericardium. Normally, the fat stripes are not readily visible because of the adjacent similar radiolucency of the air-filled lung. The delicate hairline density of the normal pericardium is not seen, except retrosternally in the lateral view (Fig. 2-33). In the presence of pericardial effusion or thickening, however, the fat stripes become distinctly visible owing to the added external density. The fat (radiolucent zone) is sandwiched between the two water densities (radiopaque zones) (24) (Fig. 2-34).

When diagnosing effusion, it is important to note that a bold contrast exists between the inner, vigorously pulsating fat stripe and the outer, immobile band of pericardial fluid. The degree of motion of the fat stripe reflects the contractility of the myocardium. Diminished excursion strongly suggests the possibility of cardiac tamponade. Absent motion means the sudden onset of cardiac arrest, which calls for immediate resuscitation measures. The pulsation of the outer border of the heart is always absent when there is a large effusion. In a patient with pericardial thickening without effusion, however, the thickened pericardium (including the parietal layer of the pericardium at the outer border of the heart) pulsates synchronously with the fat stripe. In this con-

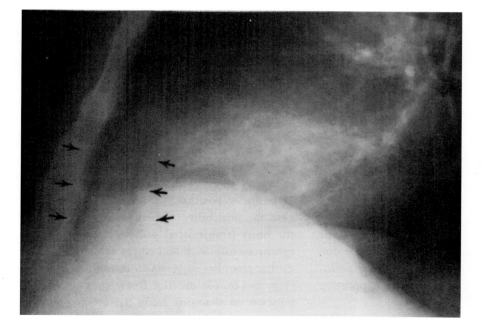

FIG 2-34. Lateral view of a patient with pericardial effusion. Note that the normal hairline density of the pericardium has been markedly widened by the pericardial fluid. Anterior arrows mark the mediastinal fat, and posterior arrows mark the subepicardial fat.

dition, diminished pulsation of the fat stripe or the outer border of the heart suggests constrictive pericarditis.

Since the advent of echocardiography, cardiac fluoroscopy has largely been replaced by ultrasound in the diagnosis of pericardial disease. However, when not clinically suspected, a pericardial effusion may first be recognized on the radiograph and confirmed by fluoroscopy, making other procedures unnecessary. For the detection of a small anterior pericardial effusion, cardiac fluoroscopy is superior to echocardiography. The effectiveness of echocardiography may be markedly diminished or nullified and the use of cardiac fluoroscopy preferred in patients with severe emphysema, those who are extremely obese, those with marked chest deformity, and any who are unable to cooperate.

While the abundance of air and fat surrounding the heart in the retrosternal area helps delineate the pericardium radiographically and fluoroscopically, a blanket of air over the heart acts as a barrier to the transmission of ultrasound. The sternum is another barrier to the sound waves. Mediastinal and subepicardial fat can be mistaken for pericardial effusion during sonography. Therefore, the echocardiographer prudently avoids making a diagnosis of anterior pericardial effusion without first securing evidence of posterior effusion.

Differentiating Cardiac from Noncardiac Lesions

By virtue of their dynamic nature, cardiovascular structures always show rhythmic excursions under the fluoroscope. When respiration is temporarily suspended, any structures that are still moving are likely to be cardiovascular structures. Conversely, noncardiovascular structures are immobile. A pulmonary arteriovenous fistula shrinks with a Valsalva maneuver, with rebound active pulsations on release of the breath. An enlarged azygos node, on the other hand, does not change with a Valsalva or Müller maneuver (16). There are, of course, exceptions to the rule. For instance, a clot-filled aneurysm may not pulsate, and a tumor adherent to the aorta may transmit pulsations. Under these circumstances, more sophisticated diagnostic imaging techniques should be used.

Evaluating Pacemakers, Prosthetic Valves, and Foreign Bodies

The position and behavior of pacemaker wires and electrodes can be promptly determined under the fluoroscope, if they have not been adequately evaluated by radiography (25). Improper placement of a pacing catheter can cause dislodgment of the electrodes, stimulation of the phrenic nerve, perforation of the heart, and, rarely, cardiac tamponade. Normally the electrodes should pulsate synchronously with the atrial or ventricular wall and with the same amplitude. Excessive movement of the electrodes within the heart may indicate dislodgment of the pacer with loss of function.

If the tip of the electrode from a right ventricular pacer is outside the subepicardial fat stripe, it means that the myocardium has been perforated (25) and the pacing electrode is probably within the pericardial cavity. This phenomenon is best seen by watching the electrode protrude beyond the fat stripe with each ventricular systole. If the tip is outside the myocardium but still within the subepicardial fat stripe, it might have entered the coronary sinus and lodged in the middle cardiac vein embedded within the fat in the posterior interventricular groove (25). Sometimes breakage of the pacing lead or the epicardial electrode may escape detection in radiographs that are taken in ventricular diastole. The fracture, however, will become obvious when the two fragments of the broken wire detach at the site of a kink seen only during systole under the fluoroscope (26).

A prosthetic valve can be promptly assessed under the image intensifier for function and stability. A tilt of the valve for >12° between the two phases of the cardiac cycle is strong evidence of valve instability (Fig. 2-35). An unstable prosthesis implies loosening of the sutures around the base of the valve and resultant valvular insufficiency. Severe valvular insufficiency, however, can occur without signs of valvular instability. The leaking may be due to ball variance or multiple small basilar perforations without rupture of the major supportive sutures.

Fluoroscopy is probably the simplest and most versatile imaging technique for detecting and localizing radiopaque foreign bodies in or outside the heart. By noting the ampli-

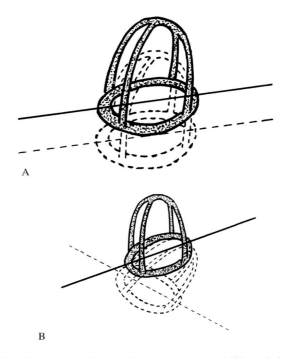

FIG 2-35. Schematic drawings depict normal (**A**) and abnormal (**B**) movements of prosthetic valves. In A, the bases of the valves between the two phases of the cardiac cycle are parallel. In B, the bases of the valves form a >12° angle between end-systole and end-diastole.

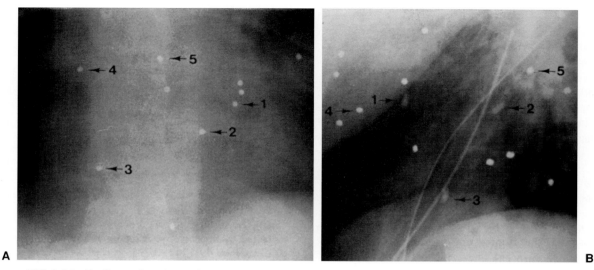

FIG 2-36. Radiographs of a patient with bullets inside and outside the heart. The PA view (**A**) shows no evidence of motion of any of the bullets. On the lateral view (**B**), however, bullets 1, 2, and 3 are blurred, implying an intramural position within the heart. Eventually fluoroscopy was performed. Bullets 1, 2, and 3 were found to pulsate synchronously with the heart in both PA and lateral views. In addition, bullets 4 and 5 moved only slightly with each heartbeat. They were thought to be transmitting the cardiac pulsation because of their position close to, but outside the heart. Both were rotated out of the cardiac silhouette by turning the patient leftward and rightward, respectively.

tude and direction of the movement or the lack of it, the depth of the foreign body can be inferred in the following ways: (a) lack of motion indicates an extracardiac position; (b) feeble pulsations suggest the possibility of being close but outside the heart (transmitted pulsations); (c) moving synchronously with and to the same degree as a cardiac chamber implies an intramural position (Fig. 2-36); (d) moving freely to a dependent position on changing body posture signifies an intracavitary position; and (e) pulsating outside the subepicardial fat stripe indicates an intrapericardial position. Moreover, an intracardiac foreign body can also be zoned according to its relation to the subepicardial fat stripes in different cardiac grooves.

Studying Juxtaposed Noncardiac Structures

By watching juxtaposed noncardiac structures under the fluoroscope, some insights may be gained into the characteristics of a cardiac disease. For example, severe mitral insufficiency is implied by abrupt systolic elevation and compression of the left mainstem bronchus (Fig. 2-37). The inapparent poststenotic dilatation of aortic coarctation can be easily identified by its abrupt anterior and rightward movement, displacing the barium-filled esophagus or the nasogastric tube. In the absence of barium or tube in the esophagus, the left mainstem bronchus is swiftly deviated by the same poststenotic aorta in anterior, inferior, and rightward directions. The abrupt displacement of the esophagus by an enlarging left atrium in mitral insufficiency and in prolapsing mitral valve is a familiar scenario. In the patient

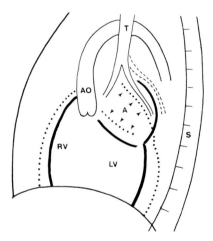

FIG 2-37. A schematic drawing depicts fluoroscopic findings on LAO view of a patient with severe mitral insufficiency. In each ventricular systole, the enlarging left atrium expanded superiorly, posteriorly, and leftward, causing elevation and compression of the left mainstem bronchus. Heavy solid lines outline the cardiac silhouette in systole and the position of the left atrioventricular groove (lucent stripe) in systole. Dotted lines outline the cardiac silhouette in diastole and the position of the left atrioventricular groove in diastole. The upper arrows point to the expanding outer border of the left atrium, displacing and compressing the left mainstem bronchus more markedly in systole. The lower arrows point to the direction of movement of the left atrioventricular groove (lucent stripe) during systole. A, left atrium; AO, aorta; LV, left ventricle; RV, right ventricle; S, spine; T = trachea.

with left-sided atrial myxoma, intermittent left-sided atrial enlargement may be seen when the tumor returns to the left atrium from the left ventricle in systole. At that moment, the barium-filled esophagus is suddenly and transiently indented. Fluoroscopic evidence of mediastinal lymphadenopathy rightfully suggests that a coexisting pericardial effusion is malignant. In children, before the era of CT and MRI the diagnosis of a right-sided aorta depended on a barium study under the fluoroscope.

Assisting Cardiac Catheterization and Angiocardiography

The modern fluoroscope, equipped with an image intensifier, has greatly facilitated the procedure of cardiac catheterization. Precise placement of the catheter in a predetermined site of the cardiovascular system ensures the accuracy of blood sampling and pressure measurement. Satisfactory catheter positioning is also crucial in maintaining a normally functioning pacemaker and in securing an unobstructed angiographic view.

REFERENCES

1. Chen JTT. The chest roentgenogram and cardiac fluoroscopy. In: Schlant RC, Alexander RW, eds. *The heart*, 8th ed. New York: McGraw–Hill, 1994:357–374.
2. Towbin JA, Roberts R. Cardiovascular diseases due to genetic abnormalities. In: Schlant RC, Alexander RW, eds. *The heart*, 8th ed. New York: McGraw–Hill, 1994:1725–1760.
3. Deleon AC Jr., Perloff JK, Twigg H, et al. The straight back syndrome. *Circulation* 1965;32:193–203.
4. Elliott LP, Jue KL, Amplatz K. A roentgen classification of cardiac malpositions. *Invest Radiol* 1966;1:17–28.
5. Elliott LP, Schiebler GL. *The x-ray diagnosis of congenital heart disease in infants, children, and adults*, 2nd ed. Springfield, Ill.: Thomas, 1979:255–326.
6. Eddleman EE Jr., Frommeyer WB Jr., Lyle DP, et al. Critical analysis of clinical factors in estimating severity of aortic valve disease. *Am J Cardiol* 1973;31:687–695.
7. Lachman AS, Roberts WC. Calcific deposits in stenotic mitral valves. *Circulation* 1978;57:808–818.
8. Torrance DJ. Demonstration of subepicardial fat as an aid in the diagnosis of pericardial effusion or thickening. *AJR Am J Roentgenol* 1955;74:850–855.
9. Stewart JR, Kincaid OW, Titus JL. Right aortic arch: plain film diagnosis and significance. *AJR Am J Roentgenol* 1966;97:377–389.
10. Higgins JA, Juergens JL, Bruwer AJ, et al. Loculated interlobar pleural effusion due to congestive heart failure. *Arch Intern Med* 1955;96:180–187.
11. Alexander GH. *The heart and its action: roentgenkymographic studies.* St. Louis: Warren H. Green, 1970:2–135.
12. Dinsmore RE, Wernikoff RE, Miller SW. Evaluation of left ventricular free wall asynergy due to coronary artery disease: use of an interlaced ECG-gated radiography system. *AJR Am J Roentgenol* 1979;132:909–914.
13. Roentgen WB. New forms of radiation. Würzburger Physical Medical Society, Dec. 28, 1895.
14. Deutschberger O. *Fluoroscopy in diagnostic roentgenology.* Philadelphia: Saunders, 1955:152–494.
15. Bartel AG, Chen JTT, Peter RH, et al. The significance of coronary calcification detected by fluoroscopy: a report of 360 patients. *Circulation* 1974;49:1247–1253.
16. Felson B. *Chest roentgenology.* Philadelphia: Saunders, 1973:1–11.
17. Green CE, Kelley MJ. A renewed role for fluoroscopy in the evaluation of cardiac disease. *Radiol Clin North Am* 1980;18:345–353.
18. Margolis JR, Chen JTT, Kong Y, et al. The diagnostic and prognostic significance of coronary artery calcification: a report of 800 cases. *Radiology* 1980;137:609–616.
19. Kelley MJ, Huang EK, Langou RA. Correlation of fluoroscopically detected coronary artery calcification with exercise testing in asymptomatic men. *Radiology* 1978;129:1–6.
20. Langou RA, Kelley MJ, Huang EK, et al. Predictive accuracy of coronary artery calcification and positive exercise test in asymptomatic nonhyperlipidemic men for coronary artery disease [abstract]. *Am J Cardiol* 1980;45:400.
21. Cooley RN. *Radiology of the heart and great vessels*, 3rd ed. Baltimore: Williams & Wilkins, 1978.
22. Chen JTT, Lester RG, Peter RH. Posterior wedging sign of mitral insufficiency. *Radiology* 1974;113:451–453.
23. Chen JTT, Robinson AE, Goodrich JK, et al. Uneven distribution of pulmonary blood flow between left and right lungs in isolated valvular pulmonary stenosis. *AJR Am J Roentgenol* 1969;107:343–350.
24. Jorgens J, Kundel R, Lieber A. The cinefluorographic approach to the diagnosis of pericardial effusion. *AJR Am J Roentgenol* 1962;87:911–916.
25. Hewitt M, Chen JTT, Ravin C, Gallagher J. Radiographic considerations of coronary sinus atrial pacing. *AJR Am J Roentgenol* 1981;135:323–328.
26. Sorkin RP, Schuurmann BJ, Simon AB. Radiographic aspects of permanent cardiac pacemakers. *Radiology* 1976;119:281–286.

Essentials of Cardiac Imaging,
James T. T. Chen,
Lippincott–Raven Publishers, Philadelphia © 1998.

CHAPTER 3

Computed Tomography in Cardiac Imaging

William Stanford

Conventional computed tomography (CT), helical (spiral) CT, and electron beam CT (EBT) (sometimes called EBCT and also known as ultrafast CT or cine CT) all have applications in cardiac imaging. Because the electron beam scanner was primarily developed for cardiac imaging and because it has the widest applicability, this chapter will concentrate primarily on EBT. Conventional CT and helical CT will be discussed in the areas where these technologies have uses.

SCANNER COMPARISONS

Conventional CT has an image resolution of 0.1 mm^2, and a 1- to 10-mm slice thickness is possible. The disadvantage of conventional CT is a 2- to 4-second scan time, which is too prolonged for most cardiac imaging applications. The lack of sharpness of the image due to motion artifacts can be a major problem. However, conventional CT can be used to evaluate overall heart and chamber size, pericardial disease, intracardiac thrombi and tumors, central pulmonary embolism, and coronary calcification.

Helical CT is better suited to cardiac imaging. It has 0.6- to 1-second scan acquisition times and the ability to obtain a volume data set that is conducive to three-dimensional image processing. As with conventional CT, helical CT has applicability in the evaluation of heart size, cardiac chamber size, intracardiac thrombi and tumors, pericardial disease, coronary artery calcification, and central pulmonary embolism. It also appears to be promising for assessing peripheral pulmonary embolism. Still, 0.6- to 1-second scan times are unsuitable for many cardiac imaging applications.

The advantages of EBT are subsecond scan times and the ability to produce high-resolution images—all important features in cardiac imaging. EBT is capable of obtaining 50- to 100-msecond images with resolutions of 0.25 to 0.5 mm^2 in the imaging plane and 1.5 mm to 10.0 mm slice thick-

nesses. Imaging can be done with a temporal resolution of 17 frames/second. These features allow EBT to play an important role in defining cardiac anatomy, evaluating cardiac wall motion abnormalities, and quantitating cardiac function. It is also possible to determine coronary artery bypass graft patency, assess pericardial disease, evaluate coronary artery calcification, define intracardiac tumors, and diagnose intracardiac central and peripheral pulmonary artery thromboembolism. Conventional CT has widespread availability, helical CT less so, and EBT considerably less.

EBT SCANNER CHARACTERISTICS AND TECHNICAL CONSIDERATIONS

The Imatron C-150 EBT scanner (Imatron, Inc., South San Francisco, CA, U.S.A.) is the updated version of the C-100 model. Both versions operate using electron beam technology, whereby moving electrons are bent electromagnetically onto one of four tungsten target rings lying in the gantry below the patient (Fig. 3-1). The x-rays generated from the sweep of the target rings are tightly collimated and pass through the patient onto a double ring of detectors lying in the gantry above the patient. An electron sweep of the target ring can take place in as little as 50 mseconds and produce two contiguous images 8 mm in thickness with a 4-mm gap between images from adjacent target rings; there is an 8-msecond time delay to reset the electron beam. The newer C-150 scanner has two volumetric imaging options, step volumetric scanning and continuous volume scanning, both of which are applicable in cardiac imaging. In addition, the flow and cine mode sequences are extensively used in imaging cardiac disease.

Imaging Sequences

Volume Mode

The C-100 step volumetric scanning is similar to the volume mode imaging sequence of conventional CT scanners.

Department of Radiology, University of Iowa College of Medicine, Iowa City, Iowa 52242, U.S.A

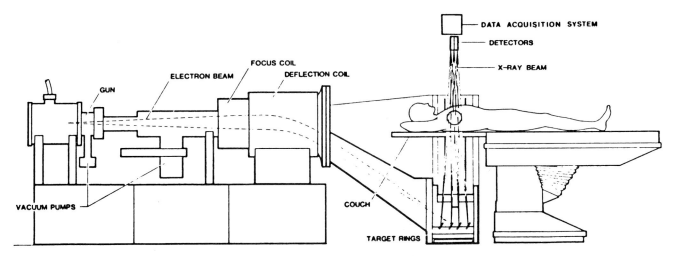

FIG 3-1. Longitudinal view of the EBT scanner. Electrons are bent electromagnetically to sweep tungsten target rings. The x-rays generated from the electron sweep of the tungsten target rings pass through the patient onto detectors located in the gantry above the patient.

This sequence is used in defining of cardiac anatomy and vessel relationships and in the evaluation of the aorta and pericardium. In this sequence, a volumetric data set is acquired by firing electrons at one target ring at a rate of 100 mseconds per sweep. This sequence produces axial images 1½ to 10 mm in thickness. Acquisition times are 100 or 400 mseconds—depending on the number of averages. A complete 40-slice study of the entire thorax requires ~76 seconds.

The C-150 scanner has continuous volume scanning capabilities. This feature permits faster image acquisition than with the step volumetric scanning mode primarily as a result of improvements in software, table speed, and bulk memory storage. While the time required for the electron beam sweep stays the same (100 mseconds), these improvements allow 40-slice data sets to be obtained in 17 seconds. Slice thickness options range from 6 mm through 10 mm. Both modes allow for image manipulation, such as reformatting and region-of-interest density measurements.

Flow Mode

In the flow mode sequence, each target ring is swept sequentially every 50 mseconds; the image acquisitions are triggered from the R wave of the ECG. Eight images 8 mm in thickness are produced in 224 mseconds. The sequence can be repeated following a short programmed delay. Since the scanner memory is limited to 80 images, an eight-level, 10-image sequence is typically programmed. If additional temporal resolution is desired, 13 or 20 images can be acquired at six or four levels, respectively. When imaging is performed during contrast administration, the images can demonstrate progressive vascular enhancement and subsequent washout as the contrast bolus traverses the cardiac

chambers (Fig. 3-2). Using this technique, time-density curves can be generated that temporally document the enhancement of a particular cardiac structure. This sequence is most useful in assessing coronary bypass graft patency and in evaluating intracardiac shunts and myocardial perfusion. It may also be useful in differentiating flow between the true and false lumina of aortic dissection and in measuring blood flow to organs such as the kidney or spleen. In the C-100 and C-150 scanners, the flow mode sequences operate identically.

Movie Mode

This sequence is used to evaluate myocardial contractility. In this mode, the scanner is programmed to sweep a single target ring at a rate of 17 images/second (50 mseconds per sweep). Initiation of the sequences is done from ECG gating. In this sequence, the electron beam sweeps a single target ring a designated number of times before it moves to the next target ring. A typical sequence consists of 10 sweeps at each level. This is sufficient to encompass ventricular contraction from diastole to systole. A complete eight-level 10-image per level sequence would require ~3 second. The images can be played back in a closed-loop movie mode to allow both atrial and ventricular contractions to be seen. In this sequence, the slice thicknesses are 8 mm and are initially triggered from the R wave of the ECG. This is the preferred sequence for quantifying ventricular function and for assessing regional wall motion.

Radiation Dosage

Radiation exposure for the EBT scanner is significantly less than for conventional CT, primarily because of the faster

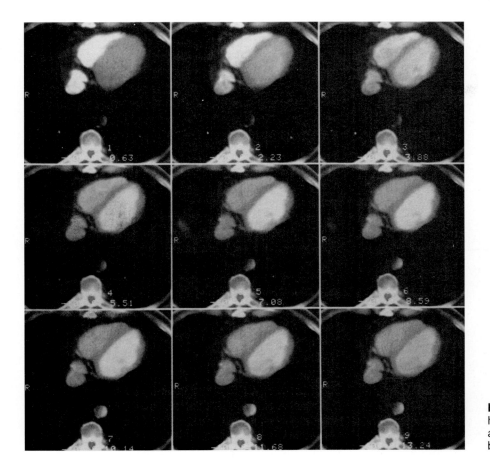

FIG 3-2. Flow mode sequence of the heart shows progressive opacification and washout of the ventricular chambers.

image acquisition times. The entrance dose for a volume study 10 mm in thickness and an exposure of 100 mseconds is 0.9 cGy/slice. This compares with a 2- to 4-cGy/slice exposure for conventional CT. Multiple exposures using the flow or movie mode sequences deliver a dose of 0.58 cGy/image. Because the target source is located posterior to the patient, the calculated exit doses anteriorly are ~17% of the entrance dose. This has important implications, since thyroid and breast doses are much smaller (0.06 cGy/slice for a 100-msecond scan).

Contrast Administration

The use of nonionic contrast material is preferred for all CT imaging because of better tolerance on the part of patients and the higher dosage limit. To ensure optimal vascular enhancement, especially in EBT, correct timing of the bolus is critical. To optimize contrast administration, a circulation time is usually obtained by injecting 10 ml of a 0.5% magnesium sulfate solution and determining as the end point a sensation of heat in the patient's throat. An alternative method is to inject indocyanine green dye solution and determine the time between injection and the appearance of the dye in the systemic circulation by noting its arrival time in a tracing from an earlobe densitometer. It is not uncommon

for patients with cardiac disease to have a prolonged circulation time, and in these circumstances the duration of the contrast medium injection may have to be prolonged.

In movie sequences, it is important to achieve maximal opacification of the cardiac chambers. This is done by delaying imaging until one half of the total contrast dose is infused. The contrast material is usually administered at a rate of 1.0 to 1.5 ml/second, and ~60 to 150 ml of 76% nonionic contrast material is used in a typical study. In a flow study, 40 ml of contrast material is administered as a bolus at 10 ml/second. For a volume study, ~ 180 ml of contrast material is administered, again at a rate of 1.0 to 1.5 ml/second.

Scanning Planes for Cardiac Images

Standard CT images show the pericardium and great vessels in a transaxial plane. However, because the position of the heart within the thorax is not parallel to the axial plane, it is often advantageous to modify the positioning. For long-axis positioning (views similar to the four-chamber views of echocardiography), the scanning platform (table) is slewed 25° to the patient's left (Fig. 3-3A). The table remains horizontal. For short-axis views (cross section), the table is slewed 25° to the patient's right, and the head is elevated 15°. This brings the ventricular chamber perpendicular to

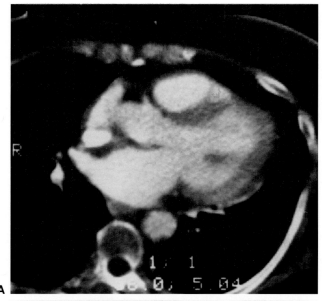

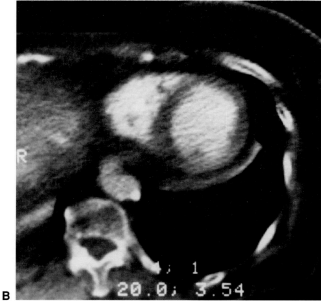

FIG 3-3. Representative EBT images from the mid-left ventricle of a normal patient positioned for the cardiac horizontal "long"-axis (**A**) and "short"-axis (**B**) projections. Proper timing of the contrast bolus and coordination of imaging are dependent upon knowledge of the "circulation time." This affords excellent simultaneous opacification of both the right and left ventricular cavities.

the scanner gantry (Fig. 3-3B). A complete cardiac examination to define anatomy and function generally includes both short- and long-axis multilevel images.

Advantages/Disadvantages

The major advantage of EBT imaging is the subsecond scan times that help minimize cardiac and respiratory lack of sharpness. Moreover, the fast image acquisitions allow scans to be completed during contrast bolus optimization, thereby providing superior vascular enhancement. This vascular enhancement is often not possible with conventional scanners. The disadvantages are the necessity to transport the patient to the scanner, scanner table weight limitations, and the need for venous access, since most patients require contrast administration.

CARDIAC STRUCTURE AND FUNCTION

Cardiac Anatomy

Axial CT images readily show the relationships of the great vessels, atria, and ventricles. The images are displayed without the superimposition of overlying structures, and calcification, fluid collections, and myocardial and pericardial thickening are readily identifiable. Conventional CT, helical CT, and EBT images are all comparable; however, contrast enhancement is often better with helical CT or EBT.

Chamber Size

EBT measurements of radiopaque casts have shown that the volumes of casts of the four cardiac chambers [left atrium, right atrium, left ventricle (LV), and right ventricle (RV)] can be accurately assessed to within 2% to 5% of the true cast volume over a broad range of chamber sizes (1,2). Conventional and helical CT will show overall chamber size, but the accuracy in measuring true volume size has not been reported.

Stroke Volume

The stroke volume for the LV and RV can be determined with a high degree of accuracy with EBT. These determinations are not possible with conventional CT or helical CT. Reiter et al. (3) compared the EBT quantification of left ventricular stroke volume and right ventricular stroke volume using thermodilution techniques and electromagnetic flow probe measurements in instrumented dogs. Using these techniques, the EBT and the electromagnetic/thermodilution, left ventricular stroke volume determinations showed excellent correlation [$r = 0.99$, standard error of the estimate (SEE) = 1.47 ML] (Fig. 3-4). For right ventricular stroke volume, similar agreement was found. LV mass can also be measured with remarkable accuracy by EBT (Fig. 3-5) (4), as can the mass of the free wall of the RV, if 3-mm-thick, high-resolution CT images are used (5).

Global Myocardial Contractility

High-resolution EBT cross-sectional tomographic images of the beating heart can provide excellent qualitative and quantitative information about global ventricular contractil-

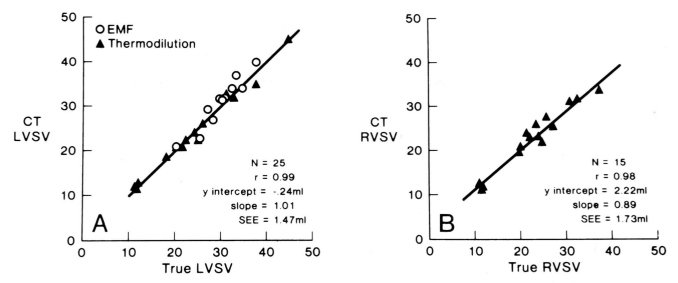

FIG 3-4. Relationship between the EBT measurements of left ventricular stroke volume (LVSV) and right ventricular stroke volume (RVSV) versus true stroke volume measured with either an electromagnetic flow meter (EMF) or thermodilution cardiac output divided by heart rate. These studies were done in chronically instrumented, closed-chest, anesthetized dogs. Note that stroke volume in both the right and left ventricles was estimated accurately with EBT. The open circle represents electromagnetic flow. The closed triangle represents thermodilution. (Reprinted with permission from Reiter SJ, Rumberger JA, Feiring AJ, et al. Precision of right and left ventricular stroke volume measurements by rapid acquisition cine computed tomography. *Circulation* 1986;74:890–900.)

ity. The cine display of images in near real time allows the observer to identify and localize areas of hypokinesis, akinesis, and dyskinesis. Myocardial thinning often occurs in conjunction with a wall motion abnormality, and its presence provides additional documentation of previous myocardial infarction.

Regional Ventricular Function

In addition to providing global contractility information, EBT can be used to measure regional and segmental ventric-

ular function. Using EBT imaging, Feiring et al. (6) looked at regional wall motion in normal volunteers and found large regional variations in ventricular contractility. This heterogeneity varied not only from segment to segment but also between the cardiac apex and base. Specifically, regional contractility was found to be greatest near the apex and decreased in a fairly predictable manner toward the base (Fig. 3-6). Moreover, serial studies in these patients were found to be an excellent way to monitor the progression-regression of these disease processes. Serial scans have also been used to document the effects of cardiotoxic medications.

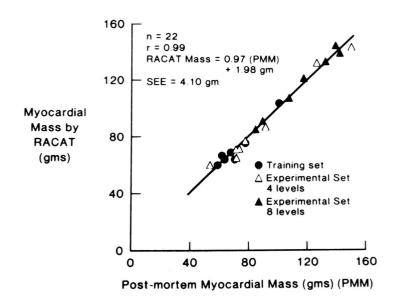

FIG 3-5. Relationship between myocardial mass measured with EBT and postmortem LV mass (PMM). These studies were performed in closed-chest, anesthetized dogs. The CT images were obtained after the intravenous administration of contrast material. There was a close relationship between cardiac mass as determined by EBT and postmortem LV mass (RACAT, rapid acquisition computed axial tomography). Solid circles represent the training set. Open triangles represent four-level experimental set. Closed triangles represent eight-level experimental set. (Reprinted with permission from Feiring AJ, Rumberger JA, Reiter SJ, et al. Determination of left ventricular mass in dogs with rapid acquisition cardiac CT scanning. *Circulation* 1985;72:1355–1364.)

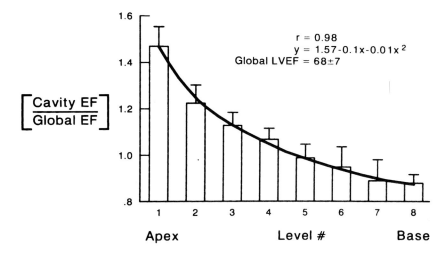

FIG 3-6. Regionalized variations of normalized ejection fraction (cavity EF) related to the global ejection fraction (global EF) at various ventricular levels in normal volunteers. (Reprinted with permission from Feiring AJ, Rumberger JA, Reiter SJ, et al. Sectional and segmental variability of left ventricular function: experimental and clinical studies using ultrafast computed tomography. *J Am Coll Cardiol* 1988;12:415–425.)

Regurgitant Volume

In healthy individuals, the SV for the RV and LV should be nearly identical; therefore, any differences would be the result of valvular insufficiency. Under experimental conditions, close correlations were found between EBT and electromagnetic flow meter measurements of regurgitant volumes. In patients with univalvular insufficiency, serial quantification of regurgitant volume was found to be useful in optimizing the time for surgical intervention. Unfortunately, the quantification of regurgitant volumes imparts little information regarding the location of the insufficient valve or its morphology. Thickened and calcified leaflets, however, are readily seen, and valvular function can be qualitatively evaluated. In patients with two or more insufficient valves or in patients with tricuspid regurgitation, the quantification of regurgitation is less meaningful.

Ejection Fraction

The cardiac ejection fraction is the most universally used measure of cardiac performance. The quantification of the ejection fraction using EBT requires planimetry of the RV and LV to determine end-diastolic volume and end-systolic volume at each level. In the hands of an experienced operator, this requires ~ 30 minutes. Once planimetry is accomplished, the ejection fraction is computed from software inherent within the scanner.

Diastolic Function

There are a number of disease processes that affect ventricular compliance and yet have little effect on global systolic function. Specifically, amyloidosis, small-vessel coronary disease, and ventricular hypertrophy may all have initial signs of abnormal diastolic filling despite a quantitatively normal EF. The assessment of ventricular diastolic function is especially applicable to patients with congestive heart failure and to patients with suspected constrictive pericardial disease. Because ventricular compliance is measured by the rate of diastolic filling, the majority of which occurs within the first 300 to 450 mseconds of diastole, multiple images taken during the early diastolic filling period are required to quantify effective RV compliance. The EBT scanner has proved extremely useful for this application (7).

CORONARY ARTERY BYPASS GRAFT PATENCY

Coronary artery bypass grafting (CABG) is performed in 165,000 Americans annually (8). Unfortunately, 10% to 30% of these grafts occlude within 1 to 2 years and 45% to 55% are occluded at 10 to 12 years. Therefore, the follow-up and subsequent treatment of these patients constitute significant medical and surgical problems.

With EBT imaging, a patent CABG is seen as an opacified conduit lying in the distribution of the bypassed artery (Fig. 3-7). The largest EBT-CABG study reported a 93.4% sensitivity in detecting angiographically patent grafts, 88.9% specificity in detecting angiographically occluded grafts, and 92.1% overall accuracy (Fig. 3-8) (9). This multicenter study also reported that technically successful examinations could be performed in 94.2% patients in whom the study was requested. Bypass grafts to the left anterior descending circulation had the best accuracy rates; however, there were no significant differences in the interpretive accuracies when comparing the left anterior descending, right, or circumflex coronary arteries.

One might expect that the detection of graft patency in patients with multiple conduits might be more difficult than in patients with fewer conduits. However, the data from the multicenter study suggest that the number of grafts placed did not interfere with interpretive accuracies. Also, internal mammary artery (IMA) conduits are smaller in diameter and more likely to have significant numbers of surgical clips, and these can produce artifacts and obscure patent grafts.

For these reasons, it was postulated that the sensitivity, specificity, and accuracy of determining conduit patency might not be as high for IMA grafts as for saphenous vein grafts. However, the sensitivity, specificity, and accuracy of EBT in determining IMA graft versus saphenous vein graft patency have not been significantly different.

Partially obstructed grafts are sometimes less well opaci-

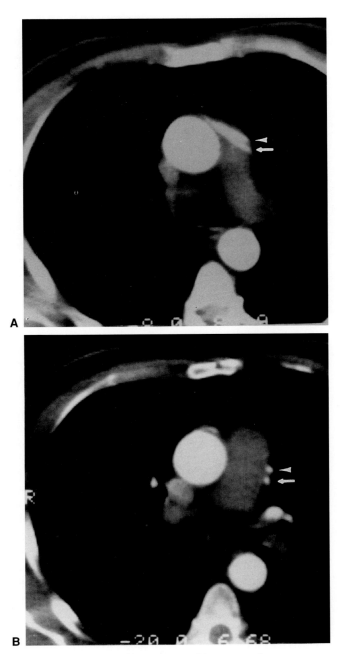

FIG 3-7. Representative tomographic scans of coronary artery bypass grafts. **A:** The left anterior descending coronary artery graft (*arrowhead*) and circumflex coronary artery graft (*arrow*) are seen tangentially as they exit the aorta. **B:** Grafts in the left anterior descending coronary artery distribution (*arrowhead*) and left circumflex artery distribution (*arrow*) are seen in cross section.

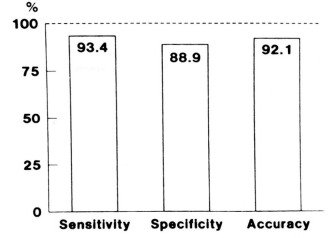

FIG 3-8. Sensitivity, specificity, and accuracy of EBT estimates of graft patency compared with graft patency determined by cardiac catheterization. In this study of 127 bypass grafts in 62 patients, it was noted that both the sensitivity and the specificity of determining bypass graft patency were excellent using EBT. (Reprinted with permission from Stanford W, Brundage BH, MacMillan R, et al. Sensitivity and specificity of assessing coronary bypass graft patency with ultrafast computed tomography: results of a multicenter study. *J Am Coll Cardiol* 1988;12:1–7.)

fied than comparable nonstenotic conduits. Hence, EBT detection of patent but partially obstructed grafts may be more difficult than that of widely patent grafts. In a small subset of patients in the multicenter study, however, the sensitivity of detecting stenotic but open grafts was similar to that of unobstructed grafts. However, it is important to realize that graft visualization provides no information concerning blood flow nor can it assess whether there is a stenosis either within the graft or at its proximal or distal anastomotic site.

When assessment of graft patency by EBT was evaluated on a per-patient basis instead of on a per-graft basis, the multicenter study showed that patency of all grafts was determined correctly in 52 of 62 (84%) patients. In nine of 62 (14.5%), there was one error, and in one of 62 (1.6%), there were two errors. The multicenter study also examined the interobserver and intraobserver variability for determining bypass graft patency by EBT. Interobserver variability was 5.8%, and intraobserver variability was 8.6%. Thus, EBT has proved extremely useful as a minimally invasive method to assess CABG patency. CABG patency can also be evaluated with conventional CT and helical CT (10); however, IMA grafts are more difficult to assess by these imaging techniques. Because of the lack of sharpness due to motion and a lesser ability to visualize the kinetics of the contrast bolus, conventional CT and helical CT are not routinely used in the evaluation of CABG patency.

CORONARY ARTERY CALCIFICATION

Coronary artery calcification is a recognized marker of atherosclerotic disease. Its detection is important because

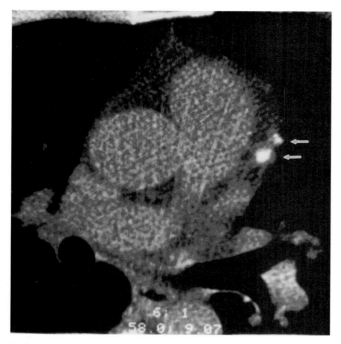

FIG 3-9. Calcifications are visible in the coronary artery (*arrows*) of a 60-year-old man undergoing balloon angioplasty for a left anterior descending artery stenosis.

the calcification is often visible before sufficient narrowing has occurred to be detectable on other tests, such as stress thallium or stress ECG (Fig. 3-9). CT is considerably more accurate than fluoroscopy or the plain chest film in detecting coronary calcification. While the calcified plaques can be detected on all CT images, only EBT has the speed to allow the quantification of them. This is important in following the progression of possible regression of the coronary disease in response to treatment.

INTRACARDIAC THROMBI

Cardiac embolic events are responsible for 15% of all ischemic strokes. The risk is increased in patients with non-rheumatic atrial fibrillation (45%), ischemic heart disease (25%), rheumatic mitral stenosis (10%), and prosthetic cardiac valve replacement (10%) (11). Since the presence of an intracardiac thrombus frequently requires treatment, the early identification of thrombus is of considerable importance. Conventional CT, helical CT, and EBT can all detect intracardiac thrombi, and, at times, these thrombi are extremely well visualized (Fig. 3-10). However, because of faster scan times, helical CT and EBT appear to be superior (12).

In patients suspected of having intracardiac thrombi, the movie mode EBT sequence is preferred because the images not only define the thrombus but also show any associated abnormalities of wall motion. In most cases, three eight-level movie sequences, including the short- and long-axis projections, are performed. The movie sequence defines wall

motion abnormalities and improves thrombus detection. In cases with indeterminate lesions, higher resolution 3-mm-thick slices can be obtained.

Ventricular thrombi may be solitary or multiple and are identified as filling defects within the opacified cardiac chambers (Fig. 3-11). The thrombi may be sessile, convex, or pedunculated; at times they may be calcified. Sessile, or flat, thrombi are the most difficult to diagnose. They characteristically appear as curvilinear filling defects along the wall of the contrast-opacified ventricle; as a result, they often go undetected or are confused with trabeculae. Alternatively, thrombi may look like a convex filling defect projecting into the ventricular cavity. When a thrombus is pedunculated, differentiation from papillary muscle is sometimes difficult and is best accomplished through knowledge of the normal location and configuration of the papillary muscles. A problem can arise when the papillary muscles are prominent or when there is thickening of the subvalvular structures as might occur in mitral stenosis. In these instances, the chordal thickening may extend almost to the valve leaflet and can be confused with a thrombus.

Thrombi are commonly associated with abnormalities of wall motion and are generally located adjacent to areas of myocardial infarction or otherwise poorly contractile myocardium. If an abnormality of wall motion is not present, one should be cautious in diagnosing a thrombus. Thrombi along the inferior wall of the ventricle are best seen on short-axis views, whereas apical thrombi are best seen on long-axis views. Atrial thrombi often arise in the left atrial appendage, which is a difficult area to visualize with transthoracic echocardiography. They appear as filling defects (Fig. 3-12).

Several reports have shown that EBT has a sensitivity similar to or greater than that of two-dimensional echocardiography (2-DE) in the detection of intracardiac thrombi. In a study comparing EBT with 2-DE in the detection of intracardiac thrombi in 41 stroke patients, Love et al. (13) found agreement between the two techniques in 86% of patients; both tests were negative in 76%, and both were positive in 10%. In the six patients (14%) in whom there was disagreement, 2-DE was positive and EBT was equivocal in four patients, 2-DE was equivocal and EBT was negative in one patient, and 2-DE was equivocal and EBT was positive in one patient; in the latter patient autopsy confirmed an LV thrombus. From this study, Love et al. concluded that EBT is an important imaging technique for detecting intracardiac thrombi. This was especially true for patients in whom 2-DE was difficult to perform or gave equivocal results because of chest deformity, extreme obesity, severe emphysema, etc.

In our series of 260 patients in whom the indication for the EBT examination was to exclude intracardiac thrombi, we selected 34 in whom another imaging technique, autopsy, or surgery had been performed at or near the time of the EBT study (14). In 28 of these 34 EBT examinations, there was agreement with the other imaging method (usually echocardiography). In the remaining six examinations, the EBT examination was positive and the echocardiographic study

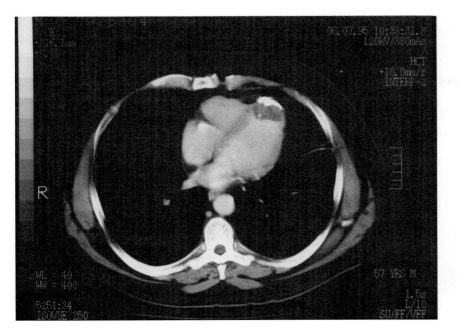

FIG 3-10. Helical CT image of an apical thrombus (T) lying adjacent to a calcified ventricular wall. The patient had had an apical infarct. The helical scan time was 1.5 seconds.

was negative. In each of these six, the EBT findings were substantiated by surgery or cardiac catheterization.

INTRACARDIAC TUMORS

Atrial myxomas account for 50% of primary cardiac tumors. They are often pedunculated and may be ≤8 cm in diameter; they generally arise within the left atrium along the interatrial septum (15). Myxomas may be sessile or pedunculated and appear as a filling defect within the opacified cardiac chambers. If the myxoma is on a pedicle, it may prolapse through the mitral valve and abut the anterior leaf-

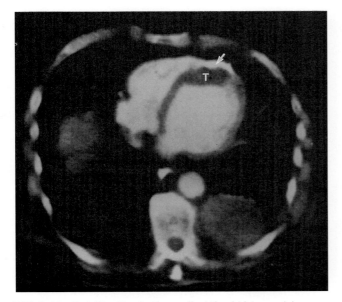

FIG 3-11. Calcification in the wall of the LV (*arrow*) in a patient who previously had myocardial infarction. There is a large thrombus (T) adjacent to the infarct. (Reprinted with permission from Stanford W, Rooholamini SA, Galvin JR. Ultrafast computed tomography for the detection of intracardiac thrombi and tumors. In: Elliott LP, ed. *The fundamentals of cardiac imaging in infants, children, adults.* Philadelphia: Lippincott, 1991.)

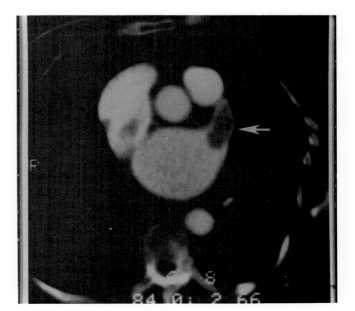

FIG 3-12. Image from an EBT study of a 77-year-old woman with atrial fibrillation, to rule out a left-sided atrial thrombus. The transthoracic 2-DE examination gave negative results. The EBT study shows a large lobulated thrombus within the left atrial appendage (*arrow*). (Reprinted with permission from Stanford W, Rooholamini SA, Galvin JR. Ultrafast computed tomography for the detection of intracardiac thrombi and tumors. In: Elliott LP, ed. *The fundamentals of cardiac imaging in infants, children, adults.* Philadelphia: Lippincott, 1991.)

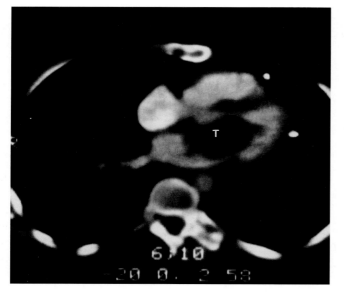

FIG 3-13. Long-axis view of a left atrial myxoma (T) prolapsing through the mitral valve in diastole. The tumor abuts the anterior leaflet of the mitral valve. A left atrial myxoma was found at operation. (Reprinted with permission from Rooholamini SA, Galvin JR, Stanford W. CT for the detection of intracardiac and proximal pulmonary artery thromboembolism [Abstract]. *Radiology* 1989;173:240.)

let, causing thickening or deformity of the valve (Fig. 3-13). Sessile tumors appear as a solid mass and may be located on the right side of the interatrial septum. Ventricular myxomas may be attached to the ventricular free wall, interventricular septum, or a papillary muscle. Rhabdomyomas, fibromas, and lipomas complete the group of benign cardiac tumors. Although they are less common than myxomas, they are often readily identified with EBT.

Tumors can also metastasize to the heart. Melanoma, lung carcinoma, and breast carcinoma are the tumors that most commonly do so. They appear as mass lesions within the cardiac chambers, as localized thickenings along the wall or ventricular septum, or as nodules on the epicardial surface. Lymphomas and renal cell carcinomas may grow intraluminally within the inferior vena cava and, at times, may extend up and into the right atrium and RV. In most cases, the size, location, attachment, and configuration of the tumor can be seen on CT, but EBT can better define any movement occurring during the cardiac cycle. CT does not suffer from the superimposition of other tissues and, therefore, is very useful for defining cardiac tumors.

PERICARDIAL DISEASE

Conventional CT, helical CT, and EBT all have applicability in evaluating pericardial disease. EBT retains the advantages of conventional CT and, in addition, can scan cardiac contractions at a rate of 17 images/second and play them back in a closed-loop movie sequence, thus allowing

visualization of the contraction pattern of the ventricles and the quantification of the diastolic filling. As mentioned earlier, it is possible to calculate LV and RV end-diastolic and end-systolic volumes, stroke volume, EF, LV mass, and cardiac output from EBT images. These determinations are important in patients suspected of having constrictive physiology. The most frequently used sequence is the short- and long-axis movie mode sequence. Additional 3-mm high-resolution images in the volume mode sequence may also be helpful in defining the pericardial anatomy.

On CT images, the pericardium is commonly seen as a 1- to 2-mm structure of soft-tissue density lying between mediastinal fat ventrally and epicardial fat dorsally. Some part of the anterior pericardium may be visualized in virtually 100% of patients; however, the posterior pericardium is seen only 25% of the time. In and around the attachment to the great vessels, there is often little or no fat; therefore, the pericardium is frequently not visible. The same is true of the pericardial cavity, unless it is distended by air, fluid, or a mass lesion.

Pericardial thickening occurs as a response to trauma, inflammation, or tumor or following pericardiotomy or radiation injury. The thickening may be localized or generalized and may measure from a few millimeters to >5 cm. CT is extremely sensitive in determining pericardial thickening, especially when calcification is present. If the thickening results in constriction, it is important not only to diagnose the thickening but also to assess ventricular function. EBT

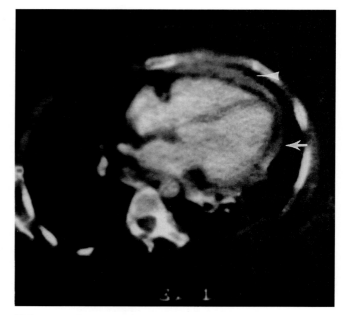

FIG 3-14. Thickened pericardium encases the RV (*arrowhead*) and LV (*arrow*), producing constriction. The cause of the constriction was thought to be an inflammatory process. (Reprinted with permission from Stanford W. Computed tomography and ultrafast computed tomography in pericardial disease. In: Elliott LP, ed. *The fundamentals of cardiac imaging in infants, children, adults.* Philadelphia: Lippincott, 1991.)

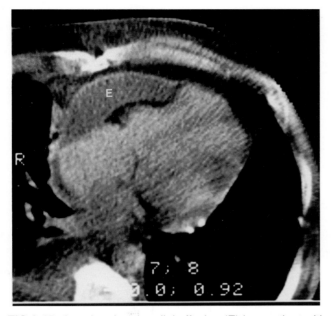

FIG 3-15. Loculated pericardial effusion (E) in a patient with shortness of breath. The effusion was compressing the right ventricle. After aspiration the patient's symptoms resolved.

can do both; hence, it is used extensively for the evaluation of patients with constrictive pericarditis (Fig. 3-14) (7).

Effusions are commonly seen on CT. They may be free flowing or loculated. If the effusion is thin and serous, it can be diagnosed readily; however, exudates and blood may have CT densities that approach those of soft tissue, and in these cases it may be difficult to differentiate fluid from a thickened pericardium. CT is important in identifying the amount of fluid and in evaluating the physiologic effect. The normal pericardium may become enormously distended and yet produce little or no hemodynamic alteration. Conversely, a small effusion can cause cardiac tamponade if the fluid accumulates rapidly or accumulates in an area in which a thickened pericardium limits distensibility (Fig. 3-15).

CONCLUSIONS

CT has many applications in cardiac imaging. Conventional CT, helical CT, and EBT delineate cross-sectional anatomy and evaluate cardiac chamber size, intracardiac thrombi and tumors, and pericardial disease. EBT is superior in assessing global and regional function, coronary artery calcification, and CABG patency. Overall, CT has many applications and is an important imaging tool in the evaluation of cardiac disease.

REFERENCES

1. Vandenberg BF, Weiss RM, Kinzey J, et al. Comparison of left atrial volume by two-dimensional echocardiography and cine-computed tomography. *Am J Cardiol* 1995;75:754–757.
2. Pietras RJ, Wolfkiel CJ, Veselik K, et al. Validation of ultrafast computed tomographic left ventricular volume measurement. *Invest Radiol* 1991;26:28–34.
3. Reiter SJ, Rumberger JA, Feiring AJ, et al. Precision of right and left ventricular stroke volume measurements by rapid acquisition cine computed tomography. *Circulation* 1986;74:890–900.
4. Feiring AJ, Rumberger JA, Reiter SJ, et al. Determination of left ventricular mass in dogs with rapid acquisition cardiac CT scanning. *Circulation* 1985;72:1355–1364.
5. Hajduczok ZD, Weiss RM, Stanford W, et al. Determination of right ventricular mass in humans and dogs with ultrafast cardiac computed tomography. *Circulation* 1990;82:202–212.
6. Feiring AJ, Rumberger JA, Reiter SJ, et al. Sectional and segmental variability of left ventricular function: experimental and clinical studies using ultrafast computed tomography. *J Am Coll Cardiol* 1988;12:415–425.
7. Oren RM, Grover-McKay M, Stanford W, et al. Accurate preoperative diagnosis of pericardial constriction using cine computed tomography. *J Am Coll Cardiol* 1993;22:832–838.
8. Trafford A. America's $39 billion heart business. *US News & World Report* March 15, 1982:53–57.
9. Stanford W, Brundage BH, MacMillan R, et al. Sensitivity and specificity of assessing coronary bypass graft patency with ultrafast computed tomography: results of a multicenter study. *J Am Coll Cardiol* 1988;12:1–7.
10. Tello R, Costello P, Ecker C, Hartnell G. Spiral CT evaluation of coronary artery bypass graft patency. *J Comput Assist Tomogr* 1993;17:253–259.
11. Cerebral Embolism Task Force. Cardiogenic brain embolism. *Arch Neurol* 1988;43:71–84.
12. Stanford W, Rooholamini SA, Galvin JR. Ultrafast computed tomography for the detection of intracardiac thrombi and tumors. In: Elliott LP, ed. *The fundamentals of cardiac imaging in infants, children, adults.* Philadelphia: Lippincott, 1991.
13. Love BA, Struck L, Stanford W, et al. Two-dimensional echocardiography and ultrafast cardiac computed tomography for evaluating intracardiac thrombi in cerebral ischemia. *Stroke* 1990;7:1033–1038.
14. Rooholamini SA, Galvin JR, Stanford W. CT for the detection of intracardiac and proximal pulmonary artery thromboembolism [Abstract]. *Radiology* 1989;173:240.
15. Scholz TD, Boskis M, Roust L, et al. Noninvasive diagnosis of recurrent familial left atrial myxoma: observations with echocardiography, ultrafast computed tomography, nuclear magnetic resonance imaging and in vivo relaxometry. *Am J Cardiac Imaging* 1989;3:142–145.
16. Stanford W. Computed tomography and ultrafast computed tomography in pericardial disease. In: Elliott LP, ed. *The fundamentals of cardiac imaging in infants, children, adults.* Philadelphia: Lippincott, 1991.

Essentials of Cardiac Imaging,
James T. T. Chen,
Lippincott–Raven Publishers, Philadelphia © 1998.

CHAPTER 4

Cardiac Magnetic Resonance Imaging

General Discussion

Jean-Paul Vallée, *Donald P. Frush, and †H. Dirk Sostman

Magnetic resonance imaging (MRI) is a noninvasive, multiplanar technique that accurately depicts cardiac, pericardial, and great-vessel anatomy; ventricular systolic function and wall motion; and blood flow. However, imaging of the heart with MR in routine clinical practice has lagged behind clinical applications of MRI to other parts of the body. The reasons for this lag include the moderately high cost of MRI procedures, the relative lack of availability of MRI when compared with ultrasound and scintigraphy, and issues of medical politics and reimbursement of costs. It is of greatest importance, however, that MRI has not yet been able to make a meaningful assessment of coronary atherosclerosis and myocardial ischemia. Developments in fast imaging techniques and MR angiography suggest that the so-called "one-stop shopping" that has been considered implicit in cardiac MRI can be achieved. Accordingly, it is likely that MRI of the heart will become increasingly important.

The plethora of MRI techniques that can be applied to the heart makes it necessary to choose carefully which to develop and which to use for particular types of patients. In this chapter, we review the basic techniques of MRI and relate them to present and future clinical uses of this important imaging method.

MAGNETIC RESONANCE IMAGING TECHNIQUES

Physical Principles

Magnetic resonance imaging is a type of emission tomography. It is based upon magnetization of the patient's tissue,

Center of Advanced Resonance Magnetic Development and *Division of Pediatric Radiology, Department of Radiology, Duke University Medical Center, Durham, North Carolina 27710, and †New York Hospital–Cornell Medical Center, New York, New York 10021, U.S.A.

generation of a weak electromagnetic signal by the application of a radiofrequency pulse, and spatial mapping of that signal by manipulating its frequency and phase in a location-dependent manner using magnetic field gradients. Unlike computed tomography (CT), MRI does not require mechanical motions of the scanner and therefore can image directly in nontransaxial planes.

Although electromagnetic radiation is used, the energy levels in MRI are well below the levels needed to ionize molecules and thus MRI appears to be remarkably free of significant bioeffects. Safety concerns in MRI relate to the extremely strong static magnetic field and rapidly switched gradient magnetic fields and to the possibility of tissue heating from radiofrequency energy absorbed by the body. Tissue heating is a theoretical concern, but in practice it does not achieve levels greater than those associated with vigorous exercise when normal techniques are employed. The rapid time-varying gradient magnetic fields could possibly stimulate electrically excitable tissue, but this does not occur at the levels used in clinical devices.

In contrast, the strong magnetic field is a major safety hazard, since the magnetic forces near a whole-body MR imager are strong enough to cause significant projectile hazards. For example, an oxygen cylinder brought into an MRI exam room will fly into the bore of the magnet with a *terminal velocity of ~ 45 mph.* The possibility of displacements or torques on metallic implants within patients must also be considered. Although the margin of safety usually is quite high, there are documented instances of harm to patients from the effects of dislodging intracranial aneurysm clips or intraocular metallic foreign bodies. Finally, the magnetic field can operate reed relays in cardiac pacemakers and cause a change in the pacing mode. Accordingly, strict security around MRI facilities is essential to prevent patients with certain types of metallic implants from entering the scanner and to prevent medical personnel from carrying into the scan room objects that could become projectiles.

Magnetic resonance imaging produces extremely high contrast between different types of soft tissue. This soft-tissue contrast is based upon intrinsic properties of the tissues and also upon operator-selectable machine parameters. The tissue properties are the tissue concentration of protons available to produce an MRI signal ("proton density"), the presence of motion or blood flow, and two tissue properties known as T1 and T2, time constants that describe how quickly an MRI signal can be generated (T1) from a tissue and how quickly the MRI signal, once generated, decays away (T2). In general, pathologic tissues have long T1 times and appear dark on those MR images whose appearance is conditioned primarily by T1 effects ("T1-weighted images"). Usually, pathologic tissues also have long T2 times and appear bright on T2-weighted images. The reason for this opposite behavior is that T1 and T2 describe processes that have opposite effects on the intensity of the MRI signal. Flowing blood also can appear either bright or dark on MR images, depending upon the examination technique. The art of performing an MRI examination depends upon appropriate manipulations of imaging techniques to capitalize upon differences in proton density, flow, T1, and T2 between different types of normal tissues and lesions that must be distinguished from normal tissues and other lesions.

Magnetic resonance images are displayed in a fashion analogous to that used for CT images. Window and level controls are as essential with MRI as they are with CT. In both cases, the image is a two-dimensional map of some property of the patient's tissues. With CT it is the tissues' x-ray attenuation, while with MRI it is the tissues' MRI signal intensity. In both instances, a higher value normally is displayed as a brighter white.

Imaging Techniques

Magnetic resonance imaging is quite complicated, and its methods are still evolving rapidly. Accordingly, specific imaging protocols are beyond the scope of this chapter. In the thorax, diagnostic images are readily obtained using field strengths of 0.35 T to 1.5 T; the images with lower field strength have the advantage of fewer motion-related artifacts but the disadvantage of a lower intrinsic signal-to-noise ratio.

Magnetic resonance images take a long time to acquire, and motion during imaging causes both discrete periodic artifacts ("ghosts") and image blurring, which can degrade MR image quality severely. Motion compensation techniques therefore are paramount to obtaining satisfactory image quality in thoracic MRI. Several techniques are available to reduce respiratory artifacts, and without exception one or more of these techniques must be used in all thoracic MRI protocols (1). Synchronizing images to the ECG is necessary in all cardiac MRI procedures (1). This can be done

by using the R-wave to trigger the start of an MRI sequence ("prospective gating") or by recording both the ECG and the MR image data and retrospectively synchronizing them ("retrospective gating").

Direct imaging in sagittal, coronal, and oblique planes is a clinically advantageous capability of MRI. Sagittal and coronal MR images can provide superior depiction of structures oriented in the long axis of the body, such as the aorta. Oblique planes can be oriented along the major cardiac axes, as is done in ultrasound and tomographic nuclear cardiac imaging.

Flow is a profound modifier of the MR image. There are two basic types of effects from flow: time-of-flight effects and spin-phase effects. Both types can be manipulated by the choice of pulse sequence; single versus multislice imaging; imaging plane; selectable machine parameters, such as pulse repetition time (TR) and echo time (TE); cardiac gating; saturation pulses; and gradient moment nulling. The manifestations of flow effects in MR images also strongly depend upon the type of flow present. The clinical implication is that one can make blood in MR images either bright ("white-blood images") or dark ("black-blood images") more or less at will. Most types of vascular pathology can be demonstrated with either white-blood or black-blood images, but there are usually clinical advantages to using one approach or the other in specific situations. Flow velocity can be quantified with MRI techniques, and thus noninvasive estimates of blood flow potentially are available. Tomographic MR images of blood vessels can be displayed with reprojection techniques to produce projection "angiographic" images.

One of the major disadvantages with MRI to date is that it is a very slow procedure. In clinical MRI, one often wants to scan rapidly enough to follow dynamic events, such as the passage of a bolus of contrast material through tissue; or fast enough to stop motion (for example, cardiac and respiratory motion); or more efficiently, in order to achieve a higher signal-to-noise ratio per unit of scan time. Conventional spin-echo and gradient-echo techniques are not capable of fulfilling these requirements and thus place limitations upon the scope of clinical MRI. This has been a particular problem in cardiac imaging.

The imaging time in MRI is given by the following equation: imaging time = TR × number of phase encoding lines × number of signal averages. Accordingly, to scan faster, one can make the TR shorter or acquire fewer phase-encoding lines or use fewer signal averages. Making the TR shorter enables one to acquire a complete image in 1 to 2 seconds, but it has the disadvantages of low signal-to-noise ratio, poor soft-tissue contrast, and the possibility of reducing the signal from slowly flowing blood. Acquiring fewer phase-encoding lines reduces spatial resolution, while acquiring fewer signal averages reduces the signal-to-noise ratio. Thus these approaches are quite limited, although they sometimes may be used adjunctly with other techniques.

A better solution to fast imaging is to acquire more than one phase-encoding line with each TR. In conventional MRI, a single phase-encoding line is acquired with each TR. If we can acquire many phase-encoding lines with each TR, we can scan much faster. The most extreme example of this approach is echo-planar imaging. In this method, all the phase-encoding lines are acquired in a single "shot" using only one TR time. The total time required to make a complete image may be 25 to 50 mseconds with this technique. Although practical hardware constraints limit the signal-to-noise ratio and spatial resolution, this method offers the fastest data acquisition time. It has great promise for cardiac MRI.

Sedation and Monitoring for MRI Examinations

Technical considerations of pediatric and, occasionally, adult MRI include the use of sedation. The goals of sedation are to maximize the patient's welfare while obtaining the best possible diagnostic examination. The first goal cannot be understated, and contemporary practice of diagnostic imaging must address the need for appropriate minimal standards for sedation (2). The approach to conscious sedation in diagnostic imaging includes determination of the need for sedation, definition of the goals of sedation, and use of a standard protocol for administration of agents, monitoring of patients, and discharge. Conscious sedation is sufficient for the vast majority of cardiac MRI examinations and can be performed by qualified radiology staff. Deep sedation of patients should be carried out under the supervision of a qualified anesthesiologist.

Successful conscious sedation can be achieved by a variety of agents and routes of administration. However, prudent use of a limited selection of agents can cover most needs. One highly successful and established protocol for sedation uses chloral hydrate, sodium pentobarbital, and fentanyl citrate (3). Newborns may not require more than swaddling or feeding. Children <2 years of age are given 75 to 100 mg/kg p.o. chloral hydrate (total dose limit of 2 g). Older children receive sodium pentobarbital i.v. (3 to 6 mg/kg) with or without limited supplemental doses (1.0 μg/kg) of fentanyl citrate.

Careful assessment during administration of agents will indicate when additional amounts or types of agents are needed to achieve a successful level of conscious sedation. It is equally important to monitor sedation during the diagnostic procedure. Strict use of equipment to monitor physiologic parameters is requisite, particularly in cases where direct visualization of the patient is limited, such as when using a head or knee coil as a body coil. Constant display of oxygen saturation and heart rate is mandatory. A number of MRI-compatible pulse oximeters can be used in infants, children, and adults. These minimal standards of monitoring may be supplemented with respiratory monitoring or other physiologic measures as needed. Adequate monitoring provides for the safety of the patient and indicates when additional sedation may be needed for completion of the procedure.

Although fast and ultrafast MRI techniques can reduce the duration of the study (often substantially), these advancements will not, as they currently exist, eliminate the need for sedation in cardiac MRI. Familiarity with the principles and practice of sedation in MRI is an essential technical skill for the radiologist.

CURRENT CLINICAL APPLICATIONS

In Pediatric Patients

Role of MRI in Diagnostic Evaluation

The outlook for the infant or child with congenital or acquired heart disease has improved dramatically in the past decade with advances in medical and surgical management. At the same time, noninvasive diagnostic imaging of these cardiac abnormalities has flourished with the development of Doppler echocardiography and MRI. These technical advances also make imaging algorithms more complex. An understanding of the indications for various imaging techniques helps in developing strategies for the diagnosis and care of individuals with congenital cardiac disease.

The imaging methods used in pediatric heart disease are chest radiography, echocardiography, MRI, and angiography (4). Scintigraphy has only limited application in children. In adults, however, myocardial ischemia is the dominant disorder scintigraphy is used to assess. After chest radiography, echocardiography is the most frequently performed imaging exam. Echocardiography is generally the test of choice in evaluating intracardiac defects and juxtacardiac vessels, but it is often limited in evaluating the central right and left and perihilar pulmonary arteries; the right ventricle (or anterior chamber), particularly in children where the lung interdigitates between the heart and chest wall; the descending thoracic aorta and arch branch vessels; and in the acute postoperative period where chest dressings or some surgical hardware may limit the acoustic window (5–7). Cardiac catheterization and angiography contribute physiologic information on pressure, cardiac output, and oxygen saturation in addition to the dynamic anatomic evaluation. Angiocardiography is obviated in cases where only structural information (echocardiography and MRI) or functional information, such as wall motion, ejection fraction, flow gradients, and intracardiac shunts (primarily echocardiography), is necessary for evaluation and follow-up.

Magnetic resonance imaging is particularly effective in the anatomic evaluation of disease in the cardiovascular system both before and after surgery (5,8–10). There is excellent characterization of the aorta and branch vessels, including collateral pathways, pulmonary arteries, venae cavae, vascular shunts and conduits, and the pericardium and extracardiac regions. Aggregate information from MRI has an important role in evaluation of the patient with complex structural disease, which is insufficiently understood using other imaging methods, such as echocardiography or angiog-

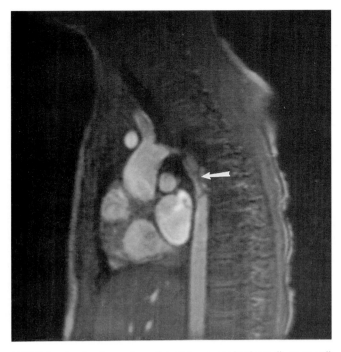

FIG 4-1. Aortic dissection. An oblique sagittal gradient-recall sequence shows the intimal flap (*arrow*) in the descending aorta after angioplasty for recurrent aortic coarctation.

raphy. Functional evaluation includes assessment of wall motion abnormalities, ejection fraction, regurgitant fraction, myocardial mass, presence and size of native and surgical shunts, pressure gradients, and metabolism with MRI spectroscopy. Although MRI can be applied to answer almost any

question in congenital or acquired pediatric heart disease, the emphasis of this section is on applications where MRI affords sufficient information either alone or in combination with other tests, usually echocardiography, to answer the specific clinical questions.

MRI Technique in Children

The MRI examination should be designed with knowledge of the clinical history and previous imaging data. Structural information is best obtained using an ECG-gated spin-echo technique in a strategy where sequences are obtained in an order that addresses prioritized clinical questions. A knee coil can be used in small infants, the head coil in small children, and the standard body coil or the new torso coil in larger individuals. Matrix size varies from 128 to 256 × 256 with slice thicknesses ≤10 mm. High-resolution images are obtained using four excitations and 3- to 5-mm-thick sections with minimal interslice gap. Respiratory compensation is generally ineffective in the infant because the shallow respirations are not consistently detected. Occasionally, "white blood" gradient-recalled-echo sequences with a cine format are helpful in evaluating the patency of small vessels or the separation of intracardiac or intravascular flow artifacts from masses (11). These same sequences may also be useful in distinguishing thrombus from flow artifact, which may not be discernible with spin-echo techniques.

Vascular Abnormalities in Children

The entirety of the thoracic aorta and its branch vessels are well depicted with MRI. Magnetic resonance imaging

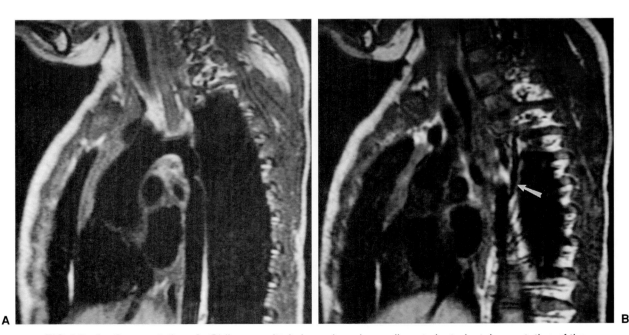

FIG 4-2. Aortic coarctation. **A:** Oblique sagittal plane view shows discrete juxtaductal coarctation of the descending thoracic aorta distal to the left subclavian artery. **B:** The descending aortic collateral vessel in the same patient (*arrow*).

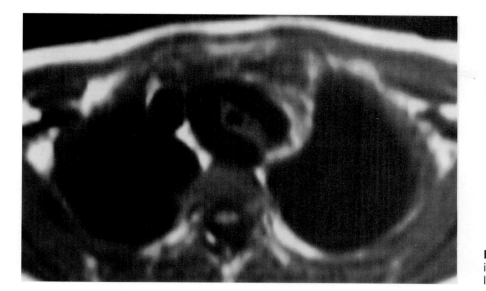

FIG 4-3. Double aortic arch. A transaxial view pinpoints a larger right and small left arches encircling the trachea.

of the aorta can be useful for detecting aneurysms, dissection (Fig. 4-1), coarctation (Fig. 4-2), and vascular rings (Figs. 4-3 to 4-5). Aneurysms of the ascending aorta may occur in a variety of disorders (including Marfan syndrome, Noonan and Turner syndromes, pseudoxanthoma elasticum, and Ehlers-Danlos) or may accompany bicuspid aortic valve or acquired conditions related to trauma, infection, or vasculitis.

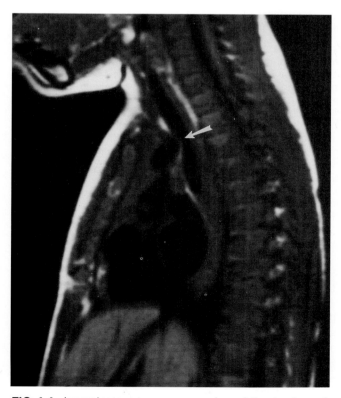

FIG 4-4. Innominate artery compression of the trachea. A sagittal view evidences the anterior impingement of the trachea by the innominate artery (*arrow*).

A yearly screening MR examination is probably sufficient for evaluation. Repair is usually undertaken when the transverse diameter of the ascending aorta approaches 6.0 cm in the adolescent (9). Dissections may be found after trauma, including aortic valve and aortic coarctation angioplasty. In the stable patient, dissections of the aorta can be adequately detected using black-blood (spin-echo) and white-blood (gradient recalled echo) sequences, including a cine display (12). In the unstable patient, transesophageal echocardiography has been advocated (12).

Aortic coarctation and atresia can often be assessed with echocardiography in the newborn, but MRI alone (or in combination with echocardiography) is usually sufficient in the older infant and child. For native coarctation, which is generally of either the discrete juxtaductal or diffuse infantile type, the degree of narrowing, the length of coarctation and its relationship to the left subclavian artery, the caliber of the transverse aorta, and the presence of collateral vessels are the most important parameters. Each of them is well demonstrated with MRI. High-resolution oblique sagittal and axial sequences result in a quick but thorough diagnostic anatomic study. If needed, gradient-recalled-echo sequences can help with determination of the severity of the coarctation and the presence of collateral vessels (13–15). MRI is also very useful alone or as an adjunct to other tests in the follow-up of complications of surgical repair or angioplasty of native or repaired coarctations. These complications include re-coarctation, anastomotic aneurysms, and, sometimes, dissections or transections.

Vascular rings typically accompany respiratory symptoms in the child. The constellation of anomalies includes circumflex aorta, double aortic arch, right arch with aberrant left subclavian artery and ligamentum arteriosis, and brachiocephalic artery compression of the trachea. In addition to the excellent anatomic display of the aorta and branch arteries, the representation of the degree and extent of airway

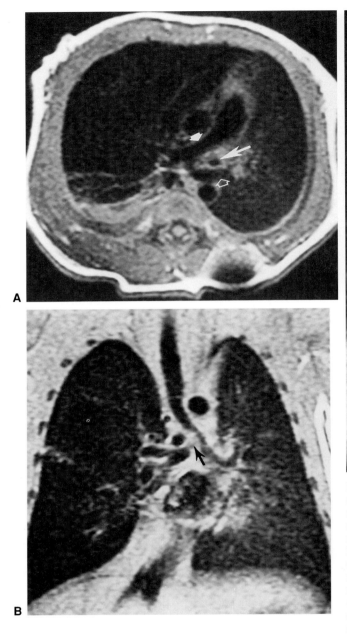

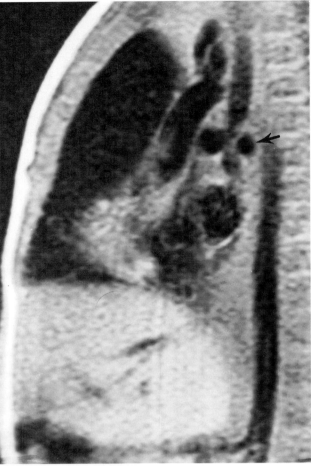

FIG 4-5. Pulmonary artery sling. **A:** Transaxial image at the level of the main pulmonary artery shows the course of the normal right pulmonary artery (*arrow*) and the origin of the left pulmonary artery from the right pulmonary artery (*open arrow*), which surrounds the narrowed and displaced trachea (*large arrow*). There is hyperinflation of the right-upper lobe with a compensatory shift of the mediastinum as well as postobstructive collapse of the right-lower lobe. **B:** The distal trachea is displaced leftward and narrowed, with a markedly narrowed right mainstem bronchus (*arrow*) due to the adjacent aberrant origin of the left pulmonary artery. The right-upper-lobe bronchus and bronchus intermedius are normal. **C:** A sagittal view demonstrates the aberrant left pulmonary artery (*arrow*), which travels between the esophagus and the trachea, narrowing the trachea.

compromise is a valuable and unique feature of MRI (16). The barium esophagogram has a diminishing role in the evaluation of suspected vascular rings, since MRI or angiography is still necessary for surgical planning. In the context of a double aortic arch, knowing the sides of the dominant and smaller, often atretic, arches may help in determining the appropriate thoracotomy site. Finally, aberrant origin of the left pulmonary artery from the right, or pulmonary sling, is a rare cause of airway compromise, which is also well represented by MRI.

Magnetic resonance imaging is very useful after heart sur-

gery to determine the status of pulmonary blood flow (7,10). It may be used as the sole study if only the pulmonary artery anatomy is being looked at (Fig. 4-6). Right ventricle to pulmonary artery conduits (Rastelli procedure), pulmonary artery outflow patches, and anastamoses with the right atrium (modified Fontan) or superior vena cava (classic and bidirectional Glenn), are amenable to MRI evaluation. Magnetic resonance imaging is also effective for assessing pulmonary artery caliber following great vessel switches (Jatene) and the patency and caliber of systemic-to-pulmonary shunts (e.g., a modified Blalock–Taussig shunt).

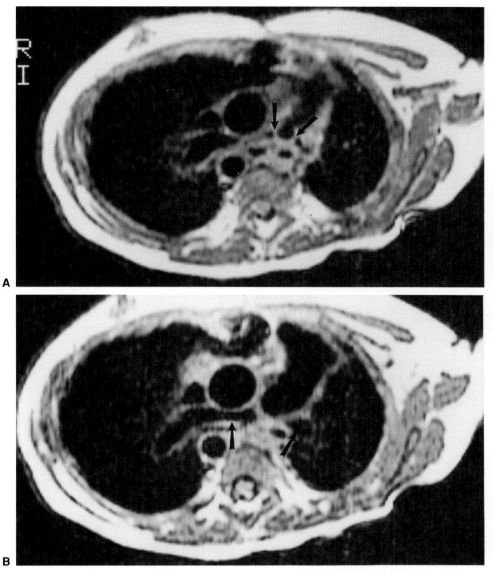

FIG 4-6. Postoperative pulmonary artery stenosis after transannular patch repair for tetralogy of Fallot. **A:** oblique axial view at the level of the main pulmonary artery shows bilateral marked narrowing at the origins of the right and left pulmonary arteries (*arrows*). **B:** An oblique axial view 4 mm caudal shows the transannular patch scars down, causing proximal narrowing; the distal main pulmonary arteries are wide open (*arrows*).

Magnetic resonance imaging is superior to other tests in evaluating the pulmonary artery in some circumstances. The appearance of the prehilar pulmonary arteries before and after surgery is better demonstrated with MRI than with echocardiography. Angiography may not be able to adequately show the presence of branch pulmonary artery confluence or the caliber of the branch pulmonary arteries in situations where pulmonary arterial blood flow may be derived from systemic collateral vessels. However spin-echo MRI is limited in the depiction of arterial vascularity distal to the hila, since there is insufficient contrast for dark-blood–filled vessels to stand out from the dark, air-filled lungs. In this situation, bright-blood gradient-recall acquisi-

tion sequences may improve the detection of flow in more distal vessels. Magnetic resonance imaging is not yet a proven technique for characterizing peripheral pulmonary stenoses.

There are occasionally situations where evaluation of the superior and inferior venae cavae (Fig. 4-7) and pulmonary veins is warranted. For the systemic veins, MRI has a primary role in the evaluation of thrombosis or stenosis, including venous anastomoses after surgery. Venous anomalies, such as left superior vena cava, can be confirmed if echocardiography gives inconclusive findings. MRI information on the status of pulmonary veins is primarily supplemental to that of echocardiography. Light can be shed on anomalous

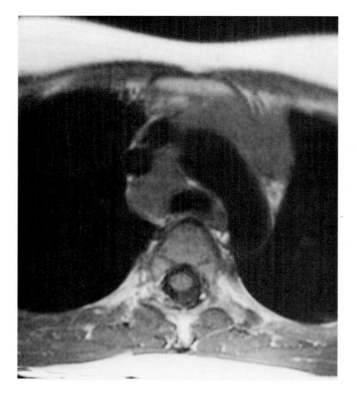

FIG 4-7. Normal thymus. A transaxial MR image at the level of the aortic arch demonstrates the unusual position of a portion of the right lobe of the thymus between the trachea and the normal superior vena cava. Echocardiographic evaluation suggested thrombus in the superior vena cava.

venous connections, the presence of venous stenosis or atresia in larger children (17), or left ventricular inflow obstruction such as is found in cor triatriatum (18).

Cardiac Abnormalities in Children

Magnetic resonance imaging is also indicated when there is complex cardiac disease and other diagnostic techniques have given inconclusive results (19–21). In addition to routine MRI sequences, there has been some limited use of three-dimensional reconstructions (6,7). Multiplanar display of structural relationships can provide useful information for preoperative planning (9). Magnetic resonance imaging has a primary role in evaluation of the pericardium and paracardiac masses. This role is extensively discussed elsewhere. Briefly, examples of clinical problems for which MRI may be useful include differentiating constrictive pericarditis from restrictive cardiomyopathy and distinguishing pseudotumors from masses that may be identified by echocardiography (22).

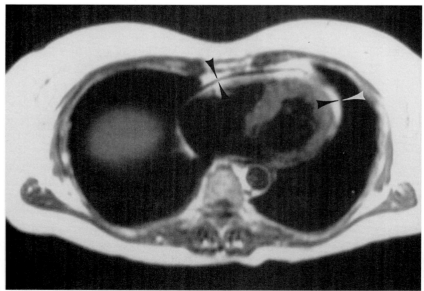

A

FIG 4-8. Differing appearances of normal pericardium, pericardial thickening, and pericardial effusion. **A:** Normal pericardium (*thin line between arrowheads*) is visible on a spin-echo (black blood) image.

FIG 4-8. *Continued.* **B:** Thickened pericardium (*arrowheads*) can be seen on a spin-echo (black blood) image. **C:** Pericardial effusion (*arrow*) is evident on a spin-echo (black blood) image; note that the pericardium itself (*arrowheads*) is normal in thickness. **D:** Pericardial effusion (*arrow*) in the same patient as C, but viewed on a gradient-echo (white blood) image. The patient illustrated in C and D also has metastasis of a melanoma (M) to right atrium.

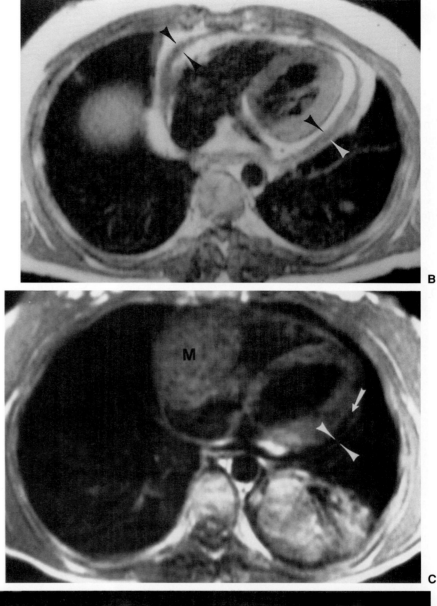

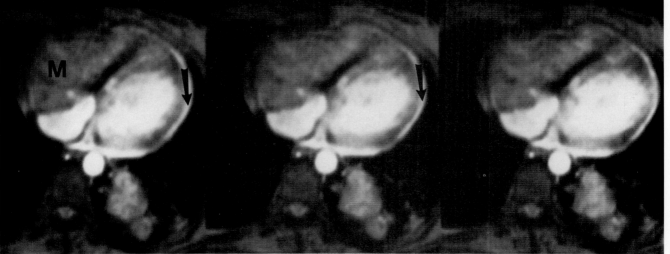

The second category of applications of cardiac MRI is assessment of function. In particular, cine display of gradient-acquired images gives a dynamic perspective on cardiac function (8,23). Functional information can be obtained relating to the ejection fraction, myocardial mass, and wall motion (24). Determination of the presence and size of intracardiac shunts (25,26) and pressure gradients across stenotic valves (27) is particularly suited to MRI. The majority of this functional information is more readily obtained with echocardiography, but MRI is better able to give a global perspective, which can be helpful if echocardiography is technically limited or otherwise provides inconclusive results.

Use of MRI has been increasing in the evaluation of ischemic heart disease and ventricular failure. Although most efforts are directed toward acquired ischemic heart disease

in adults, potential uses in children include the assessment of myocardial function in an effort to intervene surgically (such as with valve replacement or transplant) before permanent ventricular failure occurs. Spectroscopy can yield information on ventricular metabolism (28), and ultrafast techniques (29,30) can be used to appraise myocardial perfusion. MRI has also been used to determine oxygen saturation in blood (31). These applications are compelling but still under investigation.

In summary, MRI currently plays an important role in the diagnosis and management of congenital heart disease. The most dramatic impact has been made in structural evaluation. Based on the rapid evolution of the technique to date, its future contributions to assessment of function, in particular metabolism, are promising.

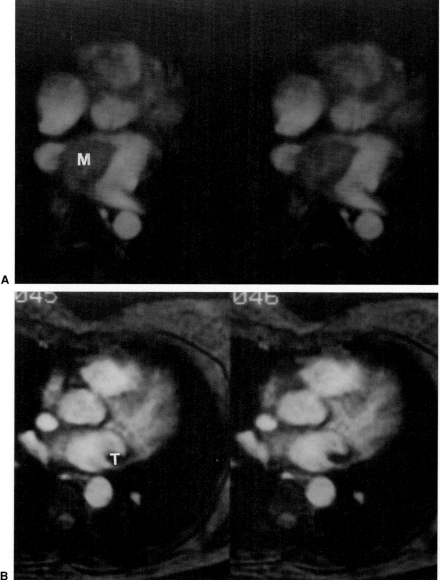

FIG 4-9. Cardiac masses visible on gradient-echo (white blood) images. A: Left atrial myxoma (M). B: Left atrial thrombus (T).

In Adult Patients

Pericardial Disease

The normal pericardium (Fig. 4-8) is thin (1 to 2 mm) and has low MRI signal intensity, reflecting its fibrous histology (32). It is most easily delineated anterior to the heart and on slices near the diaphragm. Regions of minimal pericardial thickening may be seen normally near the right ventricle. The anterior and posterior superior pericardial recesses are seen normally on MR images and must not be mistaken for lymphadenopathy or for regions of aortic dissection.

Pericardial effusions (33) are detected by MRI with great sensitivity; even small normal collections of pericardial fluid are visible. Simple effusions (Fig. 4-8) have low intensity on T1-weighted images because of both the long T1 of simple fluid and the fluid motion due to cardiac pulsation. Simple effusions are hyperintense on T2-weighted images and gradient-echo images (Fig. 4-8) with flow compensation (gradient moment nulling). Complicated effusions and pericardial thickening (Fig. 4-8) usually have higher intensity on T1-weighted and lower intensity on T2-weighted images, and they may be loculated. Hemorrhagic effusions have signal intensity characteristic of blood products in various stages of evolution.

Magnetic resonance imaging is useful in making the dis-

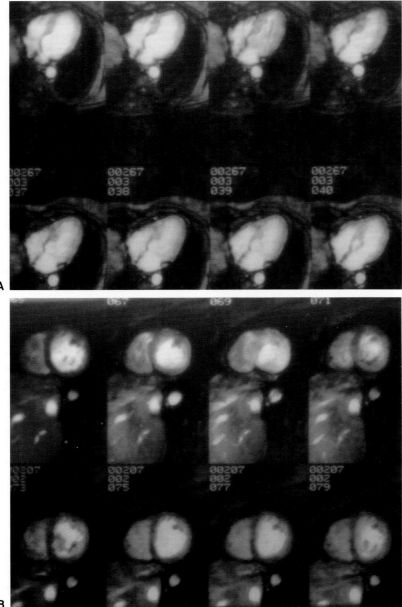

FIG 4-10. Cine gradient-echo (white blood) images taken to assess ventricular function. **A:** Images in the transaxial plane (eight of the 16 images throughout the cardiac cycle at this level are shown). **B:** Images in the oblique sagittal (short axis) plane.

tinction between constrictive pericarditis and restrictive cardiomyopathy (34,35). Normal pericardial thickness excludes constrictive pericarditis for all practical purposes, but even focal thickening can suggest this diagnosis. In addition, restrictive myopathy often shows ventricular wall thickening (36), while in constrictive pericarditis, narrowing and deformity of the right ventricle and abnormal interventricular septal shape and motion can be observed. Areas of pericardial calcification have low intensity on all pulse sequences and are better delineated by CT scanning.

Disease that has metastasized to the pericardium can appear as focal masses, as pericardial fluid, or as both. Breast cancer, lung cancer, melanoma, and lymphoma are the most common primary tumors to involve the pericardium (32). Primary neoplasms of the pericardium itself are rare. Direct invasion of the pericardium, usually from lung cancer, can be delineated well with MRI. Congenital lesions related to the pericardium, such as pericardial cysts and the partial or complete absence of the pericardium, can also be verified with MRI.

Cardiac and Paracardiac Mass Lesions

Primary (Fig. 4-9) and metastatic (Fig. 4-8) cardiac tumors usually are detected initially by ultrasound, but MRI also is an accurate method of delineating such lesions (37–43). It is thus appropriate to employ it as a problem-solving technique in patients with inconclusive results on ultrasound examinations, and it is of particular value in identifying false-positive results (43). Magnetic resonance imaging can show fat within cardiac lesions with good specificity (37). The more common challenge for diagnostic specificity, however, is to distinguish between intracardiac tumor and thrombus (Fig. 4-9). This problem has not been addressed conclusively in the literature; our own experience suggests that tumor and thrombus often can be distinguished. There is one important exception: atrial myxomas and atrial thrombi have variable and overlapping signal intensities and cannot be differentiated reliably. Gradient-echo (white blood) images are preferred for detecting thrombi (44). The use of contrast enhancement is helpful in evaluating tumors.

Magnetic resonance imaging has value for primary assessment of patients suspected of having combined vascular and extravascular disease, since it can demonstrate both vascular and soft-tissue processes with equal accuracy. It may be the only study required in such patients. In this respect, it can be recommended for patients with suspected paracardiac masses, although CT also is effective in most such patients and is less expensive.

Ventricular Function

Magnetic resonance imaging can encompass both ventricles in their entirety and can provide a direct measure of ventricular volumes (Fig. 4-10). Geometric assumptions

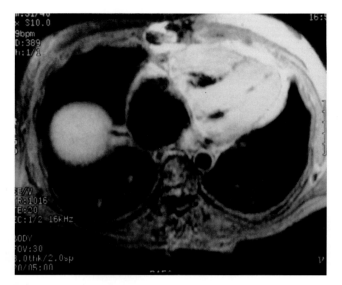

FIG 4-11. Left and right ventricular hypertrophy on spin-echo (black blood) images. In most of the image, the fat signal has been eliminated by a frequency-selective saturation pulse; thus, the signal of soft tissue, such as the myocardium and liver, is brighter than usual (a normal appearance in fat-saturated images). However, the pulse was ineffective in the upper-right portion of the image (probably due to the effect of sternal wire sutures), and subcutaneous fat and epicardial fat remain bright in this region.

used for contrast ventriculography are not necessary with MRI. The spatial resolution of MRI is superior to that of radionuclide methods. It is not possible to miss abnormal areas, as can happen with ultrasound. Accordingly, it is not surprising that MRI has been shown to have great accuracy in measuring such simple parameters as ventricular volumes and ejection fractions (45–47). The technique is particularly useful in studying the right ventricle, which is difficult to evaluate with other techniques.

The problems with MRI in ventricular function evaluation relate to its expense, which is typically greater than ultrasound and radionuclide techniques; the need for tedious manual image processing to obtain chamber volumes; and its relatively low temporal resolution (typically 16 frames per cardiac cycle), which may be inadequate to measure filling rates and diastolic function. In addition to directly measuring chamber volumes with accuracy, MRI can provide true measures of myocardial volumes (Fig. 4-11) and thus of myocardial mass (48,49). This measurement can be of particular clinical value in assessment of the right ventricle (50).

Regional wall motion can be evaluated clinically by cine MRI sequences and visual inspection. More sophisticated techniques have been developed that yield precise indexes of myocardial strain and deformation. Although they are promising for clinical evaluation of ischemia and ventricular myopathies, these methods to date have been applied primarily in basic physiologic research (51,52).

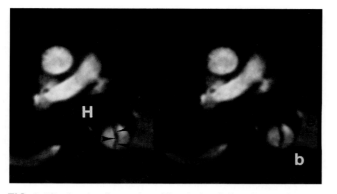

FIG 4-12. Aortic dissection. The intimal flap (*arrowheads*), mediastinal hematoma (H), pleural effusions (e), and blood in the pleural space (b) are apparent.

Acquired Aortic Disease

Aortic dissection can be imaged using aortography, CT, ultrasound, and MRI. Transthoracic ultrasound can assess the ascending aorta, but its limited field of view restricts its utility (53). There is promising experience with transesophageal ultrasound, but this technique requires sedation and carries the risk of esophageal injury (53,54). Aortography is still the standard method for picturing aortic dissection, but it is invasive and carries a small incidence of false-positive and false-negative diagnoses (53). Computed tomography can identify the intimal flap and the true and false lumen accurately, and it is used routinely for evaluating aortic dissection (53,55). Mediastinal hematoma, hemothorax, and hemopericardium can also be detected. Problems with CT include pulsation artifacts, the need to perform dynamic scans at correct anatomic levels with a compact bolus of contrast material (56), and its limited ability to assess aortic

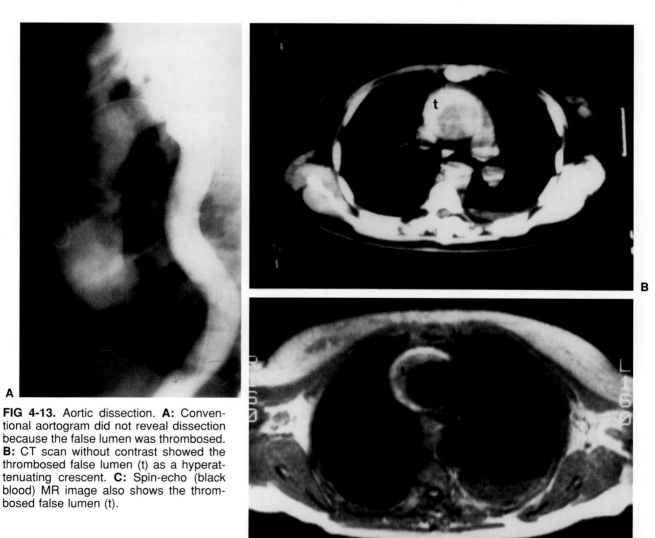

FIG 4-13. Aortic dissection. **A:** Conventional aortogram did not reveal dissection because the false lumen was thrombosed. **B:** CT scan without contrast showed the thrombosed false lumen (t) as a hyperattenuating crescent. **C:** Spin-echo (black blood) MR image also shows the thrombosed false lumen (t).

valve function and branch vessel involvement (information required by some surgeons).

Magnetic resonance imaging offers several advantages in the context of suspected aortic dissection (Figs. 4-12 and 4-13). No contrast material is required, and nontransaxial imaging is sometimes advantageous. Cine MR can assess aortic valve (57) and left ventricular function (45–47). Mediastinal hematoma, hemothorax, and hemopericardium can be identified specifically in most cases. However, MRI also has limitations in assessing dissections. Some patients are excluded from MRI for safety reasons. These examinations usually require more time than CT studies for dissection. Moreover, artifacts result in studies that do not arrive at a clear diagnosis more often with MRI than with CT (58). And greater experience is required to interpret MR images accurately (57).

The relative accuracies of aortography, transesophageal ultrasound, CT, and MRI in detecting and characterizing dissections have not been established by definitive prospective clinical trial, but numerous limited studies exist. An inclusive review of such studies (59) suggested that transesophageal ultrasound, when available, best combines speed, convenience, accuracy, and reasonable cost. The authors concluded that, overall, MRI was the most accurate technique but that cost and other practical considerations made it inappropriate as a primary diagnostic tool, while CT suffered from limitations of accuracy and aortography from high cost and limited availability. Our experience suggests, in contrast to these conclusions, that CT is an accurate test suitable for primary diagnosis (Fig. 4-13). We agree that MRI, although it is often less practical, is probably the most versatile and accurate single test—provided that artifacts can be controlled and expert interpretation is available.

Both CT and MRI have advantages over aortography for

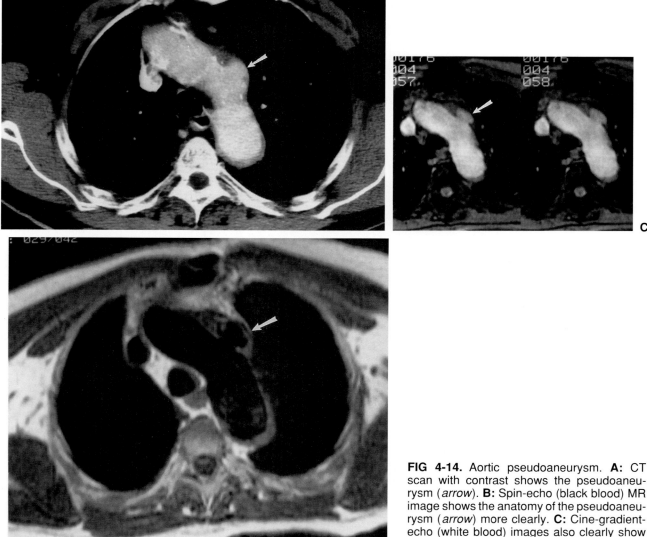

FIG 4-14. Aortic pseudoaneurysm. **A:** CT scan with contrast shows the pseudoaneurysm (*arrow*). **B:** Spin-echo (black blood) MR image shows the anatomy of the pseudoaneurysm (*arrow*) more clearly. **C:** Cine-gradient-echo (white blood) images also clearly show the pseudoaneurysm (*arrow*).

evaluating thoracic aneurysms. Both are noninvasive, can document that a mediastinal mass is an aneurysm, can assess the thickness of the aortic wall, and can accurately measure the diameter and longitudinal extent of the aneurysm. In most situations CT is sufficient for diagnosis, and since it is less expensive than MRI, it is the preferred study. Magnetic resonance imaging is particularly useful for patients with contraindications to the use of contrast material and for assessing aneurysms of the sinuses of Valsalva.

In suspected traumatic aortic rupture, the relative roles of CT and aortography are now undergoing reevaluation. It had been thought that the false-negative rate of CT was unacceptably high (60), although some studies have reported better results (61). The newest work in the field suggests that CT is sometimes a useful intermediate step between chest radiography and aortography (62,63). There has been little experience with MRI in diagnosing this condition, and the problems of monitoring and sustaining the trauma patient make MRI less practical in this context. Chronic pseudoaneurysms in survivors of traumatic or iatrogenic (Fig. 4-14) aortic injury can be evaluated appropriately by MRI or CT (64,65).

Congenital Anomalies of the Thoracic Great Vessels in Adults

In adults with congenital anomalies of the great vessels, MRI is often the procedure of choice owing to its wide field of view (compared with ultrasound) and the ability to acquire multiple image planes (Fig. 4-15) without limitation due to the volume of contrast material administered (compared with angiography or CT). Either CT or MRI can usefully depict simple vascular anomalies, such as an aberrant subclavian artery and persistence of the left superior vena cava, without the necessity of administering intravenous contrast material. The vascular supply of sequestrations (Fig. 4-16) can be identified by MRI (66) or by contrast-enhanced CT (67), permitting a more unequivocal noninvasive diagnosis.

Most of the published experience (4,6,10,12,14,16) with MRI in terms of assessing developmental anomalies of the great vessels has focused on aortic coarctation and pulmonary artery obstruction. The successful diagnosis with MRI of a variety of other congenital vascular anomalies and accurate depiction of anatomy has been reported. Systemic/pulmonary blood flow ratios have been measured by phase-contrast MRI. Comparisons of MRI with transthoracic ultrasound have, in general, shown MRI to be superior for depicting great vessel anomalies.

Coarctation is detected accurately by MRI (Fig. 4-2). Complications of treatment, including restenosis, dissection (Fig. 4-1), and aneurysm, can also be ascertained. The degree of collateral vascular supply, which affects the risk of surgery, can be established. Clinical acceptance of MRI as the sole diagnostic procedure depends, however, upon a willingness to forgo direct measurement of the pressure gradient across the lesion.

Magnetic resonance imaging is the noninvasive procedure of choice for detecting central pulmonary artery obstruction (Figs. 4-17 and 4-18), evaluating the potential for palliative shunts, and assessing the results of surgery. Currently avail-

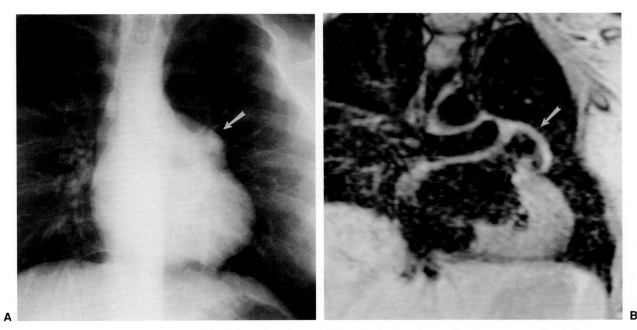

A   **B**

FIG 4-15. Partial absence of the left pericardium. **A:** Frontal chest radiograph shows a masslike bulge along the left cardiac border; this is separate from the pulmonary hilum, which is seen through the "mass." **B:** Coronal spin-echo (black blood) MR image shows that the mass (**arrow**) is composed of pulmonary vein and atrial appendage.

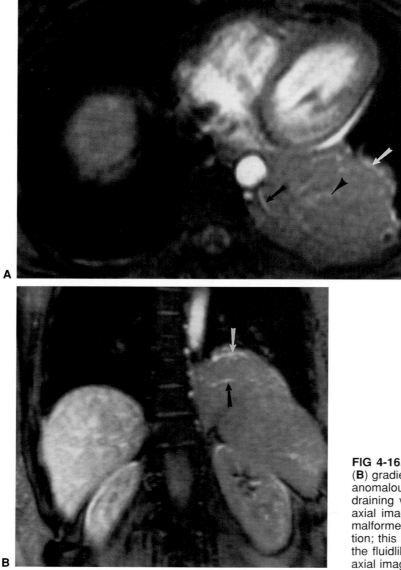

FIG 4-16. Sequestration in an adult. Axial (**A**) and coronal (**B**) gradient-echo (white blood) MR images show one of the anomalous feeding arteries (*black arrows*) and the peripheral, draining veins (*white arrows*) of the sequestration. On the axial images, a faint, branching high signal is seen in the malformed bronchi (*black arrowhead*) within the sequestration; this high signal is not due to flow but to the long T2 of the fluidlike material within these bronchi. Note also on the axial images that a small pericardial effusion is present.

able MRI techniques are not very accurate for surveying peripheral pulmonary vascular obstruction (68), but techniques are improving rapidly (69,70), and it is likely that peripheral pulmonary stenosis and arteriovenous malformations in adults will be reliably portrayed by MRI in the near future.

FUTURE CLINICAL APPLICATIONS

Coronary Angiography

Perhaps the most difficult technical challenge in MRI is to make visible normal and stenotic coronary arteries. In addition to all the usual problems of cardiac imaging, such as respiratory and cardiac motion, the need for high spatial resolution to see the small-diameter coronary arteries and

the presence of high signal intensity from blood in the neighboring heart chambers and fat surrounding the coronary vessels confound visualization of the coronary arteries. A variety of advanced MRI techniques are being developed to overcome these problems. Most of the MRI sequences used for coronary angiography are based upon white-blood time-of-flight effects. It is possible either to image contiguous slices in a two-dimensional (2D) mode or the whole volume in a three-dimensional (3D) mode. The 3D methods allow reformation of the data in any plane, free of misalignment problems that are encountered in the 2D mode. These techniques have a longer scanning time, however, so breath holding is not convenient for 3D studies. The 2D mode tends to exaggerate severe stenosis because turbulent flow dephases the MRI signal (71). Saturation of moving blood is more important in 3D, and low flow can be mistaken for occlusion.

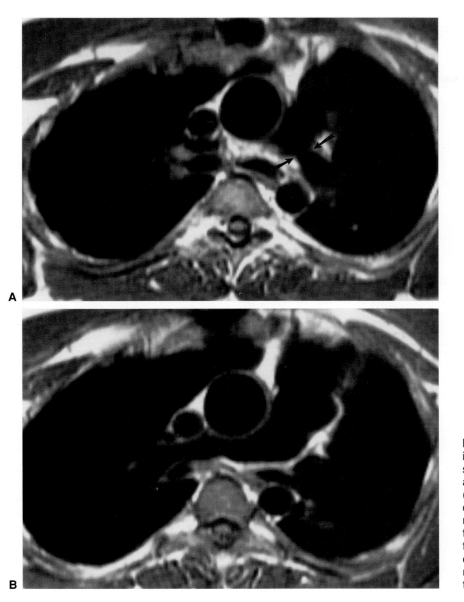

A

B

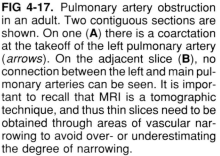

FIG 4-17. Pulmonary artery obstruction in an adult. Two contiguous sections are shown. On one (**A**) there is a coarctation at the takeoff of the left pulmonary artery (*arrows*). On the adjacent slice (**B**), no connection between the left and main pulmonary arteries can be seen. It is important to recall that MRI is a tomographic technique, and thus thin slices need to be obtained through areas of vascular narrowing to avoid over- or underestimating the degree of narrowing.

Magnetic resonance imaging can provide images of the right, the left main, and anterior coronary arteries. The circumflex coronary artery is less consistently identified, probably owing to the distance of this vessel from the surface coil. The visualized length of the coronary vessels is ≤109 mm (72,73), close to the 120 mm normally obtained from a conventional angiogram (72). The spatial resolution is about 1.6 × 0.8 × 4 mm for 2D images (72,73), and it can be smaller for 3D images. This still far larger than the submillimeter resolution of conventional coronary angiography. As a consequence, stenosis cannot be quantified as a percentage but must be classified with such designations as moderately severe or severe. Preliminary results on a small group of patients indicated the feasibility and reasonable accuracy of the method in a clinical context (74,75). It seems probable that MRI coronary angiography by itself will not supplant conventional coronary arteriography, but it could play a role in global assessment of myocardial perfusion and coronary anatomy by MRI.

Coronary Flow Measurement

A powerful application of MRI is measurement of flow in vessels. This has already been successfully applied to large vessels, like the aorta (76) or renal arteries (77), and even to smaller vessels, like native and grafted internal mammary arteries (78). However, coronary flow measurement by MRI remains challenging because of the small size of some vessels and their motion during the cardiac cycle. The reduction of the effective imaging time to one R-R cycle gives images free of motion artifacts and makes such measurements possible. The coronary flow velocity has been

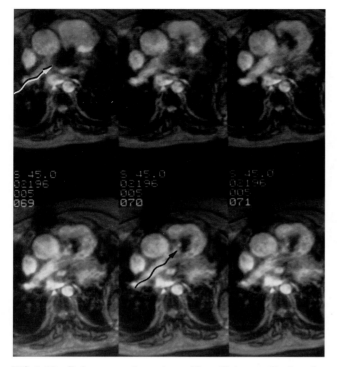

FIG 4-18. Pulmonary stenosis and insufficiency. On the cine gradient-echo (white blood) images, in systole (upper-left) there is signal dropout in the main pulmonary artery (*arrow*) owing to turbulent flow through the stenotic valve orifice, while in diastole (remaining images) there is turbulence in the out-flow tract (*arrow*) because of regurgitant jet flow.

quantified by two different approaches, one using time-of-flight effects and the other spin-phase effects.

By manipulating different parameters of time-of-flight sequences, one can progressively increase the degree of time-of-flight effects. An estimate of flow velocity can be given by an adequate fitting model (79). Cardiac images of acceptable resolution and quality are obtained by extending this method to echo planar imaging (EPI). In volunteers, flow velocity in the left anterior descending coronary artery has been measured, and a 50% increase after isometric exercise has been observed (80).

Spin-phase effects are created when flow moves through a magnetic field gradient. Faster flow experiences a greater magnetic field difference and yields more pronounced spin-phase effects. Stationary tissues always experience the same magnetic field; thus, subtraction of images acquired with or without a flow-sensitive magnetic field gradient allows for the acquisition of an image uniquely generated by flow. Segmentation of the imaging acquisition over 20 heartbeats increases the spatial resolution $\leq 1.4 \times 0.8$ mm with fewer artifacts due to movements of vessels (81). With this technique, the diastolic coronary velocity has been measured in both the right and left anterior descending coronary arteries of volunteers at rest (81,82). After adenosine administration, a fourfold increase has been observed in coronary blood flow in volunteers (81). One can indirectly measure the total

coronary blood flow and coronary flow reserve by determining the difference between the aortic blood flow above and below the coronary ostia using spin-phase effects (83). The feasibility of coronary blood flow measurement by MRI has been established. However, the sensitivity, specificity, and clinical utility of these techniques remain to be determined.

Myocardial Perfusion

Quantification of coronary blood flow is one way to assess the severity of stenosis. However, it is often insufficient to predict the functional repercussions of a lesion (84), and estimation of tissue perfusion itself is of value in determining the effects of ischemic disease. The potential of MRI to image myocardial perfusion has been well established. With the use of contrast media, two conditions can be detected: (a) failure of the contrast media to reach the ischemic area, seen in acute coronary occlusion in both animal (85–88) and human studies (89,90), and (b) increased vascular permeability for the contrast media associated with edema, which induces an accumulation of the contrast media (91) in the injured myocardium. To detect the injured myocardium, the examination needs a long delay after an infarct (86,92) and is especially marked in cases of occlusion followed by reperfusion (93,94). In acute infarction, these two effects can compete (92), but they are usually differentiated by the dose of contrast and the timing of the MRI exam after the injection.

Such contrast-enhanced images furnish information about infarct localization and extent with an unprecedented spatial resolution for a noninvasive procedure. Research has suggested that it should be possible to go a step further with quantitative estimations of myocardial perfusion by MRI (95–97). The principle of myocardial blood flow measurement is based on the analysis of signal intensity versus time curves obtained after injection of contrast media. Subsecond MRI (29) allows for the first pass of contrast media through the myocardium to be made visible (Fig. 4-19) with a temporal resolution of ~400 milliseconds or even less (98–100). With echoplanar imaging (30), transmural differences in myocardial response to the injection of contrast media have been found (101). Signal intensity versus time perfusion curves differentiate between occlusive and reperfused infarction in animal models (102).

The conversion of signal intensity into concentration, still a matter of research, is based on the assumption of a linear relationship between the concentration of the contrast agent and the signal intensity of the images. While this is a good approximation for extravascular contrast media that increase T1 (103), conversion may require corrections to be made for intravascular susceptibility agents that tend to decrease T2 (104). With intravascular agents, a relative estimation of the mean transit time between two myocardial regions is theoretically possible, and semiquantitative analysis has already been done (97,105). Absolute quantification with a pure intravascular contrast medium would require precise

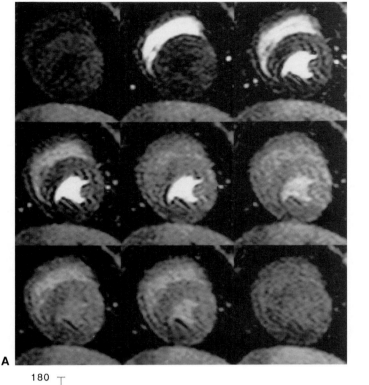

A

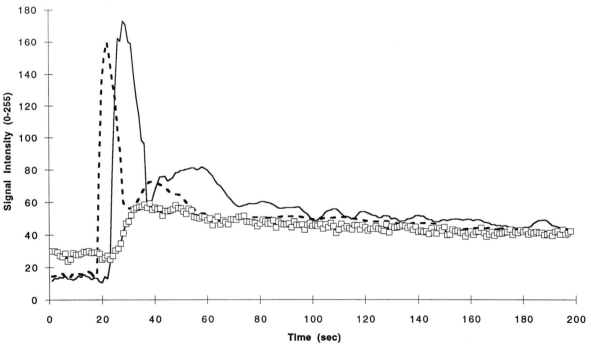

B

FIG 4-19. Magnetic resonance image of a normal dog heart after a bolus of conventional MRI contrast material (gadolinium-DTPA: 0.03 mmol/kg). With an inversion-prepared fast gradient-recalled-echo sequence [Inversion Recovery (IR)-FGRE: short axis, oblique view, with a flip angle of 25°, inversion time of 200 mseconds, TR of 6.8 mseconds, and TE of 2.5 mseconds] (**A**), images at several characteristic time points are shown from left to right, starting at the top. The first passage of the contrast media through the cardiac cavities is clearly visible. **B:** Graph of the signal intensity versus time for the blood of the right and left cavities and the left ventricular myocardium. Note the temporal resolution of about one image per second (each square of the myocardial perfusion curve represents one image). On the perfusion curve, a second pass effect is visible for the blood in both cavities. The absence of a sharp peak on the myocardial perfusion curve results from the diffusion of the contrast media outside the vessels.

knowledge of the arterial input function, which cannot be obtained without modeling the vascular architecture of the myocardium (106). With an extravascular contrast medium, myocardial blood flow quantification requires knowledge of the extraction fraction through the capillary membrane. Using an estimated extraction fraction, preliminary results have been obtained in volunteers (96). Owing to large variations, the extraction efficiency of MRI contrast media needs to be determined more precisely for a given myocardial blood flow. Procedures similar to those used for myocardial perfusion quantification by $^{13}NH_3$-positron emission tomography (107) need to be developed for MRI.

CONCLUSION

While cardiac MRI is under constant development, its ability to give both morphological and functional information about the heart in adults and children with acquired and congenital lesions has been established. The technique still needs to be compared with other available diagnostic techniques, particularly in terms of its more advanced implementations, which offer the potential of combined anatomic and physiologic information.

ACKNOWLEDGMENT

J.-P. Vallée is supported by the Swiss National Science Foundation.

REFERENCES

1. Webb WR, Sostman HD. MR imaging of thoracic disease: clinical uses. *Radiology* 1992;182:621–630.
2. Kauffman RE, Banner Jr W, Berlin CM, et al. Committee on Drugs, American Academy of Pediatrics. Guidelines for monitoring and management of pediatric patients during and after sedation for diagnostic and therapeutic procedures. *Pediatrics* 1992;89:1110–1115.
3. Ball WS, Bisset GS III. Proper sedation is essential to MR imaging in children. *Diagn Imag* 1990;12:108–112.
4. Wiles HB. Imaging congenital heart disease. *Pediatr Clin North Am* 1990;37:115–136.
5. Kersting-Sommerhoff BA, Seelos KC, Hardy C, Kondo C, Higgins SS, Higgins CB. Evaluation of surgical procedures for cyanotic congenital heart disease by using MR imaging. *AJR Am J Roentgenol* 1990;155:259–266.
6. Fellows KE, Weinberg PM, Baffa JM, Hoffman EA. Evaluation of congenital heart disease with MR imaging: current and coming attractions. *AJR Am J Roentgenol* 1992;159:925–931.
7. Gutierrez F, Mirowitz S, Canter C. Magnetic resonance imaging in the evaluation of post-operative congenital heart defects. *Semin Ultrasound CT MR* 1990;11:234–245.
8. Schlesinger AS, Hernandez RJ. Congenital heart disease: applications of computed tomography and magnetic resonance imaging. *Semin Ultrasound CT MR* 1991;12:45–60.
9. Bank ER. Magnetic resonance of congenital cardiovascular disease. *Radiol Clin North Am* 1993;3:553–572.
10. Bisset III GS. Magnetic resonance imaging of congenital heart disease in the pediatric patient. *Radiol Clin North Am* 1991;29:279–291.
11. Semelka RC, Shoenut JP, Wilson ME, Pellech AE, Patton JN. Cardiac masses: signal intensity features on spin-echo, gradient-echo, gadolinium-enhanced spin-echo and turbo FLASH images. *J Magn Reson Imaging* 1992;2:415–420.
12. Nienaber CA, Spielmann RP, Von Kodolitsch Y, et al. Diagnosis of aortic dissection: magnetic resonance imaging versus transesophageal echocardiography. *Circulation* 1992;85:434–437.
13. Ho VB, Kinney JB, Sahn DJ. Cardiovascular MR magnetic resonance imaging: strategies for congenital heart disease. Poster presentation at the 80th Scientific Assembly of the Radiologic Society of North America, Chicago, Nov. 1994.
14. Hernandez RJ, Aisen AM, Foo TKF, Beekman RH. Thoracic cardiovascular anomalies in children: evaluation with a fast gradient-recalled-echo sequence with cardiac-triggered segmented acquisition. *Radiology* 1993;188:775–780.
15. Steffens JC, Bourne MW, Sakuma H, O'Sullivan M, Higgins CB. Quantification of collateral blood flow and coarctation of the aorta by velocity encoded cine magnetic resonance imaging. *Circulation* 1994;90:937–943.
16. Bisset III GS, Strife JL, Kirks DR, et al. Vascular rings: magnetic resonance imaging. *AJR Am J Roentgenol* 1987;149:251–256.
17. Masui T, Seelos KC, Kersting-Sommerhoff BA, Higgins CB. Abnormalities of the pulmonary veins: evaluation with magnetic resonance imaging and comparison with cardiac angiography and echocardiography. *Radiology* 1991;181:645–649.
18. Bisset III GS, Kirks DR, Strife JL, et al. Cor tritriatum: diagnosis by magnetic resonance imaging. *AJR Am J Roentgenol* 1987;149:567–570.
19. Yoo S-J, Seo J-W, Lim T-H, et al. Hearts with twisted atrial ventricular connections: findings at MR imaging. *Radiology* 1993;188:109–113.
20. Geva TT, Vick GW, Wendt RE, Rokey R. Role of spin-echo and cine magnetic resonance imaging in presurgical planning of heterotaxy syndrome. *Circulation* 1994;90:348–356.
21. Link KM, Weesner KM, Formanek AG. MR imaging of the crisscross heart. *AJR Am J Roentgenol* 1989;152:809–812.
22. Kriegshauser JS, Julsrud PR, Lung JT. MR imaging of fat in and around the heart. *AJR Am J Roentgenol* 1990;155:271–274.
23. Pettigrew RI. Dynamic cardiac MR imaging: technique and applications. *Radiol Clin North Am* 1989;27:1183–1203.
24. Higgins CB, Caputo GR. Role of MR imaging in acquired and congenital cardiovascular disease. *AJR Am J Roentgenol* 1993;161:13–22.
25. Utz JA, Herfkens RJ, Heinsimer JA, Shimakawa A, Glover G, Pelc N. Valvular regurgitation: dynamic MR imaging. *Radiology* 1988;168:91–94.
26. Brenner LD, Caputo GR, Mustbeck G, et al. Quantification of left-to-right atrial shunts with velocity encoded cine nuclear magnetic resonance imaging. *J Am Coll Cardiol* 1992;20:1246–1250.
27. Sondergaard L, Stahlberg F, Thomsen C, Stenstaard A, Lindvig K, Henriksen O. Accuracy and precision of MR velocity mapping in measurement of stenotic cross-sectional area, flow rate, and pressure gradient. *J Magn Reson Imaging* 1993;3:433–437.
28. Bottomley PA. MR spectroscopy of the human heart: the status and the challenges. *Radiology* 1994;191:593–612.
29. Atkinson DJ, Edelman RR. Cineangiography of the heart in a single breath hold with a segmented Turbo FLASH sequence. *Radiology* 1991;178:357–360.
30. Edelman RR, Wielopolski P. Echo-planar MR imaging. *Radiology* 1994;192:600–612.
31. Wright GA, Hu BS, Macobski A. Estimating oxygen saturation of blood in vivo with MR imaging at 1.5 T. *J Magn Reson Imaging* 1991;1:275–283.
32. Olson MC, Posniak HV, McDonald V, Wisniewski R, Moncada R. Computed tomography and magnetic resonance imaging of the pericardium. *Radiographics* 1989;9:633–649.
33. Mulvagh SL, Rokey R, Vick GW, Johnston DL. Usefulness of nuclear magnetic resonance imaging for evaluation of pericardial effusions, and comparison with two-dimensional echocardiography. *Am J Cardiol* 1989;64:1002–1009.
34. Sechtem U, Tscholakoff D, Higgins CB. MRI of the abnormal pericardium. *AJR Am J Roentgenol* 1986;147:245–252.
35. Soulen R, Stark DD, Higgins CB. Magnetic resonance imaging of constrictive pericardial disease. *Am J Cardiol* 1985;55:480–484.
36. Sechtem U, Higgins CB, Sommerhof BA, Lipton MJ, Hucke EC. Magnetic resonance imaging of restrictive cardiomyopathy. *Am J Cardiol* 1987;59:480–482.
37. Applegate PM, Tajik AJ, Julsrud PR, Miller RA. Two-dimensional echocardiographic and magnetic resonance imaging observations in massive lipomatous hypertrophy of the atrial septum. *Am J Cardiol* 1987;59:489–491.
38. Go R, O'Donnell JK, Underwood DA, et al. Comparison of gated cardiac MRI and 2D echocardiography of intracardiac neoplasms. *AJR Am J Roentgenol* 1985;145:21–25.
39. Conces DJ, Vix VA, Klatte EC. Gated MR imaging of left atrial myxomas. *Radiology* 1985;156:445–447.

40. Barakos JA, Brown JJ, Higgins CB. MR imaging of secondary cardiac and paracardiac lesions. *AJR Am J Roentgenol* 1989;153:47–50.
41. Lund JT, Ehman RL, Julsrud PR, Sinak LJ, Tajik AJ. Cardiac masses: assessment by MR imaging. *AJR Am J Roentgenol* 1989;152:469–473.
42. Casolo F, Biasi S, Balzarini L, et al. MRI as an adjunct to echocardiography for the diagnostic imaging of cardiac masses. *Eur J Radiol* 1988;8:226–230.
43. Winkler M, Higgins CB. Suspected intracardiac masses: evaluation with MR imaging. *Radiology* 1987;165:117–122.
44. Jungehulsing M, Sechtem U, Theissen P, Hilger HH, Schicha H. Left ventricular thrombi: evaluation with spin-echo and gradient echo MR imaging. *Radiology* 1992;182:225–229.
45. Van Rossum AC, Visser FC, Sprenger M, Van Einige MJ, Valk J, Roos JP. Evaluation of magnetic resonance imaging for determination of left ventricular ejection fraction and comparison with angiography. *Am J Cardiol* 1988;62:628–633.
46. Soldo SJ, Norris SL, Gober JR, Haywood LJ, Colletti PM, Terk M. MRI-derived ventricular volume curves for the assessment of left ventricular function. *Magn Reson Imaging* 1994;12:711–717.
47. Debatin JF, Nadel SN, Paolini JF, et al. Cardiac ejection fraction: phantom study comparing cine MR imaging, radionuclide blood pool imaging and ventriculography. *J Magn Reson Imaging* 1992;2:135–142.
48. Shapiro EP, Rogers WJ, Beyar R, et al. Determination of left ventricular mass by magnetic resonance imaging in hearts deformed by acute infarction. *Circulation* 1989;79:706–711.
49. Katz J, Milliken MC, Stray-Gunderson J, et al. Estimation of human myocardial mass with MR imaging. *Radiology* 1988;169:495–498.
50. Pattynama PMT, Willems LNA, Smit AH, van der Wall EE, de Roos A. Early diagnosis of cor pulmonale with MR imaging of the right ventricle. *Radiology* 1992;182:375–379.
51. Buchalter MB, Weiss JL, Rogers WJ, et al. Noninvasive quantification of left ventricular rotational deformation in normal humans using magnetic resonance imaging tagging. *Circulation* 1990;81:1236–1244.
52. McVeigh ER, Zerhouni EA. Noninvasive measurement of transmural gradients in myocardial strain with MR imaging. *Radiology* 1991;180:677–683.
53. Petasnick JP. Radiologic evaluation of aortic dissection. *Radiology* 1991;180:297–305.
54. Shively BK. Transesophageal echocardiography in the assessment of aortic pathology. *J Thorac Imaging* 1990;5:40–47.
55. Godwin JD. Conventional CT of the aorta. *J Thorac Imaging* 1990;5:18–31.
56. Godwin JD, Breiman RS, Speckman JM. Problems and pitfalls in the evaluation of thoracic aortic dissection by computed tomography. *J Comput Assist Tomogr* 1982;6:750–756.
57. Underwood SR, Klipstein RH, Firmin DN, et al. Magnetic resonance assessment of aortic and mitral regurgitation. *Br Heart J* 1986;56:455–462.
58. Solomon SL, Brown JJ, Glazer HS, Mirowitz SA, Lee JKT. Thoracic aortic dissection: pitfalls and artifacts in MR imaging. *Radiology* 1990;177:223–228.
59. Cigarroa JE, Isselbacher EM, DeSanctis RW, Eagle KA. Medical progress. Diagnostic imaging in the evaluation of suspected aortic dissection: old standards and new directions. *N Engl J Med* 1993;328:35–43.
60. Egan TJ, Neiman HL, Herman RJ, Malave SR, Sanders JH. Computed tomography in the diagnosis of aortic aneurysm dissection or traumatic injury. *Radiology* 1980;136:141–146.
61. Heiberg E, Wolverson MK, Sundaram M, Shields JB. CT in aortic trauma. *AJR Am J Roentgenol* 1983;140:1119–1124.
62. Morgan PWE, Goodman LR, Aprahamian C, Foley WD, Lipchik EO. Evaluation of traumatic aortic injury: Does dynamic contrast-enhanced CT play a role? *Radiology* 1992;182:661–666.
63. Raptopoulos V, Sheiman RG, Phillips DA, Davidoff A, Silva WE. Traumatic aortic tear: screening with chest CT. *Radiology* 1992;182:667–673.
64. Woodard PK, Patz EF, Sostman HD. Pseudoaneurysms at aortic cannulation site after coronary artery bypass graft: MR findings. *J Comput Assist Tomogr* 1992;16:883–887.
65. Moore EH, Webb WR, Verrier ED, et al. MRI of chronic post-traumatic false aneurysms of the thoracic aorta. *AJR Am J Roentgenol* 1984;143:1195–1196.
66. Naidich DP, Rumancik WM, Ettenger NA, et al. Congenital anomalies of the lungs in adults: MR diagnosis. *AJR Am J Roentgenol* 1988;151:13–19.
67. Ikezoe J, Murayama S, Godwin JD, Done SL, Verschakelen JA. Bronchopulmonary sequestration: CT assessment. *Radiology* 1990;176:375–379.
68. Canter CE, Gutierrez FR, Mirowitz SA, Martin TC, Hartmann AF. Evaluation of pulmonary arterial morphology in cyanotic congenital heart disease by magnetic resonance imaging. *Am Heart J* 1989;118:347.
69. Foo TKF, MacFall JR, Hayes CE, Sostman HD. Pulmonary vasculature: single breath-hold MR imaging with phased array coils. *Radiology* 1992;183:473–477.
70. Wielopolski PA, Haacke EM, Adler LP. Three-dimensional MR imaging of the pulmonary vasculature: preliminary experience. *Radiology* 1992;183:465–472.
71. Haacke EM, Masaryk TJ, Wielopolski PA, et al. Optimizing blood vessel contrast in fast three-dimensional MRI. *Magn Reson Med* 1990;14:202–221.
72. Edelman RR, Manning WJ, Pearlman J, Li W. Human coronary arteries: projection angiograms reconstructed from breath-hold two-dimensional MR images. *Radiology* 1993;187:719–722.
73. Pennell DJ, Keegan J, Firmin DN, Gatehouse PD, Underwood SR, Longmore DB. Magnetic resonance imaging of coronary arteries: technique and preliminary results. *Br Heart J* 1993;70:315–326.
74. Manning WJ, Li W, Edelman RR. A preliminary report comparing magnetic resonance coronary angiography with conventional angiography [Comments]. *N Engl J Med* 1993;328:828–832. [Published erratum appears in *N Engl J Med* 1993;13;330:152.].
75. Paschal CB, Haacke EM, Adler LP. Three-dimensional MR imaging of the coronary arteries: preliminary clinical experience. *J Magn Reson Imaging* 1993;3:491–500.
76. Buonocore MH, Bogren H. Factor influencing the accuracy and precision of velocity-encoded phase imaging. *J Magn Reson Med* 1992;26:141–154.
77. Sommer G, Noorbehesht B, Pelc N, et al. Normal renal blood flow measurement using phase-contrast cine magnetic resonance imaging. *Invest Radiol* 1992;27:465–470.
78. Debatin JF, Stronng JA, Sostman HD, et al. MR characterization of blood flow in native and grafted internal mammary arteries. *J Magn Reson Imaging* 1993;3:443–450.
79. Wehrli FW, Shimakawa A, Gullberg GT, MacFall JR. Time-of-flight MR flow imaging: selective saturation recovery with gradient refocusing. *Radiology* 1986;160:781–785.
80. Poncelet BP, Weisskoff RM, Wedeen VJ, Brady TJ, Kantor H. Time of flight quantification of coronary flow with echo-planar MRI. *Magn Reson Med* 1993;30:447–457.
81. Edelman RR, Manning WJ, Gervino E, Li W. Flow velocity quantification in human coronary arteries with fast, breath-hold MR angiography. *J Magn Reson Imaging* 1993;3:699–703.
82. Keegan J, Firmin D, Gatehouse P, Longmore D. The application of breath hold phase velocity mapping techniques to the measurement of coronary artery blood flow velocity: phantom data and initial in vivo results. *J Magn Reson Med* 1994;31:526–536.
83. Bogren HG, Buonocore MH. Measurement of coronary artery flow reserve by magnetic resonance velocity mapping in the aorta. *Lancet* 1993;342:899–900.
84. Marcus ML, Harrison DG, White CW, McPherson DD, Wilson RF, Kerber RE. Assessing the physiologic significance of coronary obstructions in patients: importance of diffuse undetected atherosclerosis. *Prog Cardiovasc Dis* 1988;31:39–56.
85. Canet E, Revel D, Forrat R, et al. Superparamagnetic iron oxide particles and positive enhancement for myocardial perfusion studies assessed by subsecond T1-weighted MRI. *Magn Reson Imaging* 1993;11:1139–1145.
86. Wolfe CL, Moseley ME, Wilkstrom MG, et al. Assessment of myocardial salvage after ischemia and reperfusion using magnetic resonance imaging and spectroscopy. *Circulation* 1989;80:969–982.
87. Saeed M, Wendland MF, Yu KK, Li HT, Higgins CB. Dual effects of gadodiamide injection in depiction of the region of myocardial ischemia. *J Magn Reson Imaging* 1993;3:21–29.
88. Yu KK, Saeed M, Wendland MF, et al. Comparison of T1-enhancing and magnetic susceptibility magnetic resonance contrast agents for demarcation of the jeopardy area in experimental myocardial infarction. *Invest Radiol* 1993;28:1015–1023.
89. De Roos A, Matheijssen NAA, Doornbos J, Van Dijkman PRM, Van Voorthuisen AE, Van Der Wall EE. Myocardial infarct size after reperfusion therapy: assessment with Gd-DTPA-enhanced MR imaging. *Radiology* 1990;176:517–521.
90. De Roos A, Van Rossum AC, Van Der Wall EE, et al. Reperfused

and nonreperfused myocardial infarction: diagnostic potential of Gd-DTPA-enhanced MR imaging. *Radiology* 1989;172:717–720.

91. Ovize M, Revel D, De Lorgeril M, et al. Quantitation of reperfused myocardial infarction by Gd-DOTA-enhanced magnetic resonance imaging. *Invest Radiol* 1991;26:1065–1070.

92. Masui T, Saeed M, Wendland MF, Higgins CB. Occlusive and reperfused myocardial infarcts: MR imaging differentiation with nonionic Gd-DTPA-BMA. *Radiology* 1991;181:77–83.

93. Lim T-H, Lee DH, Kim YH, et al. Occlusive and reperfused myocardial infarction: detection by using MR imaging with gadolinium poly-lysine enhancement. *Radiology* 1993;189:765–768.

94. De Roos AR, Mohanlal RW, Van Vaals JJ, et al. Gadolinium-DTPA-enhanced magnetic resonance imaging of the isolated rat heart after ischemia and reperfusion. *Invest Radiol* 1991;26:1060–1064.

95. Diesbourg LD, Pratto FS, Wisenberg G, et al. Quantification of myocardial blood flow and extracellular volumes using a bolus injection of Gd-DTPA: kinetic modeling in canine ischemic disease. *Magn Reson Med* 1992;23:238–253.

96. Larsson HBW, Stubgaard M, Sondergaard L, Henriksen O. In vivo quantification of the unidirectional influx constant for Gd-DTPA diffusion across the myocardial capillaries with MR imaging. *J Magn Reson Imaging* 1994;4:433–440.

97. Wilke N, Simm C, Zhang J, et al. Contrast-enhanced first pass myocardial perfusion imaging: correlation between myocardial blood flow in dogs at rest and during hyperemia. *Magn Reson Med* 1993;29:485–497.

98. Eichenberger AC, Schuiki E, Kochli VD, Amann FW, McKinnon GC, Von Schulthess GK. Ischemic heart disease: assessment with gadolinium-enhanced ultrafast MR imaging and dipyridamole stress. *J Magn Reson Imaging* 1994;4:425–431.

99. Wendland MF, Saeed M, Masui T, Derugin N, Higgins CB. First pass of an MR susceptibility contrast agent through normal and ischemic heart: gradient-recalled echo-planar imaging. *J Magn Reson Imaging* 1993;3:755–760.

100. Wendland MF, Saeed M, Masui T, Derugin N, Moseley ME, Higgins CB. Echo-planar MR imaging of normal and ischemic myocardium with gadodiamide injection. *Radiology* 1993;186:535–542.

101. Edelman RR, Wei L. Contrast-enhanced echo-planar MR imaging of myocardial perfusion: preliminary study in humans. *Radiology* 1994;190:771–777.

102. Saeed M, Wendland MF, Yu KK, et al. Identification of myocardial reperfusion with echo planar magnetic resonance imaging: discrimination between occlusive and reperfused infarction. *Circulation* 1994;90:1492–1501.

103. Donahue KM, Burstein D, Manning WJ, Gray ML. Studies of Gd-DTPA relaxivity and proton exchange rates in tissue. *Magn Reson Med* 1994;32:66–76.

104. Kennan RP, Zhong J, Gore JC. Intravascular susceptibility contrast mechanisms in tissues. *Magn Reson Med* 1994;31:9–21.

105. Arteaga C, Canet E, Ovize M, Janier M, Revel D. Myocardial perfusion assessed by subsecond magnetic resonance imaging with a para-magnetic macromolecular contrast agent. *Invest Radiol* 1994;29:S54–S57.

106. Wilke NM, Jerosch-Herold M, Stillman AE, et al. Concepts of myocardial perfusion imaging in magnetic resonance imaging. *Magn Reson Q* 1994;10:249–286.

107. Schelbert HR. Consideration of measurements of myocardial blood flow with positron-emission tomography. *Invest Radiol* 1993;28:S47–S55.

Additional Case Presentation

Robert J. Optican

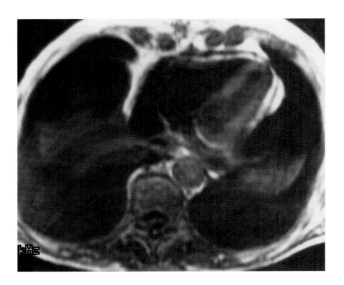

FIG 4-20. Axial gated spin-echo image of irregular thickening of the pericardium in an 80-year-old man, with "conical" deformity of the ventricles indicative of constrictive pericarditis.

Department of Radiology, Baptist Memorial Hospital, Memphis, Tennessee 38103

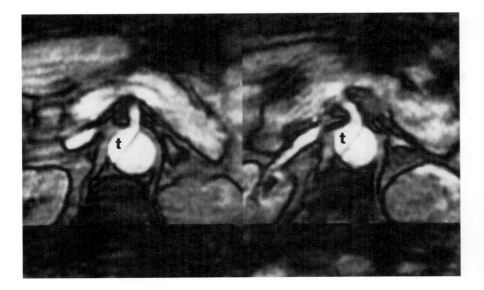

FIG 4-21. A 62-year-old man with type 3 thoracic aortic dissection extending into the abdominal aorta. Axial cine gradient-echo images at two levels show the origins of the celiac (left) and superior mesenteric (right) arteries arising from the true lumen (t).

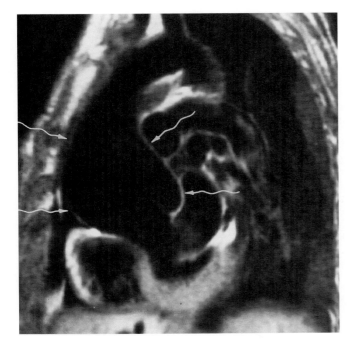

FIG 4-22. A 35-year-old woman with Marfan's syndrome. Oblique gated gradient-echo image shows marked dilatation of the aortic root and proximal ascending aorta (annulo-aortic ectasia) (*arrows*).

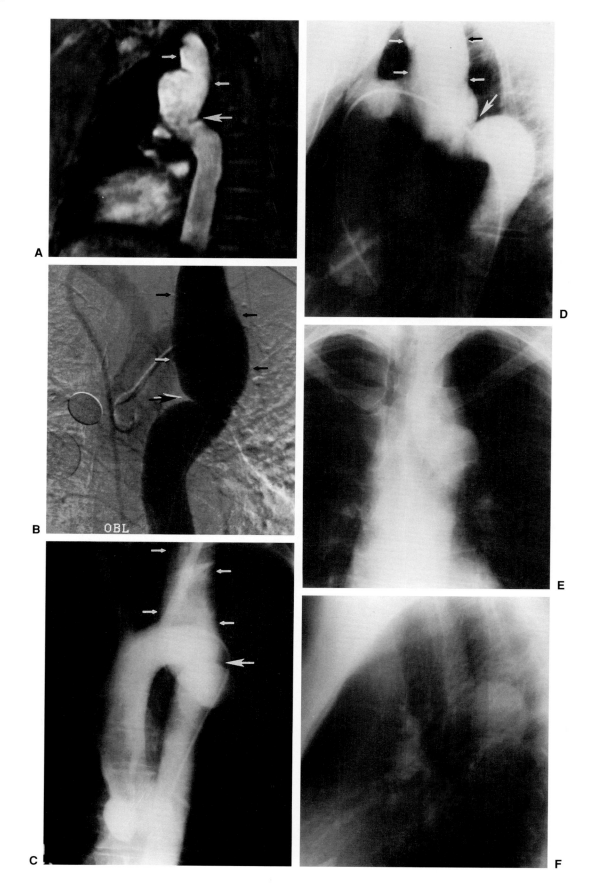

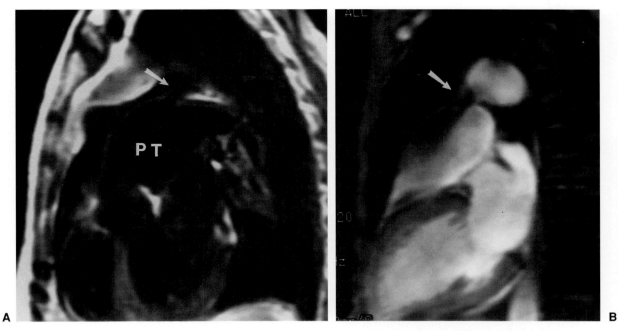

A

B

FIG 4-24. A 62-year-old woman with 3:1 left-to-right patent ductus arteriosis (PDA). This lesion was mistakenly diagnosed as an aortopulmonary window at cardiac catheterization. A near sagittal gated spin-echo image (**A**) shows the PDA (*arrow*) communicating with the roof of a markedly dilated pulmonary trunk (PT). An oblique sagittal cine gradient-echo image (**B**) shows a turbulent jet (*arrow*) of flow directed from the aorta into the pulmonary trunk through the PDA. Results from the MRI prevented the patient from undergoing median sternotomy and directed the surgeon to the appropriate approach (left thoracotomy).

FIG 4-23. Oblique cine gradient-echo image (**A**) shows marked elongation and kinking (*large arrow*) of the descending thoracic aorta of a 51-year-old man. Additionally, there is striking ectasia of the proximal left subclavian artery (*small arrows*). Corresponding intraarterial digital subtraction arteriogram (DSA) of the same patient (**B**) shows the huge left subclavian artery (*small arrows*) from the site of kinking (*large arrow*). Frontal (**C**) and lateral (**D**) aortograms of another patient, a 65-year-old asymptomatic man, show a gigantic left subclavian artery (*small arrows*) arising immediately proximal to the kink (*large arrow*). His corresponding posteroanterior (**E**) and lateral (**F**) radiographs match precisely the aortograms (C and D).

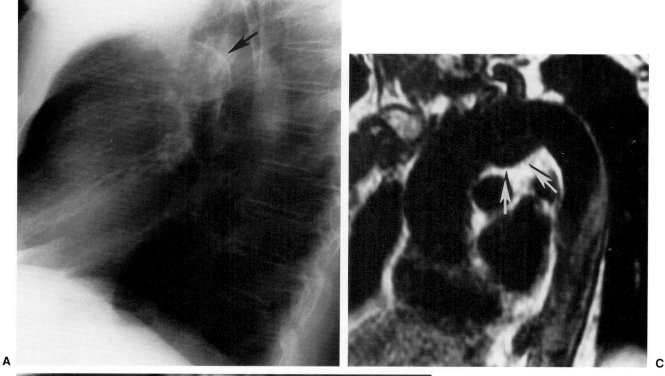

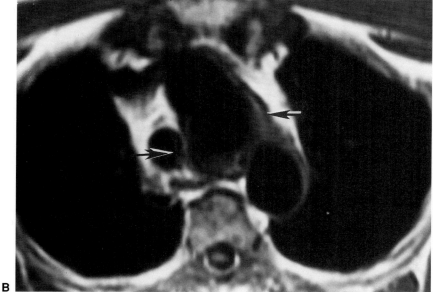

FIG 4-25. A 71-year-old former paratrooper (World War II) who had had a parachuting accident in Europe in which his chute did not deploy. The lateral chest radiograph (**A**) shows curvilinear calcification (*arrow*) superimposed over the distal aortic arch. The axial (**B**) and oblique sagittal (**C**) gated spin-echo images show a broad-mouthed saccular posttraumatic pseudoaneurysm (*arrows*) at the level of the aortic isthmus. This patient is a rare survivor of an untreated traumatic aortic injury (transection).

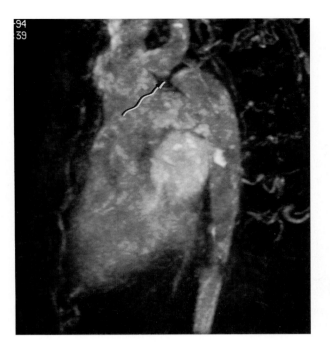

FIG 4-26. A 34-year-old man with coarctation of the aorta. Two-dimensional time-of-flight gradient-echo images displayed as maximal intensity projection (MIP) show the severe coarctation (*arrow*) and extensive collaterals (internal mammary and intercostal arteries).

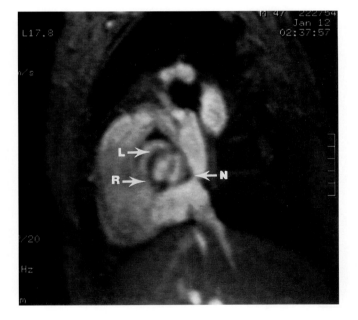

FIG 4-27. A 47-year-old man with a bicuspid aortic valve. Cine gradient-echo image through the plane of the aortic valve shows the typical configuration of a bicuspid valve with fusion of the right (R) and left (L) cusps. N, noncoronary cusp.

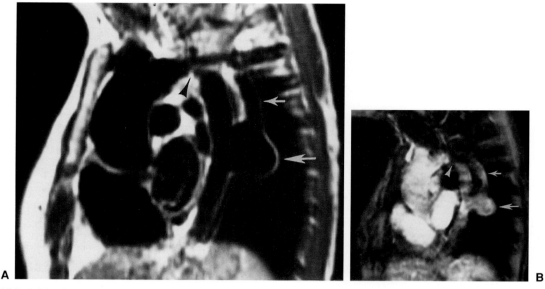

FIG 4-28. A 43-year-old woman who had had graft bypass of severe aortic coarctation as a child. A mediastinal mass is evident on chest film. The oblique sagittal gated spin-echo image (**A**) shows a large pseudoaneurysm (*large arrow*) at the distal anastomosis of the bypass graft (*small arrow*) into the descending aorta. The arrowhead points to the site of coarctation. Cine gradient-echo image in the same plane (**B**) shows bright flow within the graft and pseudoaneurysm.

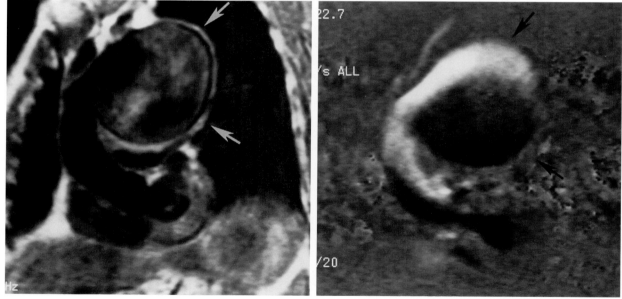

FIG 4-29. An 80-year-old man with huge saccular aneurysm of the aortic arch. The oblique sagittal gated spin-echo image (**A**) shows the aneurysm (*arrows*); the abnormal signal represents slow flow. The oblique sagittal cine phase-contrast image (encoded for right to left flow) (**B**) confirms the presence of swirling flow within the aneurysm (*arrows*).

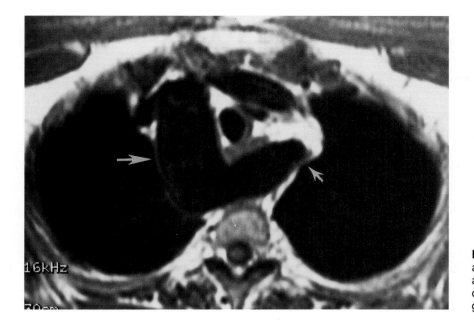

FIG 4-30. Axial gated spin-echo image of a 55-year-old man shows right-sided aortic arch (*large arrow*) with an aberrant left subclavian artery. Note mild ectasia of the origin of the subclavian artery (*small arrow*).

Essentials of Cardiac Imaging,
James T. T. Chen,
Lippincott–Raven Publishers, Philadelphia © 1998.

CHAPTER 5

Nuclear Cardiology and Pulmonary Radionuclide Imaging

Michael W. Hanson and R. Edward Coleman

NUCLEAR CARDIOLOGY

Nuclear imaging techniques provide an accurate, safe, and relatively inexpensive noninvasive way to assess the cardiovascular system. These tests are commonly performed to shed light on a wide variety of known or suspected cardiovascular disorders. Imaging can be accomplished with the patient at rest and during or after physical or pharmacologic stress procedures. Standard nuclear cardiology testing is done, in general, to evaluate either regional myocardial perfusion or ventricular function. Myocardial perfusion and cellular viability can be assessed by administering radioactive tracers that are distributed intracellularly within the myocardial tissue, such as thallium 201 and technetium 99m Sestamibi (1–5). Myocardial performance and ventricular function are more commonly assessed by the administration of radioactive tracers that remain within the intravascular space during the acquisition of the study and include the first-pass radionuclide angiogram and the multigated equilibrium techniques. Myocardial perfusion images acquired using a gated technique can also provide functional information that is derived from the administration of tracers that localize within the myocardial tissues.

Myocardial Perfusion Imaging

Imaging Methods

There are two types of imaging used for the acquisition and display of myocardial perfusion images. Regional myocardial perfusion can be assessed by planar imaging or by single photon emission computed tomography (SPECT).

Division of Nuclear Medicine, Department of Radiology, Duke University Medical Center, Durham, North Carolina 27710, U.S.A.

Recognizing the limitations of each of these studies, either technique is acceptable for evaluating the distribution of tracer in the myocardium. For each technique, a standardized protocol for imaging is important for the comparison of rest and stress images.

Three standardized views are obtained in planar imaging. The first view obtained is a 45° left anterior oblique (LAO) projection, or the degree of anterior obliquity that best demonstrates a circle or an elipse. The other two views include an anterior view (or a projection acquired 45° toward the patient's right from the first view) and a 70° LAO view (or a projection that is 25° further to the left of the first view). Some laboratories prefer to acquire a 90° view (or a true left-lateral projection). Owing to variations in the size and position of the heart within the thorax of individual patients, imaging can be inadequate if projections are based only on the degree setting of the camera angle relative to the patient. In general, there is less image contrast with planar imaging compared with SPECT, but planar imaging is less technically demanding than SPECT.

Planar images can be interpreted directly or with the assistance of a semiquantitative computer software analysis program, such as a circumferential profile analysis program, which is available on many nuclear medicine computer systems. Count density is determined within angular sections of the myocardium and compared with a normal patient database for deviations. The semiquantitative techniques have improved the sensitivity of thallium 201 imaging for the detection of significant coronary artery disease and the recognition of multivessel disease.

Single photon emission computed tomography collects data from multiple projections around the patient using standard gamma cameras that rotate around the patient. These cameras can have from one to four rotating cameras. By increasing the number of cameras gathering data, the acquisition time of the completed study can be reduced or a greater number of counts per slice can be acquired each time. The rotating camera can move continuously as data are acquired, or the camera can stop momentarily to acquire the data and resume rotation. Although there is some controversy as to the optimal SPECT technique, images have been successfully acquired and interpreted over a range of 180° or 360° around the patient. A standard SPECT study can be acquired in ~ 15 to 20 minutes. This technique offers the advantage of eliminating the superimposition of activity that occurs in planar imaging, and image contrast is improved.

Single photon emission computed tomography images are most commonly displayed in short-axis, vertical long-axis, and horizontal long-axis planes. Semiquantitative computer programs are also available for analyzing SPECT myocardial perfusion images. Most of the programs use a polar map (bull's eye) for display and analysis, wherein the short-axis images from the apex to the base of the heart are displayed as progressively enlarging concentric circles in a single image. The extent of the perfusion defect, relative to the entire ventricle, can be determined and expressed as a percentage of abnormal myocardium.

Radiopharmaceuticals

Thallium 201

Thallium 201 (Tl-201), a cyclotron-produced radionuclide that is a potassium analog, is administered intravenously as thallous 201 chloride. Tl-201 has a half-life of 73 hours and decays by electron capture to mercury 201. Tl-201 emits two gamma rays with energies of 135 keV (2.7% abundant) and 167 keV (10% abundant). As Tl-201 decays to mercury 201, characteristic x-rays (90% abundant) are emitted with photon energies of 69 to 83 keV. It is these characteristic x-rays that are primarily imaged when acquiring the Tl-201 scan.

An average dose of 3.0 mCi (111 MBq) of Tl-201 is injected at the peak of physical exercise, and the patient continues to exercise for ~1 minute. Tracer may also be injected at time of the peak effect of a pharmacologic stress agent. The stress image begins ~10 minutes after the injection of Tl-201. A redistribution image is acquired some 3 to 4 hours later. An additional injection of ≤1.0 mCi (37 MBq) may be given just before acquiring the redistribution image in an effort to improve the identification of the extent of viable myocardium.

Homogeneous tracer accumulation in the myocardium at stress indicates no significant difference in regional coronary blood flow. A region of diminished tracer on the stress image can be due to ischemia, infarct, a combination of infarct and ischemia, or artifact; these potential causes can be differentiated by comparing the stress image with the redistribution (or reinjection) image. With time, Tl-201 undergoes further wash-in and wash-out from the myocardium. This phenome-non results in changes that help distinguish the etiology of abnormalities seen on the stress image. A stress perfusion defect that becomes homogeneous with the remaining myocardium at redistribution (or reinjection) suggests ischemia. A defect at stress that does not change over time at redistribution (or reinjection) indicates myocardial infarction or a fixed artifact.

Technetium 99m Sestamibi

Technetium 99m Sestamibi (^{99m}Tc Cardiolite) is the first ^{99m}Tc-labeled agent approved for myocardial perfusion imaging (6). Like Tl-201, it is distributed in the myocardium relative to myocardial blood flow. It offers several advantages over Tl-201. Its higher photon energy of 140 keV and its shorter half-life of 6 hours allow for the injection of a higher dose of tracer, which results in better image quality. Technetium 99m Sestamibi can be prepared on site from a commercial kit, whereas Tl-201 must be delivered from a cyclotron production site. Because of higher doses of administered radioactivity, a first-pass radionuclide angiogram or a gated SPECT perfusion study can be acquired with ^{99m}Tc Sestamibi.

In contrast to Tl-201, ^{99m}Tc Sestamibi is fixed in the myocardium. Thus, imaging does not need to begin immediately after injection, but two separate injections are required for a rest and exercise study. This agent is excreted through the hepatobiliary tract. Imaging is typically delayed after intravenous injection while tracer clears from the liver parenchyma. The rest injection is done first using 8 to 10 mCi (296 to 370 MBq) of tracer. Images are acquired ~1 hour later. The exercise study is then performed using 24 to 30 mCi (888 to 1,110 MBq) of tracer. Images are acquired 30 to 45 minutes later. The pattern of fixed or new defects between rest and stress images are interpreted as described earlier for Tl-201.

Dual Isotope Imaging (Tl-201 and ^{99m}Tc Sestamibi)

Myocardial perfusion can be assessed with a technique that uses the separate advantages of Tl-201 and ^{99m}Tc Sestamibi (7). A rest study is made using an injection of Tl-201 followed by imaging after ~15 to 20 minutes. The stress study is then performed using ^{99m}Tc Sestamibi. Thallium 201 is a better tracer for determining myocardial viability than is ^{99m}Tc Sestamibi. Thus, the rest image provides assessment of myocardial viability, while the stress study offers better image quality for assessment of ischemia. The time for performing the dual isotope technique is less than that using either Tl-201 or ^{99m}Tc Sestamibi alone. The perfusion patterns for ischemia (Fig. 5-1) and infarction (Fig. 5-2) are the same as those for either agent used alone. False-positive and, less often, false-negative myocardial perfusion studies for the diagnosis of atherosclerotic coronary artery

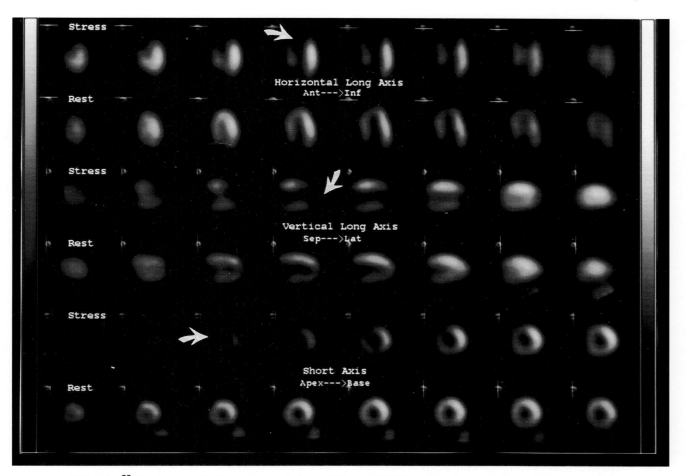

FIG 5-1. 99mTc Sestamibi stress (rows 1, 3, and 5) and Tl-201 resting (rows 2, 4, and 6) myocardial perfusion images in a 77-year-old man with a 1-month history of recurring exertional chest pain. At exercise, he had chest pain, frequent ventricular ectopy, and ST segment depression. The resting Tl-201 study is normal, with no perfusion defects. At stress, a perfusion defect (*arrows*) is seen in the anterior wall, the anteroseptum, the anteroapex, and the inferoapex. These findings are suggestive of myocardial ischemia in the distribution of the left anterior descending coronary artery. (see Color Plate 1)

disease can be seen with either Tl-201 or 99mTc Sestamibi alone or in combination (Table 5-1).

Myocardial Functional Studies

Diminished coronary artery blood flow (ischemic myocardium) or absent coronary artery blood flow (infarcted myocardium) alters myocardial performance. Assessment of right and/or left ventricular performance can be important in the assessment of several cardiovascular and/or pulmonary disorders, among them, coronary artery disease, valvular heart disease, ischemic and nonischemic cardiomyopathies, pulmonary disease, and congenital heart disease, and for cardiac or lung transplant evaluations before surgery. These studies can assess myocardial performance at baseline and during chemotherapy in oncology patients who are receiving chemotherapeutic agents that have cardiotoxic properties.

Multigated Acquisition Equilibrium Blood Pool Imaging

The multigated acquisition equilibrium blood pool study (MUGA) can be acquired on most all of the commercially available standard gamma cameras equipped with the appropriate computers. A MUGA study is acquired after radiotracer labeling of the circulating blood pool, which can be accomplished by employing one of two standard techniques that include 99mTc human serum albumin and 99mTc-labeled red blood cell techniques.

The circulating blood pool can be easily labeled by the administration of a single intravenous injection of 99mTc-labeled human serum albumin, which remains within the blood pool long enough to acquire a MUGA study. However, owing to significant accumulation of albumin in the liver and a relatively faster tracer clearance than with labeled red blood cells, the preferred method for radiolabeling of the blood pool is to label a portion of the circulating red blood cells with 99mTc sodium pertechnetate. Red blood cells are

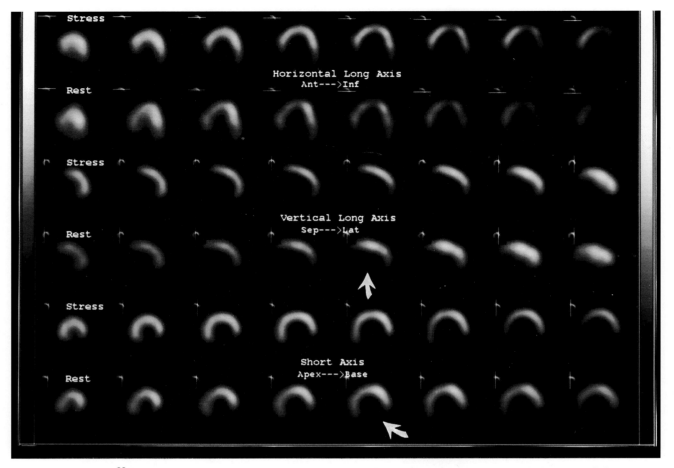

FIG 5-2. ^{99m}Tc Sestamibi stress (rows 1, 3, and 5) and Tl-201 resting (rows 2, 4, and 6) myocardial perfusion images in a 70-year-old man with a history of CAD, previous myocardial infarction, and coronary artery bypass graft surgery. At exercise, he exceeded his target heart rate without chest pain or EKG changes. A fixed perfusion defect is seen at rest (*arrows*) that is unchanged at stress in the inferior, posterobasal, and aposterolateral walls and the inferoapex. This defect is suggestive of previous infarct. There is no evidence for myocardial ischemia. (see Color Plate 2)

labeled by the in vivo, in vitro, or modified in vitro technique, with the in vivo technique being the most widely used, owing primarily to its simplicity and its satisfactory labeling of the blood pool. The in vivo technique calls for the administration of ~6 mg stannous pyrophosphate containing ~1 mg tin.

The commercial preparation of stannous pyrophosphate is convenient for the administration of the stannous ion, which crosses the red cell membrane, where it then acts as a reducing agent. Approximately 20 minutes after administration of stannous pyrophosphate, 20 to 30 mCi (740 to 1,110 MBq) of ^{99m}Tc sodium pertechnetate is given intravenously, which crosses the red cell membrane, is reduced inside the red blood cell by the stannous ion, and labels the hemoglobin. The in vitro technique requires blood to be withdrawn from the patient, and the labeling is done externally in a sterile vial using the same agents. The modified in vitro technique requires the intravenous injection of stannous pyrophosphate followed in ~15 to 20 minutes by withdrawal of blood into a

shielded syringe containing the ^{99m}Tc sodium pertechnetate, which is then gently agitated for ~15 minutes; the radiolabeled blood sample is the reinjected into the patient. The two in vitro techniques have a slightly higher labeling efficiency (~95%) than the in vivo technique (~85 to 90%). However, the simpler in vivo technique is associated with only a minimal difference in labeling efficiency that is negligible for image quality. Thus, the in vivo technique is preferred in most nuclear cardiology laboratories.

Cardiac blood pool imaging is performed in synchrony with the electrocardiogram, where the R-R interval divides the acquisition into 16 to 24 equal time frames. Rest studies are performed with a high-resolution collimator with the patient upright or supine. Images are acquired for 200,000 to 250,000 counts per frame. The rest acquisition generally requires 7 to 10 minutes per view. The resting image includes a 45° LAO (best septal) view and anterior [or 20° right anterior oblique (RAO)] view and a 70° LAO (or left-lateral) view. A left ventricular time–activity curve is generated from the

TABLE 5-1. *False positive/negative results of myocardial perfusion studies*

Causes of false-positive results of perfusion studies
    Attenuation artifact from breast tissue, diaphragm, or enlarged right ventricle
    Instrumentation artifacts
    Left and right bundle branch block
    Coronary artery spasm
    Underestimation of CAD by coronary angiography
    Misinterpretation of images due to apical thinning or decreased tracer at the base of the heart or in the membranous septum
Causes of false-negative results of perfusion studies
    Inadequate exercise—failure to achieve target heart rate
    Single-vessel or small tertiary distal vessel disease
    Small regions of ischemia
    Coronary artery disease with an adequate collateral blood flow
    Overestimation of the extent of CAD by coronary angiography
    Delay in acquisition of the T1-201 stress image

CAD, coronary artery disease

best septal view for calculation of the left ventricular ejection fraction. Counts obtained during the acquisition of the study are proportional to volume. The ejection fraction is calculated from the difference between counts at end-diastole and end-systole divided by the counts at end-diastole, and the counts are background corrected.

Rest-exercise studies are performed with an all-purpose, high-sensitivity collimator to obtain more counts in a shorter time period, although there is some loss of image resolution and the counts acquired per frame are reduced to 150,000. These variations allow a study to be acquired in ~2 minutes, an acceptable length of time for an exercise acquisition. The resting wall motion analysis and ejection fraction are then compared with the stress data. The normal response to exercise is a ≥5% increase in calculated left ventricular ejection fraction and an increase in myocardial contractility. The development of exercise-induced myocardial ischemia usually results in a wall motion abnormality that is hypokinetic, akinetic, or dyskinetic compared with the rest study, and the ejection fraction usually, though not always, will decline (Fig. 5-3).

First-Pass Radionuclide Angiography

First-pass radionuclide angiography (RNA) can be performed on some of the newer digital, single-crystal cameras, but ideally this study is performed on a multicrystal gamma camera especially designed to accept higher count rates than the standard single-crystal gamma camera. The technique varies from the MUGA study in that the images are created in a very brief time over only several heartbeats. The technique creates an image of the tracer within the blood pool as it traverses the right and left ventricles during its first pass through the heart and lungs (Fig. 5-4). Tracer is administered intravenously as a compact bolus, preferably through an external jugular vein. The studies can be performed with an antecubital venous injection as long as the bolus stays relatively intact through the cardiopulmonary circulation, since a diluted infusion results in erroneous data.

Technetium 99m sodium pertechnetate, an eluate from the ^{99}MO-^{99m}Tc generator that requires no further preparation, is a commonly used radiopharmaceutical for RNA studies. The usual administered dose is 15 mCi (555 MBq). Other radiopharmaceuticals that can be used include ^{99m}Tc diethylenetriamine pentaacetic acid (^{99m}Tc DTPA) and ^{99m}Tc sulfur colloid. A commonly used radiopharmaceutical for RNA studies is ^{99m}Tc Sestamibi, when a left ventricular function study is performed at the time of tracer injection for a subsequent myocardial perfusion image (see earlier discussion on ^{99m}Tc Sestamibi) (8). When a rest–exercise RNA study is done in conjunction with perfusion imaging using ^{99m}Tc Ses-

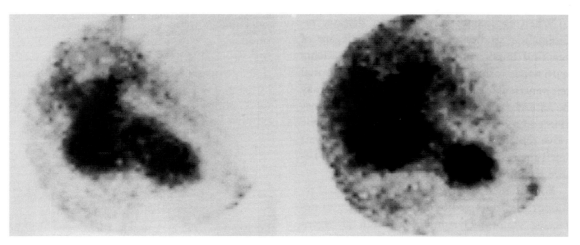

FIG 5-3. End-diastolic (left) and end-systolic (right) frames from a gated-equilibrium (MUGA, or multigated acquisition imaging) study of a patient with a left ventricular aneurysm show a dyskinetic segment in the apex.

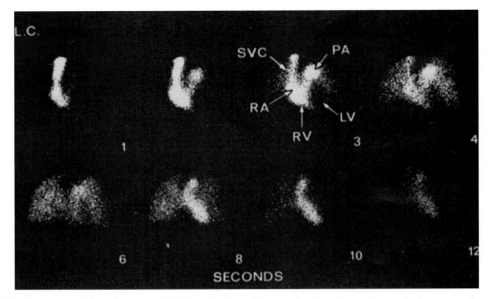

FIG 5-4. Sequential visualization of right and left cardiovascular structures from a first-pass radionuclide angiocardiogram performed on a normal person. LV, left ventricle; PA, pulmonary artery; RA, right atrium; RV, right ventricle; SVC, superior vena cava. (Reproduced with permission from Treves S, Maltz D, Adelstein S. Intracardiac shunts. In: James AE, Wagner HN, Cooke RE, eds. *Pediatric nuclear medicine*. Philadelphia: Saunders, 1974.)

tamibi, the resting study is done in the anterior projection with the patient standing (if physical exercise is to follow) or supine (if pharmacologic stress is to follow). The stress RNA study is done at the peak of physical exercise or at the peak effect of the pharmacologic stress agent. A patient's motion during physical exercise is a somewhat greater problem with treadmill exercise than with bicycle exercise, but motion-correction programs can be used to correct for patient motion.

Global and/or regional ventricular ejection fractions, wall motion analysis, left ventricular end-diastolic volumes, and stroke volumes can be determined with RNA studies. The anterior projection allows for segmental wall motion analysis of the anterior and inferior walls and apex of the left ventricle. Rest–exercise studies can be viewed simultaneously to evaluate for changes in ejection fraction and wall motion (Fig. 5-5). The peak exercise left ventricular ejection fraction by RNA has been shown to be a powerful prognostic indicator in patients with coronary artery disease. Survival rates decline as the peak exercise ejection fraction decreases. For this reason the study is often requested in the clinical prognostic assessment of patients with known coronary artery disease.

Gated Myocardial Perfusion SPECT

Another method for acquiring functional information at the time of myocardial perfusion imaging studies is by the use of gated myocardial perfusion SPECT images (9). The patient is injected at rest and at stress in the usual manner,

as described earlier, under 99mTc Sestamibi perfusion imaging. The acquisition of the stress SPECT image is changed, however, in that the images are acquired in a gated fashion, much like a MUGA study, although the frame rate is reduced to about eight frames per R-R interval on the electrocardiogram. Either the rest SPECT acquisition or the stress SPECT acquisition can be acquired by a gated technique. One needs to be aware that the gated study is acquired ~30 minutes to 1 hour following the injection of tracer administered at peak exercise. Thus, any wall motion abnormalities that may have existed during stress may have resolved by the time the gated study is acquired.

However, the gated perfusion study has been found to be helpful, particularly in the assessment of areas that show fixed defects that may be due either to infarction or to attenuation artifact. Analysis of the gated SPECT study includes evaluation of wall motion and wall thickening during the cardiac cycle. Infarcted myocardium fails to evidence either of these functions, while normal myocardium has normal wall motion and wall thickening. Transiently ischemic myocardium at peak exercise may also demonstrate normal wall motion and wall thickening at the time of image acquisition. The usefulness of this technique is under investigation, but the additional information obtained by wall motion analysis can, at times, be helpful in drawing final conclusions about SPECT perfusion images.

Positron Emission Tomography

Positron emission tomography (PET) is an alternative to Tl-201 or 99mTc Sestamibi for the evaluation of myocardial

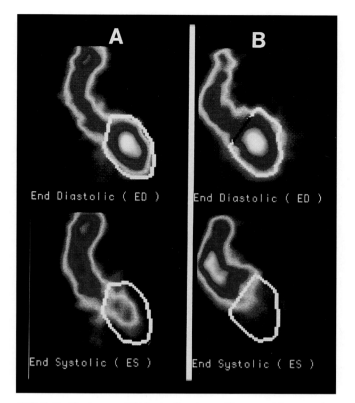

FIG 5-5. First-pass RNA studies in a 49-year-old man who is a smoker with hypertension, a family history of coronary artery disease, and a standard treadmill test that showed ST segment changes suggestive of ischemia. At exercise, he exceeded his target heart rate without chest pain. His myocardial perfusion study was normal. His resting study (**A**) shows normal wall motion and an ejection fraction of 62%. At peak exercise (**B**), wall motion remains normal, and the ejection fraction increases to 76%. (see Color Plate 3)

ischemia and/or viability (10). The many complexities and costs of PET imaging have limited the development of this technique, which offers advantages of attenuation correction and the ability to acquire absolute measurements of myocardial blood flow. It is the only method currently available for evaluating in vivo myocardial metabolism.

Myocardial perfusion can be evaluated with either nitrogen-13-labeled ammonia or rubidium 82. Metabolism in corresponding areas of myocardium can be evaluated with F-18 fluoro-2-deoxyglucose, the uptake of which requires viable myocardial cells. Thus, one of the indications of this study is identification of viable myocardium. Normally, the heart does not metabolize glucose for its energy needs. However, when a myocardial segment is ischemic, it will preferentially shift to the anaerobic metabolism of glucose, which results in a second indication for this study—the identification of ischemic myocardium. Positron imaging generally provides images with higher resolution than those provided by standard nuclear medicine imaging. However, availability continues to be limited.

RADIONUCLIDE STUDIES OF LUNG DISEASE

The primary use for radionuclide imaging in pulmonary disease is in the evaluation of patients with suspected pulmonary embolism. Scintigraphy for the evaluation of nonembolic disease is less common. Scintigraphic techniques are available for evaluating pulmonary function (aerosol clearance), inflammation (gallium 67 citrate accumulation), metabolic disorders (I-123 iodoamphetamine (IMP) and metaiodobenzylguanidine (MIBG), and tumors (F-18 fluoro-2-deoxyglucose), but in clinical practice these techniques are employed less often than ventilation/perfusion (V/Q) imaging in the assessment of suspected pulmonary embolism. This discussion will focus on radionuclide imaging in the detection of pulmonary embolism.

Pulmonary Imaging

Chest Radiography

The chest radiograph is an essential component in the evaluation of a patient who is suspected of having pulmonary embolism (12). A chest radiograph is obtained to evaluate a patient for clinical diagnoses that simulate pulmonary embolism and to compare with the V/Q scan. The conditions that may simulate pulmonary embolism and can be detected on a chest radiograph are pneumonia, rib fracture, and pneumothorax. The radiographic findings of pulmonary embolism are nonspecific and include consolidation, atelectasis, small pleural effusion, and elevation of a diaphragm. Focal oligemia and proximal pulmonary artery enlargement are uncommon, extremely subtle, and difficult to detect without good comparison films. High-quality posterior–anterior and lateral radiographs obtained at the time of lung scan are important for comparison with the lung scan. The chest radiograph should be obtained within a few hours in a patient with acute symptoms, but a chest radiograph obtained within 24 hours of the V/Q scan is acceptable in a patient who has no intervening symptoms.

Ventilation Imaging

The two radiopharmaceuticals most commonly used for ventilation imaging are xenon 133 (^{133}Xe) gas and ^{99m}Tc DTPA aerosol. The use of ^{133}Xe requires an apparatus for administering the gas and trapping the exhaled gas. For this ventilation study, the apparatus includes a tightly sealed face mask or mouthpiece, a spirometer, tubing with intake and exhaust valves, and a shielded charcoal trap. A large-field-of-view gamma scintillation camera fitted with an all-purpose collimator is employed. The procedure consists of obtaining a single-breath image of 100,000 counts in ~ 10 seconds with 20 mCi (740 MBq) ^{133}Xe administered through the intake port as the patient inspires (Fig. 5-6). Equilibrium images are then obtained while the patient rebreathes the gas in a closed spirometer system. Serial washout images are

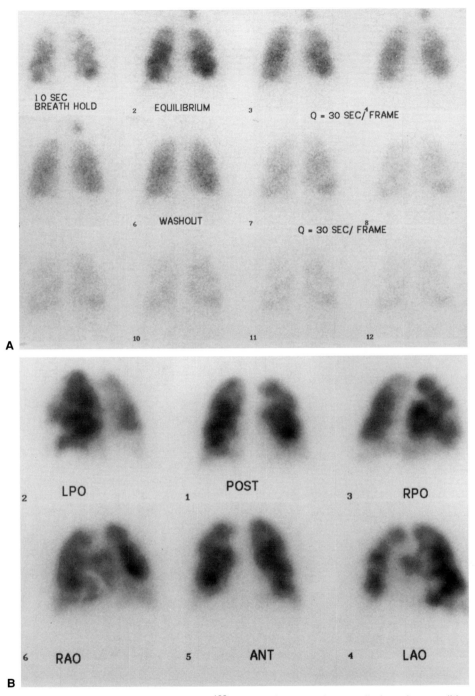

FIG 5-6. Ventilation study (**A**) obtained using ^{133}Xe reveals extensive ventilation abnormalities on the breath-hold (multiple areas of decreased accumulation) and washout (multiple areas of retention) images. The chest radiograph is normal. The perfusion study (**B**) obtained using ^{99m}Tc MAA shows multiple perfusion defects that correspond to the ventilation abnormalities. The matched ventilation and perfusion abnormalities with a normal chest radiograph place this scan in a low probability category for pulmonary embolism.

acquired as the patient breathes in air and the radioactivity is washed out of the lungs. The single breath and washout images reflect ventilation, whereas the equilibrium image corresponds to lung volume. In the single-breath image, the ventilatory abnormality appears as a deficit in radioactivity in the lung, whereas abnormal ventilation appears as a focal area of retention on washout images (Fig. 5-6). The ^{133}Xe ventilation study is best obtained before the perfusion study, which is done after the intravenous administration of ^{99m}Tc macroaggregates of albumin (MAA).

The other radiopharmaceutical used for imaging the distribution of ventilation is radiolabeled aerosol. The radioaerosol ventilation study using ^{99m}Tc DTPA is usually performed before the perfusion study. The ventilation study is best done with the patient in the supine position to provide ventilation to the apexes. For the radioaerosol study, 30 mCi (1,110 MBq) of ^{99m}Tc DTPA is placed in the nebulizer, and inhalation of the aerosol is continued until 1 mCi (37 MBq) is deposited in the lungs. The patient then can be imaged in multiple projections. This amount of radioaerosol in the lung will not result in any diagnostic problems in interpreting the perfusion study, which is obtained after the administration of 4 to 5 mCi (14 to 185 MBq) 99mTc MAA.

Perfusion Imaging

The radiopharmaceutical that is used for perfusion imaging is 99mTc MAA. To obtain an even distribution of radioactivity throughout the vascular bed, >60,000 particles need to be administered. Usually, 4 mCi (148 MBq) of ^{99m}Tc MAA is given, consisting of ~500,000 particles. The radiopharmaceutical is administered slowly over 5 to 10 seconds with the patient supine and taking moderately deep breaths. This administration technique ensures even distribution of the particles. Perfusion scintigraphy is performed with a large-field-of-view gamma camera fitted with a all-purpose collimator, the same camera–collimator setup that is used for the ventilation study. Eight views of the chest, including anterior, posterior, right and left posterior and anterior oblique, and right and left lateral views, are taken. All views are obtained for 750,000 counts, except for the lateral view. In that case, one view is imaged for 500,000 counts, and the second lateral view is acquired over the same length of time. The lateral views are least helpful, and other six images are frequently necessary.

Ventilation/Perfusion Lung Scan Interpretation

The diagnosis of pulmonary embolism is difficult even with all the imaging methods available today. Perfusion lung imaging is sensitive but not specific for pulmonary embolism, and it can be abnormal from nearly all pulmonary diseases that produce decreased pulmonary arterial blood flow to affected lung zones. Ventilation imaging is used to im-

prove the specificity of the perfusion scan for diagnosing pulmonary embolism.

Previous studies have shown that abnormalities in the perfusion scan that are matched by zones of abnormal ventilation do not represent pulmonary emboli (Fig. 5-6), whereas mismatched abnormalities, in regions with a normal chest radiograph, have a strong correspondence with the angiographic diagnosis of pulmonary embolism (Fig. 5-7) (13–15). The diagnostic accuracy of scintigraphic detection of pulmonary embolism is significantly improved when ventilation studies supplement perfusion scans and chest radiographs.

Biello and colleagues (16) provided a categorization of lung scans based on size of perfusion defects and comparison with the ventilation study and chest radiograph. They categorized perfusion defects as small (<25% of a segment), moderate (25% to 75% of a segment), and large (>75% of a segment). They compared the location of the perfusion abnormality with the findings on the ventilation study and chest radiograph and were able to accurately define criteria obtained from the V/Q scan that categorized the likelihood that the findings represented pulmonary embolism. Neumann and colleagues (15) introduced the concept of segmental equivalents and showed that two subsegmental perfusion defects may be added to produce the same diagnostic significance as a single segmental defect.

To determine the sensitivity and specificity of V/Q scintigraphy in the evaluation of patients with suspected pulmonary embolism, a multicenter prospective study was performed (17). The Prospective Investigation of Pulmonary Embolism Diagnosis (PIOPED) study of more than 700 patients is the largest existing study of the accuracy of lung scintigraphy in the diagnosis of acute pulmonary embolism. Six tertiary-care medical centers participated in the study. Patients were randomized to enter the study and, if selected, were asked to consent to having a pulmonary angiogram if the lung scan result was not normal. Perfusion scans were obtained for all patients and ventilation studies for almost all patients. Chest radiographs were taken in all patients within 12 hours of the lung scan.

These patients all underwent pulmonary arteriography. The prevalence of pulmonary embolism was 30% for the entire study, a rate that was very similar among the six institutions participating in the study. The images were interpreted according to a set of criteria that remained constant throughout the trial. A standardized, detailed description of each image set was derived by consensus of two teams of two readers blinded to clinical and arteriographic findings. The data collection and tabulation aspects of the study have been published (18). The scan description form is likely to have several uses for the medical community. The form breaks scan interpretation into many small achievable tasks, a process that may be daunting to the uninitiated. It provides a useful framework for organizing one's thoughts and is a good teaching tool. This form would be expected to improve

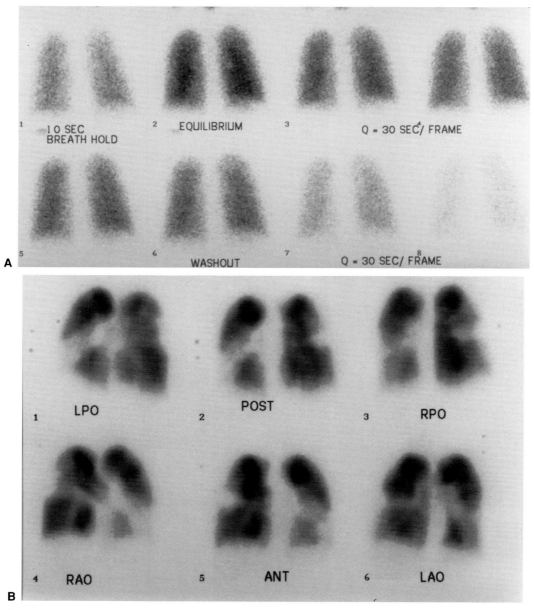

FIG 5-7. Ventilation study (**A**) displays normal ventilation. The chest radiograph also gives normal results. The perfusion study (**B**) shows multiple segmental defects in both lungs. This mismatch pattern has a high probability for pulmonary embolism.

internal consistency in interpretation between members of a group and would be helpful in reaching a consensus.

The original criteria used in the PIOPED study have been evaluated, and the correlation of percentage probability estimates with the actual prevalence of pulmonary embolism has been defined (19). Most of the criteria originally used in the PIOPED study were appropriately categorized. Three criteria need to be reconsidered:

1. A single moderate perfusion defect is appropriately categorized as intermediate, rather than as low probability.
2. Extensive matched V/Q abnormalities are better defined as low probability, provided that the chest radiograph is clear. On the other hand, single matched defects may be better categorized as intermediate probability. Owing to the small number of cases, no definite, statistically based recommendation can be made concerning this finding.
3. Two segmental mismatches may not be in the category for high probability and in some cases should be considered of intermediate probability. However, owing to the small number of cases, no definite, statistically well founded recommendation can be made concerning this finding.

The percentage probability estimates made by the physicians reading the V/Q scans in the PIOPED study correlated with the prevalence of pulmonary embolism on angiography. Receiver operating characteristic (ROC) curve analysis of the PIOPED data reveals that the use of percentage probability is slightly better than the use of the categories. Experienced readers should incorporate percentage estimates into the scan interpretation report along with the scan category interpretation.

Studies based on the PIOPED data have suggested criteria that are easier to apply and more sensitive for the detection of pulmonary embolism. These data suggest that the segmental equivalent concept does not add to diagnostic accuracy and that the total number of large or moderate defects is the important finding (20). Furthermore, patients who have cardiopulmonary disease need to have more mismatched perfusion defects to achieve the same positive predictive value as those patients who have no history of cardiopulmonary disease. A recent study by Worsley et al. (21) demonstrated that the location of abnormalities could be used as a criterion to reduce the number of intermediate probability studies. They found that radiographic opacities with matched V/Q abnormalities in the upper and middle lung zones have a lower likelihood of being associated with pulmonary embolism in the same zone whereas those in the lower zones have a higher likelihood. These results most likely relate to the distribution of pulmonary embolism, which is more common in the lower zones. These results need to be validated before

incorporation into a diagnostic scheme for interpretation of V/Q scans. The criteria that we are using for interpreting V/Q scans are noted in Table 5-2.

REFERENCES

1. Iskandrian AS, Chae SC, Heo J, Stanberry CD, Wasserleben V, Cave V. Independent and incremental prognostic value of exercise single-photon emission computed tomographic (SPECT) thallium imaging in coronary artery disease. *J Am Coll Cardiol* 1993;22:665–670.
2. Dilsizian V, Perrone-Filardi P, Arrighi JA, et al. Concordance and discordance between stress-redistribution-reinjection and rest-redistribution thallium imaging for assessing viable myocardium: comparison with metabolic activity by PET. *Circulation* 1993;88:941–952.
3. Maddahi J, Rodrigues E, Berman DS, et al. State-of-the-art myocardial perfusion imaging. *Cardiol Clin* 1994;12:199–222.
4. Berman DS, Kiat HS, Van Train KF, et al. Myocardial perfusion imaging with technetium-99m Sestamibi: comparative analysis of available imaging protocols. *J Nucl Med* 1994;35:681–688.
5. Heo J, Walmer I, Kegel J, Iskandrian S. Sequential dual-isotope SPECT imaging with thallium-201 and technetium-99m Sestamibi. *J Nucl Med* 1994;35:549–553.
6. Wackers FJT. The maze of myocardial perfusion imaging protocols in 1994. *J Nucl Cardiol* 1994;1:180–188.
7. Borges-Neto S, Coleman RE, Potts JM, Jones RH. Combined exercise radionuclide angiocardiography and single photon emission computed tomography perfusion studies for assessment of coronary artery disease. *Semin Nucl Med* 1991;21:223–229.
8. Mannting F, Morgan-Mannting MG. Gated SPECT with technetium-99m Sestamibi for assessment of myocardial perfusion abnormalities. *J Nucl Med* 1993;34:601–608.
9. Wackers FJT. Artifacts in planar and SPECT myocardial perfusion imaging. *Am J Cardiac Imaging* 1992;6:42–58.
10. The Council on Scientific Affairs Positron Emission Tomography Panel. Applications of positron emission tomography in the heart. *JAMA* 1988;259:2438–2445.
11. Treves S, Maltz D, Adelstein S. Intracardiac shunts. In: James AE, Wagner HN, Cooke RE, eds. *Pediatric nuclear medicine*. Philadelphia: Saunders, 1974:231–245.
12. Greenspan RH, Ravin CE, Polansky SM, McLoud TC. Accuracy of the chest radiograph in diagnosis of pulmonary embolism. *Invest Radiol* 1982;17:539–543.
13. McNeil BJ, Holman L, Adelstein J. The scintigraphic definition of pulmonary embolism. *JAMA* 1974;227:753–756.
14. Alderson PO, Rujanavech N, Secker-Walker RH, et al. The role of 133-xenon ventilation studies in the scintigraphic detection of pulmonary embolism. *Radiology* 1976;120:633–640.
15. Neumann RD, Sostman HD, Gottschalk A. Current status of ventilation-perfusion imaging. *Semin Nucl Med* 1980;10:198–217.
16. Biello DR, Mattar AG, McKnight REC, et al. Ventilation-perfusion studies in suspected pulmonary embolism. *AJR Am J Roentgenol* 1979;133:1033–1037.
17. The PIOPED Investigators. Value of the ventilation/perfusion scan in acute pulmonary embolism *JAMA* 1990;263:2753–2759.
18. Gottschalk A, Juni JE, Sostman HD, et al. Ventilation-perfusion scintigraphy in the PIOPED study: data collection and tabulation. *J Nucl Med* 1993;34:1109–1118.
19. Gottschalk A, Sostman HD, Juni JE, et al. Ventilation-perfusion scintigraphy in the PIOPED study: evaluation of the scintigraphic criteria and interpretations. *J Nucl Med* 1993;34:1119–1126.
20. Stein PD, Gottschalk A, Henry JW, Shivkumar K. Stratification of patients according to prior cardiopulmonary disease and probability assessment based on the number of mismatched segmental equivalent perfusion defects. *Chest* 1993;104:1461–1467.
21. Worsley DF, Kim CK, Alavia A, Palevsky HI. Detailed analysis of patients with matched ventilation-perfusion defects and chest radiographic opacities. *J Nucl Med* 1993;34:1851–1853.

TABLE 5-2. *Current Duke V/Q scan criteria*

High probability (>80%)
    No previous cardiopulmonary disease: ≥2 mismatched moderate or large perfusion defects
    Previous cardiopulmonary disease or uncertain: ≥4 mismatched moderate or large perfusion defects
Intermediate probability (20% to 80%)
    Difficult to categorize or not described as low or high
Low probability (<20%)
    Nonsegmental perfusion defects (e.g., cardiomegaly, enlarged hila, elevated diaphragm)
    Perfusion defect with a substantially larger chest radiographically evident abnormality
    Perfusion defects matched by ventilation abnormality of equal or larger size provided that there are:
        Clear chest radiograph
        Some areas of normal perfusion in the lungs
    Any number of small perfusion defects with normal results on chest radiograph
Normal
    No perfusion defects—perfusion outlines exactly the shape of the lungs seen on the chest radiograph (normal hilar and aortic impressions may be seen, and the chest radiograph and/or ventilation study may be abnormal)

Essentials of Cardiac Imaging,
James T. T. Chen,
Lippincott–Raven Publishers, Philadelphia © 1998.

CHAPTER 6

Echocardiography

Michael W. Hanson

BASIC PRINCIPLES OF ECHOCARDIOGRAPHY

Physics of Ultrasound

Ultrasound is by definition sound that has a frequency of >20,000 cycles per second, well beyond the audible range for humans. The successful use of ultrasound for imaging purposes is based upon the properties of an ultrasonic beam and its interactions with tissues as it passes through the body. Sound waves behave differently in different media, such as water, blood, muscle, bone, air, and lung. When the sound passes through a homogeneous medium, it typically travels in a straight line. However, as it passes from one medium to another, the course of the sound waves is altered at the interface between the two mediums and is either reflected away from the interface or proceeds into the next medium on an altered path (refracted). This principle of the reflection of ultrasound waves as they pass from one medium to another (e.g., blood to muscle) is the basis for the use of ultrasound as a medical imaging tool; the degree of reflection is dependent upon the differences in acoustic impedence from one medium to the other. The greater the difference in the acoustical properties of the interfaced media, the greater is the reflection of the ultrasound waves.

An ultrasound wave is composed of a series of rarefactions and compressions, often depicted as a sine wave. The *wavelength* of the ultrasound wave is the distance from one peak compression to the next, and the combination of one rarefaction and one compression represents one *cycle* of the sound wave. The *frequency* of a sound wave is a property determined by the number of cycles generated in a given time and is usually expressed as a number of cycles per second [given in hertz (Hz)]. The higher the frequency of an ultrasonic beam, the greater its reflection from smaller objects

and the greater its resolving power (the ability to distinguish objects that are close to each other as being separate objects). Echocardiography typically uses ultrasound with a frequency of approximately two million cycles per second (2 MHz), which can generate high-resolution images.

Instrumentation for Echocardiography

The ability to use ultrasound for medical imaging is based upon the development of the piezoelectric transducer. A substance that has piezoelectric properties can change its shape when struck by alternating electrical current. Examples of substances that possess piezoelectric properties include quartz and certain ceramics (e.g., barium titanate). When an electrical current strikes a piezoelectric crystal, alternating expansions and contractions, or sound waves, are produced and directed into the cardiac structures. As these sound waves encounter various interfaces, they are reflected back toward the transducer. The piezoelectric crystal also functions in reverse, that is, when the crystal is struck by a returning sound wave, the crystal produces an electrical impulse in response to this interaction. Therefore, the piezoelectric transducer serves both as the transmitter and as the receiver of ultrasound waves to create the echocardiographic images.

For echocardiography, a standard 2.25-MHz transducer directs the ultrasound beam through the human body at a velocity of 1,540 m per second. Unlike x-rays, ultrasound waves require matter in which to propagate, and they may be viewed as compression and relaxation of the propagating medium in the direction of the beam. At any interface between tissues of different densities and elasticities (different acoustic impedances), the ultrasound waves are reflected back to the transducer. Since blood has a different acoustic impedance from that of the soft-tissue structures inside the heart (e.g., the cardiac valves), these structures can be readily imaged with ultrasound.

When these reflected sound waves return to the piezoelec-

Division of Nuclear Medicine, Department of Radiology, Duke University Medical Center, Durham, North Carolina, 27710, U.S.A.

tric transducer, the electrical current that is created from the interaction of the sound wave with the crystal can be represented and displayed on an oscilloscope. The format for the presentation of the returning sound wave echoes reflected from the cardiac structures has undergone significant transition since the initial development of echocardiography. The earliest echocardiogram, using a single crystal, presented a one-dimensional display of the cardiac structures, the appearance of which did not resemble the anatomic appearance of the heart at all. The spikes or dots or lines that were created represented the returning sound waves from only a small segment of the heart at any given position and time.

Imaging Methods in Echocardiography

One method of representing the returning echo is in the "A mode" ("A" referring to amplitude of the echo), which displays the echo as a spike with a height and width determined by the structure responsible for creating the reflected, returning echo. The positions of the various echoes on the oscilloscope are determined by the distance of the interface from the ultrasound transducer. A second way to display the returning echoes is the "B mode" presentation, which involves the use of intensity modulation. This technique converts the amplitude of the returning echo to intensity, and the display is changed from a spike to a dot, the brightness of the individual dot being dependent upon the amplitude of the initiating echo ("B" referring to brightness).

The heart is constantly in motion, and the structures that create the echoes for display are continually changing in a repetitive sequence in relationship to the transducer. Thus, the dots in the B-mode format change in position with time. What is desired is to have the ability to capture the echo as it changes in the B-mode format. This concept led to the "time motion" or "M mode" display format ("M" referring to motion). With this technique, the temporal aspect of cardiac motion adds another dimension to echocardiographic imaging. By passing strip chart paper that is light sensitive past the moving B-mode dots, an image is inscribed on the paper that represents the movement of the B-mode dots over time and generates an "ice pick" view of the heart in a single line, as structures changing during cardiac contractility (Fig. 6-1).

The M-mode echocardiogram inscribes motion patterns of the cardiac structures over time, yet does not resemble the actual cardiac anatomy. The pattern of motion must be extrapolated into what is actually occurring in the three-dimensional heart. The transducer must be moved from one part of the heart to the next to incorporate all of the valvular levels in the myocardium from the base to the apex. Each of the regions through the ventricle has a normal pattern of motion (e.g., the mitral and aortic valves) to which the acquired echocardiogram (see **Fig. 11-23**) must be compared for evidence of abnormality. Currently, M-mode echocardiograms are not taken routinely, but they are occasionally use-

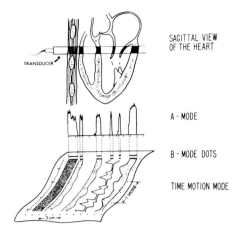

FIG 6-1. Three means of presenting echocardiographic information. A sound beam passes through the right ventricular wall, interventricular septum, mitral valve, and left ventricular wall. The echoes arising from the intracardiac structures are presented as moving spikes (A mode), as moving dots (B mode), and as moving lines (M mode). The M-mode record is obtained by passing a light-sensitive strip chart paper past the B-mode dots. A B-mode presentation is obtained by electronically turning the A-mode spikes on end. (Reproduced with permission from Johnson ML, Kisslo JA. Basic diagnostic echocardiography. *Disease-A-Month* 1976;23:7.)

ful as an adjunct to the more standard two-dimensional echocardiographic imaging study (described in the next section).

TWO-DIMENSIONAL ECHOCARDIOGRAPHY

In order to obtain a cardiac image that, when displayed, conforms more closely to the actual anatomic structure of the heart, a technique was developed to acquire a "cross sectional" view of the heart. By rapidly spatially tracking B-mode echoes, a real-time image can be created that provides a tomographic view of the cardiovascular structures that lie within the confines of the sector defined by the emitted ultrasonic beam. Referred to as "two-dimensional echocardiography," this technique has become the standard imaging technique in cardiac ultrasound.

The two-dimensional echocardiographic scanner is designed as either a mechanical or an electronic scanner. In a mechanical scanner, the ultrasonic beam is moved by an electrical motor. In an oscillating type of mechanical scanner, the active element of the ultrasound transducer moves back and forth through a defined angle that creates the sector to be imaged (1). In a rotating type of mechanical scanner, active elements (usually three or four) of the ultrasound transducer are mounted on a wheel and emit the ultrasound beam in a defined sector as they rotate within a housing unit at the end of the probe.

In electronic scanners, the transducers do not move in space; the ultrasonic beam is directed electronically. There are also two types of electronic two-dimensional echocardiographic scanners. One of them, the multi-element linear array scanner, is made up of a series of small active elements mounted side by side. These elements are electronically activated in a sequential manner, which moves the ultrasonic beam in a linear fashion (2). Because of the diagnostic acoustic window needed for this type of scanner, its use in cardiovascular ultrasound has diminished, although it is popular in other areas of diagnostic ultrasound, such as abdominal imaging and peripheral vascular imaging. The second type of electronic scanner is the phased-array scanner (3,4). This scanner also uses a multi-element transducer. The direction of the single ultrasonic beam that is created by this instrument can be rapidly and randomly altered by controlling the timing when each active element in the transducer is activated. Each of these mechanical or electronic two-dimensional echocardiographic scanners has advantages and disadvantages. The phase-array scanner is probably the most popular of the scanners used in cardiovascular ultrasound.

Standard two-dimensional echocardiography is performed via a transthoracic approach. With the patient generally placed in the left-lateral decubitus position, the transducer is most commonly set along the left sternal border to begin the examination and subsequently moved to other positions, such as the apical, subcostal, or suprasternal location, in order to image the cardiovascular structures from different vantage points. The transducer is optimally placed in these locations relative to the individual patient's anatomy (i.e., cardiac size and orientation). The three basic orthogonal views used for two-dimensional echocardiographic imaging include the parasternal long-axis view, which is oriented parallel to the heart or the left ventricle; the parasternal short-axis view, which is perpendicular to the parasternal long axis view; and the apical four-chamber view, which is orthogonal to the other two views (5) (Fig. 6-2). By manipulating the transducer through various tomographic levels from the base of the heart to the apex of the heart and from the interventricular septum to the lateral walls in each of these three basic planes, the majority of cardiovascular structures can be adequately evaluated.

Transthoracic echocardiographic imaging is technically adequate in the majority of patients. Difficulties in obtaining optimal images can occur in patients who are obese or in those with chest wall deformities or unusual orientations of the cardiovascular structures. Air within the lungs can disperse the echocardiographic signals, which can present a problem for adequate imaging, particularly in those patients with obstructive pulmonary disease.

Echocardiography has broad applications in the study of the cardiovascular system. One of the most common applications is the assessment of valvular heart disease. Two-dimensional echocardiography is very useful for evaluating native or prosthetic cardiac valves. The two-dimensional echocardiogram, in conjunction with Doppler ultrasound studies (see discussion under Doppler Ultrasound), can provide information relative to the location, the underlying cause, and the severity of various types of valvular dysfunction. In the study of anatomy, two-dimensional echocardiography can

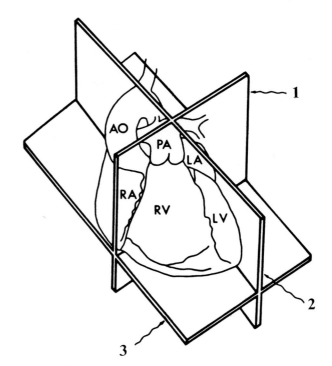

FIG 6-2. Diagram of the three orthogonal imaging planes used to visualize the heart with two-dimensional echocardiography. AO, aorta; RA, right atrium; PA, pulmonary artery; RV, right ventricle; LA, left atrium; LV, left ventricle; 1, short-axis plane; 2, long-axis plane; 3, four-chamber plane. (Reproduced with permission from Henry WL, DeMaria A, Gramiak R, et al. Report of the American Society of Echocardiography Committee on Nomenclature and Standards in Two-dimensional Echocardiography. *Circulation* 1980;62:213.).

identify thickening or calcifications of the valve leaflets (Fig. 6-3) or their supporting structures (mitral valve annular calcifications). Abnormal motion of valve leaflets (see **Fig. 11-15C,D**) or the presence of vegetations on the valve leaflets (subacute bacterial endocarditis) can be distinguished, and ruptured chordae tendineae can also be detected. Indirect evidence of regurgitant lesions (mitral regurgitation, aortic insufficiency) can be pinpointed, and the presence and severity of regurgitant lesions can be analyzed functionally with Doppler ultrasound techniques.

The aortic root and a portion of the ascending aorta can often be evaluated by transthoracic echocardiography, and the presence of a dilated aortic root that may have concomitant aortic insufficiency can be documented. Evaluation for a dissection of the aorta is better performed using transesophageal echocardiography (see discussion under Transesophageal Echocardiography).

The contour and orientation of the left ventricle can be assessed by two-dimensional echocardiography, and the wall thickness and size of the left ventricular cavity can be accurately measured by echocardiography. An adjunctive M-mode echocardiogram is helpful in left ventricular assessment. Indexes, such as the mean velocity of circumferential fiber shortening and the percentage fractional shortening,

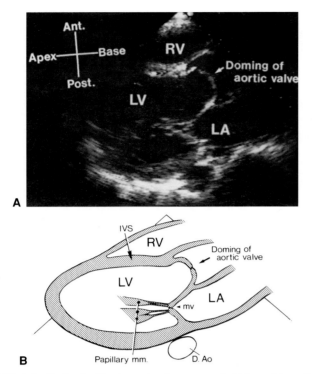

FIG 6-3. Patient with stenosis of a congenital bicuspid aortic valve. Two-dimensional long-axis echocardiogram (**A**) and corresponding diagram (**B**), taken in systole, show pronounced doming of the aortic valve, poststenotic dilatation of the aorta, and hypertrophy of the left ventricle (LV). Ant., anterior; D. Ao, descending aorta; IVS, interventricular septum; LA, left atrium; mm., muscles; mv, mitral valve; Post., posterior; RV, right ventricle.

can be calculated. The etiology of cardiac enlargement detected on chest radiography can be evaluated by two-dimensional echocardiography, which can distinguish a dilated from a symmetrically or asymmetrically hypertrophied left ventricle (see **Fig. 11-8F,G**) as well as identify the presence or absence of a pericardial effusion.

The tomographic format of two-dimensional echocardiography allows for analysis of segmental wall motion of the left ventricle. Areas of impaired contractility can be distinguished, such as hypokinesis, akinesis, or dyskinesis of specified segments of the left ventricle, which can be helpful in the evaluation of patients with known or suspected coronary artery disease. The segmental wall motion abnormalities characteristic of patients with ventricular dysfunction caused by coronary artery disease can often be detected. Patients with significant coronary artery disease may have normal left ventricular contractility at rest, but when the demand for oxygen exceeds the ability to provide adequate coronary artery blood flow to a specific region, segmental contractility of the left ventricle can become impaired and dysfunctional. Thus, baseline echocardiograms can be obtained and compared with an echocardiogram that reflects the findings of left ventricular contractility in response to physical or pharmacologic stress, in a manner similar to the rest and exercise

multigated equilibrium cardiac blood pool imaging study, an accepted, long-standing technique in nuclear imaging for evaluating the left ventricular ejection fraction and wall motion response to exercise.

The physical exercise echocardiographic study is performed with either bicycle or, more commonly, treadmill exercise testing. Ideally, imaging should be done at the peak of exercise, but image quality is adversely affected at that point by hyperventilation and the patient's motion, particularly on treadmill testing. This motion is somewhat less of a problem on bicycle exercise. With this technique, the patient stops treadmill exercise and is transferred to an imaging table, and postexercise images are acquired within a few minutes of the termination of physical exercise. This delay, although brief, may result in resolution of some transient wall motion abnormalities that were present at the peak of exercise.

A common alternative to exercise stress is the use of pharmacologic stressors, such as intravenous dipyridamole or, more often, dobutamine. The administration of dobutamine primarily increases cardiac contractility and, to a lesser degree, heart rate. Dobutamine simulates physical exercise and produces hemodynamic responses similar to those attained during physical exercise. The applications of stress echocardiography that have been investigated include the detection of coronary artery disease (6,7), prognosis and risk stratification (8), postmyocardial infarction evaluation (9), and the assessment of cardiac risk before noncardiac surgery (10).

The pericardium can be evaluated for the presence of effusion, and the echocardiogram can provide an estimate of the size of a pericardial effusion (Fig. 6-4). Evidence of pericardial thickening can sometimes be found on echocardiography. In large pericardial effusions, fibrous strands or tumor masses can be seen within the pericardial fluid.

A typical application for two-dimensional echocardiography is in the evaluation of known or suspected intracardiac masses (tumors, thrombi, or vegetations). A myxoma is the most common intracavitary cardiac tumor, most often found in the left atrium (see **Fig. 18-10**). The two-dimensional echocardiogram (Fig. 6-5) can be helpful in the identification of a left atrial myxoma and in differentiating it from mitral stenosis, which may be indistinguishable on clinical examination. Patients with typical subacute bacterial endocarditis usually have echocardiographic evidence of vegetations, which take the form of mobile masses typically attached to valve leaflets (see **Fig. 11-14**). Redundant or thickened valve leaflets can present diagnostic problems and, at times, can be misinterpreted as vegetations.

In addition to assessing congenital valvular heart disease (stenosis and/or regurgitation), two-dimensional echocardiography is also useful in the evaluation of other types of congenital abnormalities and of cardiovascular space relationships and orientations that may be altered in some of the more complex forms of congenital heart disease. The anatomy, orientation, and connections of the atria, ventricles, and great vessels can be reliably assessed in this group of

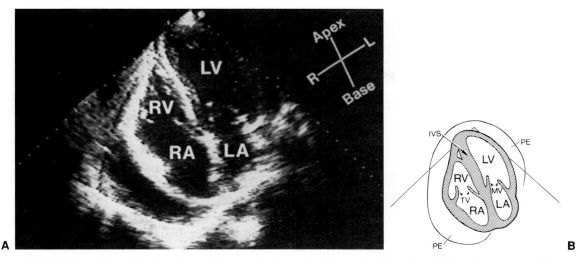

FIG 6-4. Two-dimensional echocardiogram in the apical four-chamber view (**A**) and corresponding diagram (**B**) shows a large pericardial effusion (PE) surrounding the heart. IVS, interventricular septum; LA, left atrium; LV, left ventricle; MV, mitral valve leaflets; RA, right atrium; RV, right ventricle; TV, tricuspid valve leaflets.

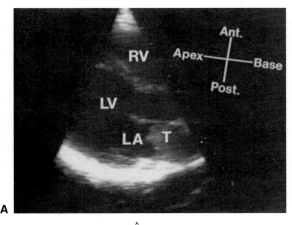

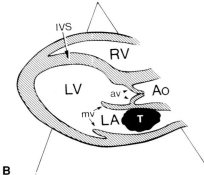

FIG 6-5. Two-dimensional echocardiogram in long-axis view of patient with left atrial myxoma (**A**) and corresponding diagram (**B**) demonstrate a large tumor mass (T) attached to the interatrial septum. In real-time display the tumor was seen to prolapse through the mitral valve orifice into the left ventricle. Ant., anterior; Ao, aorta; av, aortic valve; IVS, interventricular septum; LA, left atrium; LV, left ventricle; mv, mitral valve; Post., posterior; RV, right ventricle.

patients (see **Fig. 16-56**). Evidence of right ventricular volume overload (right ventricular enlargement and paradoxical motion of the interventricular septum) may be seen on standard two-dimensional echocardiography or M-mode echocardiography (Fig. 6-6) as a result of an atrial septal defect. The shunting of blood through an atrial septal defect or a ventricular septal defect can be further evaluated by contrast echocardiography or Doppler ultrasound (see discussions under the individual sections).

CONTRAST ECHOCARDIOGRAPHY

Visualization of various structures throughout the body with the use of contrast agents is widespread in medical imaging (e.g., cardiovascular, renal, or gastrointestinal opacification with radiopaque agents). This concept is based on the differential penetration of an x-ray beam through these agents relative to the surrounding soft tissues, which makes the structures of interest visible.

In ultrasonic imaging, the contrast agent is a medium that reflects sound waves in a manner that is different in character from the reflections of surrounding soft tissues, which allows for the identification and location of the administered contrast agent. The agent used for producing ultrasonic contrast is microbubbles. Contrast agents that have been used in echocardiography include normal saline and indocyanine green dye. When fluids are injected intravenously, microbubbles appear. A maximal contrast effect can be produced by adding small amounts of gas to the liquid before injection. Rapidly injecting normal saline that has first been vigorously agitated provides optimal visibility of the contrast effect of the microbubbles. The contrast effect results in a region of increased brightness in the location of the microbubbles,

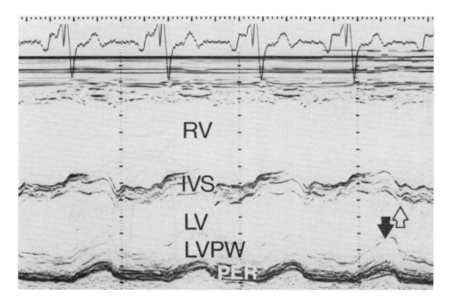

FIG 6-6. The M-mode echocardiogram of a patient with a large atrial septal defect. The right ventricle (RV) is notably enlarged. Also noted is a paradoxical septal motion: The most posterior motion of the interventricular septum (IVS) (*open arrow*) occurs after the greatest anterior displacement of the left ventricular posterior wall (LVPW) in systole (*closed arrow*). LV, left ventricle; PER, pericardium.

localized on the anatomical two-dimensional echocardiographic display.

The diagnostic usefulness of this technique is related to the physical characteristics of the microbubbles. Once injected, standard microbubbles are most readily seen as they traverse the right-sided cardiovascular structures, their contrast effect diminishing over time as the bubbles are absorbed into the blood or filtered out by dissolving at the level of the pulmonary capillary bed. After a peripheral intravenous injection in normal subjects, standard microbubbles do not traverse the lungs and do not appear on the left side of the heart, a property that is the basis of one of the more common applications of this technique, that is, the detection of cardiac shunts.

Contrast echocardiography provides accurate imaging of cardiac shunts using standard microbubbles (11). Since standard microbubbles do not traverse the lungs, the appearance of microbubbles in the atrium and the left ventricle after peripheral intravenous injection almost certainly indicates the presence of a right-to-left shunt. The apical or subcostal four-chamber views are optimal for this evaluation since the atria, ventricles, and the interatrial and interventricular septa are simultaneously visible, and the shunting of a small number of microbubbles can be detected (see **Fig. 16-14**). Contrast echocardiography can detect right-to-left shunts as small as 3% at the atrial, ventricular, or aortic levels and small right-to-left shunts in patients with patent foramen ovale or postoperative atrial septal defect repair (12).

Left-to-right shunts can also be evaluated by contrast echocardiography. Many patients with predominantly left-to-right shunts through an atrial septal defect will have transient right-to-left shunting of blood to a lesser degree, which can be confirmed by altering cardiothoracic pressures with a Valsalva maneuver, causing transient right-to-left shunting of microbubbles at the atrial level. In patients with exclusively left-to-right shunts, a negative contrast effect has been reported (13). In this context, the microbubbles will opacify a region of the right side of the heart (e.g., the right atrium) with the exception of an area near the site of shunting from the left to the right, producing a contrast-free area within the microbubbles.

Contrast echocardiography has been useful in the detection of tricuspid valvular regurgitation. The inferior vena cava is imaged on a subcostal view. After peripheral intravenous injection of contrast medium in normal subjects, a transient, minor reflux of microbubbles into the inferior vena cava may be observed during atrial contractility. However, the appearance of a larger number of refluxed microbubbles in the inferior vena cava and/or the hepatic vein during ventricular systole is good evidence for significant tricuspid regurgitation (14,15) (see **Fig. 11-25**).

The use of contrast echocardiography in the evaluation of valvular regurgitation and cardiac shunts has diminished with the increasing use of cardiovascular Doppler ultrasound (discussed later herein). However, there is still interest in the use of contrast echocardiography in other areas of cardiovascular evaluation, particularly that of myocardial perfusion imaging. The entrapment or dissolution of standard microbubbles at the pulmonary capillary level has limited their noninvasive use to the right side of the heart. Left-sided cardiovascular evaluation by contrast echocardiography can be performed by injecting the microbubbles directly through a catheter into the left cardiac chamber, the aortic root, or the coronary arteries. This technique has been applied to evaluate myocardial perfusion by injecting a variety of contrast agents (e.g., Renograffin-76 or sonicated albumin) directly into the coronary arteries while simultaneously taking a two-dimensional echocardiogram. Areas of perfused myocardium display enhanced, brightened echoes during the transit of microbubbles, while the appearance of underperfused or nonperfused myocardium remains unchanged

(16,17). These techniques have been applied to assist in the evaluation of left ventricular wall motion and to investigate myocardial ischemia and reperfusion hyperemia (18,19).

There has been long-term interest in the possible use of echocardiography to make visible the left cardiac chambersand myocardium with a contrast agent administered by peripheral intravenous injection (20,21). The achievement of this goal—transpulmonary contrast echocardiography—will depend upon the development of novel contrast agents in which the microbubbles are of such a size and stability that they can pass through the pulmonary capillary bed and remain intact to traverse the left cardiac chambers, aorta, and coronary arteries and be distributed in the myocardium in a manner that provides optimal contrast that reflects myocardial blood flow (22–25).

DOPPLER ULTRASOUND

Two-dimensional echocardiography provides thorough information on the anatomic structures of the pericardium, myocardium, and cardiac valves. Conventional two-dimensional echocardiography, however, does not furnish any direct hemodynamic information. The advent of Doppler echocardiography has added yet another important dimension to the use of the principles of ultrasound in the evaluation of cardiovascular disease. Doppler ultrasound can evaluate the pressure gradients across stenotic valves and provide an estimate of valve areas. Regurgitant blood flow and cardiac shunts can be analyzed with Doppler techniques. The combination of conventional two-dimensional echocardiographic imaging and Doppler ultrasound evaluation can provide a thorough noninvasive assessment of many cardiac disorders.

A Doppler ultrasound signal is created when an emitted high-frequency sound beam is directed to various regions of the heart and the emitted sound wave is reflected back to the transducer by the flowing red blood cells in that location. When an emitted sound wave is reflected back to the transducer, the frequency of the reflected wave is altered from its original frequency if the reflecting object is in motion. The difference in the frequency of the emitted and the reflected sound wave is referred to as the *Doppler shift*. If the reflecting surface is stationary, there is no Doppler shift. However, if the reflecting surface (i.e., the red blood cell) is moving away from or toward the point of origin of the emitted sound wave, the reflected frequency is shifted to a lower frequency or to a higher frequency, respectively.

These alterations, which represent the Doppler shift of the emitted sound wave, are detectable by the ultrasound system and are displayed as a positive deflection for a shift to a higher frequency and as a negative deflection for a shift to a lower frequency. The magnitude of the shift in frequency is proportional to the velocity at which the red blood cell is moving toward or away from the source of the emitted sound. Thus, the direction and velocity of the red blood cell flow toward or away from the transducer can be determined.

The frequency shift of the emitted sound wave is not only related to the direction and velocity of blood flow but is also dependent upon the angle at which the sound wave strikes the flowing red blood cells. The emitted ultrasound beam needs to be closely parallel to the direction of the flowing blood to generate an accurate assessment of the velocity of the blood flow. There is acceptable deviation of ~20° from parallel for determining velocity, but as the angle of intersection becomes greater, the velocity of blood flow will be underestimated accordingly.

Two forms of complementary Doppler ultrasound are available. *Continuous wave Doppler* has a very high pulse repetition frequency and continuously emits and receives ultrasound data to and from the red blood cells. The advantage of this form of Doppler ultrasound is its ability to accurately measure high-velocity blood flow. It is used to measure blood flow across an anatomical lesion, and, using a modification of the Bernoulli principle, it can be employed to calculate a pressure gradient across an anatomical lesion. *Pulsed wave Doppler* has a low pulse repetition frequency, and the transducer alternates between transmitting and receiving ultrasound waves, which makes depth discrimination possible. With pulsed wave Doppler, the ultrasound operator can define a region along the path of the ultrasound beam for analysis (the sample volume).

Pulsed wave Doppler is frequently performed under guidance of the echocardiogram, and the sample volume is positioned at varying depths in different regions of interest. The sampling rate (the number of transmitted pulses per second) in pulsed wave Doppler is limited by the depth of the sample volume. When high-velocity flows are encountered by the relatively slow sampling rate in pulsed wave Doppler, the velocity cannot be accurately measured, and an ultrasound artifact known as aliasing occurs. Aliasing creates ambiguous information regarding flow velocity and direction by misplacing data from one side of the reference baseline to the other. The Nyquist limit of a pulsed wave Doppler system refers to the maximal blood flow velocity that can be recorded without aliasing, which is generally 1.5 to 2.0 mseconds. Pulsed wave Doppler can detect stenotic, regurgitant, and certain shunt lesions by its ability to locate, in time, regions of abnormal, turbulent blood flow. Conventional continuous wave Doppler and pulsed wave Doppler are displayed in a graphic format, with time on the x-axis and the flow velocity (or the degree of frequency shift) on the y-axis. Signals above the baseline usually indicate flow toward the transducer, whereas signals beneath the baseline represent flow away from the transducer (Fig. 6-7).

Color flow Doppler is an ultrasound technique that is analogous to pulsed wave Doppler, although it is multigated. With this technique, flow velocity and direction data are visible in real time, superimposed on the structural two-dimensional echocardiographic images (Fig. 6-8). Multiple sampling sites are analyzed simultaneously within any given sector and assigned a color that is determined according to blood flow direction and velocity relative to the transducer.

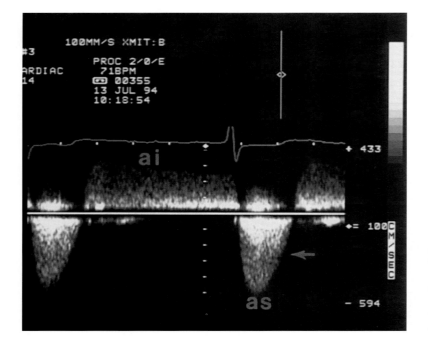

FIG 6-7. Continuous wave Doppler ultrasound study acquired with the transducer at the apex of the left ventricle in a patient with aortic stenosis (as) and aortic insufficiency (ai). Normal blood flow is moving away from the transducer. There is a high-velocity jet (*arrow*), attributed to the aortic stenosis, moving away from the transducer that peaks at ~5 mseconds (aortic valve gradient = 100 mm).

Although any color scheme can be created, conventionally, blood flow toward the transducer is designated as red, and blood flow away from the transducer is labeled blue. Turbulent, erratic blood flow is denoted as green or mosaic-patterned (the admixture of red, blue and green). The higher the velocity, the brighter the hue of each color. However, color flow Doppler is subject to aliasing in the same way as pulsed wave Doppler, which can result in a reversal of color. Color flow Doppler has an advantage over conventional Doppler techniques in that it provides instantaneous two-dimensional anatomical visual localization of any abnormal blood flow in the imaged sector. The technique is extremely useful in the detection and evaluation of valvular regurgitant lesions (Fig. 6-9), where it has shown sensitivity and specificity equal to conventional Doppler imaging (26,27); it is superior to conventional Doppler in grading the severity of these lesions.

TRANSESOPHAGEAL ECHOCARDIOGRAPHY

The soft tissues (adipose tissue, muscle, breast, and lung) of the thorax and the ribs can be obstacles in the routine transthoracic echocardiographic study and can compromise the extent and quality of the information obtained by this approach in some patients. Having the ability to place an ultrasound transducer within the esophagus and acquire images from within the thorax from a retrocardiac position avoids the interference imposed by these structures. The proximity of the esophagus to the posterior aspect of the heart usually allows for high-resolution images of the cardiovascular structures. This technique, known as *transesopha-*

geal echocardiography (TEE) has gained acceptance among cardiologists as well as anesthesiologists as a beneficial technique in ultrasonic cardiovascular evaluation, and indications for its use continue to grow (28). It can be performed on ambulatory patients, during surgery, or in the intensive care unit.

The TEE procedure requires intubation of the patient's esophagus with a specially designed flexible endoscope equipped with a high-frequency (5 MHz) transducer and a complete two-dimensional color flow Doppler system. The probe is designed to allow rotation and considerable anteroposterior and right–left lateral flexibility to perform monoplane, biplane, or multiplane imaging. Unlike transthoracic echocardiography, TEE is an invasive procedure that requires informed consent and certain precautions. The patient's medical history, allergies, and medications must be reviewed. Absolute contraindications to TEE include esophageal malignancy or stricture, active upper-gastrointestinal hemorrhage, perforated viscus, and lack of cooperation on the part of the patient. Relative contraindications include esophageal varices or diverticulum, cervical spine immobility, and severe oropharyngeal distortion (29).

Intravenous sedation is commonly used (e.g., a benzodiazipine), but institutional protocols vary—they can range from no sedation to high doses of intravenous agents. Following topical anesthesia to the pharynx, the TEE probe is inserted into the esophagus with the patient in the left-lateral decubitus position with the neck slightly flexed. The probe is gently advanced into the mid- to distal esophagus and fundus of the stomach in a retrocardiac location, where multiple images of the cardiovascular structures can be acquired (Fig. 6-10). Transesophageal echocardiography has applica-

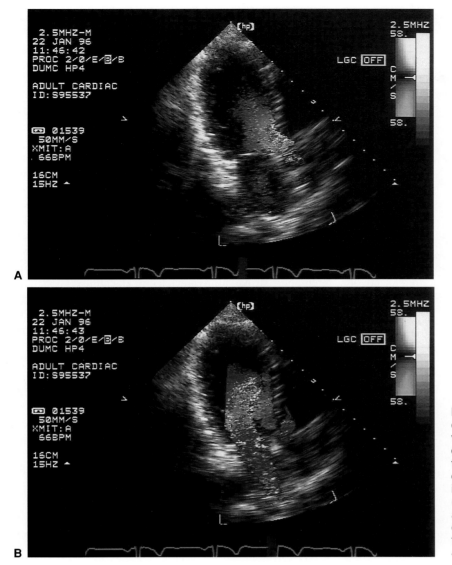

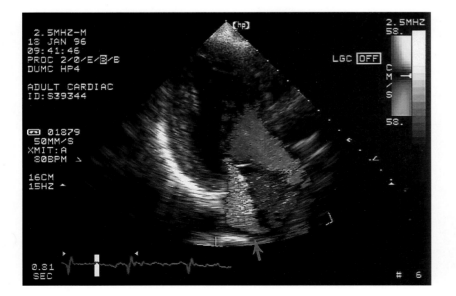

FIG 6-8. Transthoracic two-dimensional echocardiogram in the apical long-axis view with color flow Doppler ultrasound demonstrates (A) normal blood flow through the left ventricular outflow tract during ventricular systole (blue representing flow away from the transducer) and (B) normal blood flow from the left atrium across the mitral valve into the left ventricle during diastole (red representing flow toward the transducer). (see Color Plate 4)

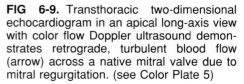

FIG 6-9. Transthoracic two-dimensional echocardiogram in an apical long-axis view with color flow Doppler ultrasound demonstrates retrograde, turbulent blood flow (arrow) across a native mitral valve due to mitral regurgitation. (see Color Plate 5)

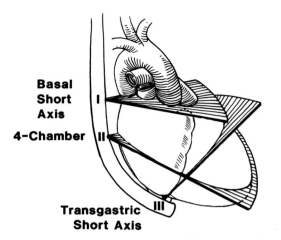

Basal Short Axis

4-Chamber

Transgastric Short Axis

FIG 6-10. Three tomographic planes for transesophageal echocardiography. (I) Basal short-axis planes obtained at a distance of 25 to 30 cm of transducer tip from incisors. (II) Four-chamber (frontal) planes obtained by retroflexion or slight advancement of tip of endoscope (or both) from position I (~30 cm from incisors). (III) Transgastric short-axis planes obtained from fundus of stomach, 35 to 40 cm from incisors. (Reproduced with permission from Sewrd JB, Khandheria BK, Oh JK, et al. Transesophageal echocardiography: technique, anatomic correlations, implementation, and clinical applications. *Mayo Clin Proc* 1988;63:654.).

tions in both nonoperative (Figs. 6-11 and 6-12) and intraoperative contexts.

This direct imaging technique provides real-time intraoperative assessment of myocardial and valvular performance, which has been a useful adjunct in the evaluation of patients during surgical procedures. Intraoperative TEE can be used to monitor changes in left ventricular contractility and to detect regional wall motion abnormalities in patients who

are at high risk of intraoperative myocardial ischemia or infarct. It has also been valuable in detecting mitral regurgitation after mitral valve repair or replacement, which can then be corrected before termination of the surgical procedure (30). TEE has been shown to be more sensitive and more specific than transthoracic echocardiography for the detection of vegetations in patients with suspected bacterial endocarditis (31,32) and in the evaluation of left atrial masses, such as tumors, thrombi, or vegetations (33).

Atrial thrombi occur most commonly in the atrial appendage and are a potential source of peripheral embolization. The left atrial appendage is more accessible for imaging by TEE than by transthoracic echocardiography, and, thus, TEE has found application in identifying or excluding a potential cardiac source of embolization (34). In patients with atrial fibrillation of uncertain duration, there is a possibility of the presence of fresh atrial thrombi, which could result in an embolic stroke following electrical cardioversion. Transesophageal echocardiography can be used to identify thrombi in the left atrium, including the left atrial appendage, and may lead to a modification of the use of precardioversion antithrombotic therapy if no thrombi are seen (35).

In selected patients with mitral stenosis, the desired therapy may be balloon valvuloplasty. Patients need to be evaluated for the presence of left atrial thrombi or mitral regurgitation before undergoing this procedure. In these patients TEE is used to optimally evaluate the mitral valve and the left atrium before attempting valvuloplasty, and it can also be used to assess results of the procedure (36).

In the evaluation of patients with congenital heart disease, TEE is particularly useful in examining the atrial septum (Fig. 6-13). Primum and secundum atrial septal defects are usually adequately detected by routine transthoracic echocardiography. However, sinus venosus atrial septal defects

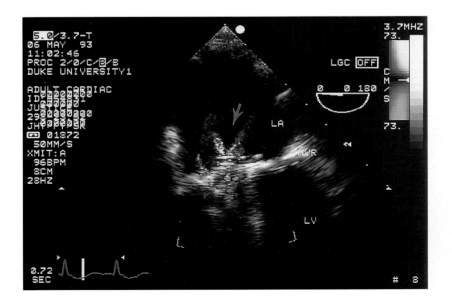

FIG 6-11. Transesophageal two-dimensional echocardiogram with color flow Doppler ultrasound demonstrates retrograde, turbulent blood flow (*arrow*) across an incompetent mechanical prosthetic mitral valve. LA, left atrium; MVR, plane of the prosthetic mitral valve;, LV, left ventricle. (see Color Plate 6)

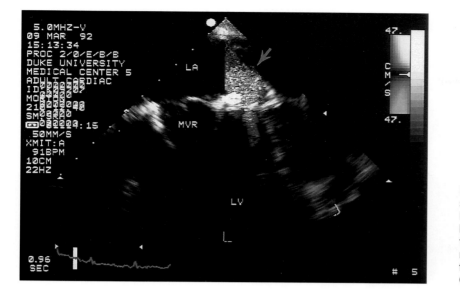

FIG 6-12. Transesophageal two-dimensional echocardiogram with color flow Doppler ultrasound shows retrograde, turbulent blood flow (*arrow*) around a porcine prosthetic mitral valve, due to perivalvular mitral regurgitation. LA, left atrium; MVR, prosthetic mitral valve; LV, left ventricle. (see Color Plate 7)

are frequently missed by transthoracic echocardiography. Because the transducer is located in proximity to the posterior aspect of the heart in TEE, this technique provides a better vantage point for visualizing sinus venosus atrial septal defects than does a transthoracic approach. By manipulating the transducer, the operator can make visible all four of the pulmonary veins, which offers an advantage in identifying anomalous pulmonary venous drainage.

Transesophageal echocardiography provides a bedside procedure that can be used for evaluation of patients with suspected aortic dissection. It can pinpoint entry and exit sites of the aneurysm as well evaluate aortic root dilatation and aortic insufficiency. In one study of 61 patients, TEE had a 97% sensitivity and 100% specificity for the diagnosis of aortic dissection, documented by angiography, surgery, or autopsy (37). A subsequent study of 110 patients has shown comparable sensitivity of 98%, but a lesser specificity of 86% in the diagnosis of aortic dissection. The lower specificity was due to false-positive findings caused by extensive atherosclerotic plaque or echo reverberations in an ectatic ascending aorta (38). The diagnosis of aortic dissection by TEE relies predominantly on the visualization of the intimal flap (Fig. 6-14) Another, less specific finding is the central displacement of intimal calcifications when there is thrombosis of the false lumen—color flow Doppler mapping can be used to differentiate the true from the false lumen. Over-

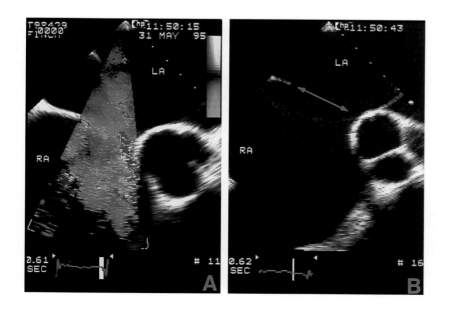

FIG 6-13. Transesophageal two-dimensional echocardiogram with color flow Doppler ultrasound (**A**) demonstrates left-to-right interatrial blood flow (blue representing flow away from the transducer) across an interatrial septal defect (**B**) (*arrow*). LA, left atrium; RA, right atrium. (see Color Plate 8)

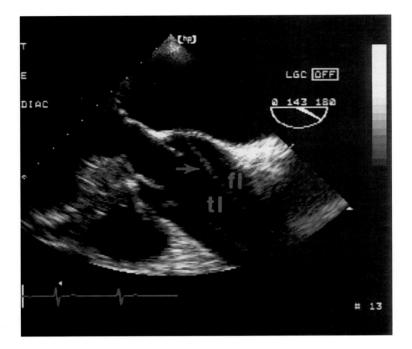

FIG 6-14. Transesophageal two-dimensional echocardiogram demonstrates a dissection of the ascending aorta. The intimal flap is identified (*arrow*) starting just above the leaflets of the aortic valve, creating a false lumen (fl) around the true lumen (tl) of the ascending aorta.

all, the advent of TEE has given us an additional useful technique in cardiovascular ultrasound to assess patients with known or suspected cardiovascular disease.

REFERENCES

1. Griffith JM, Henry WL. A sector scanner for real time two-dimensional echocardiography. *Circulation* 1974;49:1147–1152.
2. Bom N, Lancee CT, Van Zwieten G, Kloster FE, Roelandt J. Multiscan echocardiography. I. Technical description. *Circulation* 1973;48:1066–1074.
3. Kisslo JA, VonRamm OT, Thurstone FL. Dynamic cardiac imaging using a focused, phased-array ultrasound system. *Am J Med* 1977;63:61–68.
4. VonRamm OT, Thurstone FL. Cardiac imaging using a phased array ultrasound system. I. System design. *Circulation* 1976;53:258–262.
5. Henry WL, DeMaria A, Gramiak R, et al. Report of the American Society of Echocardiography Committee on Nomenclature and Standards in Two-dimensional Echocardiography. *Circulation* 1980;62:212–217.
6. Marcovitz PA, Armstrong WF. Accuracy of dobutamine stress echocardiography in detecting coronary artery disease. *Am J Cardiol* 1992;69:1269–1273.
7. Marwick T, D'Hondt A, Baudhuin T, et al. Optimal use of dobutamine stress for the detection and evaluation of coronary artery disease: combination with echocardiography or scintigraphy, or both? *J Am Coll Cardiol* 1993;22:159–167.
8. Krivokapich J, Child JS, Gerber RS, Lem V, Moser D. Prognostic usefulness of positive or negative exercise stress echocardiography for predicting coronary events in ensuing twelve months. *Am J Cardiol* 1993;71:646–651.
9. Ryan T, Armstrong WF, O'Donnell JA, Feigenbaum H. Risk stratification after acute myocardial infarction by means of exercise two dimensional echocardiography. *Am Heart J* 1987;114:1305–1316.
10. Lane RT, Sawada SG, Segar DS, et al. Dobutamine stress echocardiography for assessment of cardiac risk before noncardiac surgery. *Am J Cardiol* 1991;68:976–977.
11. Valdes-Cruz LM, Sahn DJ. Ultrasonic contrast studies for the detection of cardiac shunts. *J Am Coll Cardiol* 1984;3:978–985.
12. Valdes-Cruz LM, Pieroni DR, Roland JMA, Shematek JP. Recognition of residual postoperative shunts by contrast echocardiographic techniques. *Circulation* 1977;55:148–152.
13. Weyman AE, Wann LS, Caldwell RL, Hurwitz RA, Dillon JC, Feigenbaum H. Negative contrast echocardiography: a new method for detecting left-to-right shunts. *Circulation* 1979;59:498–505.
14. Lieppe W, Behar VS, Scallion R, Kisslo JA. Detection of tricuspid regurgitation with two-dimensional echocardiography and peripheral vein injections. *Circulation* 1978;57:128–132.
15. Meltzer RS, Van Hoogenhuyze D, Serruys PW, Haalebos MMP, Hugenholtz PG, Roelandt J. Diagnosis of tricuspid regurgitation by contrast echocardiography. *Circulation* 1981;63:1093–1099.
16. Feinstein SB, Lang RM, Dick C, et al. Contrast echocardiography during coronary arteriography in humans: perfusion and anatomic studies. *J Am Coll Cardiol* 1988;11:59–65.
17. Reisner SA, Ong LS, Lichtenberg GS, et al. Myocardial perfusion imaging by contrast echocardiography with use of intracoronary sonicated albumin in humans. *J Am Coll Cardiol* 1989;14:660–665.
18. Armstrong WF, Gage SW. Evaluation of reperfusion hyperemia with myocardial contrast echocardiography. *J Am Soc Echocardiogr* 1988;1:322–332.
19. Vandenberg BF. Myocardial perfusion and contrast echocardiography: review and new perspectives. *Echocardiography* 1991;8:65–75.
20. Meltzer RS, Serruys PW, McGhie J, Verbaan N, Roelandt J. Pulmonary wedge injections yielding left-side echocardiographic contrast. *Br Heart J* 1980;44:390–394.
21. Meltzer RS, Sartorius OEH, Lancee CT, et al. Transmission of ultrasonic contrast through the lungs. *Ultrasound Med Biol* 1981;7:377–384.
22. Ten Cate FJ, Feinstein S, Zwehl W, et al. Two-dimensional contrast echocardiography. II. Transpulmonary studies. *J Am Coll Cardiol* 1984;3:21–27.
23. Shapiro JR, Reisner SA, Meltzer RS. Prospects for transpulmonary contrast echocardiography. *J Am Coll Cardiol* 1989;13:1629–1630.
24. Shapiro JR, Reisner SA, Lichtenberg GS, Meltzer RS. Intravenous contrast echocardiography with use of sonicated albumin in humans: systolic disappearance of left ventricular contrast after transpulmonary transmission. *J Am Coll Cardiol* 1990;16:1603–1607.
25. Porter TR, Xie F. Visually discernible myocardial echocardiographic contrast after intravenous injection of sonicated dextrose albumin microbubbles containing high molecular weight, less soluble gases. *J Am Coll Cardiol* 1995;25:509–515.
26. Perry GJ, Nanda NC. Recent advances in color Doppler evaluation of valvular regurgitation. *Echocardiography* 1987;4:503–513.

27. Suzuki Y, Kambara H, Kadota K, et al. Detection and evaluation of tricuspid regurgitation using a real-time, two-dimensional, color-coded, Doppler flow imaging system: comparison with contrast two-dimensional echocardiography and right ventriculography. *Am J Cardiol* 1986;57:811–815.

28. Fisher EA, Stahl JA, Budd JH, Goldman ME. Transesophageal echocardiography: procedures and clinical application. *J Am Coll Cardiol* 1991;18:1333–1348.

29. Fleischer DE, Goldstein SA. Transesophageal echocardiography: What the gastroenterologist thinks the cardiologist should know about endoscopy. *J Am Soc Echocardiogr* 1990;3:428–434.

30. Stewart WJ, Salcedo EE, Cosgrove DM. The value of echocardiography in mitral valve repair. *Cleve Clin J Med* 1991;58:177–183.

31. Erbel R, Rohmann S, Drexler M, et al. Improved diagnostic value of echocardiography in patients with infective endocarditis by transesophageal approach: a prospective study. *Eur Heart J* 1988;9:43–53.

32. Birmingham GD, Rahko PS, Ballantyne F III. Improved detection of infective endocarditis with transesophageal echocardiography. *Am Heart J* 1992;123:774–781.

33. Alam M, Sun I. Transesophageal echocardiographic evaluation of left atrial mass lesions. *J Am Soc Echocardiogr* 1991;4:323–330.

34. Pearson AC, Labovitz AJ, Tatineni S, Gomez CR. Superiority of transesophageal echocardiography in detecting cardiac source of embolism in patients with cerebral ischemia of uncertain etiology. *J Am Coll Cardiol* 1991;17:66–72.

35. Grimm RA, Stewart WJ, Black IW, Thomas JD, Klein AL. Should all patients undergo transesophageal echocardiography before electrical cardioversion of atrial fibrillation? *J Am Coll Cardiol* 1994;23:533–541.

36. Chan KL, Marquis JF, Ascah C, Morton B, Baird M. Role of transesophageal echocardiography in percutaneous balloon mitral valvuloplasty. *Echocardiography* 1990;7:115–123.

37. Ballal RS, Nanda NC, Gatewood R, et al. Usefulness of transesophageal echocardiography in assessment of aortic dissection. *Circulation* 1991;84:1903–1914.

38. Nienaber CA, von Kodolitsch Y, Nicolas V, et al. The diagnosis of thoracic aortic dissection by noninvasive imaging procedures. *N Engl J Med* 1993;328:1–9.

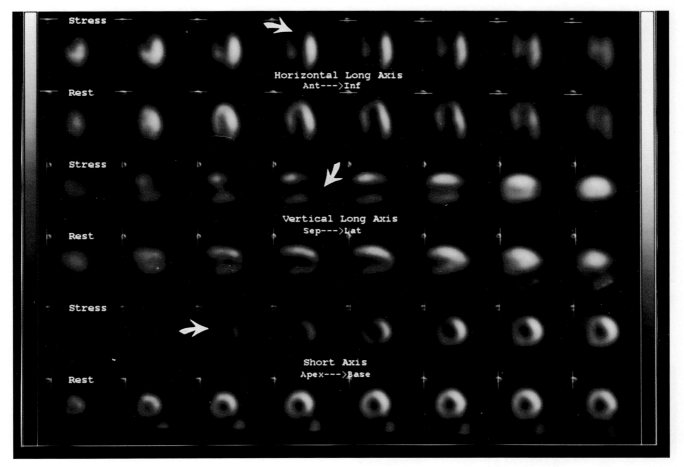

Color Plate 1. ^{99m}Tc Sestamibi stress (rows 1, 3, and 5) and Tl-201 resting (rows 2, 4, and 6) myocardial perfusion images in a 77-year-old man with a 1-month history of recurring exertional chest pain. At exercise, he had chest pain, frequent ventricular ectopy, and ST segment depression. The resting Tl-201 study is normal, with no perfusion defects. At stress, a perfusion defect (*arrows*) is seen in the anterior wall, the anteroseptum, the anteroapex, and the inferoapex. These findings are suggestive of myocardial ischemia in the distribution of the left anterior descending coronary artery. (see Fig. 5-1, p. 79)

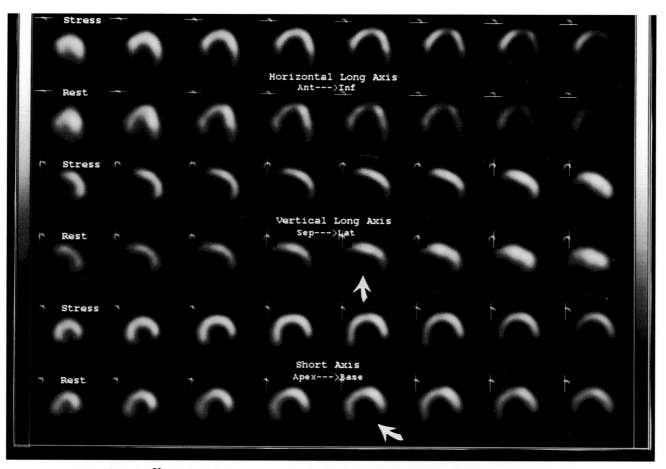

Color Plate 2. ^{99m}Tc Sestamibi stress (rows 1, 3, and 5) and Tl-201 resting (rows 2, 4, and 6) myocardial perfusion images in a 70-year-old man with a history of CAD, previous myocardial infarction, and coronary artery bypass graft surgery. At exercise, he exceeded his target heart rate without chest pain or EKG changes. A fixed perfusion defect is seen at rest (*arrows*) that is unchanged at stress in the inferior, posterobasal, and aposterolateral walls and the inferoapex. This defect is suggestive of previous infarct. There is no evidence for myocardial ischemia. (see Fig. 5-2, p. 80)

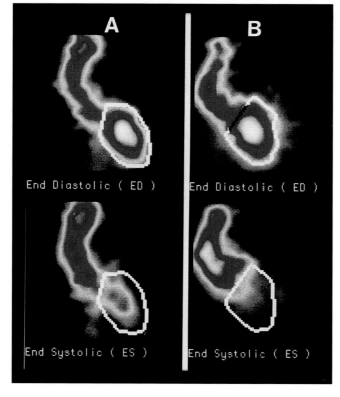

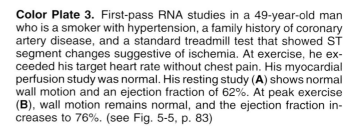

Color Plate 3. First-pass RNA studies in a 49-year-old man who is a smoker with hypertension, a family history of coronary artery disease, and a standard treadmill test that showed ST segment changes suggestive of ischemia. At exercise, he exceeded his target heart rate without chest pain. His myocardial perfusion study was normal. His resting study (**A**) shows normal wall motion and an ejection fraction of 62%. At peak exercise (**B**), wall motion remains normal, and the ejection fraction increases to 76%. (see Fig. 5-5, p. 83)

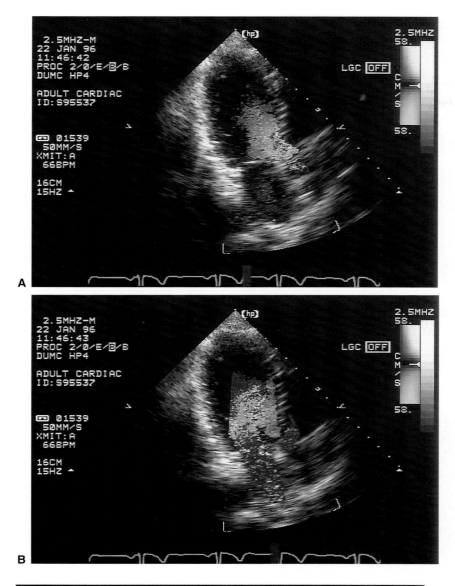

A

B

Color Plate 4. Transthoracic two-dimensional echocardiogram in the apical long-axis view with color flow Doppler ultrasound demonstrates (**A**) normal blood flow through the left ventricular outflow tract during ventricular systole (blue representing flow away from the transducer) and (**B**) normal blood flow from the left atrium across the mitral valve into the left ventricle during diastole (red representing flow toward the transducer). (see Fig. 6-8, p. 97)

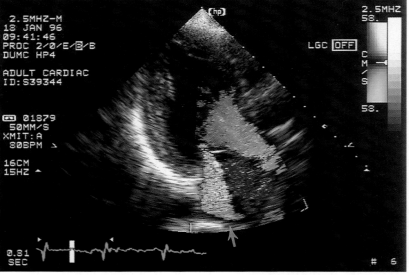

Color Plate 5. Transthoracic two-dimensional echocardiogram in an apical long-axis view with color flow Doppler ultrasound demonstrates retrograde, turbulent blood flow (arrow) across a native mitral valve due to mitral regurgitation. (see Fig. 6-9, p. 97)

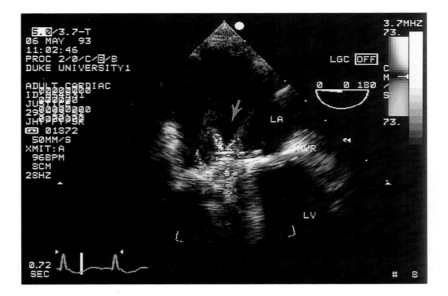

Color Plate 6. Transesophageal two-dimensional echocardiogram with color flow Doppler ultrasound demonstrates retrograde, turbulent blood flow (*arrow*) across an incompetent mechanical prosthetic mitral valve. LA, left atrium; MVR, plane of the prosthetic mitral valve;, LV, left ventricle. (see Fig. 6-11, p. 98)

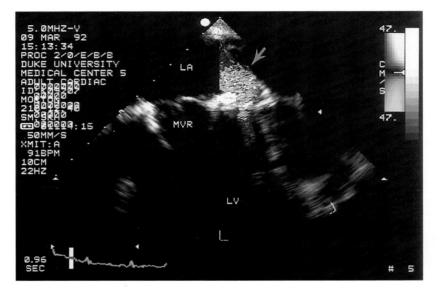

Color Plate 7. Transesophageal two-dimensional echocardiogram with color flow Doppler ultrasound shows retrograde, turbulent blood flow (*arrow*) around a porcine prosthetic mitral valve, due to perivalvular mitral regurgitation. LA, left atrium; MVR, prosthetic mitral valve; LV, left ventricle. (see Fig. 6-12, p. 99)

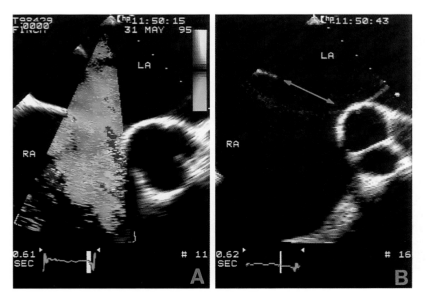

Color Plate 8. Transesophageal two-dimensional echocardiogram with color flow Doppler ultrasound (**A**) demonstrates left-to-right interatrial blood flow (blue representing flow away from the transducer) across an interatrial septal defect (**B**) (*arrow*). LA, left atrium; RA, right atrium. (see Fig. 6-13, p. 99)

Essentials of Cardiac Imaging,
James T. T. Chen,
Lippincott–Raven Publishers, Philadelphia © 1998.

CHAPTER 7

Cardiovascular Hemodynamics

James T. T. Chen

In the interpretation of cardiac images, hemodynamic data are just as important as clinical manifestations of a disease. In patients with pure mitral stenosis, for example, the presence of well-formed Kerley's B lines on the radiograph indicates a 95% probability of critical mitral stenosis with a valve area <1.3 cm^2 (1–4).

BASIC FUNCTION OF THE CIRCULATORY SYSTEM

The basic function of the circulatory system is to deliver oxygen and nutrients to, and to remove metabolic wastes from, cells throughout the body. Because various organ systems have unequal needs for blood supply and because these needs are higher during activity than at rest, a complex regulatory system is in continuous operation to adjust and distribute the cardiac output from one instant to the next.

CARDIAC OUTPUT

The cardiac output can be augmented by increasing either the heart rate or the ventricular stroke volume. The heart rate is controlled by the autonomic nervous system. Increased rate is effected by a decrease in vagal inhibition, by sympathetic stimulation of the sinoatrial pacemaker, or both. The ventricular stroke volume is a function of myocardial responsiveness, which is primarily related to the presystolic fiber length of the myocardial cells—the essence of the well-known Starling's law of the heart (5). Fiber length is determined by diastolic volume, which is proportional to venous return and filling pressure. Other factors that can increase stroke volume by augmenting myocardial contractility include hormones (epinephrine and norepinephrine) and sympathetic stimulation.

Department of Radiology, Duke University School of Medicine, Durham, North Carolina 27710, U.S.A.

REGULATION OF REGIONAL BLOOD FLOW

Regulation of regional blood flow is accomplished by adjusting the difference between the arterial and venous pressures in vessels supplying an organ and by changing the vascular resistance of that organ. Most of the vascular resistance is located at the level of small arteries and arterioles. Therefore, arteriolar constriction or relaxation is of prime importance in the regulation of regional blood flow. Changes in the capillaries and veins may at times play a role in such function. Poiseuille's formula for fluid flow in rigid tubing states:

$$\text{Flow} = \frac{\text{pressure difference} \times \text{radius}^4 \times \pi}{\text{tube length} \times \text{fluid viscosity} \times 8}$$

Reducing the radius of a vessel by one half is accompanied by a 16-fold decrease in flow or a 16-fold increase in pressure (resistance). Assuming that other factors are constant, changing the caliber of the tube has the most profound effect on the flow and resistance of the conducting system. In attempting to apply this equation to the human circulation, one must realize that our cardiovascular system is infinitely more complex than a rigid tube and that the blood vessel is not rigid nor is the blood flow streamlined.

A second useful concept of fluid dynamics relates to the geometry of the vessel and the mechanical characteristics of the vessel wall. According to the law of Laplace, the wall tension of a blood vessel is greater when the radius of the vessel is greater or when the wall is thinner. Because the wall of a vein is thinner and the radius is greater than for its arterial counterpart, the wall tension in a vein is greater than that in an artery at the same pressure. The degree of stretching of the vessel wall by wall tension depends on the elastic stiffness of the wall.

The caliber, the wall thickness, and the distensibility of a blood vessel undergo constant phasic changes owing to

TABLE 7-1. *Normal values of pressures and oxygen data*

Site	Pressures (mm Hg)	Oxygen data % Saturation	Oxygen data Content (volume %)
Right atrium	$-2-+5^a$	—	—
Right ventricle	$16-30/0-6^b$	—	—
Pulmonary artery	$16-30/5-15$	75	15
	$7-20^a$	—	—
Pulmonary artery wedge	$4-12^a$	97	19
Left atrium	$4-12^a$	97	19
Left ventricle	$90-140/4-12^b$	—	—
Aorta	$90-140/60-90$	—	—
	$70-105^a$	—	—

[a] Number represents the mean.
[b] Number represents end-diastolic pressure.

cyclic constriction and relaxation of the smooth muscle of the vessel. These changes are subject to multiple influences, the most important of which are neural, hormonal, and chemical factors. The neural influences are mediated by reflexes from the carotid sinus and the aortic stretch receptors to the brain and from the brain to the peripheral vasculature by way of the autonomic nervous system. The hormonal influences are mediated by transmitter substances at the nerve endings (i.e., norepinephrine and acetylcholine). These substances have far-reaching effects, some of which are felt even at the true capillary level (where there is no innervation). The chemical influences—hypoxia and acidosis—have different effects on the systemic vessels than on the pulmonary vessels. The systemic vessels respond to hypoxia or acidosis with vasodilatation, whereas the pulmonary vessels respond with vasoconstriction (6).

NORMAL VALUES

Normal Pressures

The pressure in the systemic arteries is five to six times higher than that in the pulmonary arteries, even though the blood flow in each system is practically equal (6) (Table 7-1). The pressure tracings from the right atrium, left atrium, and pulmonary artery wedge position have the same general characteristics. Only small variations in the phasic features are evident. Normally there are prominent A and V waves representing atrial contraction and vigorous venous inflow, respectively. The small C wave following the A wave is produced by the impact of the contracting ventricle with

bulging of the atrioventricular valve into the atrium. As the ventricle continues to contract, the atrial pressure drops temporarily, creating the X descent. When the atrium empties its contents into the ventricle, the pressure drops again, giving rise to the Y descent (Fig. 7-1). The wedge pressure is obtained through an end-hole catheter wedged in a small pulmonary artery (which is thus temporarily obstructed). The mean left atrial pressure is ~4 to 5 mm Hg higher than that in the right atrium.

The pressure tracings from the ventricles are similar, although the level of the peak systolic pressure in the left ventricle is five to six times higher than that in the right. The pressure tracings of the pulmonary artery and the aorta are also similar, except that the pressures are much higher in the aorta (Fig. 7-2).

Normal Oxygen Values

The oxygen values in the pulmonary artery are approximately 15 volume % and 75% saturation. The values in the right atrium are more variable. The contributions of blood from different organs begin to mix in the right atrium and continue to do so more completely through the right ventricle and the pulmonary artery. Therefore, in flow or shunt calculations, samples of mixed venous blood are always taken from the pulmonary artery. An oxygen step-up from the superior vena cava to the right atrium greater than 1.9 volume % is indicative of an atrial septal defect. Likewise, an oxygen step-up in excess of 0.9 and 0.5 volume % at the right ven-

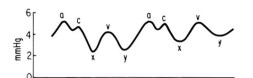

FIG 7-1. Normal right atrial pressure tracing.

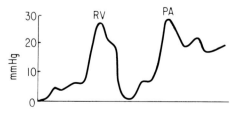

FIG 7-2. Normal pressure tracing from the right ventricle (RV) to the pulmonary artery (PA).

TABLE 7-2. *Normal values of blood flow data*

Term	Normal range
AV O$_2$ diff.	2–5 volume % (indicates O$_2$ extraction)
Fick CO	2.5–8.0 L/min (depending on body size)
Fick CI	2.6–5.0 L/min/m^2 (CO/body surface area)
CO (dye)	2.5–8.0 (dye dilution method)

AV O$_2$ diff., arteriovenous oxygen difference; CO, cardiac output; CI, cardiac index.

tricular and pulmonary arterial levels suggests a ventricular septal defect; a similar step-up in the pulmonary artery alone suggests patent ductus arteriosus (3). The oxygen content in the pulmonary wedge position and in the left side of the heart is ~19 volume % or 97% saturation. Notable systemic arterial desaturation is suggestive of a right-to-left shunt (Table 7-1).

According to Fick, the cardiac output (CO) may be calculated from the quantity of oxygen consumed per minute and the arteriovenous oxygen difference (the difference in oxygen concentration in the blood before entering and after leaving the lungs) (3):

$$CO = \frac{O_2 \text{ consumption}}{\text{arteriovenous } O_2 \text{ difference}}$$

The arteriovenous oxygen difference widens when the blood supply decreases or the oxygen demand increases, or both (Table 7-2).

Cardiac Valves

The atrioventricular valves are larger than the semilunar valves. Valve areas are calculated in terms of square centimeters using the Gorlin formula (4). The basic determinants of valve area are the pressure gradient and flow across the valve. In general, the valve area is proportional to the flow and inversely proportional to the gradient (Table 7-3).

TABLE 7-3. *Normal and abnormal valve areas*

Valve	Normal valve area (cm^2)	Stenotic valve area (cm^2)
Aortic	2.5–3.5	Mild: >0.7 Moderate: 0.5–0.7 Severe: <0.5
Pulmonary	2.5–3.5	Mild: >0.7 Moderate: 0.5–0.7 Severe: <0.5
Mitral	4.0–6.0	Mild: 1.7–2.5 Moderate: 1.3–1.6 Severe: <1.3
Tricuspid	4.0–6.0	Mild: 1.7–2.5 Moderate: 1.3–1.6 Severe: <1.3

HEMODYNAMIC AND RADIOGRAPHIC CORRELATION

Central Venous System and Right Atrium

The venae cavae and the right atrium are essentially in free communication, and the pressures in the two organs are normally identical. The mean pressure is ~3 mm Hg, although the atrial contracting wave, the A wave, can be as high as 5 mm Hg. The atrial filling wave, the V wave, falls somewhere between these two values. In the context of superior vena cava syndrome, the cava and its large tributary, the azygos vein, are markedly dilated with increased pressure in contrast to the normal intracardiac pressures. In other words, the stenosis is extracardiac, and the gradient is between the cava and the right atrium.

In tricuspid stenosis, the right atrium is dilated and the pressure in the chamber is elevated. The pressure increase is most conspicuous during atrial contraction, namely, during ventricular diastole. At the same time, vigorous pulsations of the enlarged right atrium and the venae cavae are usually

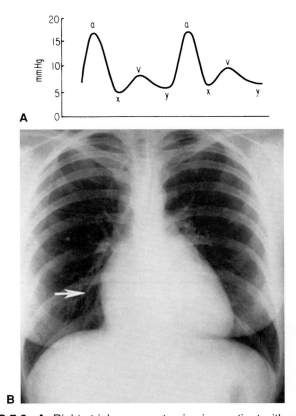

FIG 7-3. A: Right atrial pressure tracing in a patient with severe tricuspid stenosis. Note the giant a waves. **B:** Patient with rheumatic tricuspid and mitral stenosis. Note enlargement of right atrium (*arrow*) and decreased pulmonary vascularity (small size of all pulmonary vessels). The markedly reduced pulmonary blood flow owing to inflow obstruction (tricuspid stenosis) has minimized the cephalad flow pattern caused by outflow obstruction (mitral stenosis).

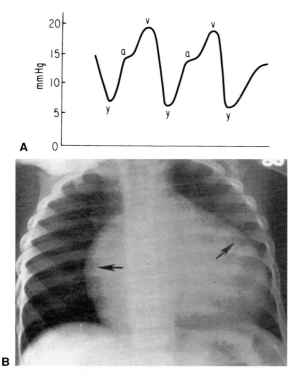

FIG 7-4. A: Right atrial pressure tracing in a patient with severe tricuspid insufficiency. Note the giant V waves with abolishment of the X descents. This is the so-called ventricularization of the atrial pressure tracing. **B:** A patient with severe valvular pulmonary stenosis, right ventricular failure, and tricuspid insufficiency. Note marked dilatation of both the right ventricle (*oblique arrow*) and the right atrium (*horizontal arrow*). Decreased pulmonary blood flow is due to a right-to-left shunt across the foramen ovale.

seen on the fluoroscopic screen. Furthermore, in the absence of atrial fibrillation, a giant A wave may be transmitted both into the neck and into the liver and can be detected by physical examination (Fig. 7-3).

In tricuspid insufficiency, both the right atrium and the right ventricle are enlarged owing to volume overload. The reactive increase in right ventricular contractility produces a tall V wave in the right atrial pressure curve. In turn, the big V wave may be visible over the neck veins and palpable over the liver during ventricular systole. By the same hemodynamic effect, vigorous systolic expansion of both the right atrium and the caval system may be found under the fluoroscope. In extreme cases, the right atrial tracing may be "ventricularized" owing to replacement of the negative X wave by the giant V wave (Fig. 7-4).

Right Ventricle and Pulmonary Valve

The right ventricular response to tricuspid insufficiency has been discussed previously. According to Starling's law of the heart, within limits, the more the cardiac muscle is stretched by increased pressure or volume, the greater the

contractility of the myocardium. Therefore, in the early stages of pulmonary stenosis, the systolic pressure in the right ventricle may be at the systemic level with the end-diastolic pressure remaining normal at 5 mm Hg (Fig. 7-5). The ventricle may be compensated but operating at its upper limits of cardiac reserve at rest. Radiographic signs indicate only right ventricular hypertrophy without dilatation. Any further increase in volume or pressure to that chamber (e.g., by exercise) will exceed its limits of compensatory capacity and lead to congestive heart failure. In this situation both the end-diastolic volume and end-diastolic pressure increase to an abnormal level. On radiography, dilatation of the right ventricle in addition to hypertrophy will be evident. On fluoroscopy, the right ventricle usually shows decreased contractility. Further progression of the disease may induce functional tricuspid insufficiency (Fig. 7-4B).

Pulmonary Vascular Bed

The pulmonary artery pressure recording is easily obtained during pulmonary arteriography. These values are extremely useful. When the pulmonary artery mean pressure is >40 mm Hg, a pulmonary arteriogram is contraindicated. Functional pulmonary stenosis with a gradient ≤20 mm Hg is sometimes found in patients with large left-to-right shunts. Such pressure gradients across normal pulmonary valves usually disappear after closure of the shunts.

In precapillary pulmonary hypertension, the pulmonary arterial pressure is elevated, but the pulmonary artery wedge and venous pressures remain normal. Radiographic signs of precapillary pulmonary hypertension include a centralized flow pattern and right-sided chamber enlargement. If hypertension is severe, particularly in the acute phase, engorgement of the venae cavae and azygos vein may also be apparent (Fig. 7-6).

In pulmonary insufficiency, the pulmonary arterial pressure increases in systole and decreases in diastole. The wide pulse pressure in the pulmonary circulation is similar to that observed in the systemic circulation with aortic insufficiency. Radiologic signs of pulmonary insufficiency are increased pulsation of the right ventricle and central pulmonary arteries and a centralized flow pattern. The pulsations of the pulmonary arteries are more dynamic than the smaller and more sustained pulsations seen in pulmonary arterial hypertension.

Left-sided Cardiac Chambers and Aorta

Left atrial pressure can be measured by a transseptal catheter guided from the right atrium through the atrial septum into the left atrium. The pressure curve of the left atrium is identical to that obtained from the pulmonary artery wedge position. The curve consists of the A wave followed by the X descent and the V wave followed by the Y descent. The A and V waves are produced by atrial contraction and the

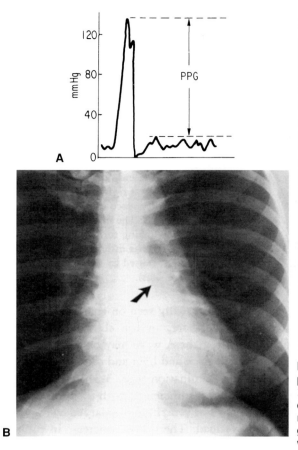

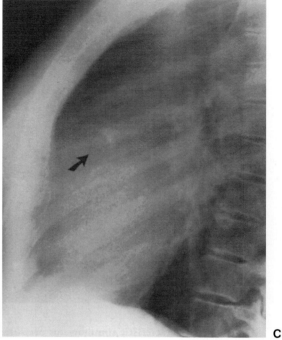

FIG 7-5. **A:** Pressure tracings of severe valvular pulmonary stenosis. The peak-to-peak gradient is >100 mm Hg. However, the right ventricle is still compensated and the end-diastolic pressure remains within normal limits. PPG, peak pulmonary gradient. **B:** Posteroanterior radiograph of a patient with severe pulmonary stenosis. Calcium is noted in the pulmonary valve (*arrow*). **C:** Lateral view of the patient shown in B. The arrow indicates the calcified valve.

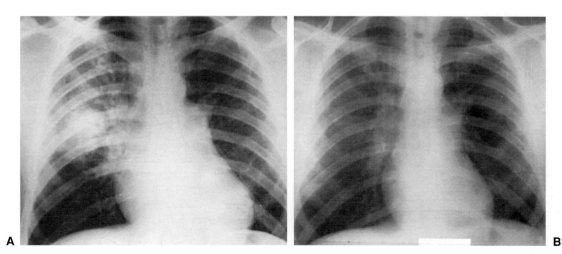

FIG 7-6. Radiograph of a 38-year-old man with chronic cor pulmonale due to recurrent thromboembolic disease. On the day before the radiograph was taken (**A**), the patient had another episode of pulmonary embolism. Note the enlarged right ventricle, right atrium, and azygos vein. The pulmonary trunk is huge, and there is a centralized pulmonary blood flow pattern. The fluffy density in the right lung represents an incomplete pulmonary infarct. A second radiograph (**B**) shows complete resolution of the fluffy density in the right lung and other signs of improvement.

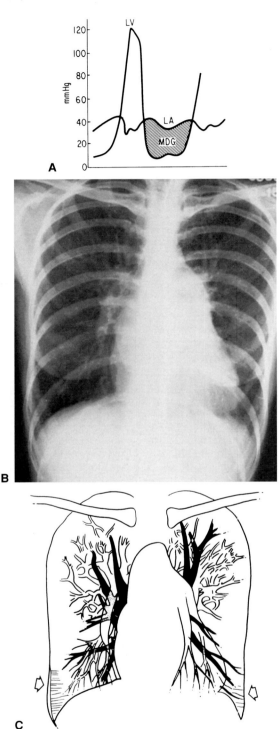

A

B

C

FIG 7-7. A: Characteristic simultaneous pressure tracings of the left ventricle (LV) and the left atrium (LA) in patients with mitral stenosis. Note the high mitral diastolic gradient (MDG) in the shaded area. In another patient with critical mitral stenosis the radiograph (**B**) and accompanying diagram (**C**) show a striking cephalic pulmonary blood flow pattern and Kerley's B lines (*arrows*).

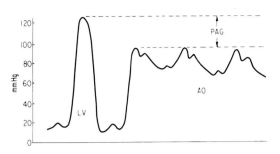

FIG 7-8. Characteristic pressure curve in patients with aortic valve stenosis. AO, aorta; LV, left ventricle; PAG, peak aortic gradient.

inflow of blood, respectively. Although mitral stenosis tends to produce a large A wave and mitral insufficiency tends to produce a large V wave, these signs may be misleading in patients with less severe conditions. The normal left atrial mean pressure is ~5 mm Hg, with an A wave of ~8 to 10 mm Hg and a V wave somewhere between these values. In severe mitral stenosis, the left atrial mean pressure can be ≥30 mm Hg, forming a high gradient with the left ventricle in diastole (Fig. 7-7A). In severe mitral insufficiency, the V wave can become systemic in magnitude. Both conditions may lead to congestive heart failure with pulmonary edema.

Both the hemodynamic findings and the radiographic signs of mitral stenosis reflect the underlying pathophysiology of left atrial failure. For example, both Kerley's lines and cephalization of the pulmonary vasculature are signs of severe mitral stenosis (Fig. 7-7B,C). They also indicate major pulmonary hypertension, with pulmonary venous mean pressure >20 mm Hg and pulmonary arterial mean pressure >30 mm Hg. The mitral valve area under these circumstances is usually <1.3 cm^2 (1).

In aortic stenosis, the left ventricle is burdened with high intracavitary pressure (Fig. 7-8). The natural compensatory mechanism induces left ventricular hypertrophy with increased contractility. The walls of the left ventricle and the papillary muscles are markedly enlarged at the expense of the lumen. The radiographic signs are increased convexity of the left ventricular contour, a positive Hoffman-Rigler sign (7), normal pulmonary vascularity, and a cardiothoracic ratio <0.5 (Seningen et al., unpublished observations) (see **Fig. 2-11A**).

After decompensation of the heart, however, both the volume and the pressure are elevated in diastole. Unlike mitral insufficiency or aortic insufficiency, the increased diastolic pressure in aortic stenosis is always indicative of cardiac failure stemming from pressure overload. By this time, radiographic signs of left ventricular dilatation (cardiothoracic ratio >0.5) and pulmonary edema are usually present (Seningen et al., unpublished observations) (see **Fig. 2-11B,C**).

In aortic insufficiency, both the left ventricle and the aorta are volume-overloaded. Although the left ventricular end-diastolic pressure is elevated, the ventricle remains effective as a pump. The pulse pressures are typically widened, partic-

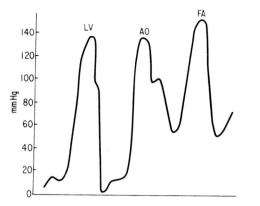

FIG 7-9. Characteristic pressure curve of severe aortic insufficiency before left ventricular failure. Note the markedly widened pulse pressure (systolic pressure − diastolic pressure), more striking in the femoral artery (FA) than in the aorta (AO). LV, left ventricle.

ularly in peripheral arteries (Fig. 7-9). After the onset of left ventricular failure, the end-diastolic pressure rises notably as the ejection fraction declines. The radiographic signs of aortic insufficiency before heart failure are marked cardiomegaly with normal pulmonary vascularity (see **Fig. 2-9A**) and increased pulsation of the left ventricle and the aorta (see **Fig. 2-25**). Following the onset of heart failure, the radiographic manifestations are a further increase in cardiac size, pulmonary edema, and decreased left ventricular contractility (see **Fig. 2-9B**).

LEFT VENTRICULAR VOLUME

During angiocardiography, the end-systolic and end-diastolic volumes of the opacified left ventricle can be determined planimetrically in two planes. The left ventricular shadow in either phase of the cardiac cycle is treated as an ellipsoid, and its surface area is measured with correction for magnification. In the meantime, the thickness of the left ventricular walls and the left ventricular mass can also be determined in diastole. For more accurate measurements of the volume, maintenance of normal sinus rhythm is essential during angiography (Table 7-4).

TABLE 7-4. Angiographic left ventricular volume data

	Calculated	Corrected	Normal
End-diastolic volume	ml	ml/m^2	≦94
End-systolic volume	ml	ml/m^2	≦40
LV stroke volume[a]	ml	ml/m^2	
Ejection fraction	%		≧60%
Angiographic CO[b]	L/min	L/min/m^2	
Wall thickness	cm		≦1.2
LV mass/BSA		gm/m^2	111

[a] LV stroke volume = end-diastolic volume − end-systolic volume.

[b] Cardiac output = LV stroke volume × heart rate.

BSA, body surface area; CO, cardiac output; LV, left ventricle.

COMMON EXPRESSIONS USED FOR SHUNTS

Ratio

A shunt can be expressed in terms of the ratio between the pulmonary and the systemic blood flows. For example, a 2 : 1 left-to-right shunt simply means that the pulmonary blood flow (PBF) is twice the systemic blood flow (SBF). A 4 : 1 right-to-left shunt means that the SBF is four times the PBF (Table 7-5).

Percentage

A shunt can also be expressed in terms of the percentage of either the pulmonary or the systemic flow, whichever is greater. A 50% left-to-right shunt means that the systemic-to-pulmonary shunt flow amounts to 50% of the PBF. A 75% right-to-left shunt means that the pulmonary-to-systemic shunt flow amounts to 75% of the SBF. For example, when the absolute value of the PBF is 12 L per minute and that of the SBF is only 6 L per minute, the patient may be said to have a 2 : 1 left-to-right shunt. Alternatively, he or she may be said to have a 12 − 6 = 6 L per minute left-to-right shunt, namely, a 6/12, or 50% left-to-right shunt. If the PBF is 18 L per minute and the SBF is 6 L per minute, the left-to-right shunt may be said to be either a 3 : 1 shunt or a (18 − 6)/18 = 67% shunt (Table 7-5).

Pulmonary Resistance

Facing torrential flow, the pulmonary arterioles usually constrict as a natural defense mechanism against the development of congestive heart failure. Prolonged pulmonary vascular spasm is accompanied by medial hypertrophy and intimal fibrosis of the arteries. Such chronic adjustments may lead to high pulmonary vascular resistance with reversing of the direction of the shunt. The degree of pulmonary

TABLE 7-5. Shunts

Direction
  Left to right
  Right to left
  Bidirectional
Ratio: pulmonary blood flow (PBF) to systemic blood flow (SBF)
  Normal: 1.0
  Below normal (right-to-left shunt): <1.0
  Above normal (left-to-right shunt): >1.0
    Mild: 1.1–1.5
    Moderate: 1.6–2.0
    Severe: >2.0
Percentage

$$\% \text{ Left-to-right shunt} = \frac{PBF - SBF}{PBF}$$

$$\% \text{ Right-to-left shunt} = \frac{SBF - PBF}{SBF}$$

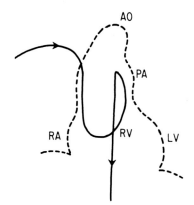

FIG 7-10. Catheter position in patients with patent ductus arteriosus. The catheter enters the right side of the heart through the superior vena cava in a normal manner. Reaching the pulmonary artery (PA), the catheter turns sharply downward into the descending aorta. AO, aorta; LV, left ventricle; RA, right atrium; RV, right ventricle.

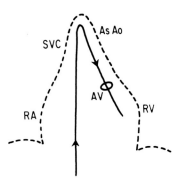

FIG 7-11. Arterial catheter position in patients with congenitally corrected (L-loop) transposition of great arteries. The retrograde aortic catheter moves upward from the descending aorta into the aortic arch. It then turns sharply to the left and downward into the ascending aorta (As Ao), which is connected to the right ventricle (RV). The right ventricle is left-sided, forming a bulge on the border of the left side of the heart. AV, aortic valve; RA, right atrium; SVC, superior vena cava.

resistance is expressed in terms of the ratio of pulmonary resistance to systemic resistance (Rp/Rs). When the ratio is >0.5, surgical closure of the shunt is usually considered risky and is contraindicated (Table 7-6).

CATHETER POSITIONS

Abnormal catheter positions in conjunction with hemodynamics and oxygen data may suggest certain diagnoses and exclude others. Both the cardiologist and the radiologist should be able to use such information as a guide for modifying or simplifying their diagnostic procedures, which may already be in progress. For example, if a forward dye curve shows only a left-to-right shunt and the venous catheter en-

ters the descending aorta from the pulmonary artery, the diagnosis of a patent ductus arteriosus is established (Fig. 7-10). What is needed to exclude other extracardiac and intracardiac left-to-right shunts is only two more dye curves: one from the pulmonary artery to the right atrium to rule out shunts at the atrial level and the other from the left ventricle to the right ventricle to rule out those at the ventricular level.

In congenitally corrected (L-loop) transposition of the great arteries, in the posteroanterior projection the retrograde aortic catheter courses to the left and inferiorly instead of to the right and inferiorly (Fig. 7-11). The venous catheter in this situation also suggests the diagnosis. Note the extreme medial position of the catheter in the region of the pulmonary

TABLE 7-6. *Pulmonary resistance*

I. Total pulmonary resistance (mm Hg/L/min or Wood units) $= \dfrac{(PA\ mean)}{CO}$
   A. Normal: 0–5
   B. Mild increase: 6–9
   C. Moderate or severe increase: >10
II. Rp = Pulmonary vascular resistance (Wood units) $= \dfrac{(PA\ mean\ -\ LA\ mean)}{CO}$
   A. Normal: 1–3
   B. Mild increase: 3–5
   C. Moderate or severe increase: >5
III. Rs = Systemic resistance (Wood units) $= \dfrac{(AO\ mean)}{CO}$
IV. $\dfrac{Rp}{Rs}$ = Resistance ratio
   A. Normal: 0.1
   B. Critical: >0.5

AO, aorta; CO, cardiac output; LA, left atrium; PA, pulmonary artery.

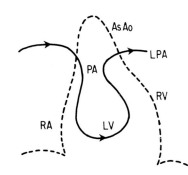

FIG 7-12. Venous catheter position in patients with congenitally corrected (L-loop) transposition of the great arteries. The catheter enters the right atrium (RA) through the superior vena cava. From the right atrium it passes through the mitral valve into the left ventricle (LV), all of which are right-sided. The left ventricle gives rise to the pulmonary artery (PA), which is abnormally posterior and medial in position. The catheter then turns outward into the left pulmonary artery (LPA). As Ao, ascending aorta; RV, right ventricle.

trunk. To enter the left pulmonary artery, the catheter must turn sharply outward (Fig. 7-12).

REFERENCES

1. Chen JTT, Behar VS, Morris JJ, et al. Correlation of roentgen findings with hemodynamic data in pure mitral stenosis. *AJR Am J Roentgenol* 1968;102:280–292.
2. Gaasch WH, O'Rourke RA, Cohn LH, et al. Mitral valve disease. In: Schlant RC, Alexander RW, eds. *The heart*, 8th ed. New York: McGraw–Hill, 1994, pp. 1483–1518.
3. Franch RH, King SB, Douglas JS. Techniques of cardiac catheterization including coronary arteriography. In: Schlant RC, Alexander RW, eds. *The heart*, 8th ed. New York: McGraw–Hill, 1994:2381–2452.
4. Gorlin R, Gorlin G. Hydraulic formula for calculation of area of stenotic mitral valve, other cardiac valves and central circulatory shunts. *Am Heart J* 1951;41:1–29.
5. Starling EH. *The Linacre lecture on the law of the heart*. London: Longmans, Green, 1918.
6. Schlant RC, Sonnenblick EH. Normal physiology of the cardiovascular system. In: Schlant RC, Alexander RW, eds. *The heart*, 8th ed. New York: McGraw–Hill, 1994:113–152.
7. Hoffman RB, Rigler LG. Evaluation of left ventricular enlargement in the lateral projection of the chest. *Radiology* 1965;85:93–100.

Essentials of Cardiac Imaging,
James T. T. Chen,
Lippincott–Raven Publishers, Philadelphia © 1998.

CHAPTER 8

Pulmonary Vascularity

James T. T. Chen

The pulmonary vasculature reflects the underlying patho-physiology of the heart (1–6). By paying meticulous attention to the volume and distribution of pulmonary blood flow, the list of diagnostic possibilities can be considerably shortened. For instance, a uniform increase in vascularity, as is manifest by enlargement of all vessels in both lungs, favors the diagnosis of a left-to-right shunt (Fig. 8-1) and militates against a left-sided obstructive lesion. A left-sided obstructive lesion is characterized by a cephalic flow pattern with dilatation of the upper-lobe vessels and constriction of the lower ones (Fig. 8-2). Clinically, a secundum atrial septal defect (2° ASD) is occasionally misdiagnosed as mitral stenosis (MS), mainly because of their similar auscultatory findings. The split-second sound of 2° ASD may be confused with the opening snap of MS. The flow murmur across the tricuspid valve in patients with ASD may be mistaken for the diastolic rumble of MS. The radiographic differences in pulmonary vascularity between the two entities are, however, unmistakable.

On the other hand, the task of deriving physiologic data from the chest radiograph is not always easy. On rare occasions, owing to the intricacies of the pulmonary circulation, it is impossible to arrive at a correct diagnosis on radiologic grounds alone. For example, a large ASD may fail to show radiographic evidence of shunt vascularity (7). There is no clear explanation. Perhaps the pulmonary vessels of these patients are unusually rigid. The large flow simply passes through them at a higher velocity without causing noticeable vascular engorgement (5). Our hemodynamic interpretive skill in terms of the pulmonary vasculature is based on a firm understanding of anatomy and physiology in health and disease.

RADIOGRAPHIC ANATOMY

The pulmonary artery (pulmonary trunk) bifurcates at the level of the carina. The right branch extends abruptly right-ward perpendicular to the pulmonary trunk. It divides within the mediastinum before reaching the hilum; therefore, its point of division is invisible on radiography. The left pulmonary artery extends backward and superiorly, almost forming a straight-line continuation of the pulmonary trunk. It bifurcates at the left hilum. Each pulmonary artery divides into an ascending and a descending branch. Further division of the arteries follows closely the distribution of the bronchial tree. On cross sections, the artery and its bronchial companion are situated side by side. Their diameters are almost equal, the artery-bronchus ratio being 1.2 : 1.0 (8). In the periphery of the lungs, the bronchoarterial bundles are in the center of the pulmonary lobules.

The pulmonary veins begin in the interlobular septa. They course centrally, converging into the left atrium in the planes of the interstitium. The lymphatics are also in the interstitium and are normally invisible. The bronchial arteries originate from the descending aorta or the subclavian artery on each side. They are not seen on radiographs in healthy individuals.

The pulmonary arteries and veins within the lungs can be distinguished by their unique anatomic relationships. The arteries come out of the mediastinum at the level of the hila. The veins return to the heart at the level of the left atrium, which is 2 to 3 cm lower than the hila. The veins can be seen to penetrate deeply into the image of the heart on either side. In the upper lung, the veins are usually lateral and inferior to the arteries, but they are frequently (40% to 50%) superimposed (9). In the lower lobe, the veins are more easily distinguished from the arteries. The veins course more horizontally, whereas the arteries extend more vertically. As a rule, the veins tend to be larger, smoother, and branch less for the same distance than their arterial counterparts (Fig. 8-3).

PHYSIOPATHOLOGIC CONSIDERATIONS

The pulmonary circulation is a low-pressure system. In response to stress, the lungs can accommodate up to eight

Department of Radiology, Duke University School of Medicine, Durham, North Carolina 27710, U.S.A.

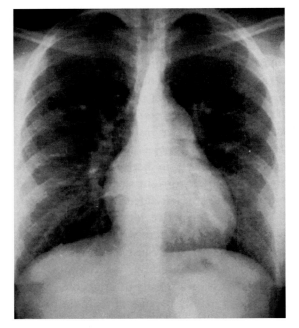

FIG. 8-1. Posteroanterior view of a patient with a large 2° ASD. Note uniform enlargement of pulmonary arteries and veins bilaterally and symmetrically. There is right-sided cardiomegaly and dilatation of the pulmonary trunk. On clinical examination the patient was suspected to have mitral stenosis because of similar auscultatory findings.

times their normal flow without developing pulmonary hypertension. During stress, the pulmonary vascular resistance may even decline (10). Such unique adaptability is thought to come about through two mechanisms. First, the pulmonary arteries are highly distensible. Morphologically, they have thinner walls with less musculature in the tunica media, compared with systemic arteries. Second, the pulmonary vascular bed capacity is enormous. Normally, a great number of small vessels are functionally inactive and can be recruited instantly on demand. Figure 8-4 shows the increased cardiovascular dimensions of a pregnant woman with greatly augmented cardiac output. Similar adjustments are often observed in athletes (see **Fig. 18-1**).

The lungs accept a dual blood supply. The venous blood comes from the right side of the heart to the pulmonary capillaries for gas exchange, and arterial blood, by way of the bronchial circulation, provides oxygen and nutrients for the bronchi and lung parenchyma. In the presence of severe pulmonary stenosis or massive pulmonary embolism, the blood supply to the alveolar capillaries may have to depend heavily on bronchial arterial collateralization. Normally, all the pulmonary arterial blood and two thirds of the bronchial arterial blood return to the heart by way of pulmonary veins (11). The volume and distribution of pulmonary blood flow are controlled by the following factors: cardiac output, gravity, pulmonary vascular resistance, neurogenic control, heart rate, and pulmonary vascular bed capacity.

Cardiac Output

The volume of the pulmonary blood flow is normally proportional to the cardiac output. During physical activity or pregnancy, the cardiac output and pulmonary blood flow increase appropriately with enhanced cardiac contractility (Fig. 8-4A). Patients with large systemic arteriovenous fistulas, including those with Paget's disease, usually show a marked increase in pulmonary blood flow (see **Fig. 18-2**). An asthenic person, on the other hand, requires only a small cardiac output with low pulmonary flow to meet biologic needs (Fig. 8-4B). Under these circumstances, more small vessels become inactive, thereby expanding the pulmonary vascular reserve. Patients with compensated aortic stenosis (see **Fig. 2-11A**) or insufficiency (Fig. 8-5) frequently show signs of decreased cardiac output with smaller than normal pulmonary vessels and unusually lucent lungs. Patients with severe tricuspid insufficiency with small cardiac output also have markedly decreased pulmonary vascularity (see **Fig. 7-4B**). At this point, we have come to realize that increased pulmonary vascularity may be present without a left-to-right shunt, and, likewise, decreased pulmonary vascularity can happen without a right-to-left shunt. It is more typical to see increased flow in a left-to-right shunt (Figs. 8-1 and 8-6) and decreased flow in a right-to-left shunt (Fig. 8-7). These entities are associated with altered cardiac outputs plus uneven distribution of blood flow between the two circulations.

Gravity

Normally the pulmonary vascular bed capacity is huge. The cardiac output or the pulmonary blood volume at any

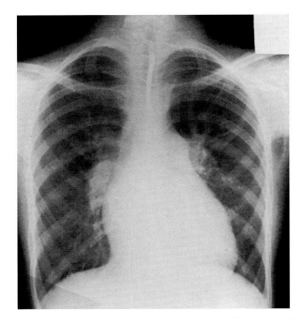

FIG. 8-2. Posteroanterior view of a patient with severe rheumatic mitral stenosis. Note the cephalic pulmonary blood flow pattern. The upper-lobe vessels are dilated, and basilar vessels are constricted.

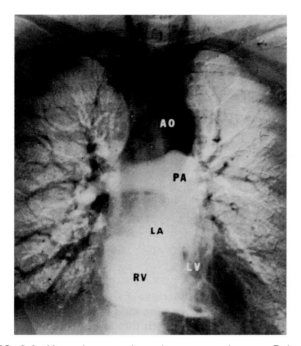

FIG. 8-3. Normal composite pulmonary angiogram. Pulmonary arteries (PA) are depicted by white and pulmonary veins by black images. AO, aorta; LA, left atrium; LV, left ventricle; RV, right ventricle.

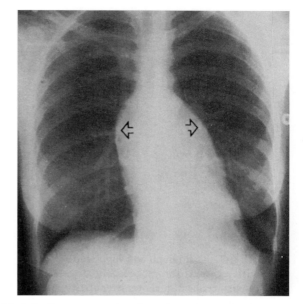

FIG. 8-5. Posteroanterior view of a patient with Marfan's syndrome and severe aortic insufficiency. Although the left ventricle contracted reasonably well, the forward cardiac output had declined significantly. Note the generalized decrease in pulmonary vascularity and unusually radiolucent lungs, reflecting the low cardiac output. Arrows mark the transverse dimension of the huge ascending aortic aneurysm.

given time is much smaller than the pulmonary vascular bed capacity. The pulmonary blood flow changes in a relatively passive manner. First, the flow is proportionate to the cardiac output. Second, the flow is influenced by the gravitational effects brought about by the weight of the blood. As long as the limits of the pulmonary vascular bed capacity are not exceeded and the pulmonary vascular resistance remains

normal, gravity is the major determinant for the distribution of flow. In the upright position, the pressure differential between the apexes and the bases of the lungs is ~22 mm Hg in the adult (12). This force increases the transmural pressure progressively from the top of the lung to the bottom. According to West (13), the blood flow to the bases is 18 times greater than to the apexes. In the classic illustration of West

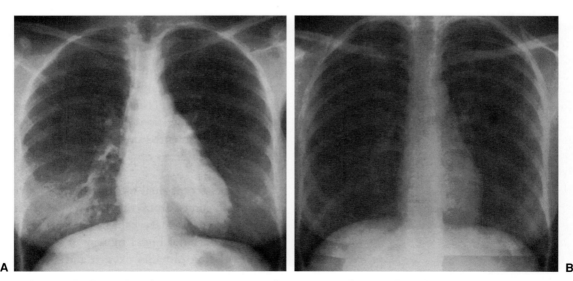

FIG. 8-4. Radiographs of a woman seven months pregnant show mild cardiomegaly with noticeably enlarged vessels throughout both lungs (**A**). Film taken before pregnancy (**B**) shows a much smaller heart with tiny vessels, as is frequently found in asthenic people.

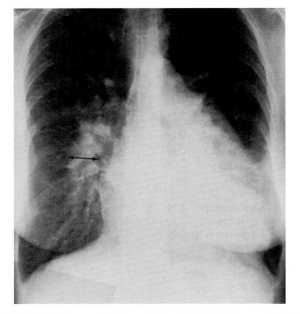

FIG. 8-6. Radiograph of a patient with ASD shows dilatation of the right descending pulmonary artery, measuring 25 mm (arrow).

(14), the lung is divided into three equal vertical zones. In the upper part, zone 1, the alveolar pressure exceeds the arterial pressure, and the vessels are collapsed. Only minimal flow occurs in the upper zone. In the middle, zone 2, the arterial pressure exceeds the alveolar pressure, which is still greater than the venous pressure. The flow through this zone is greater than that in zone 1, but smaller than the flow in zone 3. In zone 3, the lower zone, both arterial and venous

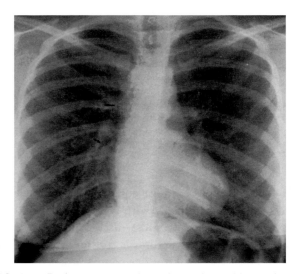

FIG. 8-7. Posteroanterior view of a patient with tetralogy of Fallot. The right descending pulmonary artery measures only 5 mm, which is far below the lower limit of 9 mm.

pressures exceed alveolar pressure; therefore, the flow is the greatest, and the vessels are fully open (5).

On radiography, the distribution of blood flow of erect human beings is entirely compatible with the aforementioned physiologic phenomena. As the transmural pressure increases down the zones, both the caliber of the vessels and the flow through them increase progressively. This normal flow pattern has been termed caudalization (2) (Fig. 8-8). Caudalization of flow can be readily abolished by changing the body posture from erect to supine, where the flow is equalized between apexes and bases. However, a new pattern of flow inequality then develops between the ventral and dorsal aspects of the chest, with the dorsal aspect receiving a greater amount of blood. Likewise, blood can be shifted to the upper lung zones by assuming an inverted position and to one side by assuming a lateral decubitus position. This kind of maneuvering could have therapeutic implications. For example, deliberately positioning a patient with unilateral lung disease so that blood flow is directed by gravity to the healthy lung may bring about dramatic clinical improvements. The rationale behind this is to eliminate the severe perfusion-ventilation mismatch in the good lung (5,15). After thoracotomy, gas exchange is better when the patient lies on the unoperated side and worse on the thoracotomy side (16).

Pulmonary Vascular Resistance

The pulmonary blood flow is inversely proportional to the pulmonary vascular resistance. Regional elevation of pulmonary vascular resistance is accompanied by diversion of

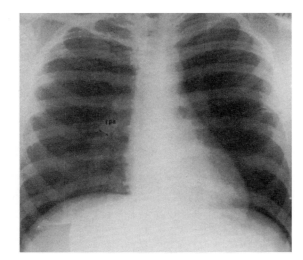

FIG. 8-8. Posteroanterior view of a healthy young man in the upright position. Note the nonuniformity of pulmonary blood flow brought about by gravitational influences. Little flow is seen in the apexes. Progressively more flow through larger vessels is evident from the apexes to the bases. The right descending pulmonary artery (rpa) measures 12.5 mm (arrows).

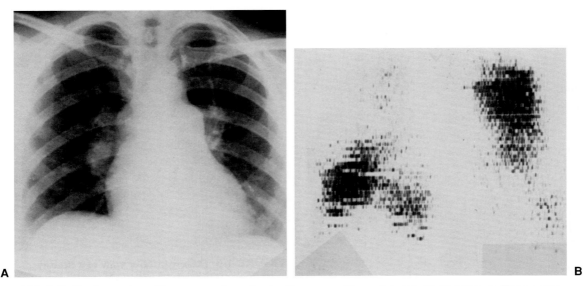

FIG. 8-9. Radiograph and lung scan of a patient with recurrent thromboembolic disease. **A:** The posteroanterior film shows irregularity in the caliber of vessels and in flow distribution. The general appearance is that of severe precapillary pulmonary hypertension. **B:** A perfusion lung scan shows multiple diversions of flow owing to regional increase in pulmonary vascular resistance caused by recurrent pulmonary emboli.

blood to the surrounding zones of lower resistance (Fig. 8-9). The pulmonary vascular resistance is controlled at the pulmonary arteriolar level. Spasm of the arterioles increases resistance, whereas their relaxation decreases resistance. The major forces causing increased pulmonary vascular resistance are hypoxia, acidosis, and the effects of some drugs (e.g., meperidine, histamine, serotonin, propranolol). Major factors causing decline in pulmonary vascular resistance include treatments for hypoxia and acidosis and some pharmacodynamic influences from isoproterenol, hydralazine, nitroglycerin, atropine, morphine, and other drugs (10).

In disease, hypoventilated or arrested ventilation causes local hypoxia. Hypoxia, in turn, induces vasoconstriction so that the 1:1 perfusion-ventilation ratio can be maintained by diverting blood from diseased to healthy areas. Uncontrolled flow through nonventilated portions of the lung results in arterial hypoxemia. Local vascular spasm under this condition actually represents the attempts of the natural defenses to minimize this shunt effect. A regional decrease in pulmonary vascular resistance, such as that caused by pulmonary arteriovenous fistulas, is associated with local increase in pulmonary blood flow through larger vessels at the expense of surrounding zones, where the flow is decreased and the vessels are smaller (Fig. 8-10).

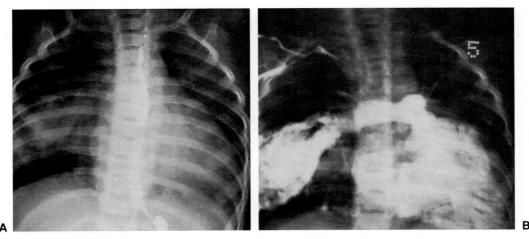

FIG. 8-10. Posteroanterior view (**A**) and angiocardiogram (**B**) of a child with a huge pulmonary arteriovenous fistula on the right side. Note the increased pulmonary blood flow through the large vascular channels with decreased flow in the remainder of the lung.

Neurogenic Control

Under certain conditions, the pulmonary vessels may tense up through a reflex-induced increase in muscle tone. This reaction transforms the pulmonary circulation into a system similar to the household plumbing unit. The vessels are then likened to rigid tubes. In this situation, the blood flow can increase only by shortening the transit time through the system (5). Therefore, the radiograph may occasionally fail to predict the volume of pulmonary blood flow, even when it is increased in response to enhanced cardiac output (7). Fortunately, this phenomenon is uncommon. In general, the pulmonary blood flow is proportionate to the caliber of pulmonary vessels and the density of the lungs as seen on the chest radiograph.

Heart Rate

In general, the size of cardiovascular structures is proportional to their volume. Cardiomegaly or vascular engorgement is primarily a problem of volume. It is well known that cardiac size is inversely related to heart rate. Cardiomegaly in patients with bradycardia results from greater cardiac volume during the prolonged diastole of the cardiac cycle. Likewise, slow transit time of flow through the pulmonary circulation allows increased amounts of blood to accumulate and to engorge the vessels. The fact that we seldom see cardiomegaly or pulmonary vascular engorgement in patients with thyrotoxicosis with high cardiac output is somewhat perplexing. Again, it is the rapid heart rate that has prevented the blood volume from building up anywhere at any time.

Pulmonary Vascular Bed Capacity

The normal pulmonary vascular bed capacity is large. The vascular reserve units can be promptly recruited when needed. Before the reserve is exhausted, and when pulmonary vascular resistance remains normal, gravity is the determinant of flow distribution. Some diseases exhaust the pulmonary vascular bed capacity, thereby nullifying the gravitational influences on pulmonary flow distribution. For example, in severe precapillary pulmonary hypertension, the centralizing flow pattern (2) cannot be abolished by changing the patient's body posture. Neither standing up nor lying down will help bring blood to the periphery of the lungs because the pulmonary vascular bed capacity has been drastically reduced by generalized pulmonary arteriolar spasm or parenchymal destruction, or both. The remaining small reserve has been fully recruited. The overwhelming pressures in the precapillary compartment of the pulmonary circulation cannot be overcome by the gravitational forces (Fig. 8-11). Likewise, the striking cephalic flow pattern of severe MS (Fig. 8-2) cannot be modified by changing the posture. The upward shifting flow pattern is not at all influenced by

assuming a supine position (17) (Fig. 8-12). Obviously the pulmonary vascular resistance is so high in the lower lung zones that flow through these areas is permanently restricted. The supine position not only fails to improve basilar flow but also facilitates apical flow, thereby exaggerating the abnormal flow pattern.

RADIOGRAPHIC EVALUATION

The volume and distribution of pulmonary blood flow are closely connected and should be studied collectively. However, for the sake of clarity and easy learning, an analytic three-stage approach is recommended (Tables 8-1–8-3). Within limits, it is possible to classify the vascular changes as primarily volume related (with normal distribution), primarily resistance related (with abnormal distribution), or a combination. In general, the volume of pulmonary blood flow is proportional to the size of the pulmonary arteries that receive blood directly from the right ventricle. The bigger the pulmonary arteries, the greater the pulmonary blood flow. This is true only when pulmonary vascular resistance remains normal, with gravity being the dominant influence to flow distribution (see the discussion in Physiopathologic Considerations). For practical purposes, two principal steps may be taken to assess the volume of pulmonary blood flow: make sure that the pulmonary vascular resistance is normal and measure the size of the pulmonary arteries.

Pulmonary Vascular Resistance

Before assessing the quantity of pulmonary blood flow, one must be certain that the pulmonary vascular resistance remains normal. Once the pulmonary vascular resistance becomes abnormal, the size of the pulmonary arteries is no longer proportional to pulmonary blood volume. Instead, it may reflect pressure and volume, or pressure alone. The normalcy of pulmonary vascular resistance is suggested by the following radiographic signs: preservation of the gradual and smooth vascular branching pattern from the hila toward the periphery of both lungs, the normal and proportionate response of the pulmonary veins to arterial flow, and the reservation of the normal caudalization or equalization flow pattern in the upright position.

At this point, some clarification is in order concerning the term equalization and the pulmonary venous response to flow. By equalization is meant the physiologically adjusted status of caudalization in response to increased flow. Equalization comes about by channeling blood from the high-pressure zone (the base) to the low-pressure zone (the apex) without causing pulmonary hypertension. The reserved channels in the low-pressure zone open up, and the pulmonary vascular resistance may actually fall. The pulmonary veins dilate passively in proportion to the flow increase in the arterial system. These changes represent a normal reaction of healthy lung (e.g., trained athletes with an enormous cardiac output and patients with a 2° ASD; see Fig. 8-1). Under

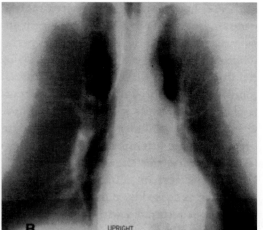

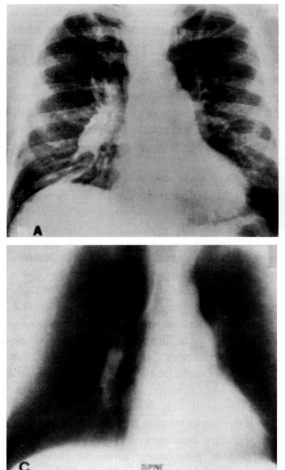

FIG. 8-11. A: Posteroanterior radiograph of a patient with Ondine's curse causing severe precapillary pulmonary hypertension. Note the striking centralized pulmonary blood flow pattern. [The term equalization is preferred by Ravin et al. (6).] The pulmonary trunk and central pulmonary arteries are enlarged, with abrupt attenuation toward the periphery of the lungs in a concentric manner. The tomogram in the upright position (B) and that in the supine position (C) both show centralization of the pulmonary flow. No change is noted in the distribution of flow between the two views. (Reproduced with permission from Ravin CE, Greenspan RH, McLoud TC, et al. Redistribution of pulmonary blood flow secondary to pulmonary arterial hypertension. *Invest Radiol* 1980; 15:29.)

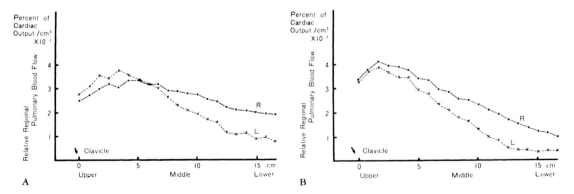

FIG. 8-12. Radionuclide studies of a patient with severe mitral stenosis show a persistent "cephalization" flow pattern regardless of body posture. A: Curve was taken when patient was upright. B: Curve was obtained when patient was supine. (Reproduced with permission from Ueda H, Iio M, Kaihara S. Determination of regional pulmonary blood flow in various cardiopulmonary disorders: study and application of macroaggregated albumin (MAA) labelled with [131]I (I). *Jpn Heart J* 1964;5:431.)

TABLE 8-1. *Principal steps in radiographic analysis of pulmonary vasculature*

Volume
  Recognition of normal pulmonary vascular resistance by noting normal flow distribution
    Gradual and smooth branching pattern
    Caudalization at rest
    Equalization on exertion or in presence of left-to-right shunt
  If normal, size of pulmonary arteries is proportional to volume of blood flow
    Right descending pulmonary artery: 10–15 mm for males; 9–14 mm for females. Values >1 mm outside the limits are abnormal
    Artery–bronchus ratio = 1.2:1.0. Artery grossly larger or smaller than bronchus is abnormal
Distribution: If abnormal, pulmonary vascular resistance (PVR) is abnormal
  Cephalization: postcapillary pulmonary hypertension
  Centralization: precapillary pulmonary hypertension
  Lateralization: unilateral increase in PVR or jet effect
  Localization: localized increase or decrease in PVR
  Collateralization: diffuse decrease in PVR provokes systemic collateral flow
Combination: combined vascular abnormalities involving volume and distribution

these circumstances, the apex-to-base flow ratio increases but never reaches 1:1, as implied by the term equalization; the gravitational influences are still in control, and the lower lung zones still receive considerably more blood than the upper. The small vessels in reserve have not been fully recruited, and there is still room for more flow.

Once the pulmonary vascular bed capacity is exceeded, however, the passive vascular engorgement will be transformed into a pattern of active vascular spasm, a generalized pulmonary arteriolar constriction. This reaction is a natural defense mechanism attempting to prevent a sudden surge of blood through the already overloaded pulmonary circulation. When this happens, the pulmonary blood flow pattern becomes distinctly abnormal. The pulmonary trunk and the central pulmonary arteries are dilated, with abrupt attenuation of the peripheral branches. The pulmonary veins constrict in sympathy. The flow may be said to be centralized. At that point the gravitational forces will be overwhelmed by the high pressures in the precapillary compartment of the pulmonary circulation. The volume of pulmonary blood flow declines and the apex-to-base flow ratio increases markedly, reaching a truly 1:1 level (Fig. 8-11). For this reason, this pattern has been called equalization by Ravin and co-workers (6) instead of centralization, which I prefer (2). For the convenience of discussion in this book and to avoid confusion between the two terms, we use equalization to denote the normal reaction of a healthy lung in response to stress and centralization to describe the abnormal reaction of a compromised vascular bed in response to stress.

Pulmonary Arteries

The size of the pulmonary arteries can be gauged in two ways. One is to measure the transverse diameter of the right descending pulmonary artery immediately above the origin of the right-middle-lobe pulmonary artery (Fig. 8-8). The other is to compare the cross sections of the bronchoarterial bundles (Fig. 8-13). Because all cross sections are not clearly defined radiographically, only those that are sharply demarcated should be used for this purpose. Normally the right descending pulmonary artery measures 10 to 15 mm for men and 9 to 14 mm for women. A value >1 mm outside these limits is considered abnormal, and either increased flow (Fig. 8-6) or decreased flow (Fig. 8-7) is suggested. The caliber of the pulmonary arteries is almost equal to that of their accompanying bronchi, with a ratio of 1.2:1.0 (Fig. 8-13). Any gross discrepancy in size between the two structures is considered abnormal. Too large an artery compared with the size of the bronchus alongside is indicative of increased pulmonary blood flow (or shunt vascularity) (Fig. 8-14) and vice versa (Fig. 8-7). Further assistance in assessing the pulmonary vascularity can be obtained by fluoroscopy. In-

TABLE 8-2. *Simplified radiographic classification of pulmonary vascularity*

Volume (example)	A/B	RDPA (mm) Male	RDPA (mm) Female	Distribution (examples)	Hemodynamics
Normal	1.2 (○●)[a]	10–15	9–14	Caudalization (normal at rest)	Normal
Increased (ASD)	>1.2 (○●)[a]	≥16	≥15	Equalization (normal on exertion, or with small left-to-right shunt)	Normal
Decreased (TOF)	<1.2 (○●)[a]	≤9	≤8	Cephalization (MS)	Postcapillary PH
				Centralization (PPH)	Precapillary PH
				Lateralization (WM, PS)	Unilateral obstruction or jet
				Localization (PE, PAVF)	Local obstruction or runoff
				Collateralization (PTA)	Pulmonary hypotension

[a] White dot indicates artery; black dot indicates bronchus.
A/B, artery–bronchus ratio; ASL, atrial septal defect; MS, mitral stenosis; PAVF, pulmonary arteriovenous fistula; PE, pulmonary embolism; PH, pulmonary hypertension; PPH, primary pulmonary hypertension; PS, pulmonary stenosis; PTA, pseudotruncus arteriosus; RDPA, right descending pulmonary artery; TOF, tetralogy of Fallot; WM, Westermark's sign.

TABLE 8-3. *Detailed radiographic classification of pulmonary vascularity*

Anatomy	Physiology							
	Site of			REC	GF → FD	PBF PA	Pressures	PBF
	PVR	A PVR	PVBC					
Volume								
Normal (at rest)	N		+ + + +	0	Yes	Yes	N	N
Abnormal								
Increased (ASD)	N		+	+ + +	Yes	Yes	N	+ + +
Decreased (TOF)	N		+ + + + +	0	Yes	Yes	—[a]	—[a]
Distribution								
Normal								
Caudalization (at rest)	N		+ + + +	0	Yes	Yes	N	N
Equalization (on exertion or with small left-to-right shunt)	N		+ +	+ +	Yes	Yes	N	+ +
Abnormal								
Cephalization (MS)	A	B	0	+ + + +	No	No	PVH	—[a]
Centralization (PPH)	A	P	0	+ + + +	No	No	PAH	—[a]
Lateralization (SJS)	A	U	+ +	+ +	Yes (OL)	Yes (OL)	Asymmetric	N
Localization (PE)	A	L	0	+ + + +	No	No	Irregular	—[a]
Collateralization (PTA)	A	D	+ + + + +	0	Yes	Yes	—[a]	—[a]
Combination	Abnormalities in volume and distribution are frequently combined. See text for examples.							

[a] Subnormal value.

0, 0% of normal capacity; +, 25% of normal capacity; + +, 50% of normal capacity; + + +, 75% of normal capacity; + + + +, normal capacity; + + + + +, supranormal capacity owing to underutilization; A, abnormal; ASD, atrial septal defect; B, basal; D, diffuse; GF→FD, gravitational forces control flow distribution; L, local; MS, mitral stenosis; N, normal; P, peripheral; PAH, pulmonary arterial hypertension; PBF, pulmonary blood flow; PBF PA, pulmonary blood flow proportional to pulmonary artery size; PE, pulmonary embolism; PPH, primary pulmonary hypertension; PTA, pseudotruncus arteriosus; PVBC, pulmonary vascular bed capacity; PVH, pulmonary venous hypertension; PVR, pulmonary vascular resistance; REC, recruitment of reserved vasculature; SJS, Swyer–James syndrome; TOP, tetralogy of Fallot; U, unilateral; Yes (OL), yes in opposite lung only.

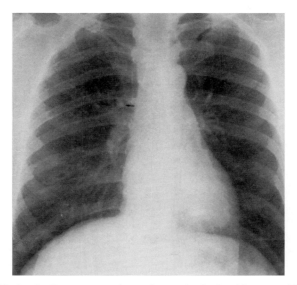

FIG. 8-13. Posteroanterior radiograph of a healthy man. The white dot represents the cross section of the pulmonary artery, and the black dot with white rim represents the end-on view of the accompanying bronchus. The artery–bronchus ratio is ~1:1.

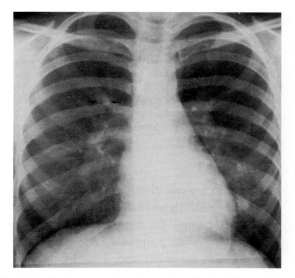

FIG. 8-14. Posteroanterior view of a patient with a small ventricular septal defect shows the artery–bronchus ratio to be far greater than unity (arrows), indicating increased pulmonary blood flow.

creased flow is generally accompanied by a greater amplitude of pulsation, and vice versa.

Resistance

Normal

Normal pulmonary vascular resistance is manifested by the smooth tapering of vessels even in response to a moderate increase in pulmonary blood flow. The distribution of flow is determined by gravity alone. Two radiographic patterns of normal distribution are caudalization and equalization. The normal flow distribution of erect human beings is represented by a caudalized flow pattern. With a moderate increase in flow, this pattern is somewhat modified into a less caudalized and more equalized form (see the discussion under Pulmonary Vascular Resistance).

Abnormal

Once the pulmonary vascular resistance becomes abnormal, the smooth tapering pattern of vessels is destroyed. Depending on the site of increased resistance, "pruning" of the arterial tree is evident either diffusely or locally. There are five radiographic patterns of abnormal distribution: cephalization, centralization, lateralization, localization, and collateralization.

Cephalization. In response to a left-sided obstructive lesion, such as MS (Fig. 8-2), the pulmonary vascular resistance increases in the lung bases, thereby diverting the flow in a cephalic direction. Cephalization of the pulmonary vascularity is the hallmark of postcapillary pulmonary hypertension. It could also be caused by a pathophysiologic obstruction, such as left ventricular failure with elevated end-

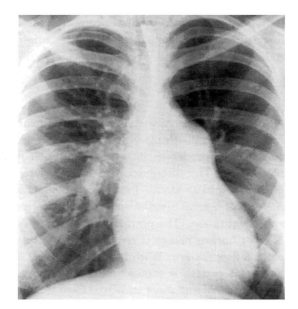

FIG. 8-16. Radiograph of a patient with Eisenmenger ventricular septal defect. Note the centralized flow pattern without evidence of preexisting shunt vascularity, reflecting a combination of pulmonary arterial hypertension and decreased cardiac output.

diastolic pressure and volume. Severe mitral insufficiency is another example of functional left-sided obstruction in which the pulmonary venous pressure is markedly elevated in systole, even before the onset of pump failure of the left ventricle.

The exact mechanism behind cephalization is obscure. The most logical explanation is as follows (5). In response to pulmonary venous hypertension, pulmonary edema first occurs in the lung bases owing to gravity in the erect position. The pathophysiologic effects of pulmonary edema are to increase the interstitial pressure or to make the interstitial pressure less negative, to decrease the pulmonary compliance, and to increase the distance traversed by oxygen from the alveoli to the pulmonary capillaries. Optimal blood flow through the lungs partly depends on the negative interstitial pressure maintained by inspiration. Therefore both increasing interstitial pressure and decreasing pulmonary compliance reduce the expansibility of the lung, diminish the tethering effect on the vessels, and allow the vessels to contract because of their inherent tonus. Increasing the alveoli-pulmonary capillary distance interferes with optimal gas exchange and, in turn, produces hypoxia. Hypoxia is a major cause of arteriolar spasm. Even when considering the mechanical factors alone, the small increase in interstitial fluid and pressure can cause a slight narrowing of the vessels but a considerable increase in resistance. This phenomenon can be explained by Poiseuille's formula, that reducing the radius of a vessel by one half is accompanied by a 16-fold increase in resistance and a 16-fold decrease in flow.

Centralization. In the presence of precapillary pulmonary hypertension, the pulmonary vascular resistance is diffusely

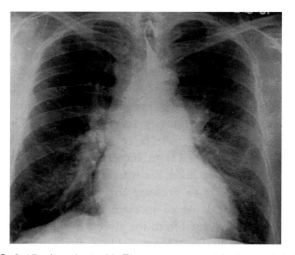

FIG. 8-15. A patient with Eisenmenger ventricular septal defect and atrial septal defect. Note that the pulmonary blood flow remains somewhat increased, with pruning of the peripheral pulmonary arteries, representing a combination of pulmonary arterial hypertension with increased cardiac output.

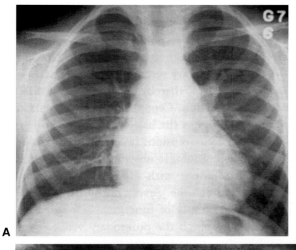

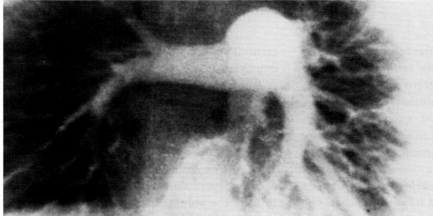

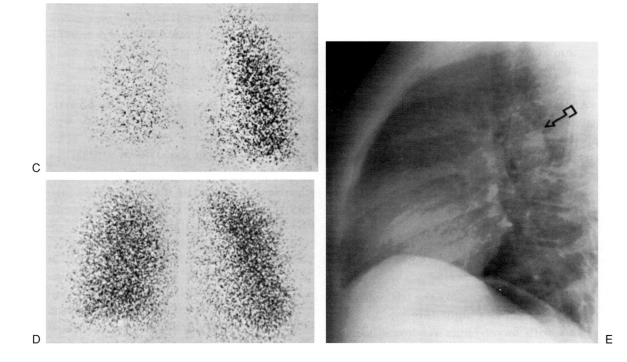

FIG. 8-17. Radiographs and scans of a child with valvular pulmonary stenosis with a peak systolic gradient of 70 mm Hg. **A:** Posteroanterior film shows a left lateralization of the flow. **B:** Pulmonary arterial phase of the study shows larger vessels on the left and smaller vessels on the right, indicative of an uneven distribution of flow between the two lungs. **C:** Radionuclide lung scan shows more uptake of radioactivity in the left lung than in the right. **D:** Postoperative lung scan shows that the abnormal flow pattern was abolished by a successful pulmonary valvulotomy. **E:** Lateral view of another patient with same disease. Note huge left pulmonary artery (arrow) and small right pulmonary artery.

elevated. The pulmonary arterial pressure is much higher than the hydrostatic pressure, and the pulmonary vascular bed capacity is exhausted. The radiographic flow pattern is that of centralization, descriptive of a concentric dilatation of the central pulmonary arteries, which taper abruptly in all directions (Fig. 8-11). When Eisenmenger syndrome develops in addition to a torrential left-to-right shunt or an admixture lesion, the picture may be of a modified shunt vascularity, a combination of increased flow and a centralization pattern (Fig. 8-15). When the cardiac output is low, Eisenmenger syndrome is no longer distinguishable from precapillary pulmonary hypertension without a preexisting left-to-right shunt (Fig. 8-16).

Lateralization. Normally, the pulmonary blood flow is symmetric and balanced, although by radionuclide perfusion scan the right-to-left lung flow ratio is ~52% to 48% (18). Under abnormal conditions, the pulmonary flow may become grossly uneven between the two lungs, which is termed lateralization of the pulmonary vascularity. Lateralization can be either leftward or rightward depending on the side that receives a greater portion of the blood.

Increased vascular resistance in the contralateral lung is the mechanism behind a lateralized pulmonary blood flow pattern in all disease processes except valvular pulmonary stenosis (Fig. 8-17). The flow disturbances causing left lateralization in valvular pulmonary stenosis are more complex. They probably operate on both mechanical and dynamic grounds (3). First, owing to the anatomic interrelationships between the pulmonary trunk and its two branches, the jet stream originating from the stenotic valve is in the direction of the left pulmonary artery and perpendicular to the right pulmonary artery. Second, when the high pressure within the right ventricle is converted at the stenosis into high velocity, a low-pressure zone is created immediately lateral to the central axis of the jet stream (19). Such reduced pressure has a suction effect, facilitating flow to the left pulmonary artery at the expense of the right. The low-pressure waves in systole distal to the stenotic valve can sometimes be recorded at cardiac catheterization as Venturi waves (19,20). Another unique feature of valvular pulmonary stenosis is the lack of lateralized flow in patients with severe obstruction when the peak gradient across the valve exceeds 100 mm Hg (see **Fig. 7-5**). This lack is due to the jet effect being progressively weakened with the rising pressure differential.

Another example of a left lateralization flow pattern is found in patients with proximal interruption, or hypoplasia of the right pulmonary artery. A unique feature of this entity is the ipsilateral smallness of the lung and the hemithorax (Fig. 8-18), an important differentiating point between this disease and Swyer–James syndrome (21).

A right lateralization pattern can be found in left-sided unilateral hyperlucent lung (Swyer–James syndrome) (Fig. 8-19) and massive pulmonary embolism occluding the left pulmonary artery (Westermark's sign) (Fig. 8-20). Most patients with Swyer–James syndrome had unilateral viral bronchitis and bronchiolitis obliterans in childhood with resultant

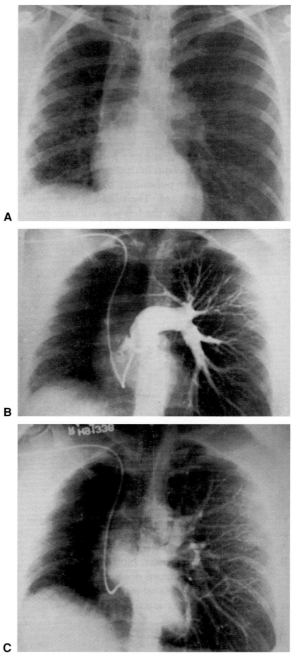

FIG. 8-18. Radiograph and arteriogram of a patient with proximal interruption of the right pulmonary artery. **A:** Posteroanterior radiograph shows smallness of the vessels, lung, and hemithorax on the right. The mediastinum is shifted to the right. **B:** Pulmonary arteriogram shows proximal interruption of the right pulmonary artery and enlargement of the pulmonary trunk and left pulmonary arteries. **C:** Levo phase of the study shows no filling of the major pulmonary veins on the right side.

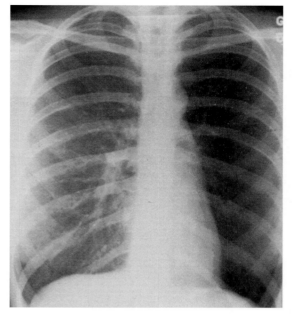

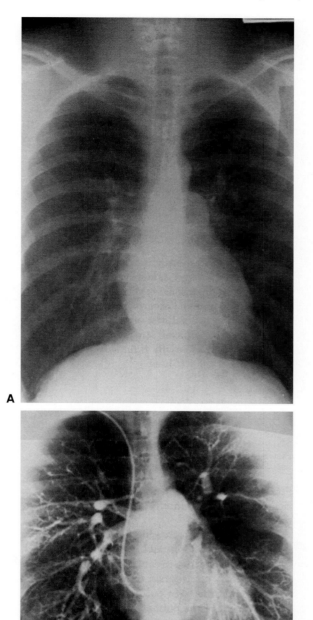

FIG. 8-19. Posteroanterior view of a 24-year-old woman with Swyer–James syndrome, who had had no recent cardiopulmonary symptoms. She had experienced recurrent episodes of pneumonia in infancy. Note the uniform smallness of all vessels in her hyperlucent left lung. The pulmonary blood flow is preferentially right sided. The left lung is markedly oligemic, without evidence of volume loss.

A

B

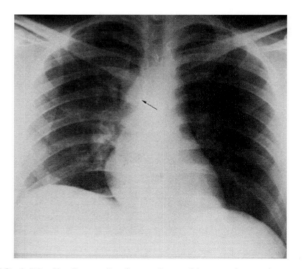

FIG. 8-20. Radiograph of a patient with massive pulmonary embolism occluding the left pulmonary artery. Note that the pulmonary blood flow is preferentially right sided. The left lung is markedly oligemic, indicative of a positive Westermark's sign. The arrow marks the dilated superior vena cava and azygos vein. The left lung volume is normal.

FIG. 8-21. Studies of a patient with multiple pulmonary artery branch stenoses. **A:** Posteroanterior radiograph. **B:** Pulmonary arteriogram. Note the multiple rounded or oval-shaped densities in both lungs, representing the dilated segments distal to the stenotic pulmonary arteries.

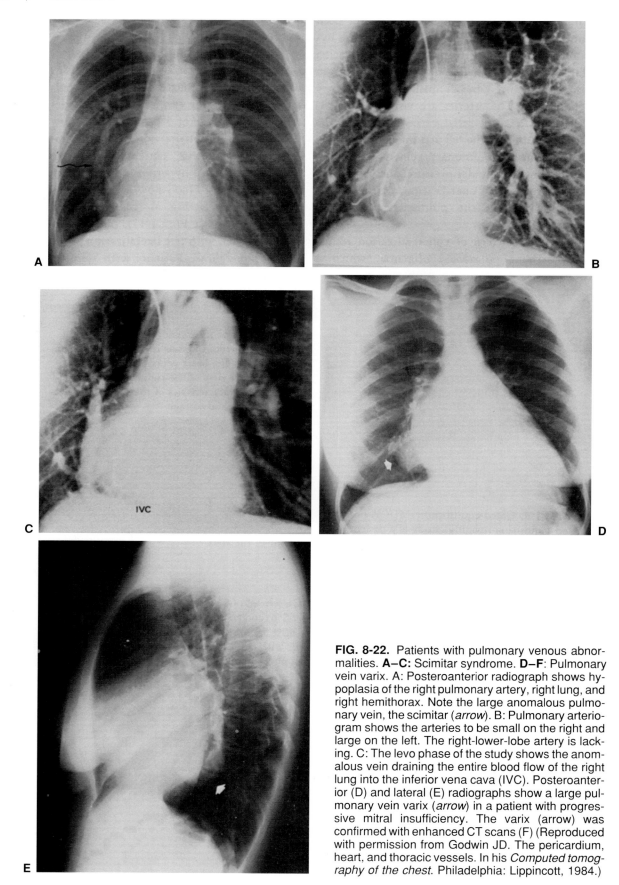

FIG. 8-22. Patients with pulmonary venous abnormalities. **A–C:** Scimitar syndrome. **D–F:** Pulmonary vein varix. A: Posteroanterior radiograph shows hypoplasia of the right pulmonary artery, right lung, and right hemithorax. Note the large anomalous pulmonary vein, the scimitar (*arrow*). B: Pulmonary arteriogram shows the arteries to be small on the right and large on the left. The right-lower-lobe artery is lacking. C: The levo phase of the study shows the anomalous vein draining the entire blood flow of the right lung into the inferior vena cava (IVC). Posteroanterior (D) and lateral (E) radiographs show a large pulmonary vein varix (*arrow*) in a patient with progressive mitral insufficiency. The varix (arrow) was confirmed with enhanced CT scans (F) (Reproduced with permission from Godwin JD. The pericardium, heart, and thoracic vessels. In his *Computed tomography of the chest.* Philadelphia: Lippincott, 1984.)

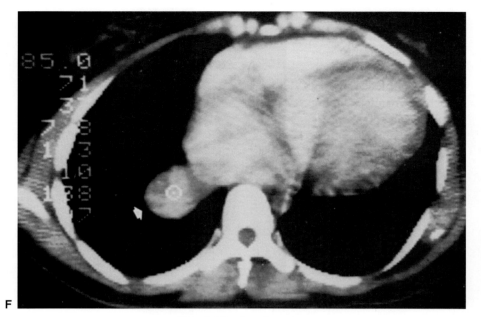

FIG. 8-22. *Continued.*

obstructive emphysema and bronchiectasis (21). Through attempts at maintaining a normal perfusion-ventilation ratio, the pulmonary blood flow is diverted away from the diseased lung. Consequently, all vessels on this side become small from the hilum to the periphery of the lung. Thus, the hyperlucent lung is caused by decreased perfusion rather than hyperinflation. In fact, the volume of the hyperlucent lung is usually normal. Westermark's sign represents an early and transient event of massive pulmonary embolism before the development of pulmonary infarction.

On inspiratory films, Westermark's sign is similar to Swyer–James syndrome except for the tendency to a greater degree of overperfusion of the contralateral lung owing to the acute nature of the disease. On expiration, however, air trapping is noted in the underperfused lung only in patients with Swyer–James syndrome (13). The clinical manifestations between the two diseases are distinctly different, which will become apparent when inquiring into the history: sudden onset of chest symptoms in patients with Westermark's sign versus complete absence of symptoms in most patients with Swyer–James syndrome. The radiologic signs of air trapping in patients with Swyer–James syndrome are manifest only during expiration. They are failure of the hyperlucent and underperfused lung to deflate, shifting of the mediastinum to the contralateral side, and failure of the ipsilateral hemidiaphragm to elevate. These signs are more striking on fluoroscopy than on radiographs.

Localization. Localized vascular changes leading to regional abnormal pulmonary blood flow patterns are, in most instances, due to localized increase in vascular resistance (e.g., pulmonary embolism). Only rarely are they caused by locally decreased vascular resistance (e.g., pulmonary arteriovenous fistulas with regional runoffs; see Fig. 8-10).

Focal constriction or dilatation or both, as well as abnormal course of the pulmonary vasculature, are seen in disorders such as pulmonary embolism, pulmonary artery branch stenosis (Fig. 8-21), anomalous origin of a pulmonary artery, extrinsic pressure on pulmonary vessels, pulmonary vein stenosis, anomalous pulmonary venous connections (Fig. 8-22A–C), and pulmonary vein varix (Fig. 8-22D–F).

Collateralization. In response to severe obstruction of flow to the lungs, the pulmonary circulation is sustained by the development of systemic arterial collateralization. Of all collaterals, the hypertrophied bronchial arteries are the most important. They arise from the descending aorta or the subclavian arteries on either side. On radiography, they are small, lacy, tortuous, and best seen near their origins in the upper medial lung zones (Fig. 8-23). By aortography or bronchial arteriography (22), narrow channels of anastomosis are visible between the collaterals, which are tortuous, and the native pulmonary arteries, which are small but appear otherwise normal. The low-pressure pulmonary arteries fill both antegrade and retrograde all the way to the hypoplastic pulmonary trunk and its bifurcation (Fig. 8-24). The small pulmonary arteries can also be seen by ipsilateral pulmonary venography. The arteries are made visible by inserting the right atrial catheter through the atrial septum into the left atrium and eventually wedging into a pulmonary vein, injecting contrast medium under pressure, and recording the retrograde opacification of the pulmonary artery from the pulmonary vein (Fig. 8-25).

The flow pattern of collateralization results from extreme pulmonary oligemia, which is most commonly encountered in pseudotruncus arteriosus, the most severe form of tetralogy of Fallot with pulmonary atresia and ventricular septal defect. This pattern is less common in severe pulmonary stenosis or atresia with intact ventricular septum, tricuspid atresia, tricuspid stenosis, and Ebstein's anomaly.

Combination. In reality, abnormalities in volume and distribution are frequently combined. For instance, patients

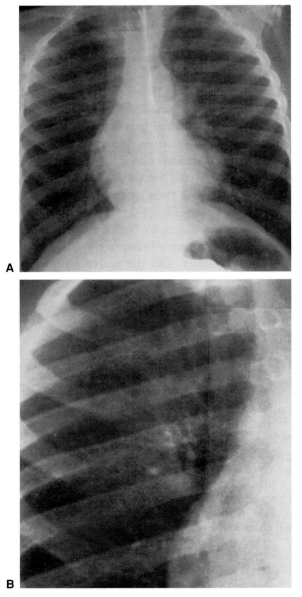

A

B

FIG. 8-23. Films of a child with pseudotruncus arteriosus. **A:** Posteroanterior radiograph shows small, lacy, and tortuous vessels in the upper medial lung zones. The heart is boot-shaped. **B:** A magnified view of the right-upper-lung zone shows the characteristics of systemic arterial collaterals to better advantage.

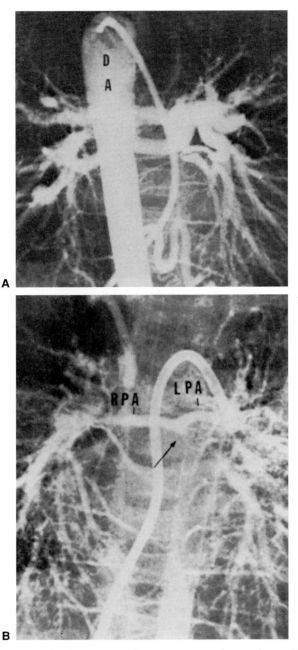

A

B

FIG. 8-24. **A:** Anteroposterior aortogram of a patient with pseudotruncus arteriosus. Note that the tortuous systemic collateral or bronchial arteries communicate in the hilar region with the true pulmonary arteries. DA, descending aorta. **B:** An aortogram in the sitting up position of another patient with pseudotruncus arteriosus. Note the seagull-like hypoplastic pulmonary arterial tree (*arrow*). LPA, left pulmonary artery; RPA, right pulmonary artery. (Reproduced with permission from Elliott LP. Axial cineangiography in congenital heart disease. In: Hipona FA, ed. *Heart: multiple imaging procedures*, vol. 5. New York: Grune & Stratton, 1983.)

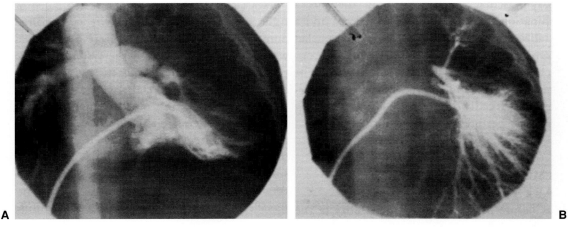

FIG. 8-25. Studies of a patient with severe tetralogy of Fallot. Right ventriculogram (**A**) shows very tight infundibular pulmonary stenosis, atretic left pulmonary artery, large right-to-left shunt at the ventricular level, and a right-sided aorta. Pulmonary vein wedge angiogram (**B**) shows that the left pulmonary artery is visualized by retrograde filling with the opacified blood from the pulmonary vein.

with severe MS (Fig. 8-2) usually have a combination of decreased pulmonary blood flow (the cardiac output can decrease from the average of 5 L/minute to as low as 2 L/minute) and cephalization of the pulmonary vascularity. Likewise, patients with severe precapillary pulmonary hypertension often have decreased pulmonary blood flow and a centralized flow pattern (Fig. 8-16). In isolated pulmonary stenosis (Fig. 8-17), cardiac output may be normal with left lateralization of the pulmonary blood flow. Patients with

scimitar syndrome actually have three abnormalities: left lateralization owing to hypoplasia of the right pulmonary artery, localization owing to a large anomalous pulmonary vein (the scimitar), and increased total pulmonary blood flow owing to a left-to-right shunt at the atrial level (Fig. 8-22). When a large left-to-right shunt is complicated by the development of rheumatic MS, the pulmonary vasculature may evidence a combination of increased flow with cephalization (Fig. 8-26; see also **Fig. 16-12**).

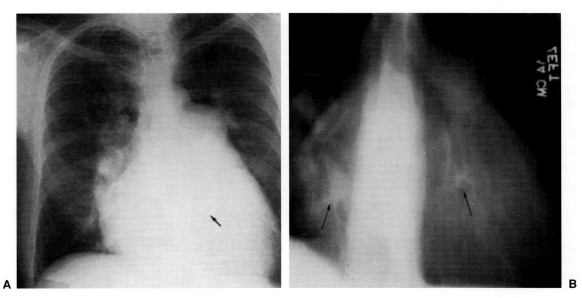

FIG. 8-26. Studies of a patient with partial anomalous pulmonary venous connection from the entire right lung to the right atrium. His condition is complicated by the development of rheumatic mitral stenosis. **A:** Posteroanterior radiograph shows cephalization of the pulmonary vascularity plus an overall increase in pulmonary blood flow, as is evident by the large pulmonary vessels that were found to be hyperpulsatile on fluoroscopy. The *arrow* points to the calcified mitral valve. **B:** Tomogram shows the calcified mitral valve (*left arrow*) and the large anomalous pulmonary vein (*right arrow*) entering the right atrium.

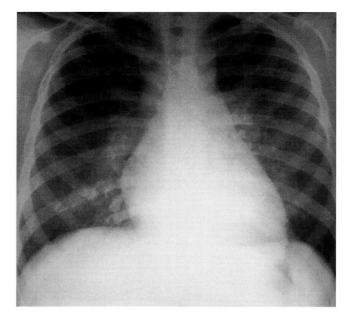

FIG. 8-27. Posteroanterior radiograph of a 14-year-old boy with veno-occlusive disease. Note right-sided cardiomegaly and a centralized pulmonary blood flow pattern, suggestive of precapillary pulmonary hypertension. Uniquely, there is also evidence of interstitial pulmonary edema, in the form of peribronchial cuffing, indistinct vascular margins, and septal lines. Since the major pulmonary veins are not dilated (on the radiograph and by selective pulmonary venography), one can confidently rule out the possibility of left-sided obstructive lesions distal to the pulmonary venules. The pressures on the left side of the heart and in the pulmonary veins were normal. The pulmonary arterial pressure was elevated to 115/65 (90) mm Hg. The patient's chief complaint had been progressive exertional dyspnea over the course of 6 months (courtesy of Dr. Eric L. Effmann).

Veno-occlusive disease (23), which is rarely diagnosed before death, may present a unique pulmonary vascular pattern. Usually there is a combination of severe pulmonary edema and a centralized flow pattern instead of a cephalic pattern. Because only the small pulmonary veins and venules are obstructed, the large pulmonary veins are not dilated. The pulmonary trunk and the central pulmonary arteries are markedly dilated with abrupt tapering toward the periphery of the lung (Fig. 8-27).

Pulmonary Vascularity in Heart Failure

Heart failure may be defined as inability of the heart to maintain one or more of its functions: adequate cardiac output, myocardial responsiveness under stress, and adequate tissue oxygenation. Heart failure may be defined as left sided or right sided according to the primary site of cardiac dysfunction. Left-sided failure is associated with a shift of blood flow from systemic to pulmonary circulation with resultant pulmonary venous hypertension. Conversely, right-sided failure is accompanied by a shifting blood flow from pulmonary to systemic circulation with resultant systemic venous

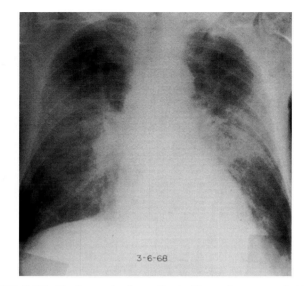

FIG. 8-28. Radiograph of a patient with acute myocardial infarction shows a bat-wing-like distribution of pulmonary edema fluid and a normal cardiac size.

hypertension. In certain diseases, both sides of the heart may be affected simultaneously, leading to bilateral heart failure, e.g., cardiac tamponade, constrictive pericarditis, multivalvular disease, and diffuse myocardial disease. Heart failure may also be classified according to the tempo of onset as acute, subacute, or chronic.

Radiographic Signs of Left-sided Heart Failure

During the acute phase of left heart failure, there is usually a combination of predominantly alveolar pulmonary edema,

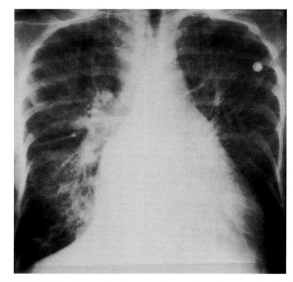

FIG. 8-29. Radiograph of a patient with subacute left-sided heart failure stemming from mitral insufficiency following an unsuccessful mitral valvulotomy. Note the apparent cephalic pulmonary blood flow pattern, the multiple ill-defined septal lines, and moderate cardiomegaly.

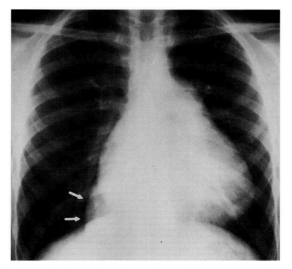

FIG. 8-30. Radiograph of a patient with severe valvular pulmonary stenosis (PS), right ventricular failure, and tricuspid insufficiency. Note the aneurysmal dilatation of the inferior vena cava (*arrows*). The typical leftward lateralization flow pattern is still present but less conspicuous than before, owing to decreased forward cardiac output from the right ventricle.

normal cardiac size, and lack of cephalization of the pulmonary vasculature (Fig. 8-28). When the left ventricle fails suddenly, as in acute myocardial infarction, volume and pressures rise abruptly in the postcapillary compartment of the pulmonary circulation. Fluid leaks quickly out of the capillaries, overwhelms the interstitium, and pours into the alveoli. On radiography, alveolar pulmonary edema has the appearance of cloudlike densities, frequently distributed in the hilar and perihilar regions bilaterally. This appearance has been likened to butterfly or bat wings. Fleishner's expla-

nation of "butterfly" pulmonary edema remains the most reasonable (24). He emphasized the morphologic and functional differences between the central (the medulla) and the peripheral (the cortex) portions of the lung. The cortex is more distensible and better ventilated than the medulla. Lymphatic drainage, which depends on movements of the adjacent tissues, is much more efficient in the well-ventilated areas (the cortex) than the poorly moving areas (the medulla). Thus, edema tends to accumulate more abundantly in the medulla of the lung.

Cardiomegaly is a function of chronic adjustments to heart failure, mediated by hypertrophy of the myocardium as well as salt and water retention by the kidneys. In the acute phase of left-sided heart failure, therefore, cardiomegaly is usually not present. Likewise, time is required for striking cephalization of the pulmonary vasculature to develop in response to sustained left-sided heart failure. Any small cephalization in acute left-sided heart failure is usually obscured by severe pulmonary edema and can be demonstrated only by the more sophisticated techniques, for example, radionuclide lung scanning.

When the onset of left-sided heart failure is subacute, the following radiographic signs are expected: noticeable cephalization of the pulmonary vasculature, predominantly interstitial pulmonary edema, hazy septal lines, and mild to moderate cardiomegaly (Fig. 8-29). Chronic left-sided failure is accompanied by the following signs: striking cephalization, interstitial pulmonary edema, sharply demarcated septal lines, and gross cardiomegaly (see **Fig. 2-7**).

Radiographic Signs of Right-sided Heart Failure

From the radiographic standpoint, right-sided heart failure may be classified into two categories according to the pri-

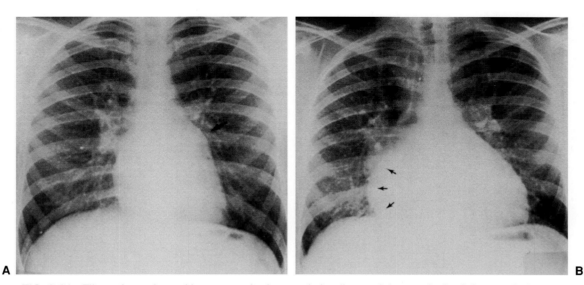

FIG. 8-31. Films of a patient with severe mitral stenosis leading to right ventricular failure and tricuspid insufficiency. **A:** Posteroanterior view shows cephalization of the pulmonary vascularity and left atrial enlargement (*arrow*). **B:** Same view taken 9 years later shows a marked increase in cardiac size, including a huge right atrium (*arrows*).

mary site of cardiac dysfunction. If the failure is caused by lesions proximal to the pulmonary valve, the following signs are likely to be present: diffuse decrease in pulmonary vascularity, hyperlucent lungs, small pulmonary vessels, right-sided chamber enlargements, dilatation of venae cavae (see **Fig. 2-6**), and some residual leftward lateralization flow pattern, provided valvular pulmonary stenosis is the cause of heart failure (see Fig. 8-30).

If right-sided heart failure is caused by elevated precapillary pulmonary hypertension (e.g., obstructive emphysema), a centralized flow pattern is always present in addition to other signs of right-sided heart failure (see **Fig. 2-12B**). If it stems from left-sided heart failure, the following signs are usually observed: decreased pulmonary blood flow; unusually radiolucent lungs; smallness of vessels, particularly in the lung bases; a persistent but less prominent pattern of cephalization; right-sided chamber enlargement and venocaval dilatation; and persistent but less prominent left-sided cardiomegaly (see **Fig. 9-5**). Severe left-sided heart failure is the most common cause of right-sided heart failure (Fig. 8-31). The symptoms of left-sided failure (e.g., dyspnea and orthopnea) usually improve because of the declining pulmonary blood flow after the development of right-sided failure.

REFERENCES

1. Chen JTT, Behar VS, Morris JJ, et al. Correlation of roentgen findings with hemodynamic data in pure mitral stenosis. *AJR Am J Roentgenol* 1968;102:280–292.
2. Chen JTT, Capp MP, Johnsrude IS, et al. Roentgen appearance of pulmonary vascularity in the diagnosis of heart disease. *AJR Am J Roentgenol* 1971;112:559–570.
3. Chen JTT, Robinson AE, Goodrich FK, et al. Uneven distribution of pulmonary blood flow between left and right lungs in isolated valvular pulmonary stenosis. *Am J Roentgenol* 1969;107:343–350.
4. Elliott LP. Stage II: Physiologic stage of analysis. In: Taveras JM, Ferrucci JT, eds. *Radiology: diagnosis-imaging-intervention.* Philadelphia: Lippincott, 1987:86–87.
5. Milne ENC, Pistolesi M. *Reading the chest radiograph: a physiologic approach.* St. Louis: Mosby-Year Book, 1993:1–50.
6. Ravin CE, Greenspan RH, McLoud TC, et al. Redistribution of pulmonary blood flow secondary to pulmonary arterial hypertension. *Invest Radiol* 1980;15:29–33.
7. Baltaxe HA, Amplatz K. Normal chest roentgenogram in presence of large atrial septal defects. *AJR Am J Roentgenol* 1969;107:322–327.
8. Wojtowicz J. Some tomographic criteria for an evaluation of the pulmonary circulation. *Acta Radiol Diagn (Stockh)* 1964;2:215–224.
9. Burko H, Carwell G, Newman E. Size, locations and gravitational changes of normal upper lobe pulmonary veins. *AJR Am J Roentgenol* 1971;111:687–689.
10. Racz GB. Pulmonary blood in normal and abnormal states. *Surg Clin North Am* 1974;54:967–977.
11. Fraser RG, Pare JAP, Pare PD, Fraser RS, Genereux GP. The normal chest. In: *Diagnosis of diseases of the chest,* vol. 1, 3rd ed. Philadelphia: Saunders, 1988:71–83.
12. Fraser RG, Pare JAP, Pare PD, Fraser RS, Genereux GP. The normal chest. In: *Diagnosis of diseases of the chest,* vol. 1, 3rd ed. Philadelphia: Saunders, 1988:128–129.
13. West JB. Regional differences in gas exchange in the lung of erect man. *J Appl Physiol* 1962;17:893–898.
14. West JB. *Ventilation/blood flow and gas exchange,* 2nd ed. Oxford: Blackwell, 1972.
15. Remolina C, Khan A, Santiago TV, et al. Positional hypoxemia in unilateral lung disease. *N Engl J Med* 1981;304:523–525.
16. Seaton D, Lapp NL, Morgan WKC. Effect of body position on gas exchange after thoracotomy. *Thorax* 1979;34:518–522.
17. Ueda H, Iio M, Kaihara S. Determination of regional pulmonary blood flow in various cardiopulmonary disorders: study and application of macroaggregated albumin (MAA) labelled with [131]I (I). *Jpn Heart J* 1964;5:431–444.
18. Perloff JK, LeBauer EJ, Miall A, et al. Differential quantification of pulmonary arterial flow in left-to-right shunt atrial septal defect using 131 I macroaggregated albumin. *Am J Cardiol* 1969;23:132.
19. Nugent EW, Plauth WH, Edwards JE, et al. Congenital heart disease. In: Hurst, JW, ed. *The heart,* 6th ed. New York: McGraw Hill, 1985:655.
20. Friedberg CK. In: *Diseases of the heart.* Philadelphia: Saunders, 1966:670–671.
21. Fraser RG, Pare JAP, Pare PD, Fraser RS, Genereux GP. Diseases of the airways. In: *Diagnosis of diseases of the chest* vol. 3, 3rd ed. Philadelphia: Saunders, 1990:2177–2186.
22. Elliott LP. Axial cineangiography in congenital heart disease. In: Hipona FA, ed. *Heart: multiple imaging procedures,* vol. 5. New York: Grune & Stratton, 1983:13–54.
23. Palevsky HI, Pietra GG, Fishman AP. Pulmonary veno-occlusive disease and its response to vasodilator agents. *Am Rev Respir Dis* 1990;142:426–429.
24. Fleischner FG. The butterfly pattern of acute pulmonary edema. *Am J Cardiol* 1967;20:39–46.

Essentials of Cardiac Imaging,
James T. T. Chen,
Lippincott–Raven Publishers, Philadelphia © 1998.

CHAPTER 9

Radiographic Anatomy

James T. T. Chen

The heart and great vessels have three dimensions. To examine all aspects of the heart, a four-view cardiac series has been used for decades, at least during the initial investigation: posteroanterior (PA) view with barium, left lateral (lateral) view with barium, right anterior oblique (RAO) view at 45° with barium, and left anterior oblique (LAO) view at 60° without barium. The obvious reason for choosing the anterior and left lateral views is to minimize magnification and distortion of the image by putting the heart closer to the film cassette or the fluoroscopic image intensifier. All radiographs are taken with the patient in the upright position at a target-film distance of 6 feet (see **Chapter 2**). Normally the heart and great vessels are outlined by the air-filled lung. The inside of the heart cannot be differentiated except where the myocardium is separated from the pericardium by the radiolucent subepicardial fat stripe (see **Chapters 2 and 14**).

THE NORMAL HEART

PA View

The PA view is the most familiar and informative of all views. It is a definite advantage to interpret cardiac findings in the light of pulmonary vascularity, which is best appreciated in this orientation (see **Chapter 8**). Because of its reproducibility, this is also the view most suited to the assessment of cardiac size (see **Fig. 2-8**).

Along the right cardiac border, from top to bottom, are seen the superior vena cava, the right atrium, and occasionally the inferior vena cava. On the left side, from top to bottom, are the aortic arch, the pulmonary trunk, and the smooth transition from the left atrial appendage to the left ventricle (1,2) (Fig. 9-1). At the apex of the heart a triangular fat pad is frequently evident. The barium-filled esophagus runs straight through the middle of the chest, displaced slightly to the right side by the aortic arch (see **Fig. 2-1A**).

Department of Radiology, Duke University School of Medicine, Durham, North Carolina 27710, U.S.A.

Lateral View

The lateral view is almost always the companion of the PA radiograph. For the detection of pericardial disease and cardiovascular calcification this view is invaluable. The anterior border of the cardiovascular silhouette is formed by the right ventricle below and by the pulmonary trunk and the ascending aorta above. In the uppermost area, the faint images of the left brachiocephalic vein and superior vena cava are occasionally visible. The right ventricle abuts the anterior chest wall for one third to one half the distance from the diaphragm to the sternal angle (the angle of Louis). Above the right ventricle, the pulmonary trunk courses posteriorly and superiorly away from the sternum. Above the pulmonary trunk and ~3 cm posterior to the sternum, the ascending aorta forms an anteriorly convex density. This convex border can be followed deep down into the shadows of the pulmonary trunk and the heart by virtue of the subepicardial fat stripe overlying the aortic root (see **Chapter 19**).

The posterior border of the cardiovascular silhouette is formed by the aortic arch and the left pulmonary artery above, the left atrium and the lower lobe pulmonary veins in the middle, and the left ventricle and the inferior vena cava below (1–4) (Fig. 9-2). The barium-filled esophagus courses behind the heart, forming a more or less straight-lined passage except for an anterior indentation caused by the aortic arch (see **Fig. 2-1B**).

RAO View

The RAO view is a valuable adjunct to the standard right-angled projections just described. As the patient turns leftward 45° from the PA projection, each atrium is effectively separated from its corresponding ventricle. This is the only view in which the left atrium and the left ventricle do not overlap (1). When the heart enlarges, each chamber extends in a different direction; therefore, the RAO view is in effect

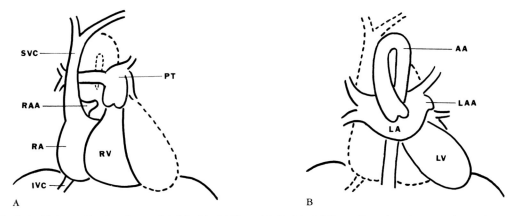

FIG. 9-1. Schematic drawings of right-sided (**A**) and left-sided (**B**) cardiac chambers and great vessels in PA view. AA, aortic arch; IVC, inferior vena cava; LA, left atrium; LAA, left atrial appendage; LV, left ventricle; PT, pulmonary trunk; RA, right atrium; RAA, right atrial appendage; RV, right ventricle; SVC, superior vena cava.

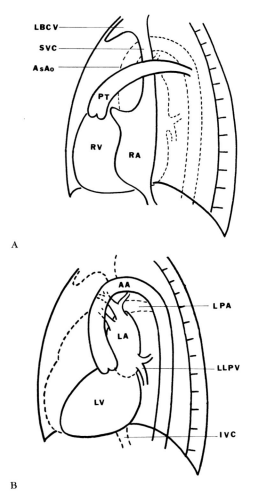

FIG. 9-2. Schematic drawings of right-sided (**A**) and left-sided (**B**) cardiac chambers and great vessels in lateral view. AsAo, ascending aorta; LBCV, left brachiocephalic vein; LLPV, lower-lobe pulmonary veins; LPA, left pulmonary artery. For other abbreviations see Fig. 9-1.

a four-chambered view (see the section entitled ''The Enlarged Heart'').

The anterior (left) border of the cardiovascular silhouette is formed, from top to bottom, by the ascending aorta, the pulmonary trunk, and the right and left ventricles. The posterior (right) border of the silhouette is formed, from top to bottom, by the superior vena cava, the descending aorta, the azygos vein at the right tracheobronchial junction, and the left and right atria (Fig. 9-3). With a standard degree of obliquity, the posterior border of the heart is shifted more anteriorly and becomes parallel to the spine with the air-containing lung positioned between (3,5). The barium-filled esophagus runs behind the cardiovascular silhouette and is displaced posteriorly by the aortic arch. The aorta folds on itself in this view and is difficult to evaluate (see **Fig. 2-1C**).

LAO View

The LAO view is ideal for evaluating the aorta, which is seen in its entirety. This view is also effective in distinguishing right ventricular enlargement from that on the left. In detecting left coronary artery calcification, the LAO view is also the projection of choice. The anterior (right) border of the cardiovascular silhouette is formed (from top to bottom) by the right brachiocephalic vein, the superior vena cava, the ascending aorta, the right atrial appendage, and the right ventricle. The posterior (left) border of the cardiovascular silhouette is formed (from top to bottom) by the left subclavian artery, the aortic arch, the left pulmonary artery, the left atrium, and the left ventricle (Fig. 9-4). To see the left atrial border clearly through the aortic window (a clear space below the aortic arch with the tracheal bifurcation astride the left atrium), a barium meal is usually omitted before this projection (3,5). When the aorta is being evaluated, however,

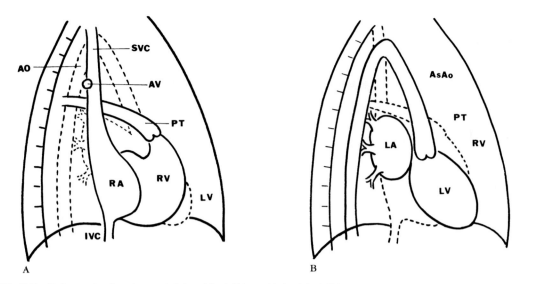

FIG. 9-3. Schematic drawings of right-sided (**A**) and left-sided (**B**) cardiac chambers in RAO view. AO, aorta; AsAo, ascending aorta; AV, azygos vein. For other abbreviations see Fig. 9-1.

barium should be given to outline the aortic arch and the anteromedial border of the descending aorta (see **Fig. 2-1D**).

THE ENLARGED HEART

As the heart enlarges, the cardiothoracic ratio will first exceed the average of 0.45 (6) (see **Fig. 2-8**). When the ratio becomes greater than 0.50, major cardiomegaly is generally present. Isolated chamber enlargement is uncommon. For the sake of clarity, however, each chamber and its vessels are described separately.

Right Atrial Enlargement

The right atrium enlarges primarily to the right side and posteriorly. Its size is best appreciated in the PA and RAO views.

PA View

In adults, the right atrium is enlarged when the right cardiac border is >5.5 cm from the midline (7) (Fig. 9-5). Right atrial enlargement is associated with greater dilatation of

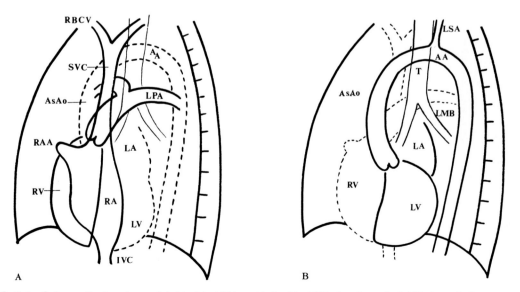

FIG. 9-4. Schematic drawings of right-sided (**A**) and left-sided (**B**) structures in LAO view. AsAo, ascending aorta; LMB, left main bronchus; LPA, left pulmonary artery; LSA, left subclavian artery; RBCV, right brachiocephalic vein; T, trachea. For other abbreviations see Fig. 9-1.

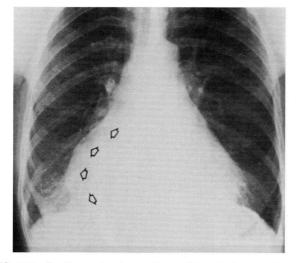

FIG. 9-5. Radiograph of a patient with mitral stenosis and tricuspid insufficiency. The right atrium is markedly enlarged (*arrows*). The right cardiac border is 10 cm to the right of the midline.

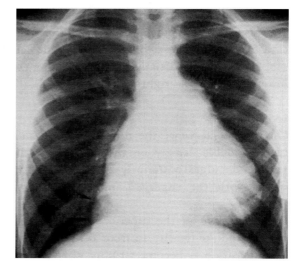

FIG. 9-7. PA view of a child with severe valvular pulmonary stenosis and tricuspid insufficiency shows aneurysmal dilatation of the inferior vena cava (*arrows*).

the inferior than the superior vena cava because of gravity. Enlargement of the superior vena cava causes a bandlike density (Fig. 9-6) or a lateral bulge in the right superior mediastinum (see **Fig. 2-13**). Enlargement of the inferior vena cava produces a lateral bulge in the right cardiophrenic sulcus partly superimposed on the lower border of the right atrium (Fig. 9-7).

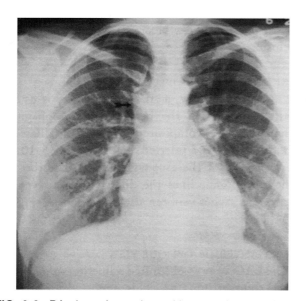

FIG. 9-6. PA view of a patient with secundum atrial septal defect and partial anomalous pulmonary venous connection from the right-upper lobe to the superior vena cava. Note dilatation of the superior vena cava (*arrow*) and increased pulmonary vasculature.

Lateral View

On the lateral view, the dilated right atrium casts a double density on the left side of the heart and bulges posteriorly and downward to merge with the engorged inferior vena cava (Fig. 9-8). Enlargement of the superior vena cava may cast a bandlike density in front of the trachea. This density may become striking when the dilated superior vena cava is superimposed on a left vertical vein or on a persistent left superior vena cava, as is commonly seen in total or partial anomalous pulmonary venous connections (see **Fig. 2-13**). A posteriorly convex contour of the inferior vena cava is suggestive of its dilatation. However, this sign by itself is not diagnostic unless the vessel has reached an aneurysmal dimension (Fig. 9-9). When in doubt, one should look for other signs of systemic venous overload in at least one more view.

RAO View

On the RAO view, a triangular density is usually seen behind the barium-filled esophagus, representing a composite shadow of the dilated right atrium and inferior vena cava (Fig. 9-10). The course of the esophagus is not disturbed, however. Sometimes the dilated superior vena cava and azygos vein can also be delineated (Fig. 9-11).

LAO View

The LAO view is of limited value in evaluating the right atrium, which is almost completely hidden in the middle of the cardiac silhouette. The right atrial appendage may form

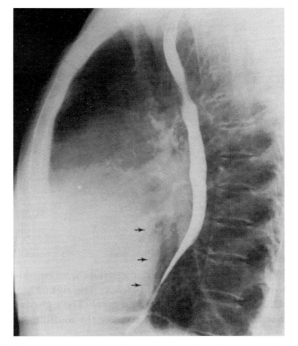

FIG. 9-8. Lateral view of a patient with mitral stenosis and tricuspid insufficiency whose PA view is shown in Fig. 9-5. The markedly dilated right atrium casts a double density (*arrows*) on the left side of the heart and bulges posteriorly and inferiorly to merge with the image of the engorged inferior vena cava.

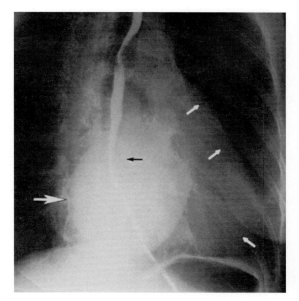

FIG. 9-10. RAO view of the patient with severe tricuspid insufficiency (TI), whose PA and lateral views are shown in Figs. 9-5 and 9-8, respectively. Note the markedly dilated right atrium and inferior vena cava forming a triangular density (*large white arrow*) behind the barium-filled esophagus. The left atrium is enlarged, displacing the barium-filled esophagus (*black arrow*). The pulmonary trunk and right ventricle (*upper white arrows*) are enlarged in the superolateral direction. The left ventricle (*lower white arrow*) is not enlarged, and the left costophrenic sulcus is not encroached on.

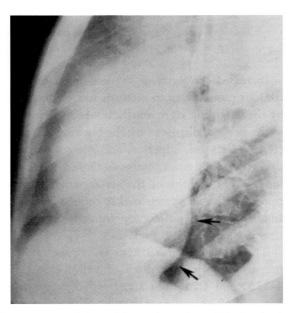

FIG. 9-9. Lateral view of the patient whose PA view is shown in Fig. 9-7. Note the aneurysmal dilatation of the inferior vena cava (*arrows*).

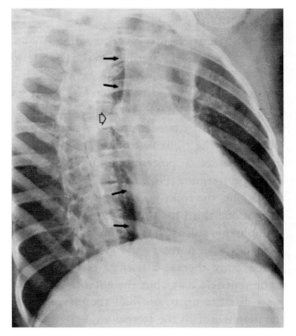

FIG. 9-11. RAO view of a patient with a right atrial myxoma shows dilatation of superior vena cava (*upper black arrows*), the azygos vein (*hollow arrow*), and the right atrium–inferior vena cava complex (*lower black arrows*).

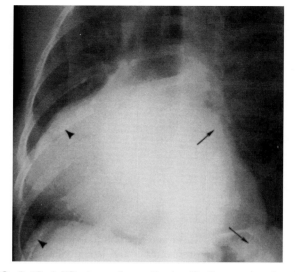

FIG. 9-12. LAO view of a patient with three-valve insufficiency whose PA view is shown in Fig. 2-7. This view shows a shelflike projection (*upper arrowhead*) from the upper anterior border representing a markedly enlarged right atrial appendage. The lower arrowhead points to multiple Kerley's B lines. The upper arrow points to the dilated left atrium, and the lower arrow points to the dilated left ventricle.

a shelflike convexity over the upper anterior cardiac border only when the right atrium is enormous (Fig. 9-12). The caval system is also obscured on the LAO view.

Right Ventricular Enlargement

The right ventricle enlarges primarily in the anterior, superior, and leftward directions. As the chamber continues to dilate, it also expands backward because of the confining sternum in front.

PA View

The right ventricle is normally not border-forming in this projection. In the early stages of right ventricular enlargement, only secondary signs are noted: dilatation of the pulmonary trunk, increased convexity of the left-upper cardiac contour, and an upturned cardiac apex. Dilatation of the pulmonary trunk is a reliable secondary sign of right ventricular enlargement (see **Fig. 8-1**) except for the following conditions: idiopathic dilatation of the pulmonary trunk without right ventricular enlargement, tetralogy of Fallot with right ventricular enlargement and a hypoplastic pulmonary trunk, and patent ductus arteriosus before the development of Eisenmenger physiology, when the pulmonary trunk is dilated but the right ventricle is not.

Increased convexity of the left-upper cardiac contour results from an intrinsic torque initiated by the enlarging right ventricle. As the left side of the heart is displaced by the

big right ventricle in the leftward, superior, and posterior directions, the whole heart rotates to the left along its long axis. In addition, the accompanying rotation of the great vessels makes the aorta appear smaller and the pulmonary trunk bigger than they actually are (see **Figs. 2-3** and 9-7). An upturned cardiac apex is frequently seen in patients with tetralogy of Fallot (see **Fig. 8-23A**) and secundum atrial septal defect (see **Fig. 2-3**). The upturned apex actually represents the normal left ventricular apex, which is markedly displaced by the enlarged right ventricle in the leftward, backward, and upward directions. In extreme cases, the left cardiac border may be formed by the huge right ventricle (see **Figs. 2-6** and **7-4B**).

Lateral View

The right ventricle first enlarges anteriorly and superiorly behind the sternum in the lateral projection. Consequently, the anterior cardiac border becomes taller and more convex. With few exceptions, the pulmonary trunk also dilates, forming a convex border on top of, but inseparable from, the right ventricle. The pulmonary trunk pursues a posterosuperior course away from the sternum (Fig. 9-13A). Under normal conditions, the right ventricle should be no taller than one-third the distance from the anterior costophrenic sulcus to the angle of Louis. With a smaller than normal anteroposterior diameter of the bony thorax, a normal but compressed right ventricle may abut the anterior chest wall for a distance up to one half that from the diaphragm to the sternal angle.

RAO View

On the RAO view the right ventricle and the pulmonary trunk enlarge in an anterosuperior direction, forming a single convexity along the upper two thirds of the anterior cardiac border (Fig. 9-14). The lower third of the border, which is occupied by the left ventricle, remains normal. The left costophrenic sulcus is preserved as long as the left ventricle is not enlarged. The only effect of right ventricular enlargement on the barium-filled esophagus is a deeper and longer anterior indentation by the aortic arch, which is displaced posteriorly.

LAO View

On the LAO view the two ventricles are effectively separated, with the right ventricle in front and the left one behind. Enlargement of the right ventricle causes anterior and superior expansion of the anterior cardiac border. The normal left ventricle is displaced posteriorly and superiorly, causing the posterior cardiac border to tilt upward. Occasionally, a notch may be seen between the enlarged right ventricle and the displaced left ventricle, marking the site of the lowermost

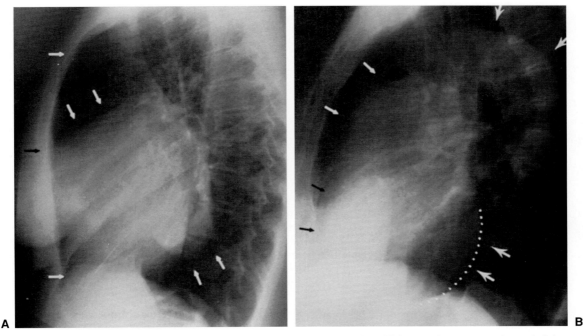

A   **B**

FIG. 9-13. A: The lateral view of a patient with severe mitral insufficiency shows an enlarged right ventricle, which is longer than one half the distance from the diaphragm (*lower horizontal arrow*) to the angle of Louis (*upper horizontal arrow*). The black horizontal arrow marks the top of the right ventricle. The dilated pulmonary trunk courses superiorly and posteriorly (*upper oblique arrows*). The lower oblique arrows point to a large pulmonary vein varix. **B:** The lateral view of a patient with patent ductus arteriosus shows that the pulmonary trunk (*upper small arrows*), the aorta (*upper large arrows*), and the left ventricle (*lower large arrows*) are enlarged. The right ventricle (*black arrows*) remains normal in size and contour.

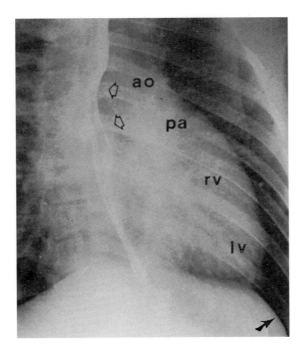

FIG. 9-14. RAO view of a patient with an atrial septal defect shows a bulging upper anterior cardiac border owing to the enlarged pulmonary trunk (pa) and right ventricle (rv). The lower anterior cardiac border, which is formed from the left ventricle (lv), remains normal. The left costophrenic sulcus (*solid arrow*) is undisturbed. The aorta (ao) is inconspicuous as a border-forming structure. The aortic arch is displaced posteriorly by the enlarged right ventricle, thereby causing a deeper and longer indentation on the barium-filled esophagus (*open arrows*).

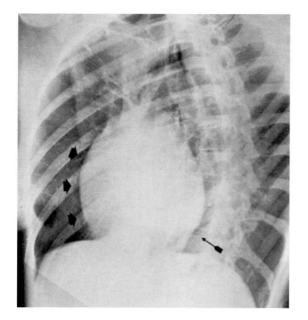

FIG. 9-15. LAO view of a patient with mitral and tricuspid stenoses shows an anterior bulge of an enlarged right ventricle (*short arrows*). The posterior border of the heart is divided by a notch (*long arrow*) representing the lowermost part of the interventricular septum. The portion of the cardiac contour above the notch is the displaced left ventricle, and the contour below is the enlarged right ventricle.

extremity of the interventricular septum (Fig. 9-15). The pulmonary trunk is invisible in this projection.

Left Atrial Enlargement

The radiographic signs of left atrial enlargement are most familiar to the diagnostician. Since the left atrium is a midline structure, its evaluation is greatly facilitated by the use of barium.

PA View

The classic signs of left atrial enlargement on the PA view are a double density (see **Fig. 2-16**) within the right cardiac contour, widening of the subcarinal angle to >75° (see **Fig. 2-17**), a bulge along the left cardiac border below the pulmonary trunk (see **Figs. 2-17** and **2-20**), and deviation of the barium-filled esophagus to the right (see **Fig. 2-22A**) as well as deviation of the descending aorta to the left (see **Fig. 2-20**). In extreme enlargement, the left atrium, with its accompanying right superior pulmonary vein, may form the right cardiac border (see **Fig. 2-20**). The double density within the cardiac contour in this case represents the enlarged right atrium, which is connected to the superior vena cava. Furthermore, in the presence of a giant left atrium, the esophagus may not be long enough to follow the right border of the atrium in the usual manner; instead, it simply flops to the left side of the chamber (see **Fig. 2-20**). This condition has been termed esophageal escape. Cephalization of the pulmonary vascularity almost always accompanies major left atrial enlargement. Occasionally, a pulmonary varix or prominent pulmonary venous confluence may be found in the right medial lung zone ~3 cm below the hilum (see **Fig.**

8-22 D, E, F). This is most commonly seen in patients with chronic severe rheumatic mitral insufficiency.

Lateral View

Left atrial enlargement causes a localized posterior deviation of the barium-filled esophagus (or the nasogastric tube)

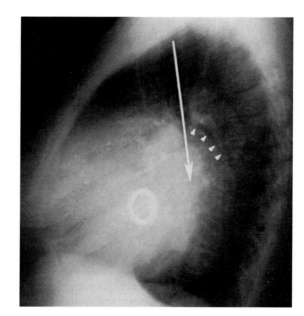

FIG. 9-16. Lateral view of a patient with recurrent severe mitral insufficiency. A disk valve is seen in the mitral position. The huge left atrium displaces the left-lower-lobe bronchus posteriorly and superiorly (arrowheads) forming a 35° angle with the axis of the trachea (*long arrow*). Compare with the PA view shown in Fig. 2-20.

below the carina (see **Fig. 2-22B**). In the absence of barium, the left-lower-lobe bronchus is displaced posteriorly and superiorly out of its normal alignment with the trachea (Fig. 9-16). The superior pulmonary veins are usually enlarged and best seen superior and anterior to the hilum. The inferior pulmonary veins or their confluences may form a rounded opacity below the hilum between the heart and the spine. Frequently this is also the site of a pulmonary varix (see **Figs. 8-22** and **9-13A**).

RAO View

On the RAO view, the enlarged left atrium casts a posterior bulge immediately below the carina. Consequently, the clear space normally present between the heart and the spine is obliterated. The barium-filled esophagus (or the nasogastric tube) is deviated posteriorly, and the subcarinal angle is widened by the dilated left atrium (Fig. 9-17).

LAO View

The left atrial enlargement is manifest by a posterior and superior bulge below the tracheal bifurcation. Consequently, the left mainstem bronchus is elevated and compressed (Fig.

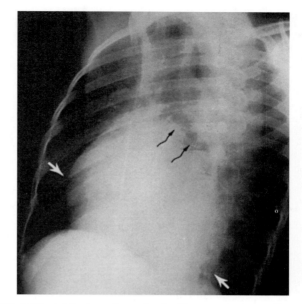

FIG. 9-18. LAO view of a patient with coronary heart disease and mitral insufficiency shows elevation and compression of the left mainstem bronchus by the enlarged left atrium (*black arrows*). The upper white arrow points to the enlarged right ventricle, the lower one to the enlarged left ventricle.

9-18; see also **Fig. 2-37**). In patients with mitral stenosis, a notch is usually visible between the dilated left atrium and the normal left ventricle (Fig. 9-19).

Left Ventricular Enlargement

The left ventricle enlarges primarily in the leftward, inferior, and posterior directions.

PA View

On the PA view, enlargement of the left ventricle causes a varying degree of prominence of the left-lower cardiac contour, depending on the underlying pathophysiology. In a patient with pressure overload, there may be only mild cardiomegaly with increased convexity of the apex. When volume overload is present, the heart extends markedly inferiorly and to the left. In fact, the cardiac apex usually protrudes below the diaphragm and compresses the gastric bubble (see **Fig. 2-9**). When the left ventricle is enormous, it may displace the right atrium laterally, giving a false appearance of right atrial enlargement (Fig. 9-20). Dilatation and tortuosity of the aorta is frequently, but not always, associated with left ventricular enlargement. Aortic insufficiency, systemic hypertension, and atherosclerosis cause generalized dilatation of the aorta; aortic stenosis and ascending aortic aneurysms (Fig. 9-20) cause localized dilatation of

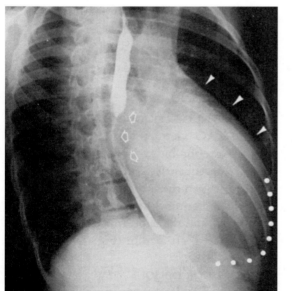

FIG. 9-17. The RAO view of a patient with severe coronary heart disease shows a posterior bulge (the enlarged left atrium) of the heart immediately below the carina. Consequently, the clear space between the heart and spine is obliterated, and the esophagus is displaced posteriorly at the same level (*open arrows*). The arrowheads mark the convex border of the enlarged right ventricle and pulmonary trunk. The dotted line marks the lower border of the enlarged left ventricle, which typically obliterates the left costophrenic sulcus.

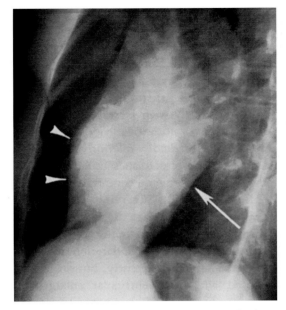

FIG. 9-19. The LAO view of a patient with mitral stenosis shows a notch (*long arrow*) along the posterior cardiac border. The bulge above the notch represents the dilated left atrium; the relatively flat cardiac border below the notch is the posterior wall of the normal left ventricle. *Arrowheads* point to the enlarged right ventricle.

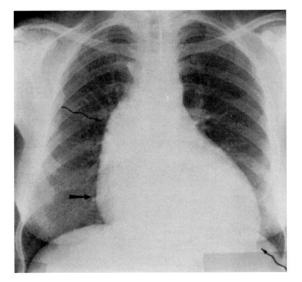

FIG. 9-20. Film of a patient with Marfan's syndrome, severe aortic insufficiency, and ascending aortic aneurysm (*thin arrow on the right*). The left ventricle is markedly enlarged (*thin arrow on the left*), displacing the normal right atrium (*thick arrow*) laterally. This film should not be interpreted as right atrial enlargement.

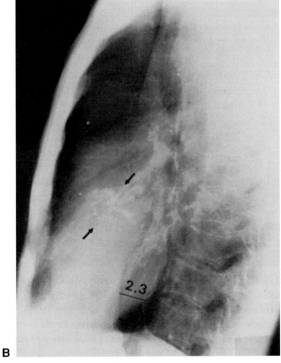

A

B

FIG. 9-21. A: Lateral view of a patient with cardiomyopathy. The enlarged left ventricle extends posteroinferiorly to compress the gastric air bubble (*arrows*). **B:** Lateral view of another patient with aortic stenosis. The left ventricle extends 2.3 cm (normally <1.8 cm) behind the inferior vena cava at a level 2 cm cephalad to the crossing point of the two structures; hence there is a positive Hoffman–Rigler sign for left ventricular enlargement. *Arrows* mark calcified valve.

the ascending aorta. When the aorta is diffusely enlarged (see **Fig. 2-9**), it buckles laterally on both sides with dilatation of all the brachiocephalic branches. Ascending aortic dilatation produces only a unilateral bulge on the right side above the right atrium (see **Fig. 2-11**). A dilated ascending aorta tends to displace the superior vena cava laterad.

Lateral View

The left ventricle enlarges posteriorly and inferiorly in the lateral projection (see Fig. 9-13B). It impinges on the gastric bubble and forms a semicircular opacity behind the inferior vena cava (Fig. 9-21A). Here a semiquantitative measurement of left ventricular size can be made according to Hoffman and Rigler (4). From the crossing point between the inferior vena cava and the left ventricle, a 2-cm line is drawn upward along the inferior vena cava. At this level another line is drawn parallel to the horizontal planes of the vertebral bodies. The distance between the inferior vena cava and the posterior border of the left ventricle normally should not exceed 1.8 cm (Fig. 5-21B). This measurement is generally reliable except under three conditions: a markedly rotated lateral view, the presence of a pectus excavatum, and the presence of predominantly right-sided cardiomegaly.

The barium-filled esophagus on the lateral view is not indented or pushed out of the way by the enlarged left ventricle, which simply casts a shadow behind the barium column. When the aorta is enlarged and uncoiled, as found in patients with aortic insufficiency and systemic hypertension, it can be seen almost in its entirety in the lateral projection. In patients with aortic stenosis or ascending aortic aneurysm, the dilated ascending aorta is clearly delineated in the retrosternal area above the normal right ventricle.

RAO View

Left ventricular enlargement is manifested by a leftward and downward protrusion of the heart, which obliterates the left costophrenic sulcus and compresses the gastric bubble (see Fig. 9-17). Evaluation of the aorta is difficult on the RAO view because of its foreshortened image. The superior mediastinum does widen, however, in the presence of severe dilatation of the aorta.

LAO View

The left ventricle enlarges backward and downward, overlapping the spine and depressing the gastric bubble in the LAO view (Fig. 9-22). Failure of the heart to clear the spine alone, however, does not always denote left ventricular enlargement. False positives are known to occur in patients with a narrow anteroposterior diameter of the chest or with a markedly dilated right ventricle. When the right ventricle is normal, the anterior border of the heart remains flat in contrast to the protruding posterior border of left ventricular enlargement (Fig. 9-22).

On this view the aortic arch is projected in profile, and all segments of the aorta are clearly delineated (Fig. 9-22). The LAO projection is particularly effective in assessing the aortic arch and the descending aorta when barium (or nasogastric tube) is present in the esophagus. The posterolateral wall of the descending aorta is outlined by air-filled lung, and the anteromedial wall is profiled by the barium-filled esophagus. Any deviation from the normal parallelism of the two walls (Fig. 9-22) will indicate disease, most notably an aneurysm or dissection of the descending aorta (Fig. 9-23).

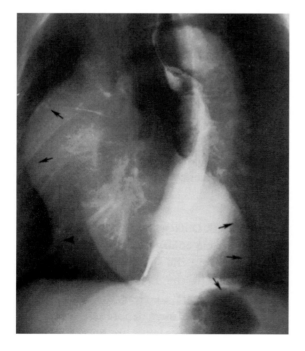

FIG. 9-22. LAO view of a patient with severe systemic hypertension and an ascending aortic aneurysm. The left ventricle protrudes posteroinferiorly (*lower arrows*). The right ventricular border is flat (*arrowheads*). The ascending aorta is aneurysmal (*upper arrows*). The aortic arch and the descending aorta are enlarged to a lesser extent; their anteromedial wall is outlined by the barium-filled esophagus and their posterolateral wall by the air-filled lung. The two walls are normally parallel.

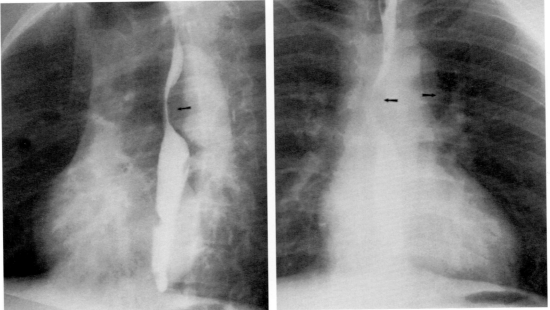

FIG. 9-23. Radiographs of a 30-year-old man with transection of the descending aorta. In the LAO view (**A**) there is loss of parallelism of the two walls of the aorta, and the barium-filled esophagus is deviated anteriorly, medially, and inferiorly (*arrow*) by the traumatic false aneurysm. The PA view (**B**) shows that the aneurysm expands both medially and laterally (*arrows*).

REFERENCES

1. Netter FH. *Heart: the Ciba collection of medical illustrations*, vol. 5. Summit, N.J.: Ciba Corporation, 1969:22–33.
2. Grollman JH. Conventional and digital angiography of the heart. In: Putman CE, Ravin CE, eds. *Textbook of diagnostic imaging*, 2nd ed. Philadelphia: Saunders, 1994:1675–1691.
3. Chen JTT. Chest radiography and cardiac fluoroscopy. In: Putman CE, Ravin CE, eds. *Textbook of diagnostic imaging*, 2nd ed. Philadelphia: Saunders, 1994:1643–1658.
4. Hoffman RB, Rigler LG. Evaluation of left ventricular enlargement in the lateral projection of the chest. *Radiology* 1965;85: 93–100.
5. Crummy AB. The cardiovascular system. In: Juhl JH, Crummy AB, eds. *Essentials of radiologic imaging*, 6th ed. Philadelphia: Lippincott, 1993: 1065–1138.
6. Keats TE. *Atlas of roentgenographic measurement*, 6th ed. St. Louis: Mosby Year Book, 1990:170–175.
7. Meszaros WT. *Cardiac roentgenology*. Springfield, Ill.: Thomas, 1969: 36–74.

Essentials of Cardiac Imaging,
James T. T. Chen,
Lippincott–Raven Publishers, Philadelphia © 1998.

CHAPTER 10

Cardiovascular Calcifications

James T. T. Chen

Calcification of the soft tissues can be classified as metastatic or dystrophic. Metastatic calcification is caused by abnormal calcium metabolism with hypercalcemia, often stemming from increased mobilization of calcium from the bone. Dystrophic calcification results from tissue injury or degeneration, without hypercalcemia. Except at a microscopic level, metastatic calcification does not involve the cardiovascular system. The heart and vessels grossly calcify only under dystrophic conditions (1). For instance, calcification of the ascending aortic aneurysm in syphilitic aortitis represents the end result of injury to the media by the spirochetes (see discussion under Calcification of the Aorta). Deposition of calcium in the mitral annulus is caused by tissue degeneration in aging (2).

Most radiologically detected cardiovascular calcifications are of practical importance. Even a tiny piece of calcium in the coronary artery, barely detectable by fluoroscopy, indicates the presence of occlusive coronary artery disease in 94% of symptomatic patients (3). The extent of coronary calcification correlates well with the severity of coronary atherosclerosis (4,5). In patients with calcific valvular stenosis, the severity of stenosis parallels the amount of calcium deposited in the valve (6,7). For practical purposes, calcification of the mitral valve is diagnostic of rheumatic mitral stenosis (8). Simple closed mitral valvulotomy or balloon valvuloplasty is contraindicated in the presence of massive valvular calcification. Instead, open valve replacement under cardiopulmonary bypass is preferred (9). Large calcifications can be seen on radiography; small ones, however, require a close scrutiny of the heart for their detection by fluoroscopy, digital subtraction fluoroscopy, computed tomography (CT) or electron beam CT (3,4,10–13). Electron beam CT (13) is the most sensitive tool for the detection of small cardiovascular calcifications (see **Chapter 3**).

Department of Radiology, Duke University School of Medicine, Durham, North Carolina 27710, U.S.A.

CARDIAC CALCIFICATION

All peripheral cardiac calcifications are not pericardial in origin. Fortunately, each type of cardiac calcification has a predilection for certain anatomic sites. Therefore, by noting the distribution of calcium deposits one can usually differentiate one from another.

Pericardial Calcification

Calcification of the pericardium represents the end result of inflammation or trauma. The more common causes include viral, tuberculous, pyogenic, and traumatic pericarditides. The presence of calcium in the pericardium strongly suggests either constrictive pericarditis (Fig. 10-1) or constrictive-effusive pericarditis. The incidence of calcification with constrictive pericarditis is 50% to 70% (8,14). However, the heart may function normally in 5% to 10% of patients with pericardial calcification (14) (Fig. 10-2).

Deposition of calcium in the pericardium tends to be more abundant on the right side and anteriorly than on the left side and posteriorly. The atrioventricular grooves and the diaphragmatic border of the heart are also fertile ground for pericardial calcification (15). The left atrium and the left ventricular apex are usually spared from encasement or calcification (14,15) (Fig. 10-1-3). The left atrium is spared, mainly because of its lack of pericardial investment and its incoming pulmonary veins. The reason for the lack of calcium over the left ventricular apex is unknown. It is conceivable that calcification is largely prevented by the vigorous apical motility. Conversely, more abundant calcification is allowed, perhaps, by the lower motility over the right side of the heart (15).

Myocardial Calcification

Calcification of the myocardium occurs in ~8% of patients after an episode of myocardial infarction (16). There are sev-

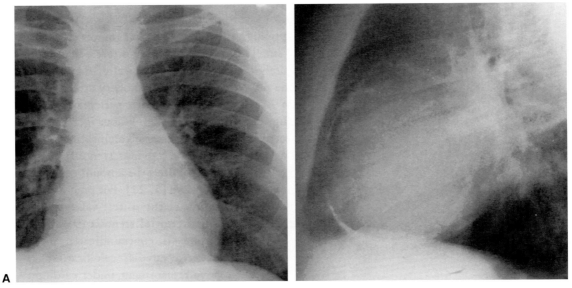

FIG. 10-1. Radiographs of a patient with calcific constrictive pericarditis showing a peculiar contour of the cardiac silhouette and mild cephalization of pulmonary vasculature on the posteroanterior view (**A**) and heavy calcification of the pericardium on the lateral view (**B**).

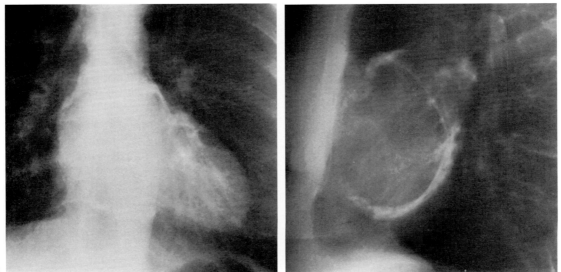

FIG. 10-2. Posteroanterior (**A**) and lateral (**B**) radiographs of a patient with heavy calcification primarily in the right and left atrioventricular grooves stemming from viral pericarditis. The patient was entirely asymptomatic, and there was no evidence of pericardial constriction.

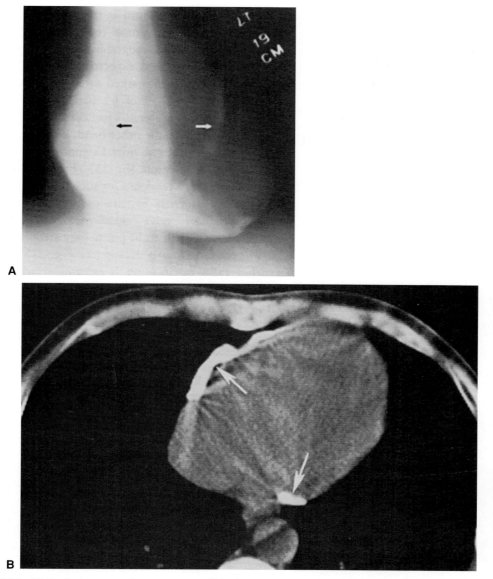

FIG. 10-3. Anteroposterior tomogram (**A**) of a patient with heavy pericardial calcification primarily on the right side of the heart, sparing the left ventricular apex. Note calcium in the right (*black arrow*) and left (*white arrow*) atrioventricular grooves. CT scan (**B**) of another, similar patient shows heavy calcium deposits in both atrioventricular grooves (*arrows*) (courtesy of Dr. Paul Silverman).

eral common features of myocardial calcification (16,17): (a) the infarct tends to be sizable (Fig. 10-4), (b) it most frequently involves the anterolateral and/or apical aspect of the left ventricle (17), as a result of anterior descending coronary artery obstruction (Figs. 10-4 and 10-5), (c) the calcium is usually present in the wall of a ventricular aneurysm, (d) survival is usually >6 years, (e) it predominates among men, and (f) most patients have a right coronary arterial preponderance, which favors a longer survival period.

The contour of myocardial calcification is usually curvilinear, consistent with a location peripheral to an area of necrosis. The calcium is almost always in the wall of a left ventricular aneurysm. However, if shaggy and laminated de-

posits are seen, one should consider the possibility of associated calcification of mural thrombi (Fig. 10-4). Coarse and amorphous myocardial calcifications are rare and have non-atherosclerotic causes, for example, trauma, cardioversion, infection, and endocardial fibrosis (8). Deposition of calcium is uncommon in inferior and posterior wall left ventricular aneurysms.

Valvular Calcification

Radiographic demonstration of calcium in a cardiac valve uniquely indicates the presence of valvular stenosis as the

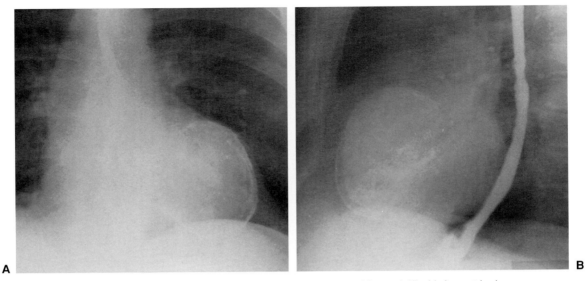

A   B

FIG. 10-4. Posteroanterior (**A**) and lateral (**B**) views of patient with a calcified left ventricular aneurysm in the most common (anterolateral–apical) location. Calcium is seen over the entire circumference of the aneurysm. The laminated contour of the calcium is suggestive of associated calcification of the mural thrombi.

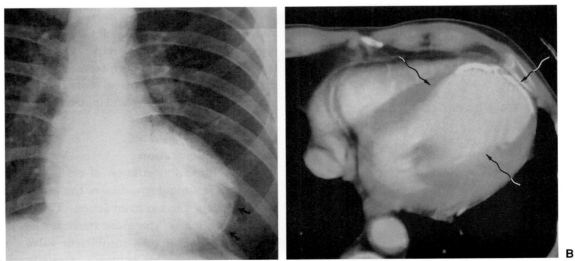

A   B

FIG. 10-5. Posteroanterior radiograph (**A**) reveals an autopsy-proved, partially calcified left ventricular aneurysm (*arrows*). Note the meager soft-tissue exterior to the calcium. Although lack of soft tissue outside the calcium has been considered evidence of pericardial calcification, its apical location militates against such a notion. Another patient's enhanced CT scan in systole (**B**) shows an akinetic and calcified apical left ventricular aneurysm (*arrows*).

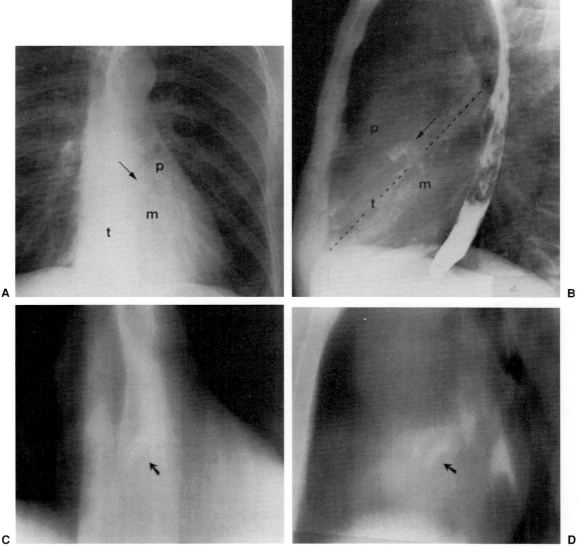

FIG. 10-6. A 50-year-old man had angina pectoris and presyncopal attacks. On the posteroanterior (**A**) and lateral (**B**) views, there is heavy calcification of the bicuspid aortic valve (*arrow*). Otherwise, no definite abnormalities are noted. The positions of other valves in relation to the aortic valve are indicated by letters: p, pulmonary valve; m, mitral valve; t, tricuspid valve. The technique of separating the aortic valve from the mitral valve by a line (*broken line in B*) drawn between the left-upper-lobe bronchus and the anterior costophrenic angle is mostly effective. Anteroposterior (**C**) and lateral (**D**) tomograms of another patient with the same disease show calcium (*arrow*) in a bicuspid aortic valve. Note the poststenotic dilatation of the ascending aorta above and anterior to the calcified valve in D.

predominant lesion. The heavier the calcification is, the more stenotic the valve becomes (Fig. 10-6). An insufficient valve does not show radiographic evidence of calcification (18). An exception to the rule is exemplified by patients with calcific aortic stenosis complicated by infective endocarditis. In this circumstance, the valve is largely destroyed, except for the calcified portion. The end result is a combination of severe aortic insufficiency with a sizable mass of residual calcium at the valve.

Valvular calcification is most commonly seen in the aortic position. Radiographic evidence of aortic valve calcification is expected in patients >40 years old who have severe aortic stenosis. In an autopsy series, 59 of 61 patients with congenital aortic valve stenosis had considerable calcification (18). On the other hand, only half of the patients with severe mitral stenosis manifest valvular calcification (1,19) (Fig. 10-7). There is, however, a tendency for such lesions to calcify more frequently in patients >50 years old. Pulmonary valve calcification is rarely evident in patients with tight congenital pulmonary stenosis who live past the fourth decade (see **Fig. 7-5**). Tricuspid valve calcification is extremely unusual, perhaps because of the rarity of pure tricuspid stenosis and the

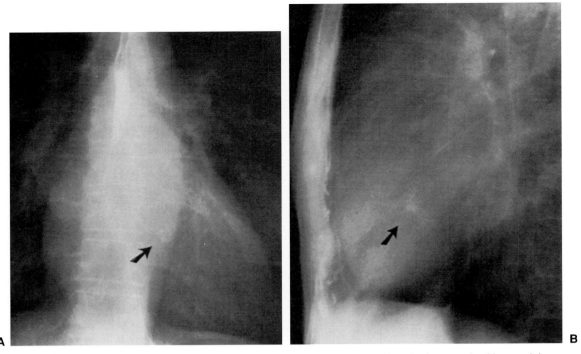

FIG. 10-7. Posteroanterior (**A**) and lateral (**B**) views of a patient with mitral stenosis. Note calcium (*arrow*) in the mitral valve.

low pressures exerted on the valve even in the presence of significant tricuspid stenosis.

The causes of valvular calcification vary with the site of the lesion and the age of the patient. Most aortic valve calcifications in patients aged ≤65 years stem from a congenital bicuspid valve (20), which is vulnerable to wear and tear resulting from tensions peculiar to the bicuspid arrangement (21). Because one cusp is larger than the other, a congenital bicuspid valve cannot open and close properly. Consequently, the valve is constantly traumatized, resulting in fibrosis, calcification, and stenosis. The average age when calcium is first detected in such valves is 25 years (21). A small percentage of patients <65 years old with calcific aortic stenosis may have a rheumatic origin of their disease. In this group, the average age when calcium is first noted in

the aortic valve is 47 years (21). In ~90% of the patients aged ≥65 years in the reported series (22–24), aortic valve calcification represented an aging process (i.e., atherosclerotic degeneration) of a normal tricuspid aortic valve. The average age at which calcium is first seen in these valves is 54 years (21) (Table 10-1). The time of clinical presentation of isolated aortic stenosis varies with differing etiologies: congenital forms appear at <30 years, rheumatic forms at 30–65 years; degenerative forms at >65 years (25) (Table 10-1).

Spindola-Franco and co-workers (26) have found the patterns of calcification to be valuable in diagnosing a bicuspid aortic valve. Twenty-six of 40 (65%) bicuspid valves were correctly recognized by plain film analysis. In contrast, only 10 of 40 (25%) were diagnosed by aortography. Among the

TABLE 10-1. *Major differences in three types of aortic valve stenosis*

	Congenital	Rheumatic	Degenerative
Clinically apparent	<30 years	30–60 years	>65 years
Ca^{++} first appearing	25 years	47 years	54 years
Ca^{++} on CxR			
40–65 years	>90%	<10%	
>65 years			>90%
Ca^{++} Contour^a	Nodular or bicuspid	Nodular	Nodular or tricuspid
Dilatation of AsAo	+ + +	+ + +	0
Diffuse aortic dilatation	0	0	+ + +

^{a} Lesser calcification is more likely to preserve the original bicuspid or tricuspid contour than greater calcification, which usually develops into a nodular form, a cluster of smaller deposits in one place.
Ca^{++}, calcification; CxR, chest radiograph; AsAo, ascending aorta.

common calcific patterns of a bicuspid valve are type 3, where both cusps and the raphe of the larger conjoined cusp are calcified (Fig. 10-8D), and type 5, where only the two cusps are calcified (Fig. 10-8B). When heavy calcification develops, the original bicuspid pattern of the valve will disappear, forming a nonspecific nodule (Fig. 10-8A). A nodular form of calcification represents the end point of all heavily calcified aortic valves—congenital, rheumatic, and degenerative (Table 10-1). Figure 10-9 shows the typical radiographic features of degenerative aortic stenosis in an elderly woman. The original well-formed tricuspid valve is outlined by relatively mild calcification. The thoracic aorta is uniformly dilated without disproportionate enlargement of the ascending aorta (Table 10-1).

Mitral valve calcification almost always represents the end stage of rheumatic valvulitis. One exception was encountered in a 14-year-old girl who had congenital calcific mitral valve stenosis (27). Pulmonary valve calcifications have been found exclusively in patients with congenital pulmonary stenosis (28,29). The gradient of the right ventricle to the pulmonary artery is usually >80 mm Hg. Most of these patients are >40 years old at the time of radiologic diagnosis. Less than 50% show evidence of healed bacterial endocarditis. Accordingly, both severity and chronicity of pulmonary stenosis are required for the development of calcification of the valve. The role of previous infective endocarditis in this regard is probably of lesser importance (28). Tricuspid valve calcification is extremely rare. It has been associated with rheumatic heart disease, septal defects, congenital tricuspid valve defects, and infective endocarditis.

Annular Calcification

The annuli, or valve rings, are the fibrous skeleton of the heart, to which the myocardial fibers attach and from which the cardiac valves are suspended. Calcification of the mitral annulus is a degenerative process associated with aging. It occurs most commonly in women >65 years old (2,30). In infants, the annuli are composed of parallel collagen fibers embedded in a clear ground substance. The collagen fibers gradually become swollen and lose their parallel arrangement from childhood through early adulthood. In the third decade of life, lipid deposits begin to make their appearance. By age 45, foci of calcification are evident in these areas (2,29,30).

Mitral annulus calcification is entirely different from mitral valve calcification, not only in terms of cause and age of appearance but with regard to radiologic appearance and clinical implications. The annular calcific deposits typically show a J, U, or reversed C-shaped opacity on radiographs. The density tends to be bandlike and of more uniform radiopacity (Fig. 10-10) than the nodular and more irregular opacity of mitral valve calcification (Fig. 10-7). In rare cases, mitral annulus calcification may form a complete circle, representing the most extensive variety of the lesion (31).

Usually, only the annulus of the posterior mitral leaflet calcifies. However, if deposition of calcium in the mitral annulus extends across the ventricular aspect of the anterior leaflet, an ''O'' configuration may develop. In most instances, calcium in the mitral annulus is believed to have little clinical importance. If the calcific deposits are massive, however, cardiac function may be impaired by the accompanying mitral insufficiency, atrial fibrillation, or conduction defects (2). Calcification of the aortic annulus is frequently seen with degenerative aortic valve calcification, because both entities are related to aging. In contrast, mitral annulus calcification is rarely associated with mitral valve calcification (8).

Tricuspid annulus calcification is rare and is usually associated with long-standing right ventricular hypertension (e.g., resulting from severe pulmonary stenosis) (29,32). Calcium in the tricuspid annulus forms a C configuration, which is anterior, inferior, and to the right of the mitral annulus (29). The presence of calcium in the tricuspid annulus may serve as a clue to the presence of valvular pulmonary stenosis. The tricuspid valve, on the other hand, is usually normal.

Another interesting aspect of annular calcification relates to the higher incidence of mitral than tricuspid involvement. In 1969, Rogers and co-workers (29) theorized that prolonged right ventricular hypertension was a major factor in the development of tricuspid annular calcification in four patients. Likewise, under normal conditions, only the mitral annulus is consistently under the influence of high left ventricular pressures, thus leading to the more frequent occurrence of mitral than tricuspid annulus calcification.

Interventricular Septal Calcification

Between the mitral and tricuspid annuli, there is a triangular fibrous area called the trigona fibrosa or the fibrous trigones. The fibrous trigones represent the basal segment of the interventricular septum, closely related to the bundle of His. When there is heavy calcification of the mitral annulus, the trigona fibrosa is occasionally involved, resulting in heart block. The degree of calcification of the trigones varies considerably. The calcific deposits may be quite small and radiographically invisible, or they may be gross, extending down to involve a large portion of the interventricular septum (8,29,33) (Fig. 10-11).

Left Atrial Wall Calcification

Calcification of the left atrium is frequently associated with a history of rheumatic fever, long-standing congestive heart failure, mitral stenosis, atrial fibrillation, mural thrombi, and systemic or pulmonary emboli or both (34). Early recognition of left atrial calcification is essential for treatment, particularly when surgery is contemplated.

Most authors believe that left atrial calcification is related to the severity of endocarditis associated with the initial or subsequent attacks of rheumatic heart disease. The calcium is usually deposited sheetlike in the endocardium and the underlying myocardium, following the contour of the left atrial wall. When the deposits are shaggy and laminated,

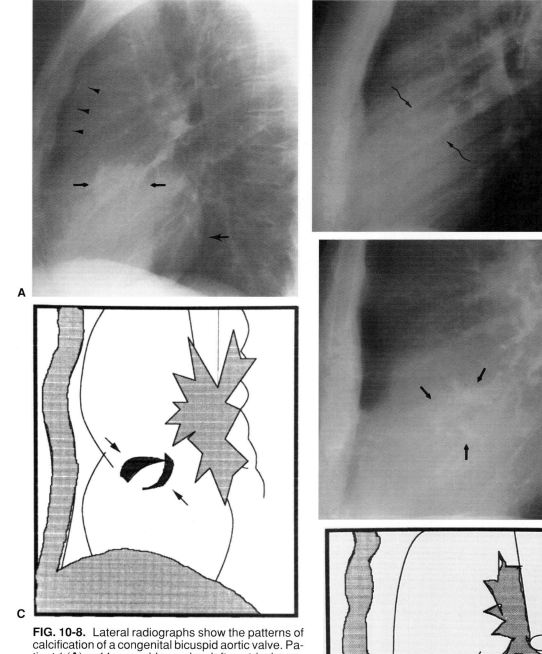

FIG. 10-8. Lateral radiographs show the patterns of calcification of a congenital bicuspid aortic valve. Patient 1 (**A**), a 44-year-old man, has left ventricular enlargement (*large arrow*) and diffuse calcification of the entire aortic valve (*small arrows*). The original bicuspid morphology has been erased by heavy calcification, and we may consider this to be the "nodular" type. Also note the isolated ascending aortic dilatation (*arrowheads*). Patient 2 (**B**), a 40-year-old woman, shows a definite bicuspid pattern (*opposing arrows*). The accompanying diagram (**C**) depicts the same pattern. Patient 3 (**D**), a 77-year-old man, shows an alternative pattern of bicuspid aortic valve, the "mushroom" type. The oblique arrows point to diffuse calcification of both cusps, and the vertical arrow points to the calcified raphe of the conjoined cusp. The accompanying diagram (**E**) depicts the same pattern.

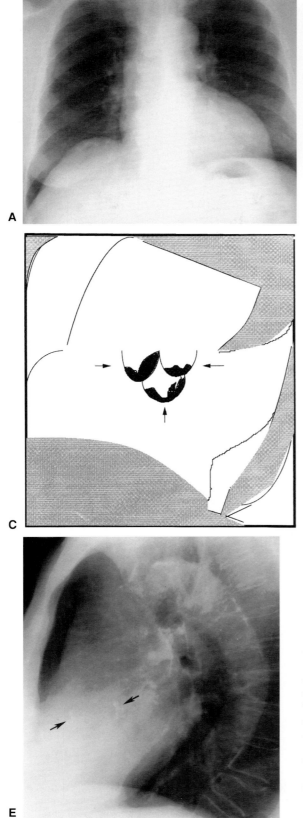

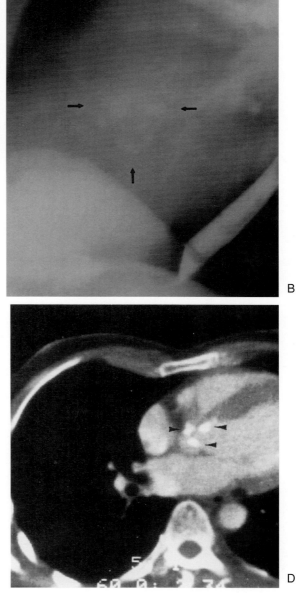

FIG. 10-9. Patients with degenerative aortic stenosis (AS). Posteroanterior radiograph (**A**) of patient 1, a 71-year-old woman, shows mild cardiomegaly with left ventricular hypertrophy and diffuse dilatation of the aorta. The lateral view (**B**) shows calcification of the normally formed tricuspid aortic valve (*arrows*). The accompanying diagram (**C**) depicts the same calcification. Electron beam CT of patient 2 (**D**) demonstrates discrete calcification of all three aortic cusps (*arrowheads*). The lateral view of patient 3 (**E**) shows curvilinear calcification of two of three cusps (*opposing arrows*). (The image in D was reproduced with permission from Stanford W, Rumberger JA. *Ultrafast computed tomography in cardiac imaging: principles and practice*. Mt. Kisco, N.Y.: Futura, 1992.)

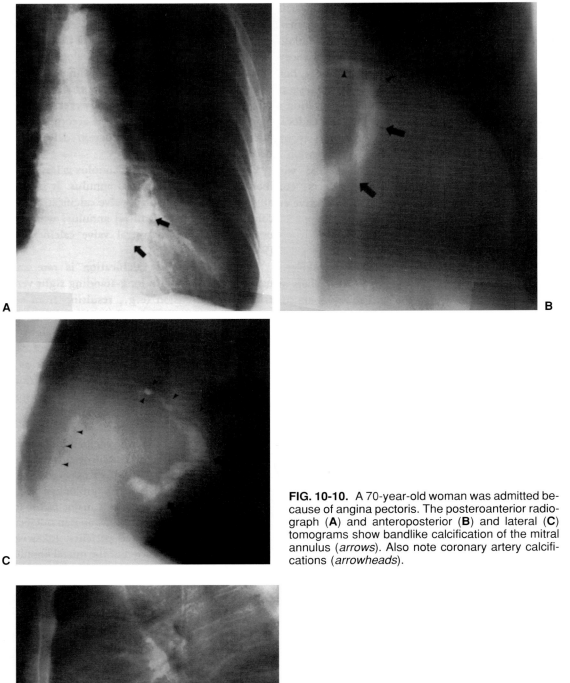

A

B

C

FIG. 10-10. A 70-year-old woman was admitted because of angina pectoris. The posteroanterior radiograph (**A**) and anteroposterior (**B**) and lateral (**C**) tomograms show bandlike calcification of the mitral annulus (*arrows*). Also note coronary artery calcifications (*arrowheads*).

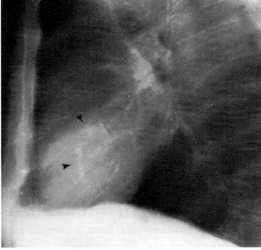

FIG. 10-11. Lateral view of an elderly man with aortic stenosis and heart block. Heavy calcification is seen in the aortic valve (*upper arrowhead*) and the interventricular septum (*lower arrowhead*).

associated calcification of the mural thrombi should be suspected. This calcification occurs infrequently, however. In one series (35), only three of 26 patients had histologic evidence of calcification in a thrombus.

A radiologic classification of left atrial calcification has been proposed (34) according to the dominant lesion in each group. In type A patients, the calcification is confined to the left atrial appendage, and the dominant lesion is likely to be a less severe mitral stenosis. As the lesion progresses, type A patients may show signs of type B disease, in which the free wall of the left atrium and the mitral valve are calcified in addition to the calcific left atrial appendage. Type B patients usually have advanced mitral stenosis (Fig. 10-12). In type C patients, the calcification is confined to the posterior

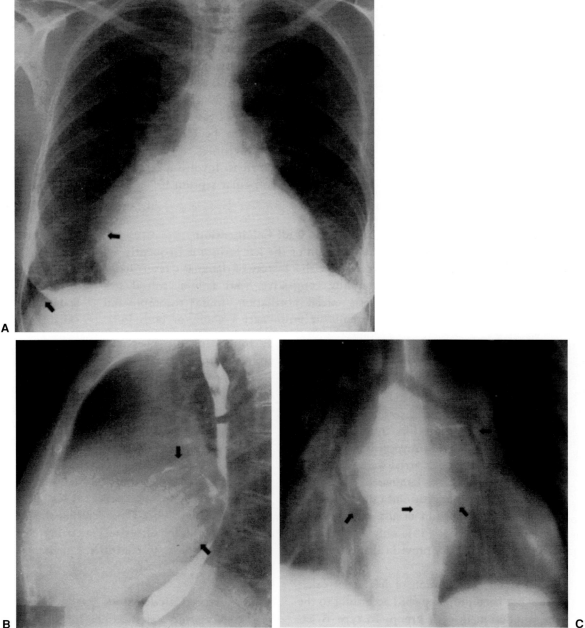

FIG. 10-12. Posteroanterior view (**A**) of a patient with severe rheumatic mitral stenosis and tricuspid insufficiency shows cephalization of the pulmonary vasculature; Kerley's B lines (*oblique arrow*); and left atrial, right atrial (*horizontal arrow*), and right ventricular enlargement. The lateral view (**B**) shows curvilinear calcifications (*arrows*) in the wall of the enlarged left atrium, which indent the barium-filled esophagus. An anteroposterior tomogram of another patient (**C**) shows a calcified left atrial wall (*oblique arrows*), left atrial appendage (*upper horizontal arrow*), and mitral valve (*lower horizontal arrow*).

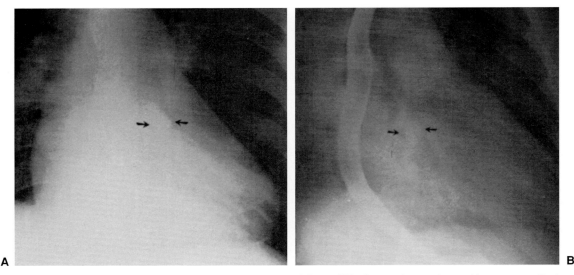

FIG. 10-13. Posteroanterior (**A**) and right anterior oblique (**B**) views of a patient with severe mitral insufficiency show a calcified MacCallum's patch (*arrows*) in the posterior wall of the left atrium.

wall of the left atrium as a result of a jet lesion inflicted by forceful regurgitant flow through an insufficient mitral valve. This jet lesion has been termed the MacCallum's patch (36) (Fig. 10-13).

The presence of left atrial wall calcification has profound clinical implications. First, patients are almost always in congestive heart failure with atrial fibrillation. Mural thrombi frequently form in the atria and become the source of systemic and pulmonary emboli. In that situation, long-term anticoagulant therapy is mandatory. Second, it is the radiologist's responsibility to inform the surgeon of the technical difficulties imposed by the presence of calcium in the left atrial wall. There are several possible surgical complications: (a) approach from the left side is likely to be difficult in closed mitral valvulotomy, (b) fatal intraoperative cerebral embolism is a real threat when the mural thrombi are dislodged, and (c) uncontrollable hemorrhage may occur when the operator has to work through a rigid wall of the chamber. Having been forewarned, the surgeon can usually circumvent the calcium by altering the approach to enter the left atrium through the noncalcified portion of the wall posterolaterally on the right side. The operation should always be done under direct vision, using cardiopulmonary bypass, to control the intracavitary clots.

Coronary Artery Calcification (CAC)

Coronary artery calcium indicates the presence of coronary atheroslerosis (4,5,12,13,37–42). The sensitivity and specificity of CAC for the diagnosis of significant coronary artery disease (CAD) depend on the tool used for detection. Gross CACs can be seen on radiographs (37) (Fig. 10-14). Small coronary calcific deposits, however, require

more sensitive tools to make them visible (see **Chapters 2 and 3**). In this regard, the following imaging methods are of increasing sensitivity: fluoroscopy (3,4,37) (see **Chapter 2**), digital subtraction fluoroscopy (10), CT (Fig. 10-15), double-helix CT (40), and electron beam CT (13) (see **Chapter 3**).

As a rule, for the purpose of identifying significant CAD, use of the more sensitive tools leads to a lower specificity than the less sensitive tools. Using the most sensitive tool, electron beam CT, patients at high risk of coronary atherosclerosis were examined for CAC, and the results were correlated with angiographic findings (41). The sensitivity was 97%, and the specificity was 41%. These results are almost the exact reverse of our statistics using fluoroscopy for identifying significant CAD in 800 symptomatic patients—we found a sensitivity of 40% and a specificity of 94% (3). The five-year survival rate was 58% for patients with calcification and 87% for those without (3).

Fluoroscopically detected CAC in asymptomatic, nonhyperlipidemic men was associated with a ninefold increased risk of a positive exercise stress test (43). More than 90% of those who had both coronary calcification and a positive exercise test harbored at least one major coronary artery with stenosis of >50% (44). In a 5-year follow-up of 100 healthy persons screened with a maximal treadmill test, Aronow and Cassidy (45) noted that 46% of those who had an abnormal response to the test later showed signs of myocardial infarction or angina pectoris. However, only 3.4% of those with a normal response to the test had the same result. In asymptomatic high-risk subjects, the presence of CAC on cine fluoroscopy was associated with an increased risk of coronary events after 1 year (10).

Electron beam CT is currently the only imaging technique that allows accurate quantification of CAC. Although find-

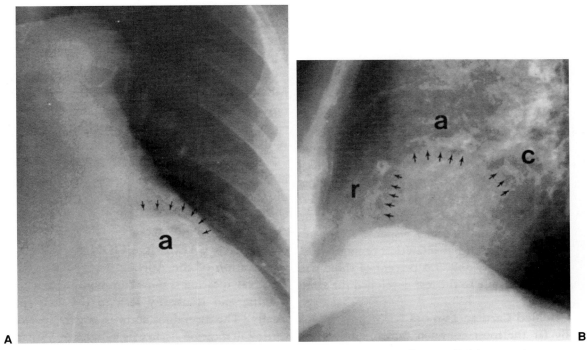

A   **B**

FIG. 10-14. Radiographs of a patient with three-vessel coronary artery disease. Calcium can be seen in the coronary artery calcification triangle in the posteroanterior (**A**) view. The calcified vessels are better seen on the lateral (**B**) view. a, anterior descending (*arrows*); c, circumflex (*arrows*); r, right (*arrows*).

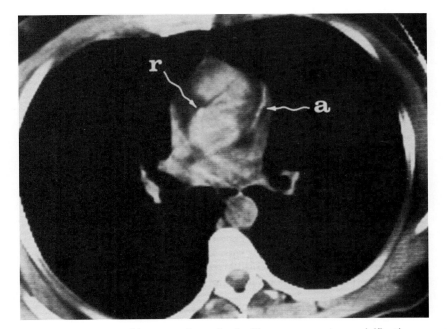

FIG. 10-15. Computed tomographic scan of a patient with coronary artery calcification. a, anterior descending artery; r, right coronary artery.

ing small calcific deposits does not necessarily mean there is obstructive disease, the heavier the calcification, the more likely it is that significant disease is present (12,13). This technique has the following potential benefits in terms of treatment: early identification of high-risk asymptomatic patients may bestow benefits from vigorous risk reduction programs (12,13,38); comparison of serial quantitative evaluation of calcified plaques may reflect the progression or regression of atherosclerosis (38); the absence of CAC by electron beam CT rules out significant CAD in ~95% of the patients (12).

Calcified Cardiac Tumors

By far the most common cardiac tumors that calcify are atrial myxomas. Myxomas have been reported in all cardiac chambers as well as in the great vessels. Most of them, however, are found in the left atrium. Approximately 10% of atrial myxomas calcify (46) (Fig. 10-16). Other calcified cardiac neoplasms include rhabdomyoma, fibroma, angioma, osteosarcoma, and osteoclastoma. Rhabdomyomas are frequently associated with tuberous sclerosis and are mainly found in children (1). Pericardial cysts also occasionally calcify (14). A thymic cyst may calcify along the margin adherent to the pericardium.

VASCULAR CALCIFICATION

Calcification of the Aorta

Aortic calcification is most commonly a result of aging and is usually seen in the arch and distally. The ascending aorta is largely spared. Aortic calcification occurs in >25% of persons between 61 and 70 years of age (47). According to Bell and colleagues (48), a relationship exists between the age at which calcium is first described and average life span. The death rates are not likely to be different among those with calcification compared with those without calcification if such a lesion is first noted during the sixth decade or thereafter. On the other hand, if calcium in the aorta is first detected in the fifth decade or before, the incidence of death would be increased because of coronary heart disease. Hyperlipidemia and diabetes are factors that predispose patients to calcific atherosclerosis at an early age (Fig. 10-17).

Luetic aortitis is a disease of the media—predominantly involving the ascending aorta, the sinuses of Valsalva, and the aortic valve—forming a huge ascending aortic aneurysm with aortic insufficiency. Accompanying the reparative process of the injured media, both the adventitia and the intima undergo fibrosis and thickening (49). This, in turn, predisposes the intima to earlier and more severe atherosclerosis, which has been likened to a wrinkled treebark appearance by pathologists. The intima eventually

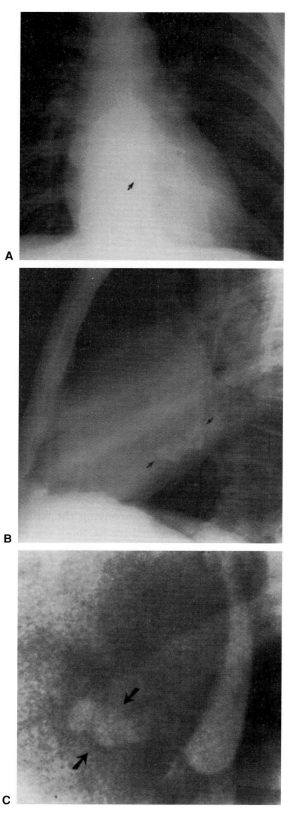

FIG. 10-16. Atrial myxoma with calcification. Posteroanterior **(A)** and lateral **(B)** radiographs and a lateral fluoroscopic spot film **(C)** show a calcified left atrial myxoma (arrows). The tumor moved widely between the atrium and ventricle at fluoroscopy.

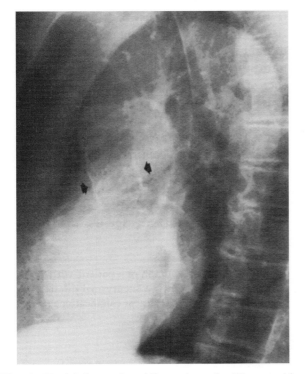

FIG. 10-17. A left anterior oblique view of a 50-year-old patient with hyperlipidemia shows extensive calcific deposition in the ascending aorta (arrows), aortic cusps, and coronary arteries.

calcify in 20% of the patients (50) (Fig. 10-18). The calcific deposits are typically linear and confined to the ascending aorta. The advanced atherosclerosis of the intima frequently involves the ostia of the coronary arteries. This is another reason, besides aortic insufficiency, for the anginal chest pain in these patients (1). In summary, the main features of luetic aortitis are calcific ascending aortic aneurysm, aortic insufficiency, angina pectoris, age 40–50 years, and positive serologic test.

In patients >65 years, calcification of the ascending aorta may be of nonsyphilitic (mostly atherosclerotic) origin (51). This is particularly true when there is neither an ascending aortic aneurysm nor aortic insufficiency. Aneurysms of the ascending aorta in patients with Marfan's syndrome may be calcified, although this is a rare finding. There are major differences between syphilitic aortitis and the aortic disease of Marfan's syndrome. Patients with the latter are much younger, usually <40 years old. The disease is often found in members of one family. Also, there is a much greater tendency for such aneurysms to dissect than their luetic counterparts.

Calcification confined to the proximal descending aorta in a young adult is highly suggestive of a post-aortic-transection false aneurysm, which is uncommon because most patients with this entity either die promptly or are treated surgically. Perhaps <2% of them survive and show signs of a calcific aneurysm. Its recognition and surgical repair are mandatory if late rupture is to be prevented.

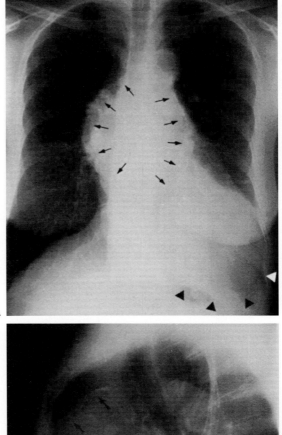

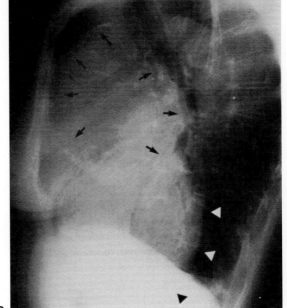

FIG. 10-18. Radiographs of a patient with syphilitic aortitis show aneurysmal dilatation of the ascending aorta with linear calcifications (*arrows*). **A:** Posteroanterior view. **B:** Lateral view. Also note the huge left ventricle (*arrowheads*), a result of aortic insufficiency.

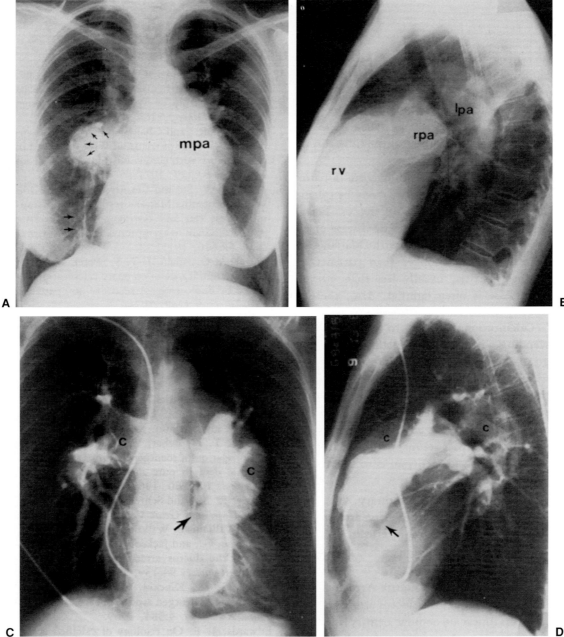

FIG. 10-19. Radiographs and arteriograms of a patient with recurrent thromboembolic disease. **A:** The posteroanterior view shows a huge main pulmonary artery (mpa) trunk and major branches. Note calcium in the right pulmonary artery (*upper arrows*) and scars (*lower arrows*) from previous pulmonary infarction in the right-lower lobe. The pulmonary blood flow shows a striking centralized pattern, representing severe precapillary pulmonary hypertension. **B:** The lateral view shows a dilated right ventricle (rv), right pulmonary artery (rpa), and left pulmonary artery (lpa). **C:** An anteroposterior pulmonary arteriogram shows multiple filling defects (c) representing thrombi in pulmonary arteries. An arrow points to the insufficient pulmonary valve. **D:** Lateral pulmonary arteriogram. The arrow points to the insufficient pulmonary valve. Thrombi are marked with a "c."

Calcification of the Pulmonary Artery

Calcification of the pulmonary arteries results from pressure or volume overload or both (1,8,52,53) (Fig. 10-19).

Calcification of the Ductus Arteriosus

Calcific deposits in the ductus arteriosus appear as a curvilinear or nodular density at the junction between the aorta and the pulmonary trunk. In adults, the ductus is usually patent, and precapillary pulmonary hypertension is usually present (Fig. 10-20). In children, calcification in the ductal area is thought to represent deposition in the ligament of Botallo (54). Its presence militates against patency of the ductus arteriosus. Calcium in the ligament usually disappears in a few years.

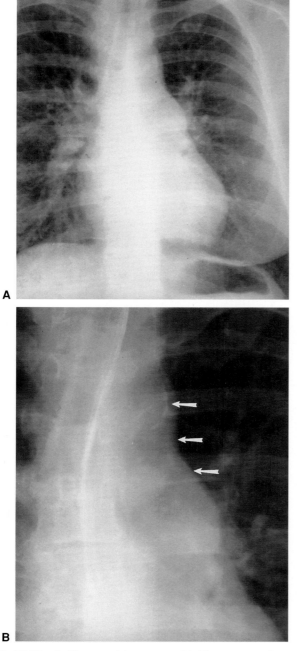

FIG. 10-20. A 40-year-old woman with Eisenmenger's syndrome stemming from a large patent ductus arteriosus. The posteroanterior (PA) radiograph (**A**) shows right-sided cardiomegaly, a centralized pulmonary blood flow pattern, and dilatation of both the pulmonary trunk and the aorta. A magnified view of another PA radiograph (**B**) shows curvilinear calcifications (*arrows*) of both great arteries and the patent ductus to better advantage.

REFERENCES

1. Freundlich IM, Lind T. Calcification of the heart and great vessels. *CRC Crit Rev Clin Radiol Nucl Med* 1975;6:171–216.
2. Sell S, Scully RE. Aging changes in the aortic and mitral valves: histologic and histochemical studies with observations on the pathogenesis of calcific aortic stenosis and calcification of the mitral annulus. *Am J Pathol* 1965;46:345–355.
3. Margolis JR, Chen JTT, Kong Y, et al. The diagnostic and prognostic significance of coronary artery calcification: a report of 800 cases. *Radiology* 1980;137:609–616.
4. Bartel AG, Chen JTT, Peter RH, et al. The significance of coronary calcification detected by fluoroscopy: a report of 360 patients. *Circulation* 1974;49:1247–1253.
5. Mautner GC, Mautner SL, Froehlich J, et al. Coronary artery calcification: assessment with electron beam CT and histomorphometric correlation. *Radiology* 1994;192:619–623.
6. Batson GA, Urquhart W, Sideris DA. Radiological features in aortic stenosis. *Clin Radiol* 1972;23:140–144.
7. Lachman AS, Roberts WC. Calcific deposits in stenotic mitral valves. *Circulation* 1978;57:808–815.
8. Cooley RN, Schreiber MH. *Radiology of the heart and great vessels*, 3rd ed. Baltimore: Williams & Wilkins, 1978.
9. Tuzcu EM, Block PC, Griffin B, et al. Percutaneous mitral balloon valvotomy in patients with calcific mitral stenosis: immediate and long-term outcome. *J Am Coll Cardiol* 1994;3:1604–1609.
10. Detrano RC, Wong ND, Tang W, et al. Prognostic significance of cardiac cinefluoroscopy for coronary calcific deposits in asymptomatic high risk subjects. *J Am Coll Cardiol* 1994;24:354–358.
11. Lippert JA, White CS, Mason AC, et al. Calcification of aortic valve detected incidentally on CT scans: prevalence and clinical significance. *AJR Am J Roentgenol* 1995;164:73–77.
12. Stanford W, Thompson BH, Weiss RM. Coronary artery calcification: clinical significance and current methods of detection. *AJR Am J Roentgenol* 1993;161:1139–1146.
13. Stanford W, Rumberger JA. *Ultrafast computed tomography in cardiac imaging: principles and practice*. Mt. Kisco, N.Y.: Futura, 1992: 77–95.
14. Schinz HR. *Roentgen diagnosis*, 2nd ed. Rigler LG, ed. New York: Grune & Stratton, 1970.
15. MacGregor JH, Chen JTT, Chiles C, et al. The radiographic distribution of pericardial and myocardial calcification. *AJR Am J Roentgenol* 1987; 148:675–677.
16. Brean HP, Marks JH, Sosman MC, Schlesinger MJ. Massive calcification in infarcted myocardium. *Radiology* 1950;54:33–41.
17. Abrams DL, Edelist A, Luria MH, Miller AJ. Ventricular aneurysm: reappraisal based on a study of 65 consecutive autopsied cases. *Circulation* 1963;27:164–169.
18. Roberts WC. Congenitally bicuspid aortic valve: a study of 85 autopsy cases. *Am J Cardiol* 1970;26:72.

19. Chen JTT, Behar VS, Morris JJ, et al. Correlation of roentgen findings with hemodynamic data in pure mitral stenosis. *Am J Roentgenol* 1968; 102:280–292.

20. Roberts WC. Valvular, subvalvular, and supravalvular aortic stenosis: morphologic features. *Cardiovasc Clin* 1973;5:97–126.

21. Edwards JE. On etiology of calcified aortic stenosis. *Circulation* 1962; 26:817–818.

22. Matthews B, Medd WE, Gorlin R. Aortic stenosis: clinical study. *Br Med J* 1955;2:759–763.

23. Roberts WC. *Congenital heart disease.* Philadelphia: Davis, 1979.

24. Roberts WC, Perloff JK, Costantino T. Severe valvular aortic stenosis in patients over 65 years of age: a clinicopathologic study. *Am J Cardiol* 1971;27:497–506.

25. Rapaport E, Rackley CE, Cohn LH. Aortic valve disease. In: Schlant RC, Alexander RW, eds. *The heart,* 8th ed. New York: McGraw-Hill, 1994:1457–1482.

26. Spindola-Franco H, Fish BG, Dachman A, et al. Recognition of bicuspid aortic valve by plain film calcification. *AJR Am J Roentgenol* 1982; 139:867–872.

27. Rodan BA, Chen JTT, Kirks DR, et al. Mitral valve calcification in congenital mitral stenosis. *Am Heart J* 1983;105:514–675.

28. Rodriguez GR, Bennett KR, Lehan PH. Calcification of the pulmonary valve. *Chest* 1971;59:160–164.

29. Rogers JV Jr., Chandler NW, Franch RH. Calcification of the tricuspid annulus. *Am J Roentgenol* 1969;106:550–557.

30. Korn D, De Sanctis RW, Sell S. Massive calcification of the mitral annulus: a clinicopathological study of fourteen cases. *N Engl J Med* 1962;267:900–909.

31. Roberts WC, Waller BF. Mitral valve "annular" calcium forming a complete circle or "O" configuration: clinical and necropsy observations. *Am Heart J* 1981;101:619–621.

32. Arnold JR, Ghahramani AR. Calcification of annulus of tricuspid valve (observed in two patients with congenital pulmonary stenosis). *Chest* 1971;60:229–232.

33. Windholz F, Grayson CE. Roentgen demonstration of calcification in the interventricular septum in cases of heart block. *AJR Am J Roentgenol* 1947;58:411–421.

34. Shaw DR, Chen JTT, Lester RG. X-ray appearance and clinical significance of left atrial wall calcification. *Invest Radiol* 1976;11:501–507.

35. Gedgandas E, Kieffer SA, Erickson C. Left atrial calcification. *AJR Am J Roentgenol* 1968;102:293–296.

36. MacCallum WG. Rheumatic lesions of the left auricle of the heart. *Bull Johns Hopkins Hosp* 1924;35:329.

37. Chen JTT. The significance of cardiac calcifications. *Appl Radiol* 1992; 21:11–19.

38. Janowitz WR, Agatston AS, Viamonte M Jr. Comparison of serial quantitative evaluation of calcified coronary artery plaque by ultrafast computed tomography in persons with and without obstructive coronary artery disease. *Am J Cardiol* 1991;68:1–6.

39. Agatston AS, Janowitz WR, Kaplan G, et al. Ultrafast computed tomography–detected coronary calcium reflects the angiographic extent of coronary atherosclerosis. *Am J Cardiol* 1994;74:1272–1274.

40. Shemesh J, Apter S, Rozenman J. Calcification of coronary arteries: detection and quantification with double-helix CT. *Radiology* 1995; 197:779–783.

41. Devries S, Wolfkiel C, Fusman B, et al. Influence of age and gender on the presence of coronary calcium detected by ultrafast computed tomography. *J Am Coll Cardiol* 1995;25:76–82.

42. Fallavollita JA, Brody AS, Bunnell IL, et al. Fast computed tomography detection of coronary calcification in the diagnosis of coronary artery disease. *Circulation* 1994;89:285–290.

43. Kelly MJ, Huang EK, Langou RA. Correlation of fluoroscopically detected coronary artery calcification with exercise testing in asymptomatic men. *Radiology* 1978;129:1–6.

44. Langou RA, Kelley MJ, Huang EK, et al. Predictive accuracy of coronary artery calcification and positive exercise test in asymptomatic nonhyperlipidemic men for coronary artery disease. *Am. J. Cardiol* 1980;45:400.

45. Aronow WS, Cassidy J. Five-year follow-up of double Master's test, maximal treadmill stress test and resting and post exercise apexcardiogram in asymptomatic persons. *Circulation* 1975;52:616–618.

46. Davis GD, Kincaid OW, Hallermann FJ. Roentgen aspects of cardiac tumors. *Semin Roentgenol* 1969;4:384–394.

47. Rescigno B, D'Alfonso G, Carratu L. Calcifications of the intrathoracic aorta and the pulmonary artery in various ages of life (statistical, clinicoradiologic and anatomicopathologic findings). *Arch Fisiol* 1965;19:800.

48. Bell MF, Schaaf RS, Jernigan TP. The prognostic import of calcification of the aortic knob. *Trans Assoc Life Insur Med Dir Am* 1963;47:33.

49. Gould SE. *Pathology of the heart and blood vessels,* 3rd ed. Springfield, Ill.: Thomas, 1968.

50. Jackman J, Lubert M. Significance of calcification in the ascending aorta as observed roentgenographically. *AJR Am J Roentgenol* 1945; 53:432–445.

51. Higgins CB, Reinke RT. Nonsyphilitic etiology of linear calcification of the ascending aorta. *Radiology* 1974;113:609–613.

52. Mallamo JT, Baum RS, Simon AJ. Diffuse pulmonary artery calcifications in a case of Eisenmenger's syndrome. *Radiology* 1971; 99:549–550.

53. Steinberg I. Calcification of the pulmonary artery and enlargement of the right ventricle. *AJR Am J Roentgenol* 1966;98:369–377.

54. Currarino G, Jackson JH Jr. Calcification of the ductus arteriosus and ligmentum botalli. *Radiology* 1970;94:139–142.

Essentials of Cardiac Imaging,
James T. T. Chen,
Lippincott–Raven Publishers, Philadelphia © 1998.

CHAPTER 11

Valvular Heart Disease

James T. T. Chen

The features of uncomplicated valvular lesions are relatively straightforward on chest radiographs as well as on images obtained with other techniques. They should be thoroughly understood and properly interpreted in the evaluation and treatment of cardiac patients.

BASIC PATHOPHYSIOLOGY

Valvular stenosis imposes pressure overload and myocardial hypertrophy of the proximal cardiac chamber. Any dilatation of that chamber is indicative of heart failure. Valvular insufficiency, on the other hand, imposes volume overload, which causes dilatation followed by compensatory hypertrophy of the involved chambers (1,2). For example, aortic stenosis (AS) provokes concentric hypertrophy of the left ventricle at the expense of volume, and this effect is particularly striking in systole. The radiographically determined cardiac size at this time is usually within the top limits of normal (with a cardiothoracic ratio still <0.5, which is only slightly larger than the mean normal value of 0.45) (Fig. 11-1A).

From this point on, even a slight further increase in left ventricular size would suggest dilatation on top of hypertrophy and would be evidence of heart failure. This is almost always accompanied by cephalization of the pulmonary vascularity and/or pulmonary edema. The same sequence of events from left ventricular compensation to decompensation can also be observed in other pressure overload situations, for example, systemic hypertension (SH) (Fig. 11-2) and coarctation of the aorta.

In the case of aortic insufficiency (AI), volume overload leads to dilatation of the left ventricle and the thoracic aorta. The heart is usually moderately enlarged (with a cardiothoracic ratio >0.5) but may be grossly enlarged (with a ratio >0.6) without signs of failure (Fig. 11-1B). In this circum-

stance, only a gigantic heart plus pulmonary venous congestion suggests the onset of myocardial insufficiency (Fig. 11-3).

AORTIC STENOSIS

Anatomic Classification

Aortic stenosis occurs most commonly (60% to 70%) at the valve, less commonly (15% to 30%) below the valve, and rarely above the valve. Valvular AS is subdivided into the bicuspid, unicuspid, and tricuspid varieties. Subvalvular AS may be further classified as membranous, tunnel-like, or functional. Functional obstruction of the left ventricular outflow tract happens in systole only and has been termed idiopathic hypertrophic subaortic stenosis (IHSS), hypertrophic obstructive cardiomyopathy, and asymmetric septal hypertrophy. Supravalvular AS can be familial and isolated or nonfamilial and associated with hypercalcemia, mental retardation, elfin facies, and pulmonary artery branch stenoses (Williams' syndrome or infantile hypercalcemia syndrome).

Etiology

Isolated valvular AS is mostly congenital or degenerative, depending on the patient's age. An age <65 years favors a congenital etiology. Isolated rheumatic AS is rare and is seen in patients aged 30 to 60 years (**see Table 10-1**). Subvalvular and supravalvular AS are mostly congenital in origin.

Pathophysiology and Clinical Presentation

Regardless of cause, AS can be classified according to its severity into three categories: mild (with a valve area >0.7 cm^2), moderate (0.5 to 0.7 cm^2), and severe (<0.5 cm^2). The normal aortic valve area ranges from 2.5 to 3.5 cm^2. With

Department of Radiology, Duke University School of Medicine, Durham, North Carolina 27710, U.S.A.

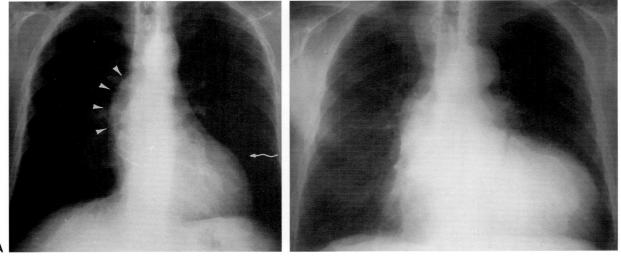

FIG. 11-1. A: Posteroanterior radiograph of a middle-aged man with congenital valvular AS. There is only mild cardiomegaly with increased convexity of the hypertrophied left ventricle (*arrow*). The ascending aorta is markedly dilated (*arrowheads*). **B:** Posteroanterior view of another middle-aged man with AI. Gross cardiomegaly primarily reflects the marked volume overload of the left ventricle. The aorta is diffusely dilated with increased volume. The lungs are clear, and there is no evidence of heart failure.

mild AS, the cardiac output can be maintained by left ventricular hypertrophy with increased contractility. The patient, therefore, remains asymptomatic. As the severity of AS increases, the cardiac output begins to decrease, as does left ventricular contractility. The clinical manifestations of severe AS are angina pectoris, syncope, and congestive heart failure. Severe AS in infancy frequently causes congestive heart failure and death.

The systolic and pulse pressures are typically lowered in

severe AS. A diamond-shaped systolic murmur accompanied by a thrill is characteristic, with the addition of an aortic ejection click in the valvular variety before calcification of the valve. Symptoms of mitral insufficiency in patients with all types of subaortic stenosis are common. Patients with membranous subaortic stenosis may show signs of AI because of a jet injury to the aortic valve. The main electrocardiographic sign of severe AS is left ventricular hypertrophy with a strained pattern. The development of arrhythmias is

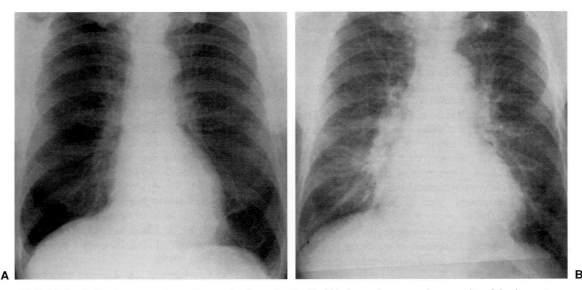

FIG. 11-2. A: Posteroanterior radiograph of a patient with SH shows increased convexity of the hypertrophied left ventricle and a tortuous aorta. Overall cardiac size is within normal limits, and the lungs are clear. **B:** A second radiograph 4 months later shows a slight increase in cardiac size and frank pulmonary edema indicative of congestive heart failure.

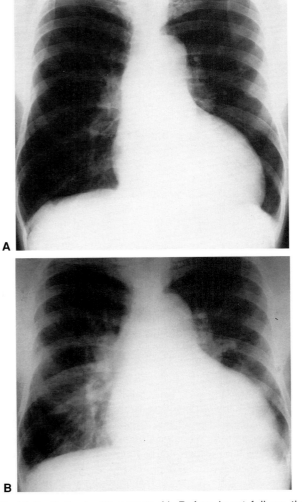

FIG. 11-3. Patient with severe AI. Before heart failure, the posteroanterior radiograph (**A**) shows moderate cardiomegaly (cardiothoracic ratio of 0.58) and clear lungs. After heart failure, 6 months later, another radiograph (**B**) shows gross cardiomegaly (cardiothoracic ratio of 0.64) and pulmonary edema.

detrimental to such patients. Infective endocarditis is a serious complication capable of converting an obstructive valve into a leaky one within a short period of time. Severe AS may be present in an asymptomatic patient with a normal electrocardiogram. The incidence of sudden death is estimated at 7.5%; it is higher in adolescents than in adults.

Surgical treatment of valvular AS consists of valvulotomy for children and valve replacement for adults. Resection of a subaortic membrane can be difficult because of its proximity to the aortic valve, the ventricular septum, and the anterior mitral leaflet. Transaortic septal myotomy and myectomy may be used for the treatment of patients with IHSS. After excision of the obstructing fibrous tissue, a prosthetic enlargement of the ascending aorta may be necessary for the treatment of patients with supravalvular AS. Balloon valvuloplasty has been used as a palliative measure in very

old patients in whom surgery is contraindicated. The results with this procedure have been disappointing (1).

Radiographic and Angiographic Signs

In response to left ventricular outflow obstruction, all types of AS go through the same two stages: left ventricular hypertrophy before congestive heart failure and left ventricular dilatation in addition to hypertrophy with pulmonary edema after heart failure. As the obstruction becomes more severe, however, the unique radiologic features of each type of AS usually emerge, and they should be promptly recognized.

Valvular AS

With mild obstruction, the chest radiographs may be entirely normal. At times, an isolated ascending aortic dilatation with increased pulsation (see **Chapter 2**) provides the only clue to the diagnosis (Fig. 11-4). With moderate AS, the left ventricle begins to enlarge with increased convexity representing hypertrophy without dilatation (Fig. 11-1A). With severe AS before left ventricular failure, the radiographic signs may remain unimpressive in patients <25 years old. In patients >40 years old, however, nodular or bicuspid calcification of the aortic valve is usually evident on the lateral chest radiograph (Fig. 11-5; see also **Figs. 2-11C, 10-6B,** and **10-8A–E**). As is applicable to all cardiac valves, the extent of valve calcification is proportionate to the severity of valve stenosis (see **Figs. 7-5 and 10-6**). Post-

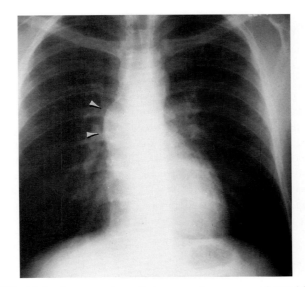

FIG. 11-4. An asymptomatic teenage boy was evaluated for a systolic murmur. The posteroanterior radiograph shows normal results, except for an enlarged ascending aorta—so-called poststenotic dilatation (*arrowheads*). The aortic valve was not calcified. On echocardiography, there was a systolic gradient of 100 mm Hg across the valve.

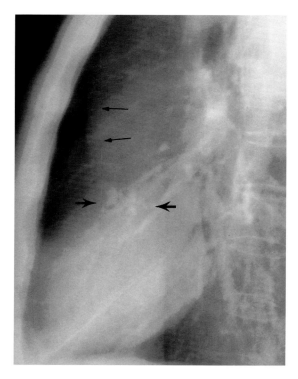

FIG. 11-5. A lateral radiograph of patient with congenital bicuspid aortic valve shows diffuse calcification of the entire valve (*thick arrows*). The original bicuspid morphology has been erased by heavy calcification of the "nodular" type. (Compare with **Fig. 10-8A,B,D**). Also note the poststenotic dilatation of the ascending aorta (*thin arrows*).

stenotic dilatation of the ascending aorta, on the other hand, correlates better with the chronicity of the disease than the severity of the stenosis.

In degenerative valvular AS of the elderly, smooth curvilinear calcifications (see **Fig. 10-9E**) may be seen outlining the well-developed tricuspid aortic valve with or without calcification of the aortic annulus. Sometimes, major intrinsic calcification is evident in each of the three cusps (see **Fig. 10-9B–D**). Since such lesions develop late in life (after age 65), isolated ascending aortic dilatation is usually absent. Instead, one sees a generalized dilatation and tortuosity of the entire thoracic aorta without a disproportionately enlarged ascending aorta (see **Figs. 10-9A,B**).

On aortography or left ventriculography, a forceful jet can usually be seen emanating from the dome of the stenotic aortic valve into the dilated ascending aorta (Fig. 11-6A). The same upward doming of the valve can be found with echocardiography (Fig. 11-6B). The poststenotic dilatation can also be imaged with a spin-echo coronal magnetic resonance (MR) image (Fig. 11-6C). On the same MR image (Fig. 11-6C) one can appreciate the heavily hypertrophied left ventricle with a reduced volume.

Subvalvular AS

The unique features of subvalvular AS include (a) absence of isolated ascending aortic dilatation (Figs. 11-7 and 11-8); (b) signs of AI (generalized dilatation of the thoracic aorta) in patients with membranous subvalvular AS as a result of injury to the aortic valve by the jet stream from the obstruct-

ing membrane (Fig. 11-7C); (c) indications of mitral insufficiency in patients with severe subaortic stenosis (Figs. 11-7D and 11-8A,B,D–G); and (d) in a minority of patients with IHSS, an isolated bulge along the upper-left ventricular border, which represents marked hypertrophy of the anterior aspect of the ventricular septum (Fig. 11-8C).

On angiography, the subvalvular membrane can be delineated by injecting contrast medium into the aorta (Fig. 11-8C) in the presence of AI, or into the left ventricle (Fig. 11-8D). The narrowed left ventricular outflow tract in patients with IHSS can be seen in systole (Fig. 11-8D). This effect is caused by the systolic anterior motion (SAM) of the anterior mitral leaflet against the hypertrophied interventricular septum. With MR images, one can see that the degree of left ventricular hypertrophy is greater in the septum than in the free wall (Fig. 11-8E). With real-time echocardiography the SAM of the mitral leaflet is evident with each heartbeat (Fig. 11-8F,G).

Supravalvular AS

Radiographically, supravalvular AS mimics its valvular counterpart closely except for the absence of a dilated ascending aorta. In fact, the image of the ascending aorta tends to be small or invisible (Fig. 11-9A). On the angiogram, the stenosis is usually situated immediately above the aortic valve. Since both sinuses of Valsalva and coronary arteries are in the high-pressure compartment, they tend to be dilated and well opacified (Figs. 11-9B,C). In Williams' syndrome (see discussion in Anatomic Classification), supravalvular

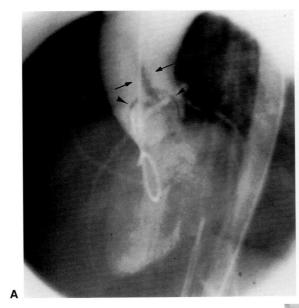

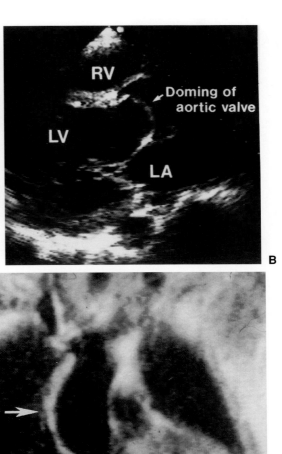

FIG. 11-6. Comparative imaging of valvular AS. Aortogram of patient 1 (**A**) shows late opacification of the left ventricle due to changing catheter position during the injection of contrast medium. Note the negative jet (*opposing arrows*) and doming of the thickened aortic valve (*arrowheads*). Echocardiogram of patient 2 (**B**) shows a similar updoming of the stenotic aortic valve (*arrow*). Coronal spin-echo MR image of patient 3 (**C**) shows considerable poststenotic dilatation of the aorta (*large arrow*), a markedly hypertrophied left ventricle (*small arrows*), and normal pericardium (*arrowheads*). Also note that the volume in the left ventricle is actually smaller than normal. RV, right ventricle; LV, left ventricle; LA, left atrium.

AS is frequently associated with pulmonary artery branch stenoses (Fig. 11-10A–C) as well as mental retardation and hypercalcemia.

Echocardiography

The type and severity of AS as well as the status of the left ventricle can be determined by echocardiography (Figs. 11-6B and 11-8F,G). Ultrasonography is also effective in ruling out AS.

AORTIC INSUFFICIENCY

Etiology and Pathology

Isolated AI most commonly results from a congenitally bicuspid aortic valve (2,3) (see **Fig. 2-24**). The larger of the two cusps tends to prolapse into the left ventricle in diastole and gradually causes the valve to leak. Such lesions usually become clinically apparent in the third or fourth decade of life, although they may occasionally appear in childhood. Rheumatic AI is common as a component lesion of combined aortic and mitral disease and less common as an isolated lesion (1,2). Uncommon causes of isolated AI include syphilitic aortitis (see **Fig. 10-18**) (4), Marfan's syndrome (Fig. 11-11), ankylosing spondylitis, relapsing polychondritis, infective endocarditis, and traumatic rupture of the aortic valve (see **Fig. 18-20**).

Pathophysiology and Clinical Presentation

The basic pathophysiology of AI is a volume overload between the left ventricle and the aorta. Over a long period of

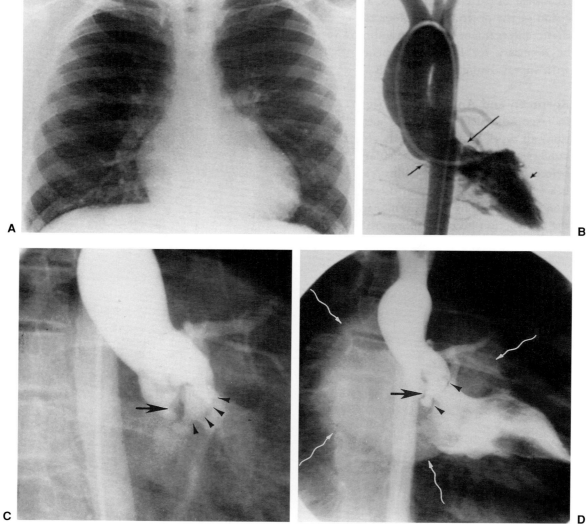

FIG. 11-7. Patients with membranous subvalvular AS. Posteroanterior view (**A**) of patient 1 shows mild left-sided cardiomegaly. Note that in contrast to valvular AS, the ascending aorta is not dilated. On the left ventriculogram (**B**), a linear filling defect (*long arrow*) is seen between the aortic valve (*medium arrow*) and the hypertrophic left ventricle (*short arrow*). (Modified with permission from Kirks DR. *Practical pediatric imaging.* Boston: Little, Brown, 1984.) Aortogram (**C**) of patient 2 shows moderate AI outlining the subvalvular membrane (*arrowheads*) and the thickened and deformed aortic valve (*arrow*). A left ventriculogram (**D**) shows the same. In addition, there is opacification of the left atrium (*white arrows*) indicative of MI.

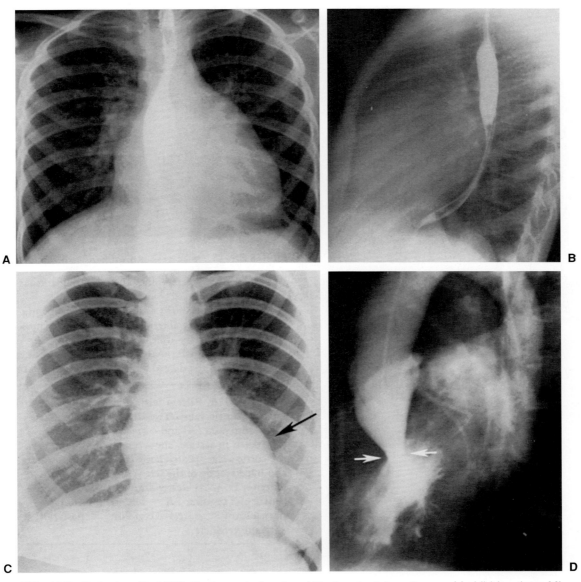

FIG. 11-8. Patients with IHSS. Posteroanterior view (**A**) of patient 1, a 6-year-old child in whom MI eventually developed, shows moderate cardiomegaly with left atrial and biventricular enlargement. The pulmonary blood flow pattern is cephalic. The lateral view (**B**) shows posterior deviation of the barium-filled esophagus indicative of MI. A posteroanterior view (**C**) shows patient 2, a 20-year-old woman with recurrent attacks of syncope. The systolic subaortic pressure gradient was 105 mm Hg. This view shows a bulge (*arrow*) along the upper-left ventricular border. Lateral systolic left ventriculogram (**D**) of patient 3 demonstrates a narrowed subaortic pathway between the hypertrophied ventricular septum and the anterior mitral leaflet (*arrows*). Also noted is evidence of MI. (*continued on page 170*)

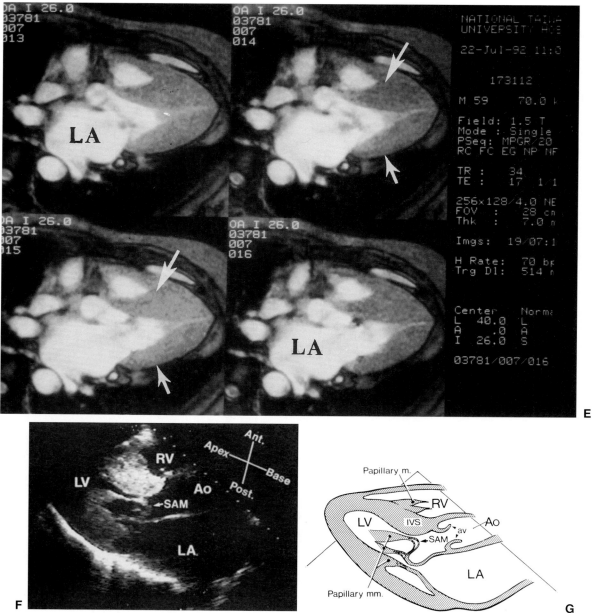

FIG. 11-8. *Continued.* Gradient-echo MR images (**E**) of patient 4 displays considerable left ventricular hypertrophy, more marked in the interventricular septum (*long arrow*) than in the free wall (*short arrow*). The left atrium (LA) is also dilated due to MI (courtesy of Dr. Yeun-Chung Chang of National Taiwan University). An echocardiogram in the long-axis view (**F**) of patient 5 shows SAM of the anterior mitral leaflet against the interventricular septum (IVS). The IVS is disproportionately thick in comparison with the posterior wall of the left ventricle (LV). The left atrium (LA) is enlarged in the presence of MI. Ant., anterior; Ao, aorta; av, aortic valve; m., muscle; mm., muscles; Post., posterior; RV, right ventricle. Accompanying diagram (**G**) shows the same echocardiographic findings as described in F.

time, the left ventricle is allowed to stretch and hypertrophy gradually without apparent dysfunction. The end-diastolic and stroke volumes are typically increased, whereas the end-systolic volume is not. The end-diastolic pressure is only mildly elevated. The radiographic manifestations of these early hemodynamic changes are gross cardiomegaly, normal pulmonary vasculature, increased left ventricular contractility, and increased aortic pulsation.

As the disease progresses, the cardiac output begins to decline in the face of widening pulse pressure, increasing myocardial hypertrophy, and gross left ventricular dilatation. Such combined derangement is detrimental to the myocardium. Since the peak coronary flow occurs during diastole, decreased diastolic pressure on top of decreased cardiac output further compromises myocardial perfusion. This is reflected clinically by the onset of angina pectoris and dyspnea on exertion. The chest radiograph may show decreased pulmonary vascularity owing to markedly reduced forward cardiac output (see **Fig. 8-5**).

After the onset of frank left ventricular failure, both the volume and the pressure are notably elevated in diastole, as is the volume in systole. Consequently, the blood becomes stagnant in the left ventricle, and symptoms of marked pulmonary venous hypertension soon follow (Fig. 11-3B; see also **Fig. 2-9B**). When aortic regurgitation develops suddenly (e.g., secondary to infective endocarditis), acute left-sided heart failure is usually unavoidable and frequently intractable without surgical intervention.

The electrocardiographic findings of severe AI include left ventricular hypertrophy, left axis deviation, ST-segment depressions, and T-wave inversions. The physical findings revolve primarily around the markedly widened pulse pressure, which causes the aorta and larger arteries to expand abruptly in systole and collapse suddenly in diastole. The outward expressions of such physiologic derangement are a water-hammer (Corrigan's) pulse, a ''pistol-shot'' sound over the femoral arteries, and a blowing diastolic murmur in the aortic area. Sometimes, a diastolic rumble of mitral valve vibration (the Austin Flint murmur) can also be heard.

In the early stages of AI, mild congestive heart failure can usually be treated medically. The proper timing of aortic valve replacement is not always easy to determine. Serial radiologic, radionuclide, and echocardiographic studies of left ventricular performance in a relatively asymptomatic patient may shed light on such dilemmas.

Radiographic and Angiographic Signs

In patients with mild AI, the chest radiograph may show mild engorgement of the thoracic aorta or no abnormalities. But on fluoroscopy, even at this early stage, the hyperdynamic nature of the aorta and the left ventricle may already be apparent, reflecting the widened pulse pressure and volume overload. On the angiogram, only a transient puff of opacified

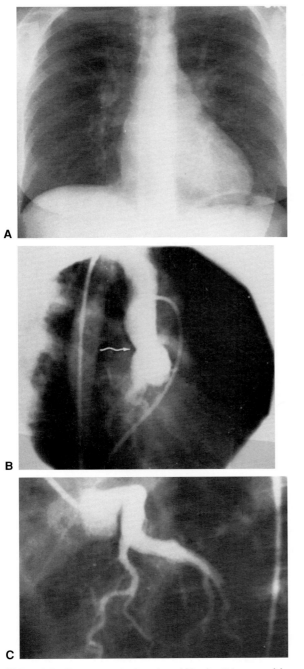

FIG. 11-9. Posteroanterior view (**A**) of a 24-year-old woman with isolated supravalvular AS shows evidence of left ventricular hypertrophy. The ascending aorta is invisible. An aortogram (**B**) shows supravalvular narrowing of the ascending aorta (*arrow*). The aortic sinuses and the coronary arteries are dilated. A left coronary arteriogram (**C**) in the right posterior oblique view shows the dilated vessels to better advantage.

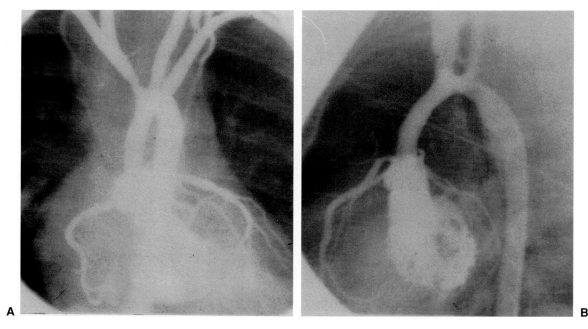

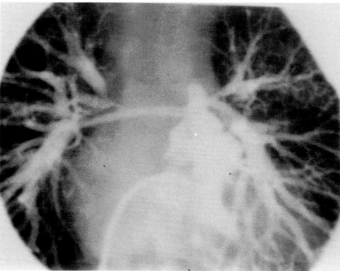

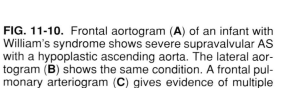

FIG. 11-10. Frontal aortogram (**A**) of an infant with William's syndrome shows severe supravalvular AS with a hypoplastic ascending aorta. The lateral aortogram (**B**) shows the same condition. A frontal pulmonary arteriogram (**C**) gives evidence of multiple bilateral pulmonary artery branch stenoses.

blood is seen to enter the left ventricle during diastole when contrast medium is injected into the ascending aorta.

With moderate AI, the chest radiograph becomes distinctly abnormal. The basic abnormalities are enlargement and increased pulsation of both the aorta and the left ventricle (see **Figs. 2-24** and **2-25**). The left ventricle is markedly hypertrophied and moderately dilated. The cardiothoracic ratio is usually >0.50. The aorta is diffusely dilated in AI in contrast to the isolated ascending aortic dilatation in AS. One exception to the rule is the absence of aortic dilatation on radiography in patients <25 years old who have no history of hypertension. The reason for this is twofold. First, the aorta is pliable in young people, tending to collapse more fully in diastole. Second, when the radiograph is taken at random, it is the diastolic image that one most frequently

obtains. In a situation such as this, fluoroscopic observation of dynamics is more specific than radiographic analysis of anatomy (see **Figs. 2-24** and **2-25**).

In severe AI the left ventricle may become gigantic, with an enormous diastolic volume; this is known as cor bovinum. Radiographic evidence of aortic valve calcification usually means there is coexistent aortic valve stenosis. As a rule, pure aortic regurgitation does not show radiographic evidence of valve calcification. On the angiogram, severe AI is manifested by immediate and sustained opacification of the left ventricle after an injection of contrast medium into the aorta (Fig. 11-11C). Consequently, the left ventricle becomes denser than the aorta (8). After the onset of frank left ventricular failure, the chamber becomes markedly dilated with decreased contractility. An aneurysmal dilatation of the

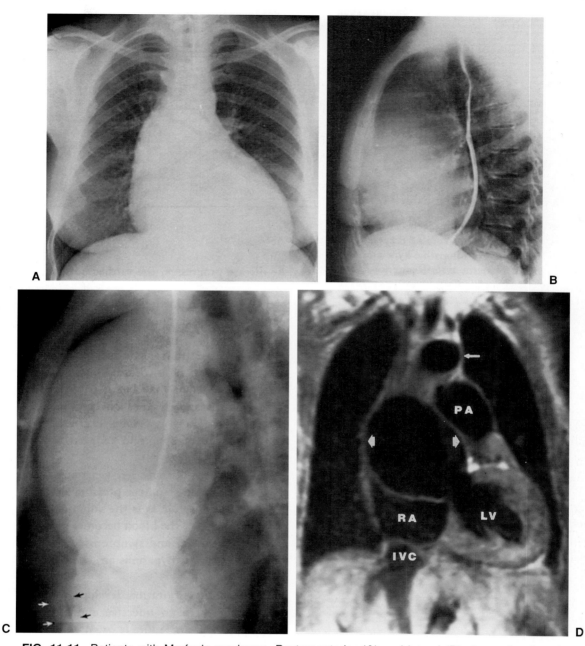

FIG. 11-11. Patients with Marfan's syndrome. Posteroanterior (**A**) and lateral (**B**) views of patient 1 show the heart and ascending aorta to be markedly enlarged. The pulmonary vascularity is decreased owing to reduced forward cardiac output. The lateral aortogram (**C**) shows a huge ascending aortic aneurysm with evidence of AI. The pericardium is widened and opacified (*white arrows*), suggesting dissection of the aneurysm into the pericardium. Note that the subepicardial fat stripe (*black arrows*) is displaced posteriorly by the pericardial fluid. Coronal spin-echo MR image (**D**) of patient 2, a 71-year-old woman, shows a huge ascending aortic aneurysm (*thick arrows*). The rest of the aorta (*thin arrow*) and the left ventricle (LV) are also dilated owing to AI. The pulmonary artery (PA), right atrium (RA), and inferior vena cava (IVC) are all dilated as a result of the rupturing of the aortic aneurysm into the RA. Sagittal MR image (**E**) again shows the huge aneurysm (*thick arrows*). Note the intimal flap (*thin arrow*) at the site of dissection. Both the LV and left atrium (LA) are markedly displaced posteriorly and inferiorly. Axial MR image (**F**) shows the huge aneurysm (*thick arrows*). Again note that the LA and PA are displaced away from the aneurysm.

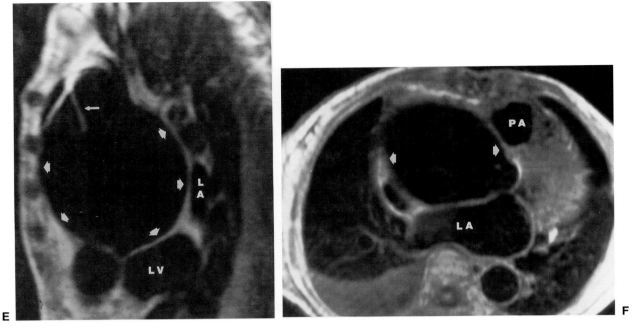

FIG. 11-11. *Continued*

ascending aorta is specific for the diagnosis of syphilitic aortitis (see **Fig. 10-18**) as well as for Marfan's syndrome with AI (Fig. 11-11). In syphilitic aortitis, calcification of the ascending aorta is an additional diagnostic feature.

Echocardiography

Echocardiography may show the diastolic flutter of the mitral valve even in mild AI. In patients with severe disease, septal and posterior wall motion is usually increased. Echocardiography is also effective in determining the cause of the disease (e.g., dilated ascending aorta in syphilitic aortitis with aortic regurgitation) as well as assessing left ventricular performance in the selection of surgical candidates (1).

SYSTEMIC HYPERTENSION

Systemic hypertension is not a valvular disease, but because its radiographic features are similar to aortic valve disease it is briefly described here. This condition may mimic AS clinically because of a similar ejection systolic murmur in the aortic area. It may also mimic AS radiographically and on electrocardiography, in that both diseases provoke left ventricular hypertrophy. The greatest similarity between degenerative AS and SH is found on the posteroanterior radiograph, where one sees in both diseases a combination of left ventricular hypertrophy and diffuse dilatation of the entire thoracic aorta. However, the presence of aortic valve Ca^{2+} on the lateral radiograph will promptly distinguish AS from SH. In addition to valve Ca^{2+}, there is one more radiographic difference between the two entities—the presence of selective dila-

tation of the ascending aorta in patients with nondegenerative AS who are <65 years old.

Systemic hypertension may also mimic AI radiographically by the presence of diffuse dilatation of the thoracic aorta. The major differences distinguishing AI from SH are that the left ventricle is much bigger in AI because of volume overload and that, on fluoroscopy or other dynamic studies, the increased amplitude of pulsation of the left ventricle and the aorta is much greater in AI, also as a result of volume overload. By the time of left ventricular failure, both AS and SH manifest identical radiographic features of the heart and the lung: moderate cardiomegaly with a cardiothoracic ratio only slightly >0.50 and frank pulmonary edema (Fig. 11-2). Even at that point the dynamic differences in the aorta are still discernible (see **Fig. 2-29**).

MITRAL INSUFFICIENCY

Etiology and Pathology

The major causes of chronic mitral insufficiency (MI) are mitral valve prolapse, coronary artery disease, rheumatic fever, cardiomyopathy, mitral annulus calcification, Marfan's syndrome, and congenital heart disease. In an acute context, rupture of chordae, papillary muscle, or the mitral leaflet may be traumatic, infectious, degenerative, or idiopathic (2,5).

Rheumatic Fever

Rheumatic fever is one of the most common causes of MI. The age incidence for acute rheumatic fever ranges from

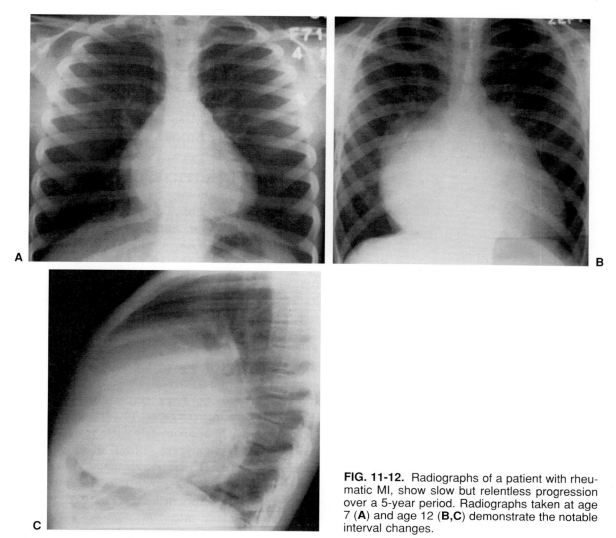

FIG. 11-12. Radiographs of a patient with rheumatic MI, show slow but relentless progression over a 5-year period. Radiographs taken at age 7 (**A**) and age 12 (**B,C**) demonstrate the notable interval changes.

5 to 15 years, with an average of 12. It has been estimated that ~19 years are required for significant mitral stenosis to develop (5,6). Therefore, rheumatic mitral disease in patients <15 years old is most likely an insufficient lesion (Fig. 11-12). At any age, rheumatic MI occurs more frequently in males. The pathologic findings of rheumatic MI consist of deformity and retraction of the valve leaflets, shortening and fusion of the chordae tendineae, and adhesion of the posterior leaflet to the left ventricular wall (7).

Bacterial Endocarditis

Bacterial infection of the mitral valve causes perforation of the leaflets or rupture of the chordae, leading to acute or subacute MI and congestive heart failure (Fig. 11-13). Echocardiography is useful for detecting valvular vegetations (Fig. 11-14) resulting from infective endocarditis.

Myxomatous Change

In patients with Marfan's syndrome and mitral valve prolapse (Fig. 11-15), MI results from myxomatous proliferation in the tissue, causing redundancy of the leaflets, spontaneous rupture of the chordae, and dilatation of the annulus (2,5).

Cardiomyopathy

Mitral insufficiency results from left ventricular failure of any cause, including dilated cardiomyopathy (Figs. 11-16; see also **Fig. 15-3**) and endocardial fibroelastosis. The mechanical factors of valve insufficiency under these circumstances are dilatation of the mitral orifice and malalignment of the tensor apparatus. In patients with IHSS, the SAM of a mitral leaflet is responsible for the valve leakage (Fig. 11-8).

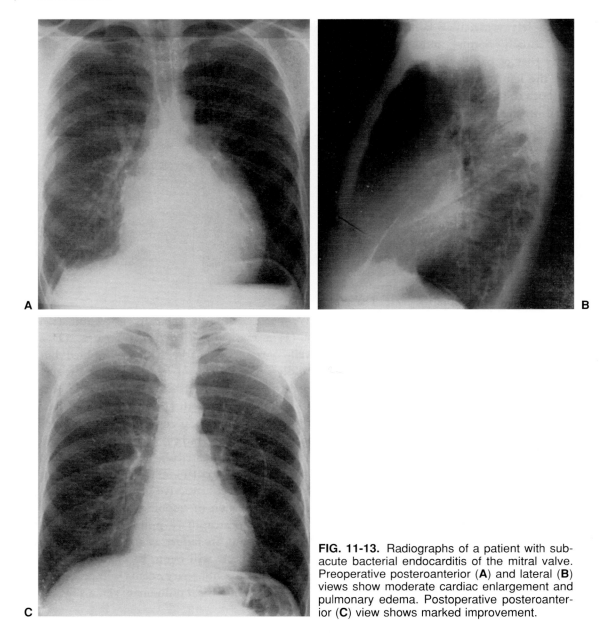

FIG. 11-13. Radiographs of a patient with subacute bacterial endocarditis of the mitral valve. Preoperative posteroanterior (**A**) and lateral (**B**) views show moderate cardiac enlargement and pulmonary edema. Postoperative posteroanterior (**C**) view shows marked improvement.

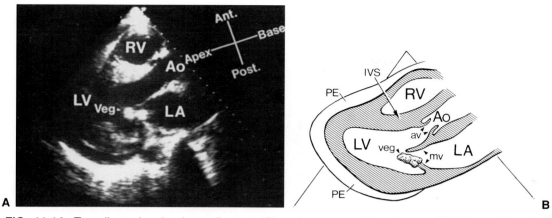

FIG. 11-14. Two-dimensional echocardiogram (**A**) and corresponding diagram (**B**) of a patient with infective endocarditis showing a large vegetation on the posterior leaflet of the mitral valve. A pericardial effusion (PE) is also noted. In real time, the vegetation (veg) appears to be shaggy and dense, but the involved leaflet moves freely. Ant., anterior; Ao, aorta; av, aortic valve; IVS, interventricular septum; LA, left atrium; LV, left ventricle; mv, mitral valve; Post., posterior; RV, right ventricle.

Myocardial Infarction

Papillary muscle dysfunction or rupture is the principal cause of MI in patients with coronary heart disease (**Fig. 13-1**).

Trauma

A rare cause of MI is rupture of the papillary muscle from blunt chest trauma (see **Fig. 18-17**).

Calcification of Mitral Annulus

Mitral insufficiency may be a complication of degenerative calcification of the mitral annulus, which becomes rigid and loses its sphincteric function (Fig. 11-17) (5).

Pathophysiology

The pathophysiology and long-term prognosis of MI revolve around two factors: the status of the left ventricular myocardium and the acuteness or chronicity of the disease. Acute MI in a previously normal heart induces severe pulmonary edema with minimal or no left atrial enlargement. The pulmonary edema tends to be of the alveolar type, sometimes with a "bat-wing" appearance (Figs. 11-3 and 11-18; see also **Fig. 18-17**). Chronic MI can be classified into two major categories: with normal myocardium and with failing myocardium.

When the myocardium is normal and the development of MI is gradual, the left ventricle can tolerate the stress of volume overload for many years with marked hypertrophy but little dilatation. On the other hand, the left atrium is a weak chamber, and it dilates considerably when subjected to volume overload under systemic pressure. This leads to pulmonary venous hypertension and reactive pulmonary arterial hypertension. Even at this stage the myocardium remains well compensated, and we are primarily dealing with the mechanical problem of a leaking valve. Once that is corrected surgically, excellent to good results are expected. This type is exemplified by MI of rheumatic etiology and MI from mitral valve prolapse syndrome.

In patients with MI stemming from left ventricular failure, the mitral valve is usually normal, and the problem is primarily that of papillary muscle dysfunction. Because the left ventricle has lost its pumping ability, both mitral regurgitant flow and left atrial size are likely to be small in contrast to the markedly dilated and poorly contracting left ventricle. This pattern is seen in patients with cardiomyopathies (Fig. 11-16; see also **Fig. 15-3**), myocarditis, and severe coronary heart disease (see **Fig. 13-1**).

Clinical Presentation

Fatigue and dyspnea are the most common complaints of patients with chronic MI. Nonrheumatic varieties of mitral MI tend to induce chest pain and palpitations. Pulmonary edema almost always accompanies acute MI (5). The murmur of chronic MI is typically holosystolic at the apex, radiating to the axilla. The murmur of acute MI tends to be louder and more harsh. In patients with mitral valve prolapse, a midsystolic click and a late systolic murmur are usually audible.

Surgical Treatment

Mitral valve replacement has been the standard treatment for severe MI for the past three decades, although mitral valve reparative procedures are being used with greater fre-

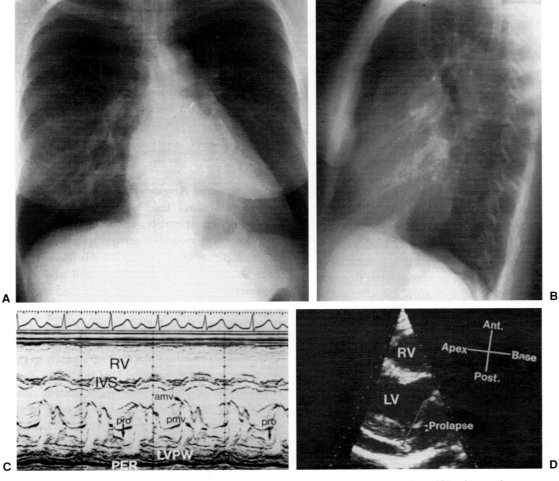

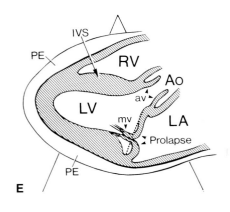

FIG. 11-15. Posteroanterior view (**A**) of a patient with mitral valve prolapse and MI shows left atrial and biventricular enlargements with cephalization of the pulmonary vascularity. Lateral view (**B**) shows a straight back (spine) and a pectus excavatum with narrowing of the anteroposterior diameter of the chest. The left-lower-lobe bronchus is displaced posterosuperiorly by the dilated left atrium. The left ventricle is obviously enlarged. An M-mode echocardiogram (**C**) of another patient shows late systolic mitral valve prolapse (pro). In addition, the mitral leaflets appear slightly thickened. A two-dimensional long-axis echocardiogram (**D**) and corresponding diagram (**E**) show prolapse of both mitral leaflets into the left atrium behind the plane (dotted lines) of the mitral valve (mv). A pericardial effusion (PE) is also evident. amv, anterior mitral leaflet; Ant., anterior; Ao, aorta; av, aortic valve; IVS, interventricular septum; LA, left atrium; LV, left ventricle; LVPW, posterior wall of the left ventricle; mv, mitral valve; PER, pericardium; pmv, posterior mitral leaflet; Post., posterior; RV, right ventricle.

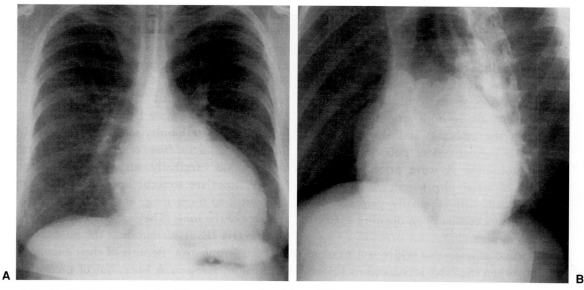

FIG. 11-16. Posteroanterior (**A**) and left anterior oblique (**B**) views of a patient with dilated cardiomyopathy and MI. Note that the left ventricle is markedly dilated while the left atrium is only mildly enlarged.

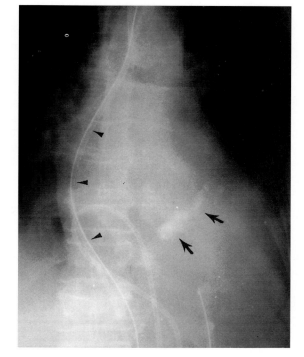

FIG. 11-17. An elderly woman with mitral annular calcification (*arrows*), atrial fibrillation, and severe MI. Note that the nasogastric tube is deviated to the right side (*arrowheads*).

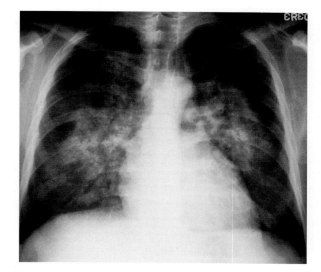

FIG. 11-18. In a patient with acute MI resulting from myocardial infarction, note the "bat-wing" type of pulmonary edema. There was no significant cardiomegaly.

quency and success (5). In selected patients with localized valvular abnormalities and/or annular dilatation, mitral valve repair has been shown to be superior to replacement in terms of long-term survival, freedom from thromboembolism, and postoperative ventricular function. A variety of reparative techniques are used to maintain the papillary muscle-chordae-annular continuity, which is crucial to preserving postoperative ventricular function. A rigid Carpentier-Edwards or a flexible Duran annuloplasty ring may be used to stabilize the annulus. One contraindication of valve repair is the presence of heavy valvular calcification (5).

Echocardiography

Echocardiography is more useful in determining the cause than in assessing the severity of MI (2). Mitral valve prolapse (Fig. 11-15), flail leaflets, vegetations (Fig. 11-14), and rupture of chordae, for example, can all be identified by this method as the basis of a leaky valve.

Radiographic and Angiographic Signs

In chronic MI with good left ventricular function, there are several typical radiographic signs: (a) a giant left atrium (Fig. 11-12); (b) a moderately enlarged, markedly hypertrophied but well-contracting left ventricle; (c) striking paradoxical movements between the left atrium and ventricle representing an enormous reciprocal volume exchange (see **Fig. 2-37**); (d) a posterior wedging sign (8) (see **Fig. 2-27**); (e) a calcified MacCallum's patch in the left atrial wall if some mitral stenosis is present (see **Fig. 10-13**); and (f) redistribution of the pulmonary blood flow toward the upper lung zones without apparent pulmonary edema. On the left ventriculogram, blood can be seen regurgitating into the left atrium and even filling the pulmonary veins (see **Fig. 18-17B**).

In MI stemming from left ventricular failure, the radiographic signs are distinctly different from the pattern just described (Fig. 11-16). It is the left ventricle instead of the left atrium that is markedly dilated. Moreover, the left ventricle contracts poorly and is unable to pump blood efficiently in either direction. The regurgitant flow is therefore small, and so is the size of the left atrium. The paradoxical movements between the left atrium and ventricle are much less conspicuous. And, last, cephalization of the pulmonary vasculature with or without pulmonary edema is usually present. The different dynamic features between the two types of chronic MI can be assessed with cine angiocardiography or noninvasively by fluoroscopy, echocardiography, cine computed tomography, or cine MR imaging.

MITRAL STENOSIS

Etiology

Rheumatic fever is the most common cause of mitral stenosis (MS). Infrequently, a myxoma or a ball valve thrombus may obstruct the mitral valve (2,5). In rare instances, MS may be congenital (9,10). With the subsidence of rheumatic pancarditis, the myocardium and pericardium usually recover satisfactorily. Healing of the endocarditis, on the other hand, may lead to permanent damage to the valve with MI or MS or both. The effects of rheumatic valvulitis may be scarring and fusion between leaflets, at commissures, and among chordae tendineae. In the early stages of the process the mitral valve leaks. After an average of ~20 years (6), a considerable number of adhesions may develop at the edges of the mitral leaflets to form a funnel-like stenotic valve (2).

Pathophysiology

Mitral valve obstruction is accompanied by left atrial hypertension, which is transmitted backward, raising pressures in the pulmonary veins and capillaries. When the intravascular hydrostatic pressure exceeds the plasma oncotic pressure of 25 mm Hg, fluid begins to leak out of the vessels, causing pulmonary edema. Since there is a pressure gradient of 22 mm Hg from the apex to the base of the lung in the upright position, pulmonary edema in these patients will understandably commence in the bases. The predictable reaction to edema and its resultant hypoxia is pulmonary vasoconstriction. The pulmonary blood flow is thus rechanneled from the bases to the apexes, forming a cephalic pattern on the chest radiograph. If MS worsens, the right ventricle may fail, and the tricuspid valve may become incompetent, as may the pulmonary valve. Subsequently, pulmonary venous congestion may improve at the expense of severe systemic venous hypertension.

Clinical Presentation

The classic symptoms of MS are dyspnea, palpitations, easy fatigue, and hemoptysis. Occasionally, the patient experiences chest pain and, rarely, hoarseness. Following the development of atrial fibrillation, mural thrombi can form in both atria and embolize both the systemic and pulmonary arteries. The jugular venous pulse typically exhibits a prominent A wave before the development of atrial fibrillation. A parasternal right ventricular lift is usually palpable. The classic murmurs consist of an opening snap and a diastolic rumble.

The normal mitral valve orifice is 4 to 6 cm^2 in adults. When the valve is reduced to ≤ 1.3 cm^2, medical treatment alone will not suffice; catheter balloon dilatation or surgical intervention becomes necessary. If the valve appears flexible on echocardiography or angiocardiography and there is no evidence of major calcification on fluoroscopy, balloon valvotomy or open surgical valvuloplasty may be preferred to valve replacement. Valve replacement with its known complications should be reserved for patients with a rigid or heavily calcified valve. Regardless of the surgical procedure used, the annular-papillary muscle continuity should be preserved for improved postoperative ventricular function (5).

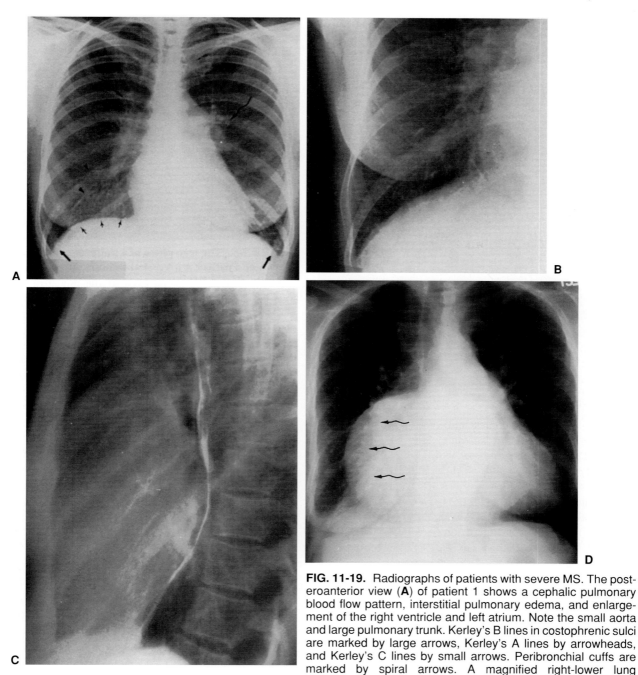

FIG. 11-19. Radiographs of patients with severe MS. The posteroanterior view (**A**) of patient 1 shows a cephalic pulmonary blood flow pattern, interstitial pulmonary edema, and enlargement of the right ventricle and left atrium. Note the small aorta and large pulmonary trunk. Kerley's B lines in costophrenic sulci are marked by large arrows, Kerley's A lines by arrowheads, and Kerley's C lines by small arrows. Peribronchial cuffs are marked by spiral arrows. A magnified right-lower lung zone (**B**) of patient 2 shows multiple Kerley's B lines and constriction of the lower zone vessels. A lateral view (**C**) of patient 3 shows a small left ventricular image behind the inferior vena cava, cephalization of the pulmonary vasculature, and enlargement of the left atrium and right ventricle. The posteroanterior view (**D**) of patient 4 shows a huge RA (*arrows*) due to TI in addition to signs of critical MS.

Radiographic Signs

The radiographic signs are subtle in the early stages of MS. Special attention should be directed to mild left atrial enlargement, of which the most sensitive evidence is a localized posterior and rightward deviation of the barium-filled esophagus (see **Fig. 2-22**) or the nasogastric tube.

The advanced stage of MS (calculated mitral valve area <1.3 cm^2) is manifested by the following signs (11): (a) moderate left atrial and right ventricular enlargements, (b) moderate pulmonary trunk dilatation, (c) cephalization of the pulmonary vasculature (see **Figs. 7-7B,C** and **8-2**), (d) septal lines or Kerley's B lines in the costophrenic sulci (Fig. 11-19B; see also **Fig. 7-7B,C**), (e) unusually small left

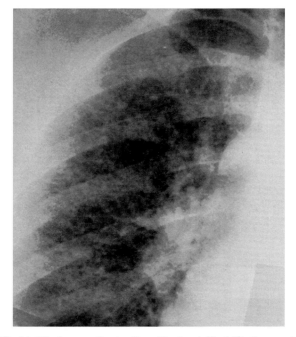

FIG. 11-20. In a patient with critical calcific MS, the posteroanterior radiograph (not shown) reveals fine stipplings throughout both lungs. A magnified view of the right-upper zone shows the classic hazy miliary pattern, a combination of hemosiderosis and interstitial pulmonary edema. The patient's sputum evidenced hemosiderin-laden macrophages.

ventricular image on the lateral view (Fig. 11-19C), (f) an unusually small image of the aortic arch on the posteroanterior view (Fig. 11-19A; see also **Fig. 7-7**), and (g) calcification of the mitral valve (see **Fig. 10-7**). Calcification of the mitral valve occurs in ~60% of patients with severe MS, with the highest incidence in patients >50 years of age (12).

Kerley's lines are believed to represent thickening of interlobular septa (hence the alternative term, septal lines) rather than engorged lymphatics, as originally suspected by Kerley (13). "A" lines are straight lines, ~1 mm thick and 2 to 6 cm long and well within the substance of the lung. They are thickened sheets of connective tissue surrounding the pulmonary veins and lymphatics. Because of their anatomic distribution, Kerley's A lines of necessity converge to the hilum on either side. Kerley's B lines represent thickened interlobular septa in the periphery of the lung. They are of the same width as A lines but much shorter, usually <2 cm long. They are straight lines abutting against and perpendicular to the visceral pleura or the edematous subpleural interstitial space, found most frequently in the right costophrenic sulcus, next frequently in the left costophrenic sulcus, and rarely in the more superior position (see **Fig. 8-29**). Kerley's C lines are fine weblike reticulations, probably representing superimposition of multiple B lines (Fig. 11-19A). Septal lines are reversible when pulmonary edema or neoplastic infiltration is the sole reason for their existence. They are irreversible when hemosiderosis, fibrosis, or pneumoconiosis is well advanced.

Rare signs of severe MS are pulmonary hemosiderosis representing the end result of alveolar and interstitial hemorrhage (Fig. 11-20); pulmonary ossification exemplifying the far-advanced stage of pulmonary venous congestion and hemorrhage, perhaps one step further than the stage of hemosiderosis (Fig. 11-21); and calcification of the left atrial wall (12) (see **Fig. 10-12**).

Angiocardiography

During cine left ventriculography, the valve is delineated by the opacified blood on one side and the nonopacified blood on the other. Since the mitral leaflets typically fuse along their edges, in diastole the valve balloons downward into the left ventricle, forming a funnel-shaped lucency. Sometimes a negative jet may be seen emanating from the apex of the funnel into the opacified chamber. In systole the valve pops back to the floor of the left atrium. The wide excursion of the valve between the two phases of the cardiac cycle denotes its flexibility. The mitral valve can also be evaluated by injecting contrast medium into the pulmonary trunk and then watching the levo phase of the study (Fig. 11-22). When the valve is diffusely fibrosed or calcified, such flexibility will be lost. A left ventriculogram is important for ruling out MI. An aortogram is used to exclude AI.

Echocardiography

Echocardiography is a useful noninvasive technique for evaluating the mitral valve. In MS the E-F slope is typically

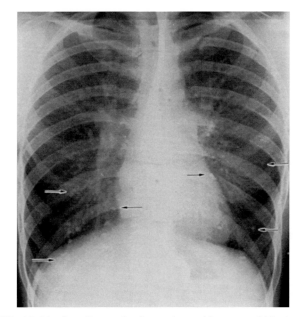

FIG. 11-21. A radiograph of a patient with severe MS shows numerous small, rounded bone densities in both lower lung zones (*arrows*). The presence of rheumatic heart disease and the absence of mediastinal, hilar, and splenic calcifications support the diagnosis of pulmonary ossification and militate against that of a granulomatous process.

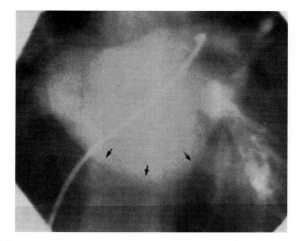

FIG. 11-22. The levo phase of a pulmonary arteriogram of a patient with MS shows a markedly dilated left atrium with the mitral valve (*arrows*) ballooning into the left ventricle in diastole. There is very little opacification of the left ventricle, suggestive of MS.

diminished (Fig. 11-23), the valve motion is decreased, and the calcified mitral valve produces thick echoes. This technique is also valuable in differentiating MS from nonrheumatic causes of mitral valve obstruction, such as left atrial myxoma (see **Figs. 18-9** and **18-10**). The domed mitral valve in diastole can be recorded in the long-axis view of a two-dimensional echocardiogram (Fig. 11-24) similar to that seen in a left ventriculogram (see the discussion under Angiocardiography). In the short-axis view, the orifice of a stenotic mitral valve can also be seen and measured.

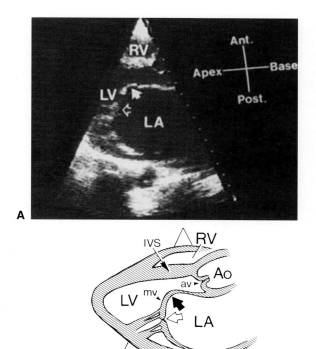

FIG. 11-24. A two-dimensional echocardiogram in long-axis (**A**) view and corresponding diagram (**B**) demonstrate the enlarged left atrium (LA) and the abnormal mitral valve configuration (mv) suggestive of MS. The tips of the mitral valve (*open arrow*) are thickened and tethered to the chordal apparatus. The mitral valve leaflet (*closed arrow pointing to the anterior leaflet*) is not thickened and has great mobility. In this diastolic frame, the aortic valve (av) is closed and appears mildly thickened. The left ventricular cavity (LV) seems small in comparison with the dilated left atrium (LA). Ant., anterior; Ao, aorta; IVS, interventricular septum; Post., posterior; RV, right ventricle.

Cardiac Catheterization

The hemodynamic variables of MS are most accurately determined by cardiac catheterization. The mitral valve gradient is measured by simultaneously tracking the left atrial and the left ventricular pressures. The mitral valve area is then calculated by correlating the pressure gradient with the cardiac output.

TRICUSPID INSUFFICIENCY

Etiology

The most common cause of tricuspid insufficiency (TI) is right ventricular failure with marked dilatation of the tricuspid annulus and major distortion of other structures of the tricuspid apparatus. This is a functional insufficiency without organic changes of the tricuspid valve. The less com-

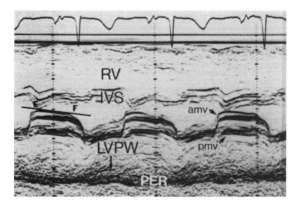

FIG. 11-23. An M-mode echocardiogram of a patient with MS shows that both the anterior leaflet (amv) and the posterior leaflet (pmv) of the mitral valve are thickened. Instead of moving in an antiparallel manner, as expected, the pmv moves in the same direction as the amv in diastole. The E-F slope is typically reduced or flat. The right ventricle (RV) is mildly dilated. E, the most forward position of amv during early ventricular filling; F, the partially closed position of amv as rapid filling decreases; IVS, interventricular septum; LVPW, posterior wall of left ventricle; PER, pericardium.

mon causes include carcinoid syndrome, traumatic rupture of the valve, and infective endocarditis in drug addicts. The congenital anomalies see in association with TI include Ebstein's anomaly (see **Fig. 2-6**), atrioventricular septal defects (see **Figs. 16-19** and **16-20**), and infantile persistence of fetal pulmonary circulation.

In patients with malignant carcinoid, the fibrous plaques are most extensively deposited on the ventricular side of the tricuspid valve, thereby causing adhesions between the valve and the right ventricular wall. The result is tricuspid regurgitation (see **Fig. 18-15**) (2). In rheumatic heart disease, tricuspid lesions do not exist in isolation. Mitral disease almost always coexists with tricuspid disease, most notably severe MS leading to functional TI (Fig. 11-19D; see also **Figs. 9-5, 9-8,** and **9-10**). Frequently, mitral, tricuspid, and aortic insufficiencies may be present in one patient, producing a gigantic heart (see **Fig. 2-20**).

Pathophysiology and Clinical Presentation

Without pulmonary hypertension (e.g., in Ebstein's anomaly), the hemodynamic impact of TI is well tolerated by the patient for a long time before the onset of right-sided heart failure. In the presence of pulmonary hypertension, however, TI rapidly leads to systemic venous congestion and pulmonary oligemia (e.g., severe MS leading to TI). In this situation, the symptoms of pulmonary venous congestion may actually improve at the price of severe abdominal distension and peripheral edema (2).

Physical findings of TI include neck vein distension with positive hepatojugular reflux, hepatomegaly, ascites, and peripheral edema. A parasternal right ventricular lift is usually present. If the foramen ovale is patent, a right-to-left shunt may develop in the face of pressure and volume overload of the right atrium, inducing clinical cyanosis. On auscultation, a blowing holosystolic murmur is usually intensified during inspiration. The treatment for TI depends primarily on whether significant pulmonary hypertension is present. If it is not, surgical intervention may be delayed. If it is, valve replacement with anticoagulation therapy becomes necessary for most patients.

Radiographic and Angiographic Signs

The radiographic signs of TI include right-sided chamber enlargement (see **Figs. 2-30, 9-5,** and **9-10**) and exaggerated systolic expansion of the right atrium and venae cavae (see **Fig. 2-30**). The azygos vein and the aortic nipple (the left superior intercostal vein) may also dilate as a result of systemic venous hypertension (see **Fig. 18-15A**). An abrupt elevation of the right hemidiaphragm during systole indicates a forceful reflux of blood from the right atrium all the way into the hepatic veins. The value of angiography in the diagnosis of TI is questionable mainly because, to reach the right ventricle, the catheter must cross the tricuspid valve. In the case of left-sided heart failure leading to right-sided heart failure with TI, the associated findings of mitral disease (see **Figs. 9-5, 9-8,** and **9-10**) and aortic disease may also be present.

Echocardiography

Echocardiography can distinguish both anatomic and functional abnormalities of the tricuspid valve. Contrast ultrasonography (Fig. 11-25) can identify the to and fro current across the valve (in TI) as well as any right-to-left shunt across the atrial septum (in atrial septal defects); the echo Doppler technique can estimate the severity of TI.

TRICUSPID STENOSIS

Etiology

Tricuspid stenosis (TS) is most commonly rheumatic in origin. Other causes, such as congenital TS, right atrial tumors, and carcinoid syndrome, are rare. Rheumatic TS is almost always associated with MS. In the congenital category, tricuspid atresia is more common than stenosis. Right atrial myxoma is the dominant neoplasm causing tricuspid valve obstruction. In carcinoid syndrome the tricuspid valve tends to be insufficient rather than stenotic (2).

Pathophysiology and Clinical Presentation

With severe TS cardiac output becomes markedly diminished when the mean diastolic pressure gradient exceeds 5 mm Hg or the tricuspid valve area is <2.0 cm^2. The clinical manifestations are primarily those of low cardiac output (fatigue) and systemic venous hypertension (abdominal distension and peripheral edema). Although MS almost always coexists with rheumatic TS, the symptoms of MS, such as dyspnea, hemoptysis, and pulmonary edema, are usually mild or absent because of the markedly reduced pulmonary blood flow.

The physical findings of TS include a presystolic pulsation of the neck veins and liver and signs of hepatomegaly and ascites. On auscultation, a diastolic murmur and an opening snap may be heard. Furthermore, a diastolic thrill that increases in intensity during inspiration is usually present. When MS coexists with TS, the auscultatory findings of TS may be overshadowed by similar but louder sounds originating from the mitral area (2). The electrocardiogram in patients with TS without atrial fibrillation frequently shows evidence of an enlarged right atrium disproportionate to the severity of right ventricular hypertrophy (2). Medical treatment for severe TS is usually unsatisfactory. Surgical inter-

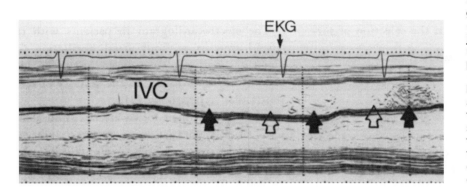

vention in the form of open commissurotomy or valve replacement is indicated when the tricuspid valve becomes tighter than 2.0 cm² (2). Anticoagulation with coumadin is usually required after valve replacement.

Radiographic and Angiographic Signs

The classic radiographic signs of TS are right atrial and systemic venous dilatation (see **Fig. 7-3B**). Before the development of atrial fibrillation, exaggerated diastolic expansion of the right atrium, venae cavae, and azygos vein is usually observed. At the same time, abrupt elevation of the right hemidiaphragm may also be seen as the liver expands in diastole. Very similar dynamic changes are also encountered in patients with right atrial myxoma. Since there is a marked decrease in cardiac output in general and in pulmonary blood flow in particular, the lungs are usually oligemic in patients with severe TS. When MS coexists with TS, the pulmonary vascularity manifests a combination of decreased flow and

mild cephalization. In the context of a low-flow situation, the other signs of MS would also be less conspicuous.

The best angiographic projection is a left posterior oblique view when the tricuspid valve is imaged tangentially and the right atrium and ventricle are effectively separated. When contrast medium is injected into the right atrium, the enlarged chamber quickly becomes densely opacified and remains distended for a prolonged period of time (Fig. 11-26). In each diastole, the stenotic valve balloons into the right ventricle with an opaque jet emanating from the apex of the funnel-shaped valve. The thickened tricuspid leaflets appear as mobile radiolucent stripes between the opacified cardiac chambers.

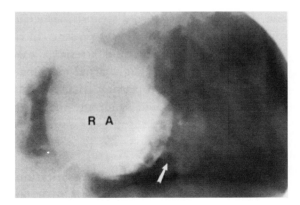

FIG. 11-26. Right atrial injection of a patient with TS. Note a densely opacified and markedly dilated right atrium (RA) emptying its contents through a small orifice with difficulty. The tricuspid valve has some pliability, and it balloons downward and leftward into the right ventricle in diastole. The arrow points to a jet of contrast medium entering the right ventricle.

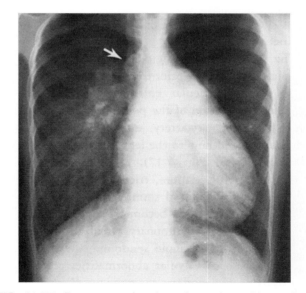

FIG. 11-27. Posteroanterior view of a patient with tetralogy of Fallot, absent pulmonary valve, and partial anomalous pulmonary venous connection from the right lung to the azygos vein. Note the markedly enlarged pulmonary trunk and central pulmonary arterial segments with a paucity of peripheral pulmonary vascularity. Also note the enlarged azygos vein (*arrow*).

Echocardiography

Echocardiography can diagnose TS and the severity of the disease. It can also recognize mural thrombi and intracavitary tumors.

PULMONARY INSUFFICIENCY

By far the most common cause of pulmonary insufficiency (PI) is severe pulmonary arterial hypertension of any derivation, such as severe MS and recurrent pulmonary thromboembolic disease (see **Fig. 10-19**). Less commonly, PI may result from conditions such as infective endocarditis, surgical treatment of pulmonary stenosis, and Marfan's syndrome. Occasionally, one may encounter a leaky pulmonary valve as a component of congenital heart disease, such as in tetralogy of Fallot (Fig. 11-27), ventricular septal defect, and valvular PS. Carcinoid syndrome and syphilis rarely produce an incompetent pulmonary valve (2).

PULMONARY STENOSIS

Valvular pulmonary stenosis (PS) is most commonly a congenital condition. Other causes include carcinoid syndrome and rheumatic inflammation, both of which are extremely rare.

Radiographic Signs

The basic radiographic findings of valvular PS before heart failure include right ventricular enlargement, poststenotic dilatation of the pulmonary trunk and the left pulmonary artery, increased pulmonary blood flow to the left, and decreased flow to the right (see **Fig. 8-17**). After the onset of right ventricular failure, TI and a right-to-left atrial shunt may develop (see **Fig. 7-4**). The heart becomes quite large and globular, and the pulmonary vascularity begins to decrease. In carcinoid syndrome, the typical combination of valvular abnormalities are TI (see the previous discussion) and PS. Pulmonary stenosis is due to deposition of fibrous tissue on the endocardium of the valve and the right ventricle, leading to fusion and constriction of these structures. Special attention should be paid to the lack of poststenotic dilatation of the pulmonary trunk in carcinoid PS (2) (see **Fig. 18-15**) as opposed to congenital PS. Calcific PS is a rarity (14) (see **Fig. 7-5**).

Echocardiography

Echocardiographic techniques can assess the anatomic and functional abnormalities of the pulmonary valve as well as the condition of the right ventricle.

COMBINED VALVULAR DISEASE

Multivalvular involvement is common in patients with rheumatic heart disease, cardiomyopathies, and such connective tissue disorders as Marfan's syndrome. In general, the proximal valve lesion tends to mask the distal one in clinical and radiographic manifestations (2). For instance, when mitral and tricuspid lesions coexist, the clinical and radiographic signs of tricuspid disease are more prominent than those of mitral disease (see **Fig. 9-5**). By the same token, signs of mitral disease tend to mask those of coexistent aortic disease.

REFERENCES

1. Rapaport E, Rackley CE, Cohn LH. Aortic valve disease. In: Schlant RC, Alexander RW, eds. *The heart*, 8th ed. New York: McGraw–Hill, 1994:1457–1482.
2. Braunwald E. Valvular heart disease. In: Braunwald E, ed. *Heart disease: a textbook of cardiovascular medicine*, 4th ed. Philadelphia: Saunders, 1992:1007–1077.
3. Nugent EW, Plauth WH, Edwards JE, et al. Congenital heart disease. In: Schlant RC, Alexander RW, eds. *The heart*, 8th ed. New York: McGraw–Hill, 1994:1761–1828.
4. Stone J. Syphilis and the cardiovascular system. In: Schlant RC, Alexander RW, eds. *The heart*, 8th ed. New York: McGraw–Hill, 1994: 1949–1952.
5. Gaasch WH, O'Rourke RA, Cohn LH, et al. Mitral valve disease. In: Schlant RC, Alexander RW, eds. *The heart*, 8th ed. New York: McGraw–Hill, 1994:1483–1578.
6. Wood P. An appreciation of mitral stenosis. *Br Med J* 1954;1: 1051–1063.
7. Edwards JE, Burchell HB. Pathologic anatomy of mitral insufficiency. *Proc Mayo Clin* 1958;33:497–509.
8. Chen JTT, Lester RG, Peter RH. Posterior wedging sign of mitral insufficiency. *Radiology* 1974;113:451–453.
9. Ferencz C, Johnson AL, Siglesworth FW. Congenital mitral stenosis. *Circulation* 1954;9:161–179.
10. Rodan BA, Chen JTT, Kirks DR, et al. Mitral valve calcification in congenital mitral stenosis. *Am Heart J* 1983;105:514–515.
11. Chen JTT, Behar VS, Morris JJ, et al. Correlation of roentgen findings with hemodynamic data in pure mitral stenosis. *AJR Am J Roentgenol* 1968;102:280–292.
12. Chen JTT. The significance of cardiac calcifications. *Appl Radiol* 1992; 21:11–19.
13. Fraser RG, Pare JAP. *Diagnosis of diseases of the chest*, vol. 1, 2nd ed. Philadelphia: Saunders, 1977.
14. Convarrubias EA, Sheikh MU, Isner JM, et al. Calcific pulmonic stenosis in adulthood. *Chest* 1979;75:399–402.
15. Stanford, W. Assessment of valvular heart disease. In: Stanford W, Rumberger JA, eds. *Ultrafast computed tomography in cardiac imaging: principles and practice*. Mount Kisco, N.Y.: Futura, 1992.
16. Kirks DR. *Practical pediatric imaging*. 2nd ed. Boston: Little, Brown, 1991:417–513.

Essentials of Cardiac Imaging,
James T. T. Chen,
Lippincott–Raven Publishers, Philadelphia © 1998.

CHAPTER 12

Pulmonary Heart Disease

James T. T. Chen

The term pulmonary heart disease means a disease of the right side of the heart caused by either structural or functional abnormalities of the lung or its vasculature (1). It is also known as cor pulmonale. Acute cor pulmonale (2) usually results from massive pulmonary embolism. Chronic cor pulmonale (1,3–5) has many causes, including structural abnormalities (e.g., emphysema, chronic bronchitis, restrictive lung disease, upper-airway obstruction, and multiple pulmonary emboli), functional abnormalities (e.g., neuromuscular and chest wall disorders and inadequate ventilatory drive), and primary pulmonary hypertension of unknown cause.

The pulmonary circulation is a high-flow, low-resistance system with considerable reserve. In most patients without cardiopulmonary disease, the cross-sectional area of the pulmonary arteries must be reduced by >50% before any hemodynamic effect can be detected (4). When the normal limits are exceeded, as by massive pulmonary embolism, the pulmonary arterial pressure rises abruptly, leading to right ventricular failure and systemic venous congestion. In addition to mechanical obstruction of the pulmonary vasculature, vasoconstriction mediated by reflex neural and humeral factors also contributes to the development of precapillary pulmonary hypertension (4–6).

PULMONARY EMBOLISM AND INFARCTION

Pulmonary embolism is one of the leading causes of death in the United States. Its incidence in unselected autopsies is ~10%. In patients with chronic cardiopulmonary disease, pulmonary emboli are found in >30% (3–6). Death occurs immediately in 10% of patients with acute pulmonary embolism. For those who survive the first hour, continued survival depends on whether appropriate therapy is initiated promptly. Unfortunately, in 70% of these individuals the diagnosis is missed, and one third of them eventually die of

Department of Radiology, Duke University School of Medicine, Durham, North Carolina 27710, U.S.A.

repeated bouts of pulmonary embolism. Patients who survive pulmonary embolism without treatment are likely to suffer chronic cor pulmonale owing to the cumulative effects of a recurrent disease (1,3). On the other hand, the death rate of patients treated for pulmonary embolism is only 8% overall and 16% for those with massive emboli (6). In patients who are adequately treated in the acute phase and with whom preventive measures are taken against recurrent episodes of pulmonary embolism, the long-term prognosis is encouraging.

Pathophysiology

Venous thrombi that eventually embolize the pulmonary arteries originate in the calves of the leg in >90% of patients (5,6). Predisposing factors for venous thrombosis are stasis of blood, damage to the venous wall, and a hypercoagulable state. Stasis of blood is by far the most serious factor fostering the development of venous thrombi. Usually, it is the result of congestive heart failure or prolonged bed rest. Damage to the venous wall occurs from inflammation, trauma, surgery, and phlebosclerosis of old age. A hypercoagulable state is encountered in pregnant women, women on oral contraceptives, and people with congenital antithrombin III deficiency. The pathogenesis of pulmonary embolism is twofold. First, gradual obstruction of the pulmonary arteries leads to progressive pulmonary hypertension and right ventricular strain. Second, such derangements are compounded by vasoconstriction in response to hypoxia and the vasoactive and bronchoactive agents (serotonin, histamine, and prostaglandins) released from platelets aggregated on the emboli (4).

Pulmonary embolism is frequently accompanied by atelectasis resulting from bronchospasm and alveolar collapse. Bronchospasm is provoked by hypocapnia and the bronchoactive agents. Alveolar collapse is due to the depletion of surfactant. Hemorrhagic pleural effusion is common and generally indicative of pulmonary infarction. The mechanism of

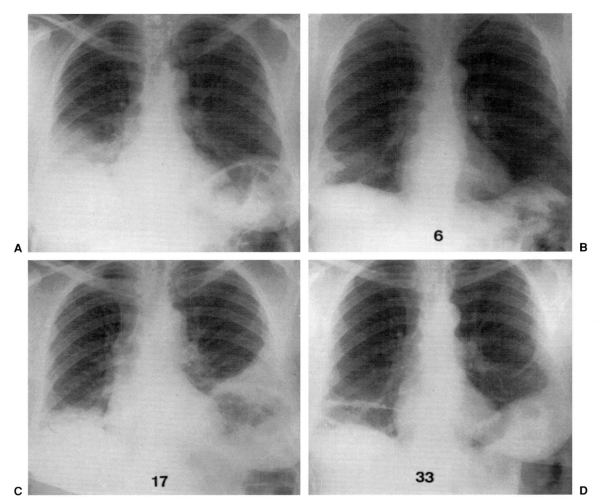

FIG. 12-1. Radiographs of a 55-year-old man with thrombocytopenic purpura. Recurrent episodes of pulmonary embolism and infarction occurred over a period of several weeks. On day 1 (**A**) hazy opacities were noted in the right base, representing a combination of hemorrhagic edema, atelectasis, and pleural effusion. The infarct itself was obscured. On day 6 (**B**), considerable clearing was noted in the right base. At that time faint infiltrates began to appear in the left base. On day 17 (**C**), no marked change was seen on the right. The left base was opacified with volume loss. By day 33 (**D**), scars had formed on both sides with pleural thickening and deformity.

its formation in the presence of pulmonary embolism is unclear.

The two types of pulmonary infarction (7) are incomplete infarct, which actually represents a hemorrhagic pulmonary edema without tissue necrosis, and complete, or true, infarct, which is associated with destruction of the lung parenchyma. Incomplete infarcts are resolved with treatment in a few days (see **Fig. 7-6**); complete ones heal by organization and scar formation over the course of ≥4 weeks (Figs. 12-1 and 12-2).

Clinical Presentation

Depending on the severity of the disease, the symptoms and signs of pulmonary embolism vary. In general, chest

pain and dyspnea are the most common symptoms. Next are anticipatory fear or anxiety and cough. Hemoptysis, diaphoresis, and syncope are seldom seen (5). The quality of chest pain may sometimes mimic angina pectoris. Rarely, acute wheezing as a result of severe bronchospasm may masquerade as bronchial asthma. The signs of pulmonary embolism are (in order of decreasing frequency) tachypnea, rales, an accentuated pulmonary component of the second heart sound, tachycardia, fever, gallop rhythms, diaphoresis, and phlebitis (5). The electrocardiographic findings are highly variable and, in most patients, not diagnostic.

Radiographic Signs

The radiographic findings per se are nonspecific. However, given the proper context of clinical implications, they can be quite useful in suggesting the diagnosis of pulmonary embolism. the first such finding is Westermark's sign (localized pulmonary oligemia) due to acute obstruction of a major pulmonary artery (see **Fig. 8-20**). This pattern is reversible with thrombolytic or vigorous anticoagulant therapy. There may also be evidence of recent development of a centralized pulmonary blood flow pattern (Fig. 12-3).

Third, there may be persistent centralization with mosaic pulmonary oligemia (8) (Fig. 12-4; see also **Fig. 8-9**). This flow pattern is associated with localized arterial constrictions and dilatations owing to recurrent thromboembolic events. Mural thrombi with calcification of the pulmonary arterial wall may be encountered in its most severe form (see **Fig. 10-19**). The mosaic oligemic flow pattern is usually irreversible despite medical treatment, but it may improved with embolectomy (8) (Fig. 12-5).

Dilatation of the right side of the heart, the systemic veins, and the central pulmonary arteries with acute cor pulmonale

(see Fig. 7-6) is the fourth possible finding. Fifth is the development of pulmonary edema, atelectasis, and plural effusion with pulmonary infarction; the infarcts, however, are usually obscured until the other opacities have cleared (Figs. 12-1 and 12-2). Last, irregularly shaped pleural-based opacities may be present, which indicate pulmonary infarcts. The triangular or truncated cone (Hampton's hump) appearance of an infarct is actually a rarity (7) (Fig. 12-2).

Nuclear Pulmonary Imaging

Radionuclide ventilation–perfusion lung scans are valuable in the detection of pulmonary embolism (see **Chapter 5**). These tests should be obtained within 24 hours of an acute episode because resolution of pulmonary emboli can be swift. In general, a normal perfusion scan rules out a clinically important pulmonary embolism. A combination of

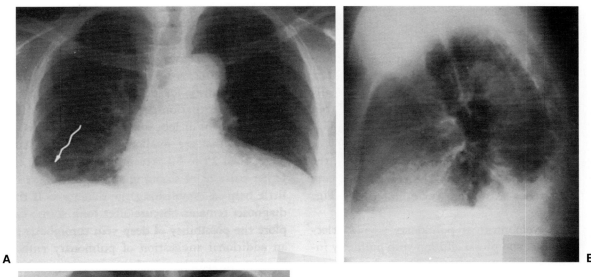

FIG. 12-2. Posteroanterior view (**A**) of a 70-year-old man recovering from bilateral pulmonary emboli shows marked hypoventilation and bilateral pleural effusions. As the acute pulmonary and pleural changes were subsiding, the pulmonary infarct in the right costophrenic sulcus began to emerge as a typical Hampton's hump (*arrow*). The lateral view (**B**) shows a residual pleural effusion and basilar atelectasis posteriorly. Posteroanterior view (**C**) of another patient with a Hampton's hump (*arrow*).

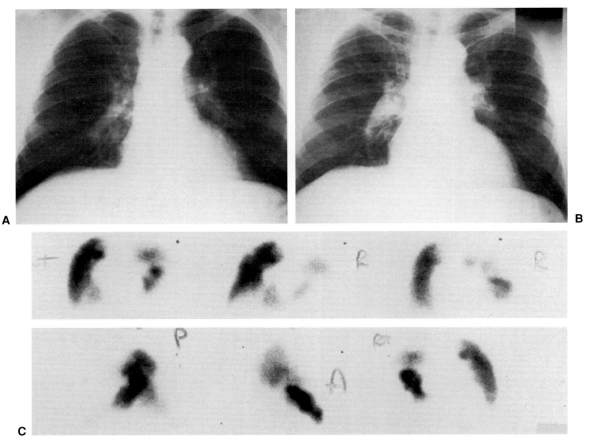

FIG. 12-3. Echocardiography of a 53-year-old man with a 5-month history of typical angina pectoris showed right-sided cardiomegaly suggesting an atrial septal defect. The patient was catheterized and found to have precapillary pulmonary hypertension, no left-to-right shunt, and no coronary or other left-sided problem. A chest film (**A**) taken 6 months previously showed normal results. The admission radiograph (**B**) reveals a striking centralized pulmonary flow pattern suggesting pulmonary arterial hypertension. A perfusion lung scan (**C**) shows multiple large defects bilaterally. The ventilation scan (**D**) gave normal results. Right (**E**) and left (**F**) pulmonary arteriograms show multiple pulmonary emboli bilaterally.

multiple perfusion defects that are greater than segmental defects, normal ventilation, and radiographically clear lungs is diagnostic of pulmonary embolism (Figs. 12-3 and 12-4). Patterns indicating a strong probability of pulmonary embolism include ventilation–perfusion mismatch of a single segment or lobe and multiple areas of mismatch that are smaller than a segment but >25% to 50% of a segment (9). Other patterns of scanning abnormalities are of little help in establishing the diagnosis. If the diagnosis remains obscure after lung scans, explore the possibility of deep vein thrombosis or go directly to pulmonary angiography.

Pulmonary and Bronchial Arteriography

Although the method is not foolproof, pulmonary arteriography remains the most reliable method of diagnosing pulmonary embolism. The angiographic signs of pulmonary embolism are filling defects in the contrast-opacified pulmonary arterial system, complete cutoff of pulmonary arteries, pruning or abrupt tapering of pulmonary arteries, prolongation of the arterial phase and delayed filling and emptying of the venous phase of the pulmonary angiogram, and regional oligemia (Figs. 12-3 and 12-4).

If pulmonary embolectomy is contemplated after an unsuccessful trial of thrombolytic therapy, a bronchial arteriogram should be performed to assess operability. In general, retrograde filling of the obstructed pulmonary artery from the bronchial arterial system is a favorable omen for surgical success (3) (Fig. 12-4).

Newer Imaging Methods

Electron beam computed tomography, spiral computed tomography, and magnetic resonance imaging have shown

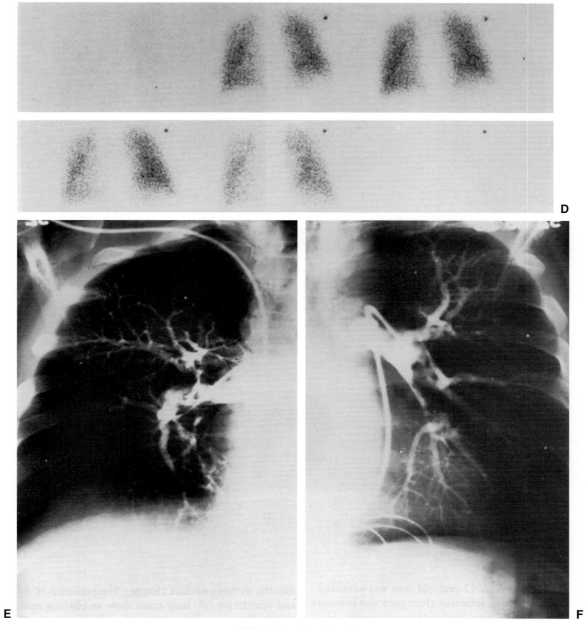

FIG. 12-3. *Continued*

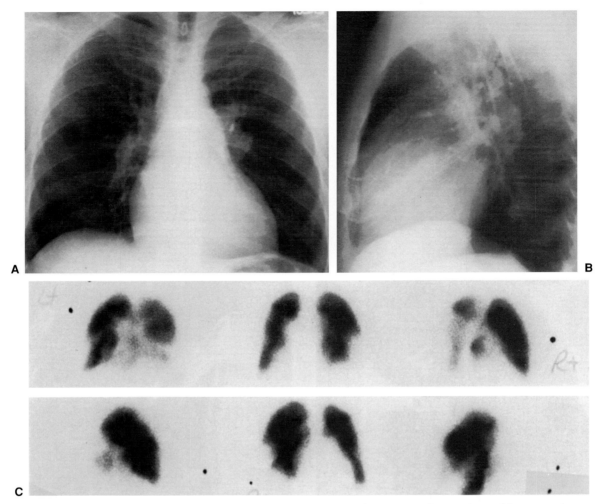

FIG. 12-4. A 42-year-old man was admitted for evaluation of recurrent chest pain and hemoptysis, which had continued for several months. His posteroanterior (**A**) and lateral (**B**) chest films show a centralized pulmonary blood flow pattern with mosaic oligemia. This pattern had persisted for months without notable change. The perfusion (**C**) and ventilation (**D**) lung scans show an obvious mismatch. The right (**E**) and left (**F**) pulmonary arteriograms confirm the diagnosis of recurrent thromboembolic disease.

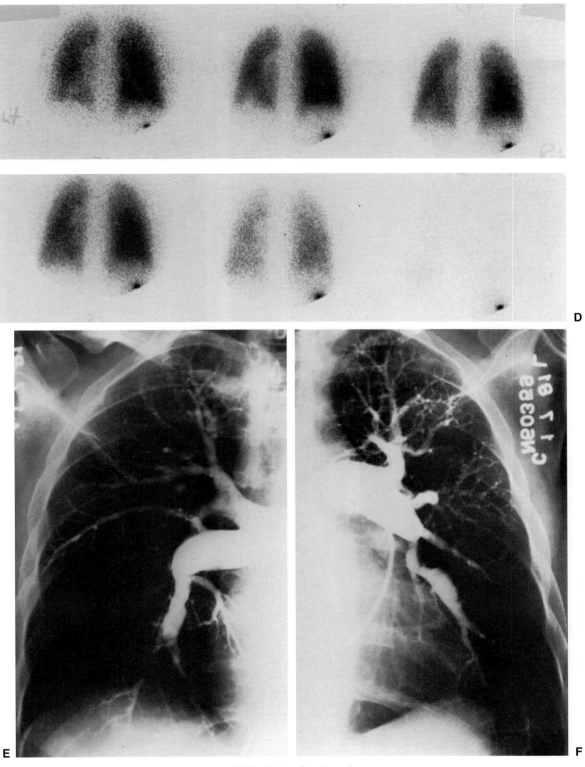

FIG. 12-4. *Continued*

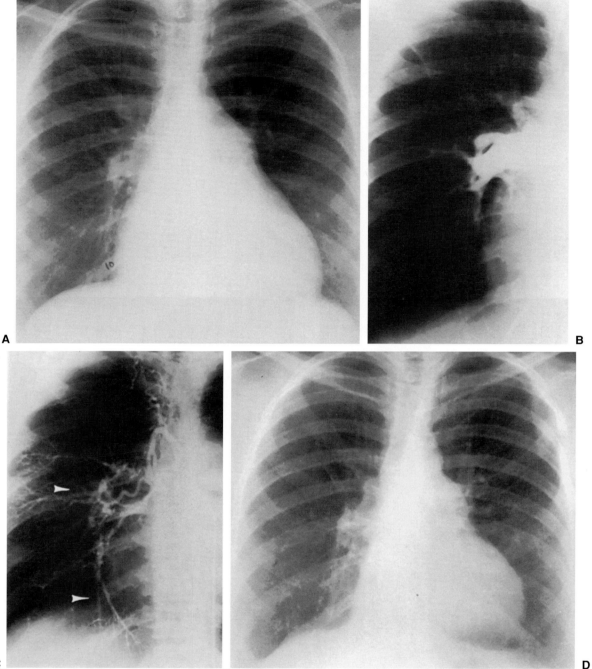

FIG. 12-5. Studies of a 40-year-old woman with bilateral massive pulmonary embolism refractory to vigorous thrombolytic therapy. Admission chest film (**A**) shows right-sided cardiomegaly, marked dilatation of the pulmonary trunk, a centralized flow pattern, and mosaic oligemia. A selective right pulmonary arteriogram (**B**) shows abrupt cutoff of all segmental branches to the right-upper lobe and occlusion of the interlobar artery. A bronchial arteriogram (**C**) shows the obstructed pulmonary arteries (*arrowheads*) to be filled from the bronchial arterial collaterals. Marked improvement is evident on the follow-up chest film (**D**) taken 1 year after embolectomy.

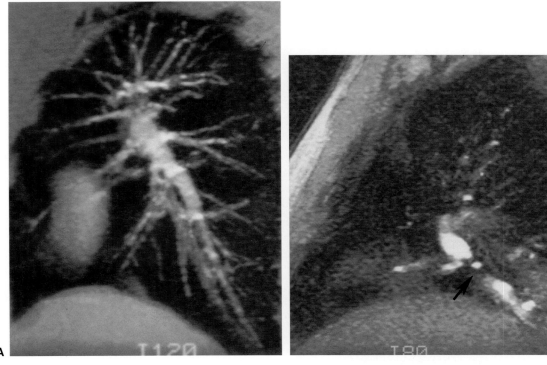

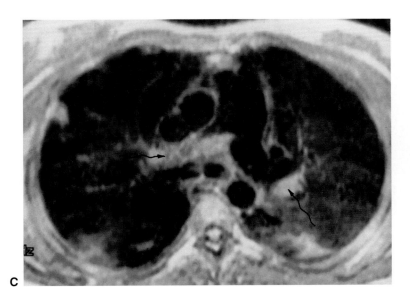

FIG. 12-6. In a normal subject, a sagittal gradient-echo magnetic resonance (MR) image (**A**) shows a normal right pulmonary arterial tree. In patient 1, a 26-year-old man, a comparable sagittal MR image (**B**) shows areas of decreased signal (*arrow*) in the right pulmonary artery, suggesting pulmonary embolus. He also had a high-probability V/Q scan and an MR image with positive signs of bilateral iliac vein thrombosis. In patient 2, a 17-year-old girl, an axial spin-echo MR image (**C**) shows a large amount of isointense material filling the right pulmonary artery (*horizontal arrow*) and a small mass in the distal left pulmonary artery (*oblique arrow*), suggestive of pulmonary emboli. Also noted are bilateral lower-lobe wedge opacities, indicative of pulmonary infarcts. The spiral computed tomography slices (**D**) and (**E**), obtained the day before, show a filling defect in the right pulmonary artery (*horizontal arrow in D*) and in the left pulmonary artery (*oblique arrow in E*). She also had a positive Westermark's sign on chest radiography and a high-probability V/Q scan. (*Continued on page 196*)

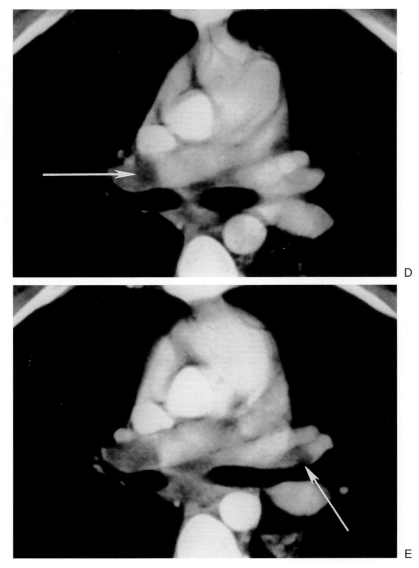

FIG. 12-6. *Continued*

potential in diagnosing central pulmonary emboli and their effects (Fig. 12-6).

Diagnostic Tests for Deep Vein Thrombosis

Both venography and Doppler ultrasound flow detection are capable of establishing the diagnosis of deep venous thrombosis. Magnetic resonance imaging has also been used effectively for this purpose, particularly in the pelvic areas.

FAT EMBOLISM

Fat embolism is most commonly a result of traumatic fracture of a lower extremity. Fat globules from the bone marrow enter the bloodstream through the damaged vein, eventually embolizing the pulmonary arteries. Within the lungs the neutral fat is converted by lipase into free fatty acids, which provoke hemorrhagic pulmonary edema (Fig. 12-7). Fat embolism typically manifests from 1 to 3 days after trauma, in contrast to lung contusion, which causes pulmonary opacity almost immediately after injury. Small fat globules may cross the pulmonary capillaries into the systemic circulation, embolizing the vessels in the brain, kidneys, and skin. The symptoms are similar to those of pulmonary embolism in general. Petechiae are frequently found, as is fat, in the urine and sputum.

PARENCHYMAL DISEASE

Cor pulmonale may be a result of chronic obstructive (Fig. 2-12), suppurative, or restrictive (Fig. 12-8) lung disease.

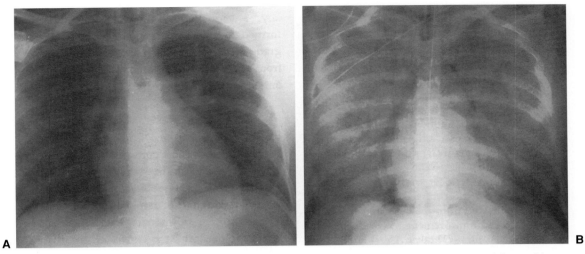

FIG. 12-7. Radiographs of an 18-year-old girl who fractured both femora in an automobile accident. Her admission chest radiograph (**A**) was normal. A second film (**B**) taken 48 hours later shows complete opacification of both lungs with air bronchograms. Fat was recovered from her urine.

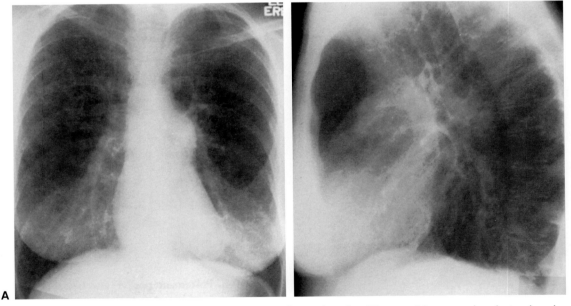

FIG. 12-8. Posteroanterior (**A**) and lateral (**B**) radiographs of a 32-year-old woman in whom chronic cor pulmonale developed from a long-standing eosinophilic granuloma. Note the dilatation of the right ventricle, pulmonary trunk, and central pulmonary arteries. Rapid attenuation of the arteries is evident bilaterally. The lungs have a honeycomb pattern.

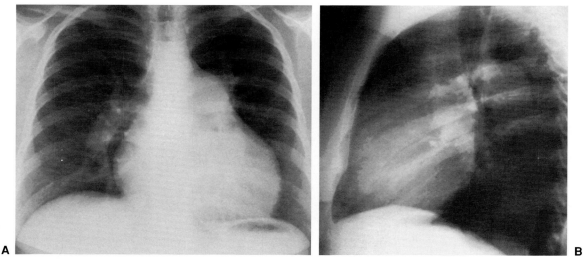

FIG. 12-9. Posteroanterior (**A**) and lateral (**B**) views of a 25-year-old woman with long-standing severe precapillary pulmonary hypertension of unknown cause. Note the right-sided cardiomegaly and striking centralized pulmonary flow pattern. However, there is no localized vascular constriction or dilatation or mosaic oligemic pattern to suggest pulmonary embolism. The blood distribution is symmetric, though centralized. All vessels are smoothly marginated.

PRIMARY PULMONARY HYPERTENSION

After all known causes have been excluded, pulmonary hypertension may be assumed to be primary or idiopathic (Fig. 12-9). However, pulmonary hypertension caused by microembolism is indistinguishable from primary pulmonary hypertension in a living patient (Fig. 12-10). Autopsy is required for final confirmation. Both diseases run a relentless course ending in death.

EISENMENGER SYNDROME

Although most authorities exclude Eisenmenger syndrome (see Figs. **8-15** and **8-16**) from the family of cor pulmonale, the radiographic appearance of the two entities can be quite similar and even indistinguishable. This is particularly true for Eisenmenger atrial or ventricular septal defect and primary pulmonary hypertension. Under the fluoroscope, Eisenmenger syndrome tends to cause bigger

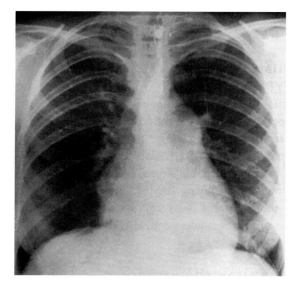

FIG. 12-10. A posteroanterior chest radiograph of a 23-year-old woman on contraceptive pills who died of relentless pulmonary hypertension. At autopsy, diffuse microemboli were found in both lungs. The pulmonary arteriogram (not shown) gave negative results for pulmonary embolism. Marked dilatation of the pulmonary trunk and moderate right ventricular enlargement are apparent. The central pulmonary arteries were only mildly dilated. A paucity of peripheral pulmonary vasculature is noted bilaterally.

and more pulsatile central pulmonary arteries than primary pulmonary hypertension because of the preexisting torrential pulmonary blood flow through a large left-to-right shunt.

REFERENCES

1. Newman JH, Ross JC. Chronic cor pulmonale. In: Schlant RC, Alexander RW, eds. *The heart*, 8th ed. New York: McGraw–Hill, 1994: 1895–1906.
2. Fontana GP, Sabiston DC. Acute pulmonary embolism. In: Sabiston DC, Spencer FC, eds. *Surgery of the chest*, 6th ed. Philadelphia: Saunders, 1995:773–802.
3. Sebastian MW, Sabiston DC. Chronic pulmonary embolism. In: Sabiston DC, Spencer FC, eds. *Surgery of the chest*, 6th ed. Philadelphia: Saunders, 1995:803–821.
4. Fishman AP. Pulmonary hypertension. In: Schlant RC, Alexander RW, eds. *The heart*, 8th ed. New York: McGraw–Hill, 1994:1857–1874.
5. Goldhaber SZ, Braunwald E. Pulmonary embolism. In: Braunwald E, ed. *Heart disease: a textbook of cardiovascular medicine*, 4th ed. Philadelphia: Saunders, 1992:1558–1580.
6. Alpert JS, Dalen JE. Pulmonary embolism. In: Schlant RC, Alexander RW, eds. *The heart*, 8th ed. New York: McGraw–Hill, 1994:1875–1894.
7. Hampton AO, Castleman B. Correlation of postmortem chest teleroentgenograms with autopsy findings. With special reference to pulmonary embolism and infarction. *AJR Am J Roentgenol* 1940;43:305–326.
8. Woodruff WW, Hoeck BE, Chitwood WR, et al. Radiographic findings in pulmonary hypertension from unresolved embolism. *AJR Am J Roentgenol* 1985;144:681–686.
9. Sullivan DC. Radionuclide studies in lung disease. *Semin Respir Med* 1983;5:31–42.

Essentials of Cardiac Imaging,
James T. T. Chen,
Lippincott–Raven Publishers, Philadelphia © 1998.

CHAPTER 13

Coronary Heart Disease

James T. T. Chen

Coronary heart disease, a major killer of humans today, is caused by severe atherosclerosis of the coronary arterial system (1–5). Radiography, fluoroscopy (see **Chapter 2**), coronary arteriography, left ventriculography (6), echocardiography (see **Chapter 6**), and radionuclide methods (see **Chapter 5**) are the basic imaging techniques used for patients with this disease. Electron beam computed tomography (CT) (7,8) and magnetic resonance imaging (MRI) (4) have also been used in the assessment of certain aspects of ischemic heart disease. Accurate interpretation of the images obtained with each technique requires a thorough understanding of anatomy and physiology of the heart in health and disease.

PATHOLOGY

Atherosclerotic lesions occur primarily in the proximal portions of major coronary arteries before their branches enter the myocardium. The affected coronary arteries, in decreasing order, are the anterior descending, the right, and the circumflex arteries. Atherosclerotic disease develops in three stages (1). Intimal fatty streaks first begin in childhood. Fibrous plaques develop during the adult years in high-risk persons. Eventually, advanced complicated lesions evolve and become increasingly commonplace with age.

Macroscopically, fatty streaks are flat, yellowish, streaky elevations over the lining of the artery. Microscopically, there is a greater than normal number of lipid-laden macrophages and smooth-muscle cells within the intima. These lesions may remain stationary and nonobstructive and therefore not clinically evident. Under the influence of risk factors, however, they may develop into fibrous plaques or complicated lesions with serious consequences. The known risk factors include family history of atherosclerotic disease, obesity, smoking, hypertension, stress, sedentary life-style, and excessive intake of saturated fat. Fibrous plaques represent an outgrowth of the fatty intimal streaks, causing narrowing of the arterial lumen with its clinical effects. Microscopically, increased cell proliferation occurs, with accelerated lipid accumulation and fibrous tissue formation.

As the disease progresses, fibrous plaques become vascularized and more bulky. Necrosis, hemorrhage, and calcification may occur in the lipid-rich center of the lesions. Consequently, disintegration, ulceration, and, finally, surface thrombosis on the intimal side of the lesion appear in the atheroma, which is termed a complicated lesion. Either the bulky atheroma or its surface thrombosis may obstruct blood flow. Other causes of acute luminal occlusion are coronary artery spasm and hemorrhage into the atheromatous plaques. Tissue necrosis usually results from uncompensated myocardial ischemia when the supplying coronary artery is suddenly occluded. This is called myocardial infarction. Myocardial necrosis may not occur if the involved artery is gradually narrowed, allowing time for adequate intercoronary collateral circulation to develop.

Myocardial infarction is said to be transmural when necrosis involves the entire thickness of the myocardium; it is defined as subendocardial when the myocardial damage is confined to the inner layer. Transmural infarction may spread to the epicardium, causing localized pericarditis or Dressler's syndrome, which is an autoimmune reaction causing fever, leukocytosis, elevated erythrocyte sedimentation rate, and pericardial and pleural effusions. The incidence of Dressler's syndrome is ~3% (5). Serious complications of myocardial infarction include cardiac rupture, perforation of the ventricular septum, left ventricular aneurysm, rupture of the papillary muscle, and, of course, sudden death.

PATHOPHYSIOLOGY AND CLINICAL PRESENTATION

As atherosclerosis progresses, the major coronary arteries become increasingly stenosed. By the time 75% of the cross-

Department of Radiology, Duke University School of Medicine, Durham, North Carolina 27710, U.S.A.

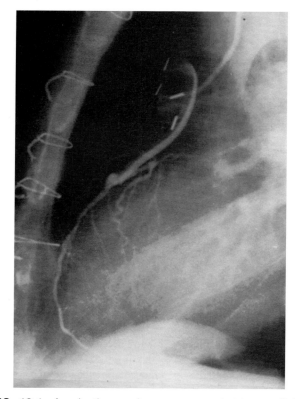

FIG. 13-1. A selective angiogram succeeded in opacifying the saphenous vein graft from the ascending aorta to the anterior descending coronary artery. The graft appears to be wide open.

sectional area or 50% of the diameter of a major coronary artery is obstructed, blood flow through the vessel will be severely compromised, and symptoms of myocardial ischemia are likely to emerge if the lost flow has not been adequately compensated. An alternative pathway of flow to the obstructed area may be established in time by collateral coronary artery circulation. Such compensation is, however, frequently inadequate to relieve the patient's symptoms or to prevent serious complications (2).

Angina pectoris is typically manifested by substernal chest pain caused by exertion or emotion, frequently radiating to the arms and less frequently to the neck and jaws. The pain is usually relieved by rest or nitroglycerin. Myocardial infarction should be suspected when chest pain is intense and prolonged, particularly when it is accompanied by weakness, sweating, dizziness, nausea, and vomiting. However, myocardial infarction causing heart failure, shock, arrhythmia, or loss of consciousness may also come about without accompanying painful symptoms.

The basic electrocardiographic findings are peaked T waves, ST-segment elevation, and marked Q waves. The exercise electrocardiogram (ECG) is more valuable than the resting ECG in the diagnosis of coronary heart disease. The cardiac enzyme levels are frequently elevated in patients with myocardial infarction.

Medical treatment of coronary heart disease is aimed at increasing the blood supply to and reducing the work of the myocardium by noninvasive means (3–5). Surgical procedures (9) include saphenous vein aortocoronary bypass (Fig. 13-1), internal mammary–coronary artery bypass, aneurysmectomy, mitral valve repair or replacement, repair of the perforated ventricular septum, and excision of the reentrant circuit in patients with ventricular tachycardia. An alternative to surgical revascularization is percutaneous transluminal coronary angioplasty (10). By way of a balloon catheter, the obstructed vessel can be selectively dilated under fluoroscopic control.

BASIC IMAGING TECHNIQUES

Radiography and Fluoroscopy

Chest radiographs in patients with major coronary artery disease may be entirely normal. Fluoroscopy is more sensitive in revealing small coronary artery calcifications (see **Fig. 2-32**), which may be the only evidence of coronary artery atherosclerosis. Sometimes dynamic abnormalities of the left side of the heart can also be detected by fluoroscopy, for example, left ventricular dyskinesia or aneurysm (see **Fig. 2-28**) and papillary muscle dysfunction with mitral insufficiency (see **Fig. 2-37**).

The most reliable radiologic sign of coronary atherosclerosis is coronary artery calcification. Even a tiny piece of calcium in the coronary artery, barely detectable by fluoroscopy, indicates the presence of occlusive disease in 94% of symptomatic patients (11). Unfortunately, the sensitivity of this test is rather low (43%), and notable coronary artery disease cannot be excluded merely because calcium is not found. In the asymptomatic population, fluoroscopic evidence of coronary calcification is associated with a ninefold increase in the risk of a positive exercise stress test (12). In the overwhelming majority of those who have both coronary calcification and a positive exercise test, at least one major coronary artery is significantly stenosed (13).

The next definitive radiologic sign of coronary heart disease is a left ventricular aneurysm. Left ventricular aneurysm seldom develops in the absence of coronary artery disease. Right ventricular and atrial aneurysms are extremely rare. A left ventricular aneurysm can be classified as anatomic or functional. An anatomic aneurysm can be further classified as true or false (14). A functional aneurysm is made up of thin scar tissue, with or without viable myocardium. A striking paradoxical movement of such an aneurysm is usually observed on fluoroscopy or other dynamic studies (15) (see **Fig. 2-28**). Since the weakened left ventricular wall protrudes only during systole, a functional aneurysm may be missed altogether on the chest radiograph, which captures mostly the diastolic image of the heart. Systolic expansion of the aneurysm puts the left ventricle, as a pump, at a mechanical disadvantage. The forward cardiac output to the systemic circulation is necessarily decreased when a large amount of blood is propelled into the expanding aneurysm.

A true aneurysm represents the end stage of the lesion made up of fibrous tissue with or without residual myocardial fibers. The mouth of the aneurysm is comparable in size to, or wider than, the maximum dimension of the aneurysm. An intracavitary mural thrombus is frequently found on angiocardiography, on CT scan, on echocardiography, or at autopsy. On fluoroscopy, a true aneurysm is motionless compared with the remainder of the left ventricular wall. Since the bulge over the ventricle is constant and unyielding, it can also be seen radiographically (see **Figs. 2-14** and **10-4**). True aneurysms with their fibrotic walls never rupture and by themselves do not impose a major functional burden on the left ventricle.

False aneurysm represents the aftermath of a localized cardiac rupture and is made up of a hematoma that has been contained by the parietal pericardium; as a result, accompanying mural thrombi are almost always present. Such aneurysms have a mouth that is very small in proportion to their maximum dimensions. They have a tendency to rupture and should be surgically removed on a semi-emergency basis. Under the fluoroscope, false aneurysms are space-occupying lesions maintaining a constant size and shape, most commonly posterobasal in location, lifting the entire heart upward (Fig. 13-2).

Left ventricular aneurysms develop at the sites of myocardial infarction in ~20% of patients. They are located, in decreasing order of frequency, in the anterolateral apical wall (71%), inferior wall (20%), and posterior wall (9%) (16). The

incidence of a calcified left ventricular aneurysm after myocardial infarction is ~8% (Figs. 13-3 and 13-4).

The last, and relatively nonspecific, finding of chronic coronary heart disease is congestive heart failure. At first, failure tends to be primarily left sided, with mitral insufficiency (Fig. 13-5A). But eventually, the entire heart will fail, showing signs of mitral and tricuspid insufficiency, poor ventricular contractility, and a cephalic flow pattern but without frank pulmonary edema (Fig. 13-5B). The radiographic appearance at this stage of the disease becomes indistinguishable from that of dilated cardiomyopathy (see **Chapter 15**).

The signs of acute myocardial infarction are generally nonspecific, but they can be useful when correlated with clinical information. They may become specific if calcium deposits are found in the coronary arterial system. Severe pulmonary edema with a normal-appearing heart is the most common finding. With proper treatment, resolution of pulmonary edema may be realized within days (Fig. 13-6). At other times, congestive heart failure becomes intractable, suggesting the development of serious complications, such as left ventricular aneurysm, mitral insufficiency, and perforation of the ventricular septum (Fig. 13-7). With the development of a left ventricular aneurysm, congestive heart failure may (Fig. 13-8) or may not improve. The timing of such a complication is during the first 2 weeks after coronary occlusion, when myocardial necrosis and softening takes place (16). With profound ischemia or rupture of the papillary muscle, worsening of heart failure is inevitable because of the resultant severe mitral insufficiency.

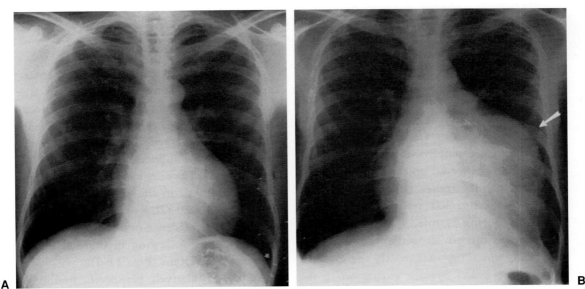

FIG. 13-2. Posteroanterior (PA) false views of a patient with postmyocardial infarction mitral insufficiency and left ventricular false aneurysm. PA view taken after the first myocardial infarction (**A**) shows moderate cardiomegaly, mild left atrial enlargement, and normal pulmonary vascularity. A second heart attack 9 months later resulted in cardiac decompensation, hypotension, and delirium. A second PA view (**B**) shows marked cardiomegaly with a cephalic pulmonary flow pattern. Also noted is the markedly elevated left ventricle with its apex tilted upward (*arrow*). At cardiac catheterization, the left ventricle was found to have ruptured, giving rise to a huge inferior wall pseudoaneurysm that pushed the heart upward.

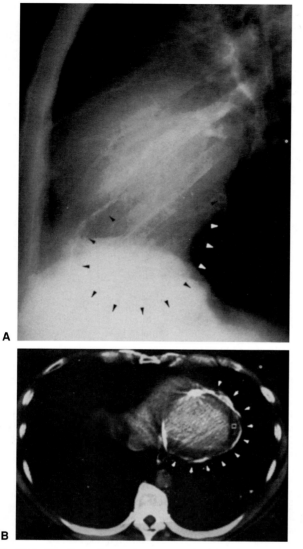

FIG. 13-3. Studies of a patient with a calcified inferior wall aneurysm of the left ventricle. The aneurysm was not seen on PA radiograph. A lateral film (**A**) and CT scan at 130 mm from the sternal notch (**B**) show a large calcified aneurysm (*arrows*) with mural thrombi (*square*).

Acute perforation of the ventricular septum is not manifested by the characteristic radiographic signs of a ventricular septal defect. Instead, it is a picture of nonspecific and profound congestive heart failure with severe pulmonary edema, generalized cardiomegaly, poor contractility of the heart, and poor pulsation of the pulmonary vessels (Fig. 13-7). The typical manifestations of ventricular septal defect may not emerge until weeks or even months after the left ventricle has regained its pumping ability.

Echocardiography

Because M-mode echocardiography can image only one small area at a time, it may miss important wall motion abnormalities, particularly those situated anteriorly in the left ventricle. Two-dimensional echocardiography, on the other hand, can clearly image a large portion of the heart in multiple views, thereby providing valuable information of anatomic and functional abnormalities, including the presence of an aneurysm, a mural thrombus, a ventricular septal defect, and mitral insufficiency (3,5). Doppler echocardiography, transesophageal echocardiography, and stress echocardiography have all been used in the workup of patients with ischemic heart disease (see **Chapter 6**).

Radionuclide Studies

Nuclear imaging techniques are valuable for the assessment of myocardial perfusion, ventricular function, and myocardial metabolism. For myocardial perfusion and cellular viability either thallium 201 or technetium 99m Sestamibi or both can be used. Either multigated acquisition equilibrium blood pool study or first-pass radionuclide angiography are helpful in evaluating ventricular function. For assessing myocardial metabolism, however, positron emission tomography with F-18 fluoro-2-deoxyglucose is the only method currently available (see **Chapter 5**).

Computed Tomographic Scanning

Computed tomographic screening, particularly electron beam CT, has been used with increasing frequency for the diagnosis of coronary heart disease (see **Chapter 3**). The detection of coronary artery and myocardial calcifications (see Figs. 3-9 and 3-10), the evaluation of graft patency (see **Fig. 3-7**), and the diagnosis of mural thrombi (see Figs. 3-11 and 3-12) are just a few of the cardiac applications of CT scanning (7,8) (see **Chapter 3**).

Magnetic Resonance Imaging

Magnetic resonance imaging has been found to be useful in the assessment of ventricular function owing to its ability to encompass both ventricles in their entirety and provide a direct measure of ventricular volumes. The spatial resolution is superior to that of radionuclide methods. The ability of MRI to estimate coronary blood flow and assess infarct size is under investigation (5) (see **Chapter 4**).

Selective Coronary Arteriography

Selective coronary arteriography (17–20) is the most reliable tool in evaluating coronary circulation. It accurately delineates the site and degree of coronary artery disease as well as the patency of coronary bypass grafts (Fig. 13-1). When this study is supplemented by cardiac catheterization and left ventriculography (Fig. 13-9), most questions regarding the advisability of surgery for a given patient with coro-

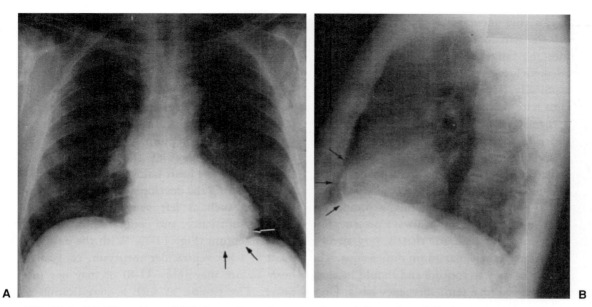

FIG. 13-4. PA (**A**) and lateral (**B**) views of a patient who showed signs of a calcified apical left ventricular aneurysm 4 years after acute myocardial infarction. Radiographs show the typical curvilinear calcification of the aneurysm (*arrows*).

nary heart disease will be answered. If the diagnosis is still uncertain, exercise radionuclide angiocardiography and thallium 201 myocardial imaging may be of help. For the detection of small mural thombi, electron beam CT, cine MRI, and transthoracic and transesophageal echocardiography may supplement left ventriculography.

Selective visualization of each coronary artery was first designed by Sones (17), employing the brachial artery cutdown technique. This method was later modified and simplified by Judkins (18), using a percutaneous transfemoral approach. The standard views of the angiogram are posteroanterior (PA), lateral, right anterior oblique, and left ante-

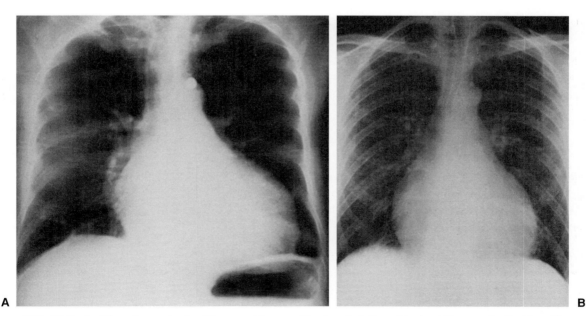

FIG. 13-5. A: PA radiograph of a 65-year-old man with chronic left ventricular failure and mitral insufficiency 5 months after acute myocardial infarction. **B:** PA view of another patient with three-vessel disease and bilateral heart failure. There is generalized cardiomegaly and a cephalic pulmonary flow pattern but no frank pulmonary edema.

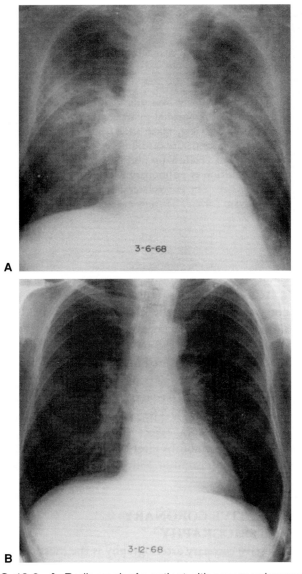

FIG. 13-6. A: Radiograph of a patient with severe pulmonary edema and mild cardiomegaly resulting from acute myocardial infarction. **B:** With appropriate medical treatment, considerable improvement was achieved in 6 days.

rior oblique (LAO) views. Cranial and caudal angulation projections have been used to modify the standard views for the purpose of separating overlapped vessels or stretching out foreshortened ones (19,20) (Fig. 13-10).

ANATOMY

In the PA view, the right coronary artery arises anteriorly from the right coronary cusp of the aorta. The left coronary artery arises posterolaterally from the left coronary cusp. The noncoronary cusp of the aorta is situated posterolaterally on the right side. The best projection for catheterizing either coronary artery is the LAO view, in which the two major vessels are widely separated (Figs. 13-10A,B and 13-11A,B).

The left main coronary artery divides into two main branches, the anterior descending and the circumflex (Fig. 13-11). The anterior descending artery courses down the anterior interventricular groove, giving rise to multiple diagonal and septal branches. The circumflex artery continues in the left atrioventricular groove to become the atrioventricular branch. A third branch courses laterally to form the obtuse marginal artery.

After passing under the right atrial appendage, the right main coronary artery courses in the right atrioventricular groove toward the crux of heart (Fig. 13-12), where both the atria and ventricles intersect. From the proximal segment of the right coronary artery two branches arise—the conal artery (anteriorly) and the sinoauricular node artery (posteriorly). Lower down come the ventricular branches, the atrial branch, and the acute marginal branch. As the right coronary artery turns posteriorly at the crux cordis, it branches superiorly into the atrioventricular node artery, anteriorly into the posterior descending artery, and posterolaterally into the left ventricular ramifications (Fig. 13-12).

The coronary arterial tree is said to have a right-sided predominance (84% of patients) when the right coronary artery is larger than the left and gives rise to the atrioventricular nodal artery. A left-sided predominance (12%) is manifested by a larger left system with the atrioventricular node artery arising from the circumflex. In the remaining 4% of patients, the coronary arterial tree is said to be balanced, with two posterior descending arteries, one from the circumflex and the other from the right coronary artery (21) (Fig. 13-13).

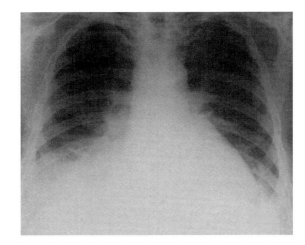

FIG. 13-7. Admission film of a patient with perforation of the ventricular septum as a result of transmural myocardial infarction. Radiograph shows moderate cardiomegaly with severe pulmonary edema. Note that the pulmonary arteries are not engorged to suggest a shunt vascularity.

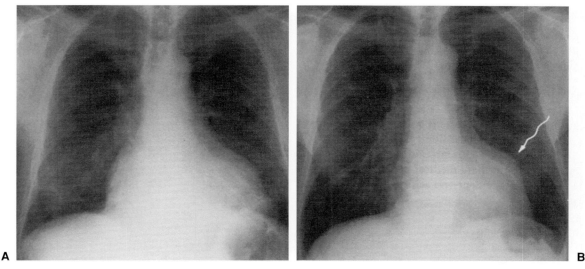

FIG. 13-8. PA view (**A**) of a patient with a post-myocardial infarction left ventricular aneurysm. This view, taken shortly after the heart attack, shows moderate cardiomegaly and mild pulmonary edema. Follow-up film 6 weeks later (**B**) shows resolution of pulmonary edema and decrease in cardiac size. The anterolateral wall left ventricular aneurysm (*arrow*) has emerged.

GRADING OF STENOSIS

The stenosis of a coronary artery is considered significant when 50% of its diameter or 75% of its cross-sectional area is obstructed. The artery is severely stenosed when >75% of its diameter or >90% of its area is obstructed. Total occlusion and subtotal occlusion mean complete and near-complete blockages of a vessel.

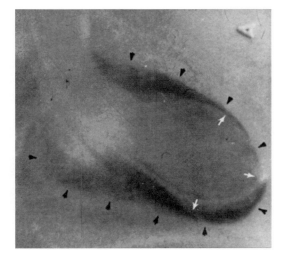

FIG. 13-9. An intercalative left ventriculogram shows a large apical aneurysm (*white arrows*). The black arrows mark the outer border of the ventricular lumen in diastole. The inner gray zone represents the systolic image of the ventricular cavity, including the immobile aneurysm. The black stripe indicates the stroke volume of the left ventricle.

COLLATERAL CIRCULATION

When the lumen of a coronary artery is narrowed by 90% of its diameter (22), the perfusion to the obstructed area may be compensated to some extent by the development of homocoronary or intercoronary anastomoses. Homocoronary anastomoses are connections between branches of the same coronary artery (Fig. 13-14D), and intercoronary anastomoses are connections between branches of the three major coronary arteries (23) (Fig. 13-14 A–C,E). In descending order, (Fig. 13-15), the common pathways of intercoronary anastomoses are located (a) over the surface of the apex, between the anterior and posterior descending coronary arteries; (b) over the surface of the pulmonary conus between the conal branch of the right coronary artery and that of the anterior descending artery; (c) in the ventricular septum between the septal branches of the anterior and posterior descending coronary arteries; (d) in the atrioventricular groove between the distal circumflex and the distal right coronary arteries; (e) on the surface of the right ventricular wall between the right ventricular branch of the right and the anterior descending coronary arteries; (f) in the atrial wall between the sinoatrial node branch of the right coronary artery and the left atrial circumflex branch of the left coronary artery; (g) in the atrial septum bridging the proximal right to the proximal left coronary arteries by way of Kugal's artery.

Kugal's artery is a vessel running in the interatrial septum. It arises either from the proximal left (by way of the left main or circumflex artery) or from the proximal right coronary artery (by way of the conal or sinoatrial node artery). Thence it passes through the atrial septum

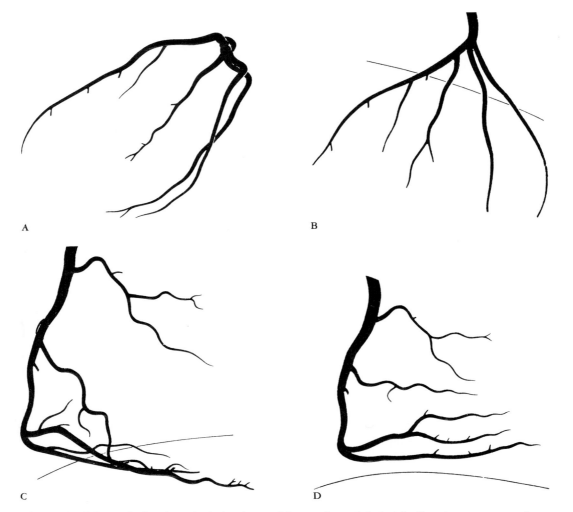

FIG. 13-10. Schematic drawings depicting the usefulness of angulated projections in coronary angiography. (Reproduced with permission from Miller RA, Warkentin DL, Felix WG, et al. Angulated views in coronary angiography. *AJR Am J Roentgenol* 1980;134:407–412.) **A:** Left coronary artery in a conventional (nonangulated) 71° LAO view. **B:** A 71° LAO view, 20° cranially angulated projection. **C:** Right coronary artery, nonangulated 40° right anterior oblique (RAO) view. **D:** A 61° RAO view, 15° caudally angulated projection.

heading to the A-V node artery. In the presence of severe obstruction of the proximal left or right coronary artery Kugal's artery becomes a common collateral pathway, for example, as a homocoronary collateral bridging the conal artery to the A-V node artery in the case of proximal right occlusion or as an intercoronary collateral bridging the A-V node artery to the left circumflex artery in the case of proximal left occlusion.

PITFALLS OF CORONARY ARTERIOGRAPHY

The angiographer and interpreter must be familiar with the pitfalls in coronary arteriography (6). First, in the context of a short left main coronary artery, a superselective injection is liable to be made in one of the two branches (the anterior descending and the circumflex),

causing nonvisualization of the other vessel. Second, an orifice lesion of the left or right coronary artery may be missed if the catheter is tightly wedged in the proximal segment of the vessel. Sometimes an injection in the aortic sinus near the origin of the vessel in question may be necessary. Third, certain coronary arteries, particularly the anterior descending, tend to dip into the myocardium and become compressed during systole. In diastole, however, the vessel will open wide (Fig. 13-16).

Fourth, spasm of a coronary artery may be spontaneous or catheter induced (Fig. 13-17). Spontaneous spasm causing Prinzmetal's angina with ECG changes may subside in minutes and then recur for no obvious reason. During cine angiography, the spasm can be provoked with ergot derivatives (e.g., ergonovine) (24). Fifth, congenital anomalies of the coronary arteries can present difficulty in interpreting coronary arteriograms. For instance, in 5% of patients with tetralogy of Fallot, the anterior descending artery arises anomalously from the right coronary artery and is therefore in danger of being severed during right ventriculotomy. Finally, totally occluded arteries or bypass grafts may escape the angiographer's attention. The clue to this situation is the visualization of the distal occluded artery by collateral channels.

DIFFERENTIAL DIAGNOSIS

Angina pectoris from coronary heart disease can be mimicked by a number of cardiac and noncardiac diseases. Fortunately, they can frequently be distinguished by the telltale signs of each on the chest radiographs.

Other Cardiac Diseases

Aortic Valve Disease

Angina pectoris is known to occur in patients with severe aortic stenosis and insufficiency without coronary artery disease. The chest pain in these patients actually represents ischemic pain from the left ventricle. In patients with aortic stenosis, myocardial ischemia is caused by a combination of decreased cardiac output and increased intracavitary pressure and muscle hypertrophy of the left ventricle. However, since about one third of patients with severe aortic stenosis also have coronary artery disease, the presence of radiographic signs of aortic stenosis should not be used to exclude coronary artery disease. In patients with severe aortic insufficiency, left ventricular ischemia

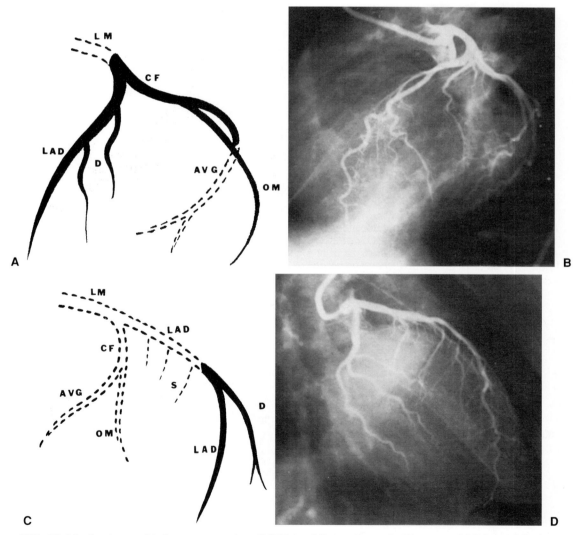

FIG. 13-11. Anatomy of left coronary artery (LCA) in oblique views. **A:** Diagram of LCA in LAO view. **B:** Arteriogram of LCA in LAO view. **C:** Diagram of LCA in right anterior oblique (RAO) view. **D:** Arteriogram of LCA in RAO view. AVG, atrioventricular groove; CF, circumflex; D, diagonal; LAD, left anterior descending; LM, left main; OM, obtuse marginal; S, septal.

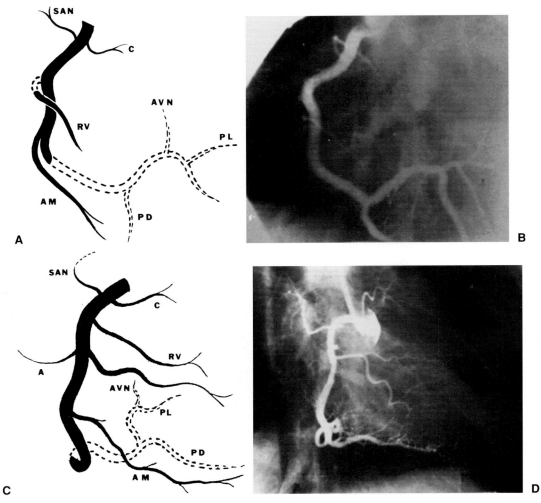

FIG. 13-12. Anatomy of the right coronary artery (RCA) in oblique views. **A:** Diagram of RCA in LAO view. **B:** Arteriogram of RCA in LAO view. **C:** Diagram of RCA in right anterior oblique (RAO) view. **D:** Arteriogram of RCA in RAO view. A, atrial branch; AM, acute marginal branch; AVN, atrioventricular node; C, conal; PD, posterior descending branch; PL, posterolateral branch; RV, right ventricular branch; SAN, sinoatrial node.

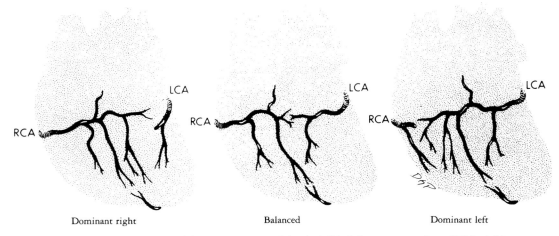

Dominant right   Balanced   Dominant left

FIG. 13-13. The three patterns of the coronary arterial tree. LCA, left coronary artery; RCA, right coronary artery. (Reproduced with permission from Peter RH. Coronary arteriography. In: Sabiston DC Jr, Spencer FC, eds. *Gibbon's surgery of the chest,* 4th ed. Philadelphia: Saunders, 1983.)

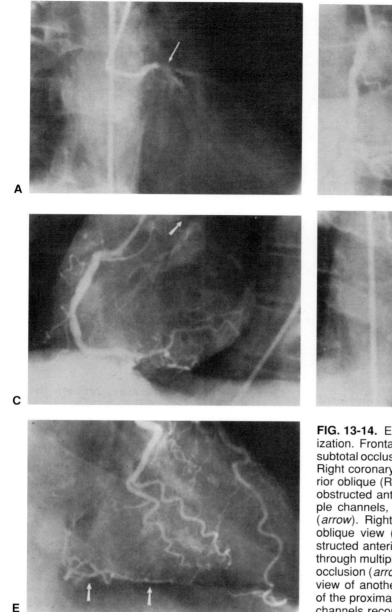

FIG. 13-14. Examples of coronary arterial collateralization. Frontal left coronary arteriogram (**A**) shows subtotal occlusion of the distal left main artery (*arrow*). Right coronary arteriogram (**B**) in shallow right anterior oblique (RAO) view shows collateral filling of the obstructed anterior descending artery through multiple channels, all the way to the site of obstruction (*arrow*). Right coronary arteriogram in left anterior oblique view (**C**) shows collateral filling of the obstructed anterior descending and circumflex arteries through multiple channels, all the way to the proximal occlusion (*arrow*). Right coronary arteriogram in RAO view of another patient (**D**) shows a total occlusion of the proximal segment with multiple homocollateral channels reconstituting the right coronary artery distally. An injection into the left coronary artery (**E**) demonstrates retrograde filling of the posterior descending artery (*arrows*) and the distal main trunk of the right coronary artery.

results from three important factors: severe left ventricular hypertrophy, marked reduction in cardiac output, and a notable decrease in myocardial perfusion pressure, which is the aortic diastolic pressure.

Severe Right Ventricular Hypertension

In patients with pulmonary stenosis, chronic cor pulmonale, Eisenmenger syndrome, pulmonary thromboembolism, and mitral stenosis, angina pectoris represents ischemic pain

from the right ventricle induced by severe right ventricular hypertrophy with marked reduction in cardiac output.

Pericarditis with Effusion

Although chest pain in patients with pericarditis with effusion is pleuritic and aggravated by breathing, it may occasionally mimic angina pectoris and cause confusion. When this is the case, the typical "displaced fat stripe" sign of pericardial effusion on the lateral radiograph is useful in the

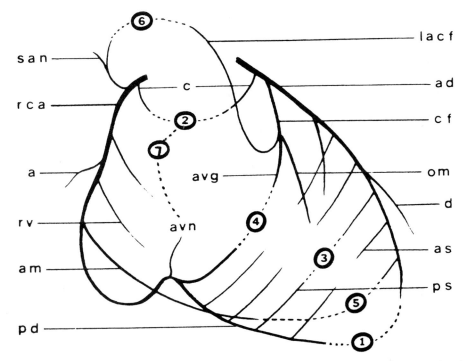

FIG. 13-15. Schematic drawing of the sites of intercoronary collateralization. See text for details. a, atrial; ad, anterior descending; am, acute marginal; as, anterior septal; avg, atrioventricular groove; avn, atrioventricular node; c, conal branches; cf, circumflex; d, diagonal; lacf, left atrial circumflex; om, obtuse marginal; pd, posterior descending; ps, posterior septal; rca, right coronary artery; rv, right ventricular; san, sinoatrial node.

differential diagnosis. If still in doubt, echocardiography is extremely helpful.

Aortic Disease

Syphilitic aortitis with severe aortic insufficiency and occlusion of the coronary ostia is known to cause angina pectoris. The typical additional radiographic sign of this disease is a calcified ascending aortic aneurysm. Patients with Marfan's syndrome may develop chronic angina pectoris owing to the presence of severe aortic insufficiency. They may also experience acute chest pain owing to dissection of the ascending aortic aneurysm into the pericardium. Atherosclerotic aortic aneurysms may dissect in any direction to cause

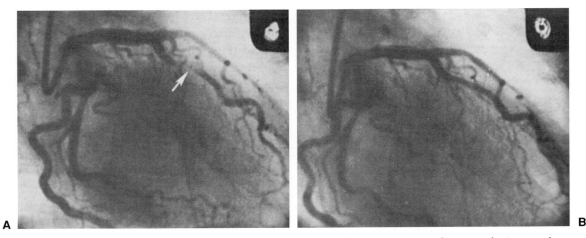

FIG. 13-16. Systolic (**A**) and diastolic (**B**) appearances of the left coronary artery show transient narrowing of the anterior descending artery (*arrow*) during systole by an overlying muscular ridge. (Reproduced with permission from Franch RH, King SB, Douglas JS. Techniques of cardiac catheterization including coronary arteriography. In: Schlant RC, Alexander RW, eds. *The heart*, 8th ed. New York: McGraw–Hill, 1994: 1107–1184.)

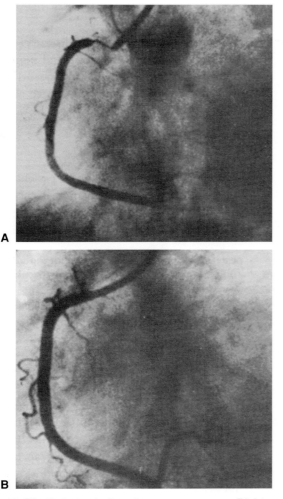

FIG. 13-17. Catheter-induced coronary spasm. Right coronary artery in left anterior oblique view (**A**) shows pericatheter spasm. Same vessel in same view (**B**) following nitroglycerin, showing relief of spasm. (Reproduced with permission from Franch RH, King SB, Douglas JS. Techniques of cardiac catheterization including coronary arteriography. In: Schlant RC, Alexander RW, eds. *The heart*, 8th ed. New York: McGraw–Hill, 1994:1107–1184.)

chest pain mimicking angina pectoris. Besides chest radiography, other imaging techniques, such as echocardiography, CT, and MRI, can all help differentiate coronary artery disease from aortic disease.

Noncardiac Diseases

Spontaneous Pneumothorax

Occasionally a spontaneous pneumothorax or pneumomediastinum may cause confusion in the differential diagnosis of coronary heart disease. The radiographic signs of these entities are, however, definitive.

Gastrointestinal Tract Diseases

Among the gastrointestinal abnormalities, pains from esophagitis, achalasia, and gallstones are the best known mimickers of angina pectoris. The so-called splenic flexure syndrome is an uncommon cause of a referred chest pain from gas distension in the splenic flexure of the colon, which is subphrenic. Since these entities have definitive radiographic signs, they should be promptly recognizable in the differential diagnosis of coronary heart disease.

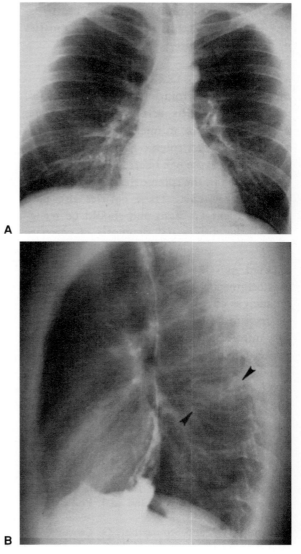

FIG. 13-18. Films of a 30-year-old man who was admitted because of a 3-week history of anginal chest pain. Five weeks before his admission, routine chest radiographs (not shown) were normal. Films taken on admission showed a normal cardiovascular system. A compression fracture in the midthoracic spine (*arrows*) was found and considered to be the source of his chest pain. This impression was verified by the normal results from cardiac catheterization and selective coronary arteriography. PA (**A**) and lateral views (**B**) are illustrated.

Skeletal Abnormalities

Pains originating from the musculoskeletal system, such as cough fracture of a rib or compression fracture of the thoracic spine (Fig. 13-18), may mimic angina pectoris. So-called Tietze's syndrome—painful swelling of a costal cartilage—is, however, not diagnosed radiographically.

REFERENCES

1. Davis MJ. The pathology of coronary atherosclerosis. In: Schlant RC, Alexander RW, eds. *The heart*, 8th ed. New York: McGraw–Hill, 1994: 1009–1020.
2. Factor SM, Bache RJ. Pathophysiology of myocardial Ischemia. In: Schlant RC, Alexander RW, eds. *The heart*, 8th ed. New York: McGraw–Hill, 1994:1033–1054.
3. Schlant RC, Alexander RW. Diagnosis and management of chronic ischemic heart disease. In: Schlant RC, Alexander RW, eds. *The heart*, 8th ed. New York: McGraw–Hill, 1994:1055–1082.
4. Théroux P, Waters D. Diagnosis and management of unstable angina. In: Schlant RC, Alexander RW, eds. *The heart*, 8th ed. New York: McGraw–Hill, 1994:1083–1106.
5. Roberts R, Morris D, Pratt CM, Alexander RW. Pathophysiology, recognition, and treatment of acute myocardial infarction and its complications. In: Schlant RC, Alexander RW, eds. *The heart*, 8th ed. New York: McGraw–Hill, 1994:1107–1184.
6. Franch RH, King SB, Douglas JS. Techniques of cardiac catheterization including coronary arteriography. In: Schlant RC, Alexander RW, eds. *The heart*, 8th ed. New York: McGraw–Hill, 1994:2381–2400.
7. Brundage BH. Computed tomography of the heart. In: Schlant RC, Alexander RW, eds. *The heart*, 8th ed. New York: McGraw–Hill, 1994: 2325–2338.
8. Stanford W, Brundage BH, MacMillan R, et al. Sensitivity and specificity of assessing coronary bypass graft patency with ultrafast computed tomography: results of a multicenter study. *J Am Coll Cardiol* 1988; 12:1–7.
9. Jones EJ, Hatcher CR. Techniques for the surgical treatment of atherosclerotic coronary artery disease and its complications. In: Schlant RC, Alexander RW, eds. *The heart*, 8th ed. New York: McGraw–Hill, 1994: 1381–1390.
10. Douglas JS, King SB. Techniques of percutaneous transluminal angioplasty and atherectomy of the coronary arteries. In: Schlant RC, Alexander RW, eds. *The heart*, 8th ed. New York: McGraw–Hill, 1994: 1345–1358.
11. Margolis JR, Chen JTT, Kong Y, et al. The diagnostic and prognostic significance of coronary artery calcification: a report of 800 cases. *Radiology* 1980;137:609–616.
12. Kelley MJ, Huang EK, Langou RA. Correlation of fluoroscopically detected coronary artery calcification with exercise testing in asymptomatic men. *Radiology* 1978;129:1–6.
13. Langou RA, Kelley MJ, Huang EK, et al. Predictive accuracy of coronary artery calcification and positive exercise test in asymptomatic nonhyperlipidemic men for coronary artery disease [Abstract]. *Am J Cardiol* 1980;45:400.
14. Cabin HS, Roberts WC. Left ventricular aneurysm, intraaneurysmal thrombus, and systemic embolus in coronary heart disease. *Chest* 1980; 77:586–590.
15. Chen JTT, McIntosh HD, Capp MP, et al. Intercalative angiocardiography: a method for recording cardiovascular dynamics on a single film. *Radiology* 1969;93:499–506.
16. Gould SE. *Pathology of the heart and blood vessels*, 3rd ed. Springfield, Ill.: Thomas, 1968:627–641.
17. Sones FM Jr. Acquired heart disease: symposium on present and future of cineangiocardiography. *Am J Cardiol* 1959;3:710.
18. Judkins MP. Selective coronary arteriography: a percutaneous transfemoral technique. *Radiology* 1967;89:815–827.
19. Miller RA, Warkentin DL, Felix WG, et al. Angulated views in coronary angiography. *AJR Am J Roentgenol* 1980;134:407–412.
20. Paulin S. Terminology for radiographic projections in cardiac angiography. *Cathet Cardiovasc Diagn* 1981;7:341–344.
21. Peter RH. Coronary arteriography. In: Sabiston DC Jr, Spencer FC, eds. *Gibbon's surgery of the chest*, 4th ed. Philadelphia: Saunders, 1983:1379–1408.
22. Gensini GG, DaCosta BCB. The coronary collateral circulation in living man. *Am J Cardiol* 1969;24:393–400.
23. Baroldi G, Scomazzoni G. *Coronary circulation in the normal and the pathologic heart*. Washington, D.C.: Office of the Surgeon General, Department of the Army, 1967.
24. Lowe JE. Prinzmetal's variant angina and other syndromes associated with coronary artery spasm. In: Sabiston DC Jr, Spencer FC, eds. *Gibbon's surgery of the chest*, 4th ed. Philadelphia: Saunders, 1983: 1458–1472.

Essentials of Cardiac Imaging,
James T. T. Chen,
Lippincott–Raven Publishers, Philadelphia © 1998.

CHAPTER 14

Pericardial Disease

James T. T. Chen

The pericardium is a delicate fibroserous membrane, occupying a negligible volume of the heart. This seemingly unimpressive organ has nevertheless fascinated the medical profession for ages because of its rather colorful clinical and radiologic panorama of manifestations (1). For example, when stretched gradually, the pericardium is able to accommodate an astounding ≥3,000 ml of fluid, whereas in acute contexts, an effusion of a mere 100 ml or even less may prove fatal (1,2). Constrictive pericarditis is known to mimic myocardial disease, right-sided heart failure, cirrhosis of the liver, and mitral stenosis (1,3). Pericardial diseases are usually classified as either congenital or acquired. The former group includes pericardial defects and pericardial cysts; the latter encompasses diseases of infectious, traumatic, metabolic, neoplastic, or other origin.

ANATOMY

Embryologically, the pericardium constitutes only a portion of the single serous cavity, the coelom. At about the fourth week of intrauterine life, the coelom develops into three isolated compartments: the pericardial, pleural, and peritoneal spaces. The pericardium, therefore, shares the common characteristics of all serous membranes. When pericarditis is associated with connective tissue disease, notably disseminated lupus erythematosus, the other two serous cavities are usually also involved. This is known as polyserositis (4). In constrictive pericarditis, renal failure, and congestive heart failure, effusion tends to collect in all three serous compartments.

The pericardium consists of two layers: the external fibrous pericardium and the internal serous pericardium. The serous pericardium lines the fibrous pericardium and is inseparable from it up to 2 to 3 cm beyond the root of the great vessels. From that point the serous pericardium folds

back on itself to envelop parts of the great vessels and the entire heart. The part that lines the fibrous sac is called the parietal layer of the serous pericardium, and that which clothes the heart and the nearby vessels is called the visceral layer of the serous pericardium or the epicardium. The epicardium is therefore a continuation of the serous lining of the fibrous pericardium (5). Between the two opposing serous surfaces is the potential pericardial cavity, filled with 15 to 50 ml of clear serous fluid as the lubricant for normal cardiac movement (6). The fibrous pericardium and its serous lining are often collectively called the parietal pericardium (Figs. 14-1–3).

The fatty connective tissue beneath the epicardium is called the subepicardial fat stripe. It is an "elastic cushion" between myocardium and pericardium. Embedded in it are coronary arteries, cardiac veins, and nerves. As a rule, greater deposition of fat is present in cardiac grooves than over the convexities of the heart. Such fat stripes cast radiolucent shadows that help separate myocardium from pericardium, atria from ventricles, and one ventricle from another. The subepicardial fat stripe is therefore the single most important landmark in the field of cardiac radiology.

The pericardial sac is anchored posteriorly by the incoming pulmonary and systemic veins, superiorly by the ascending aorta, anteriorly by the manubrium and xiphoid process of the sternum, and inferiorly by the central tendon of the left hemidiaphragm (5,7,8) (Fig. 14-4).

The essential functions of the pericardium (1,9,10) are (a) to maintain the heart in the optimum functional position and to provide lubrication for free cardiac movements; (b) to prevent acute dilatation of the heart and to equalize hydrostatic forces on the heart; (c) to protect the heart from noxious influences from the surrounding structures, such as infectious diseases of the lung or pleura; (d) to protect the lungs from injury by the beating heart; and (e) to prevent injury, pressure, or tension around the roots of the incoming and outgoing vessels during vigorous physical activities or trauma. Certain functions of the pericardium, however, are

Department of Radiology, Duke University School of Medicine, Durham, North Carolina 27710, U.S.A.

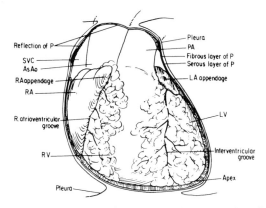

FIG. 14-1. Ventral view of the heart with the pericardial sac opened. AsAo, ascending aorta; LA, left atrium; LV, left ventricle; PA, pulmonary trunk; RA, right atrium; RV, right ventricle; SVC, superior vena cava.

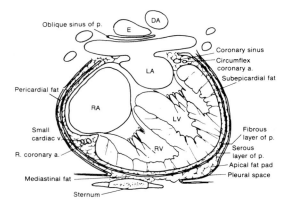

FIG. 14-3. Cross section of the heart. DA, descending aorta; E, esophagus; LA, left atrium; LV, left ventricle; RA, right atrium; RV, right ventricle.

not fully understood, for example, why a successful pericardiectomy does not cause cardiac dysfunction (9) and why total absence of the left pericardium induces no cardiac impairment of cardiac function.

NORMAL RADIOGRAPHIC APPEARANCE

The subepicardial fat stripe is visible on a lateral radiograph as a radiolucent zone molded over the anterior border of the right ventricle. The width of the stripe varies

in proportion to the differing amounts of fat present (5). Immediately anterior to the subepicardial fat and posterior to the mediastinal fat is the hairline density of a normal pericardium, which should be <2 mm wide (Fig. 14-5). Sometimes the delicate normal pericardium may fail to cast a shadow; in that case, there is only an undivided radiolucent zone between the heart and the sternum. This phenomenon is normal. Occasionally, the apical fat pad, which contains more fibrous tissue and less fat, may cast a pale triangular density in the anterior costophrenic sulcus in front of the subepicardial fat stripe. This is another normal variant (Fig. 14-6) and should not be misinterpreted as a small loculated pericardial effusion.

On the posteroanterior (PA) view, the subepicardial fat stripe and the pericardium are normally invisible, except over the left ventricular apex. Here the apical fat pad provides a relative radiopacity that allows the fat stripe

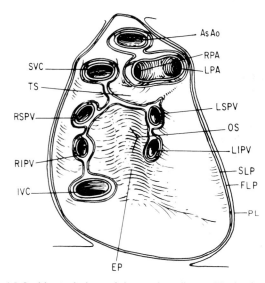

FIG. 14-2. Ventral view of the pericardium with the heart removed. AsAo, ascending aorta; EP, esophageal prominence; FLP, fibrous layer of pericardium; IVC, inferior vena cava; LIPV, left inferior pulmonary vein; LPA, left pulmonary artery; LSPV, left superior pulmonary vein; OS, oblique sinus; PL, pleura; RIPV, right inferior pulmonary vein; RPA, right pulmonary artery; RSPV, right superior pulmonary vein; SVC, superior vena cava; SLP, serous layer of pericardium; TS, transverse sinus.

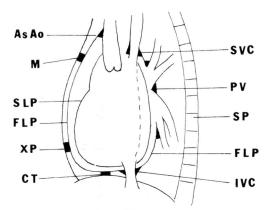

FIG. 14-4. Points of fixation of the parietal pericardium in lateral view. AsAo, ascending aorta; CT, central tendon of diaphragm; FLP, fibrous layer of pericardium or parietal pericardium; IVC, inferior vena cava; M, manubrium of sternum; PV, pulmonary veins; SLP, serous layer of pericardium or epicardium; SP, spine; SVC, superior vena cava; XP, xiphoid process of sternum.

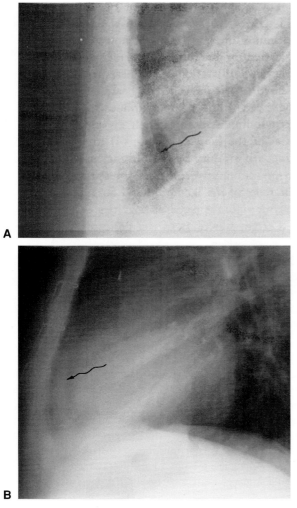

FIG. 14-5. Lateral view (**A**) of a patient with mitral insufficiency. His pericardium was perfectly normal; it is visible as a hairline density (*arrow*) between the subepicardial and mediastinal fat stripes. Lateral view (**B**) of another patient with pericardial effusion shows the dilated pericardium (*arrow*) measuring >1 cm (the upper limit of normal is 2 mm).

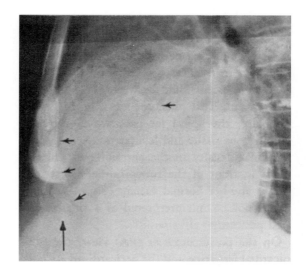

FIG. 14-6. Lateral view of a patient with calcific aortic stenosis shows a normal subepicardial fat stripe, which is touching the sternum (*three short arrows*). The long arrow marks the apical fat pad, which is a triangular density anterior and inferior to the subepicardial fat stripe and in the anterior costophrenic sulcus. The upper small arrow points to the calcified aortic valve.

to stand out in contrast (Fig. 14-7). Sometimes the apical fat pad can be unusually large, either as a normal variant or as a result of steroid therapy (11). It should be differentiated from enlarged diaphragmatic lymph nodes that accompany Hodgkin's disease (12). Today it should be relatively simple to distinguish lymph nodes or a pericardial cyst from a fat pad by computed tomographic scanning (13,14) (Fig. 14-8).

Although the subepicardial fat stripe is frequently seen on chest radiography, it is much more easily and consistently visible under the fluoroscope because of its rhythmic motion with each cardiac contraction (see **Chapter 2**). Echocardiography, conventional computed tomography (CT), spiral CT, and electron beam CT are all superior imaging methods to radiography and fluoroscopy in the study of pericardium (see **Chapters 3, 4,** and **6**).

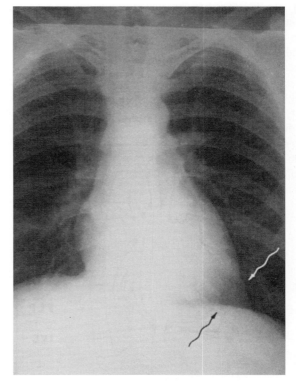

FIG. 14-7. PA view of a normal person. The apical fat pad appears as a pale triangular density (*arrows*) over the left ventricular apex. It is actually situated between the parietal layers of the pericardium and the mediastinal pleura.

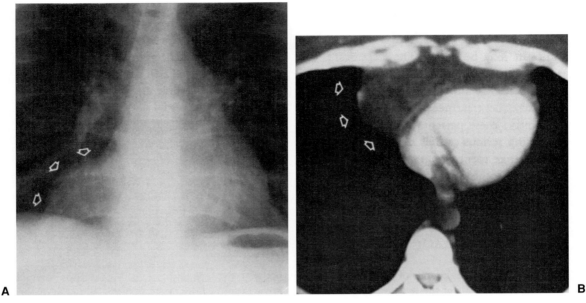

FIG. 14-8. Radiograph of a patient (**A**) with a mass (*arrows*) in the right cardiophrenic sulcus. A computed tomographic scan (**B**) revealed it to be a large fat pad (*arrows*) rather than a soft-tissue mass or pericardial cyst.

CONGENITAL ANOMALIES

Congenital Pericardial Defects

The most plausible explanation about the origin of congenital pericardial defects is the vascular atrophy theory (9). The normal development of pericardium and pleurae depends on the uninterrupted process of enfolding of the pleuropericardial membrane and closing of the pleuropericardial foramen. Premature atrophy of the left duct of Cuvier apparently jeopardizes the blood supply to the membrane and affects its smooth transition into separate serous cavities. Pericardial defects rarely occur on the right side, which is explained by the persistence of the right duct of Cuvier (which eventually becomes the superior vena cava) and the atrophy of the left duct of Cuvier (which eventually becomes the small vein of Marshall).

Congenital absence of the pericardium is traditionally classified as total or partial; total absence is more common than partial. Total absence of the pericardium, however, arises only on the left side (15–17); partial defects of the pericardium also tend to be left-sided. Right-sided or bilateral partial defects are quite rare (18,19). Other congenital cardiac lesions are seen in ~30% of patients with pericardial defects, among them, atrial septal defect, bicuspid aortic valve, and mitral valve prolapse. Congenital defects have a male predominance at a ratio of 3:1 (10).

Total Absence of the Left Pericardium

Total absence of the left pericardium is almost always associated with a defect of the left pleura. The heart is consequently displaced and jammed together with the left lung

FIG. 14-9. Radiographs of patients with absence of the left hemipericardium. PA view of patient 1 (**A**) shows the heart to be displaced and rotated to the left side. The lung wedges between the two great arteries (*upper arrow*) and between the heart and the left hemidiaphragm (*lower arrow*). The right anterior oblique view (**B**) shows the same (*upper and lower arrows*) to better advantage. A cross-table lateral view of patient 2 in the supine position (**C**) shows the heart falling backward for lack of anchorage to the sternum and diaphragm. Such anchorge is normally provided by the left hemipericardium. An enhanced CT scan of patient 2 (**D**) shows the posterior and leftward rotation of the heart with absence of pericardium from the arrow leftward. A comparable axial magnetic resonance image of patient 3 (**E**) shows the posterior and leftward rotation of the heart with lack of pericardium from the arrow leftward. A coronal spin echo (SE) magnetic resonance image of patient 3 (**F**) shows the leftward rotation of the heart with the lung insinuated between the aorta and the prominent pulmonary trunk (*oblique arrow*) and between the heart and the left hemidiaphragm (*horizontal arrow*). Also note the lack of pericardium over the left side of the heart. (The radiograph in C was reproduced with permission from Larsen RL, Behar VS, Brazer SR, Chen JTT, O'Conner C. Chest pain presenting as ischemic heart disease: absence of the pericardium. *N C Med J* 1994; 55:306–308.)

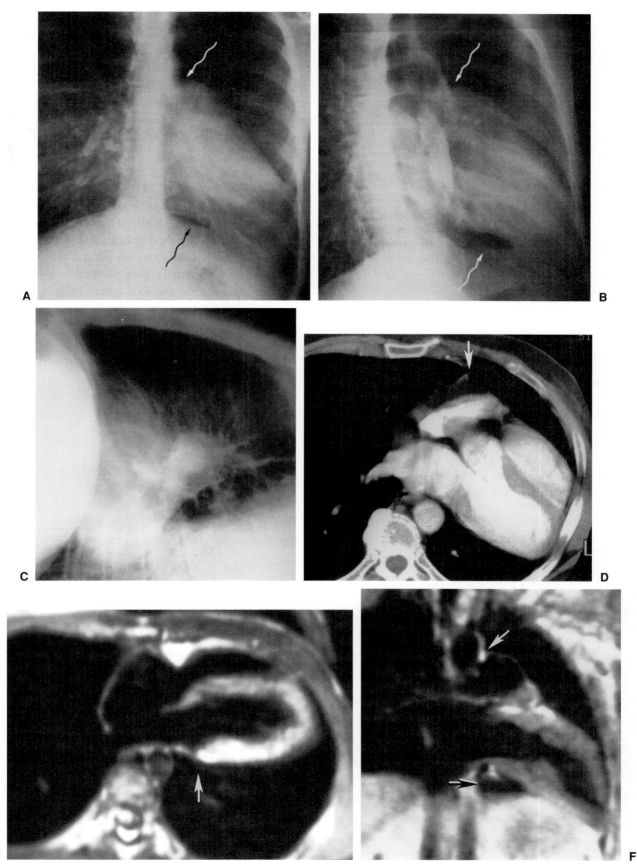

within the left pleural cavity. The patient is usually asymptomatic. Mild chest discomfort is experienced occasionally. On physical examination, the apical cardiac pulsation is in the left axilla, and a variable cardiac murmur may be heard. The electrocardiogram shows a pattern of right axis deviation. Since normal cardiac function is not affected by the anomaly, no treatment is necessary. More important, these patients should not be labeled as having serious cardiac disease simply because of a strange radiographic appearance.

On radiography the findings are unique and usually diagnostic. The heart is deviated and rotated to the left side; the PA view (Fig. 14-9A,F) therefore mimics a normal right anterior oblique view. Usually, three distinct convexities are seen along the left border, representing the aortic arch, the pulmonary trunk, and the right ventricle. In other words, the left cardiac border is formed by the right ventricle; the ascending aorta and the pulmonary trunk are displaced to the left side, while the descending aorta and the trachea remain in the normal position. As the heart and the left lung are crowded in the left pleural space, the lung tends to wedge between the aorta and the pulmonary trunk as well as between the heart and the left hemidiaphragm (Fig. 14-9A,B,F). In the supine lateral view taken with horizontal x-ray beams, the heart falls away from the sternum and the diaphragm because of the lack of anchorage normally provided by the ligments from the left hemipericardium (1,15,17) (Fig. 14-9C). Leftward and downward shift of the heart is also evident on transaxial images (Fig. 14-9D,E). On fluoroscopy, there is an increase of pulsation and movability of the heart and the great arteries on the left side, particularly during respiration and when the body posture is changed.

Partial Absence of the Pericardium

Small defects of the pericardium have no pathologic importance and are not diagnosed during life. A medium-size defect of the pericardium, however, may cause life-threatening episodes of cardiac strangulation for which emergency surgery is mandatory (20–22). On the radiograph, a left hilar mass, representing the herniated pulmonary trunk or the left atrial appendage or both, is most commonly seen through a left-sided pericardial defect (23). Rarely one may encounter a right-sided defect causing either the right atrium or the right ventricle to protrude laterally (18–20,24). The differential diagnosis of a left-sided defect includes hilar adenopathy, tumors of the lung, valvular pulmonary stenosis, and idiopathic dilatation of the pulmonary trunk.

Artificial pneumothorax has both historic and practical importance in the diagnosis of congenital pericardial defects. When pneumothorax was used for the treatment of pulmonary tuberculosis, many congenital pericardial defects were accidentally revealed. With a better understanding of the disease, total absence of the left pericardium can now be diagnosed by standard radiographic techniques without the need for artificial pneumothorax (16,17). Occasionally, artificial pneumothorax may be helpful in confirming the diag-

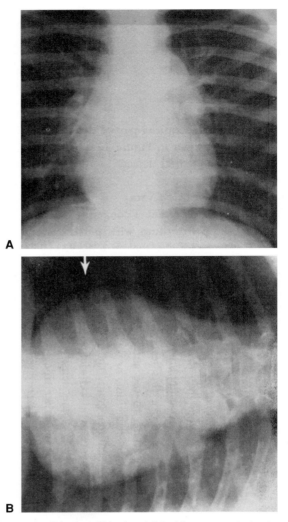

FIG. 14-10. PA view (**A**) of a child with recurrent chest pain. The left hilar mass represents the herniated left atrial appendage and the pulmonary trunk. A left-sided artificial pneumothorax in the left-lateral decubitus position (**B**) shows air in the pericardium over the right atrium (*arrow*). Air has passed through defects both in the pleura and in the pericardium on the left side (compare with **Fig. 4-15A,B**).

nosis of partial defects by showing pneumopericardium after the introduction of air into the pleural space (Fig. 14-10). A definitive diagnosis of partial absence of the pericardium can be made with echocardiography, CT, and MRI (14,15) (see **Fig. 4-15B**) (see also **Chapters 3, 4,** and **6**). A patient with an acquired partial defect of the pericardium is shown in Fig. 14-11 for comparison with a congenital defect.

Pericardial Coelomic Cysts

Pericardial cysts represent a congenital malformation of the pericardium with persistence of the ventral recess of the coelom (25,26). The pericardial coelom develops by fusion of many disconnected mesenchymal lacunae. Failure of one

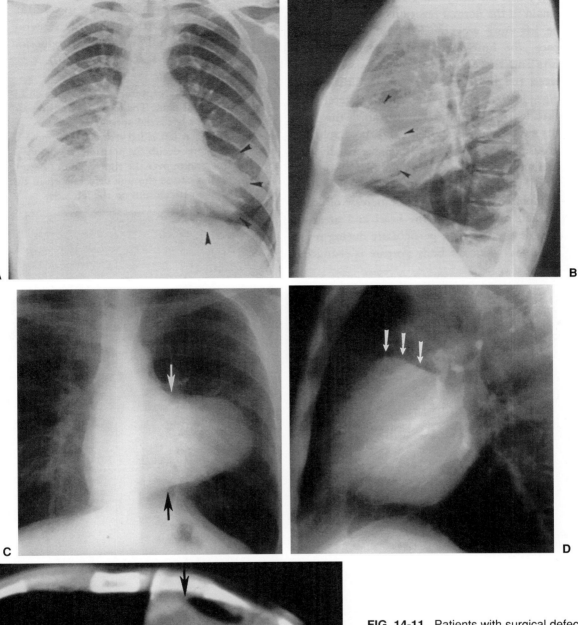

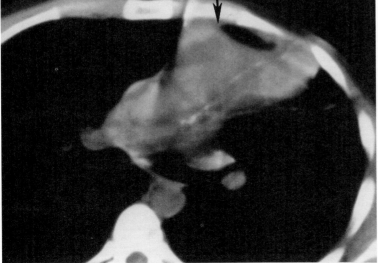

FIG. 14-11. Patients with surgical defects of the pericardium. Patient 1 has a partial pericardial defect as a complication of myocardial biopsy. The PA (**A**) view shows a "mass" (*arrows*) over the cardiac apex, representing the left ventricle herniating through the defect. The lateral view (**B**) shows a density (*arrows*) in the lower retrosternal region. In patient 2, a healed surgical window (surgery was done for recurrent pericardial effusions due to chronic renal failure) is visible in the lower-left pericardium. The PA view (**C**) shows herniation of the left ventricle through the defect leftward and superiorly (*opposing arrows*). The lateral view (**D**) shows an anterior double density with a sharp superior border (*arrows*). A CT scan (**E**) shows herniation of the left side of the heart from the arrow leftward.

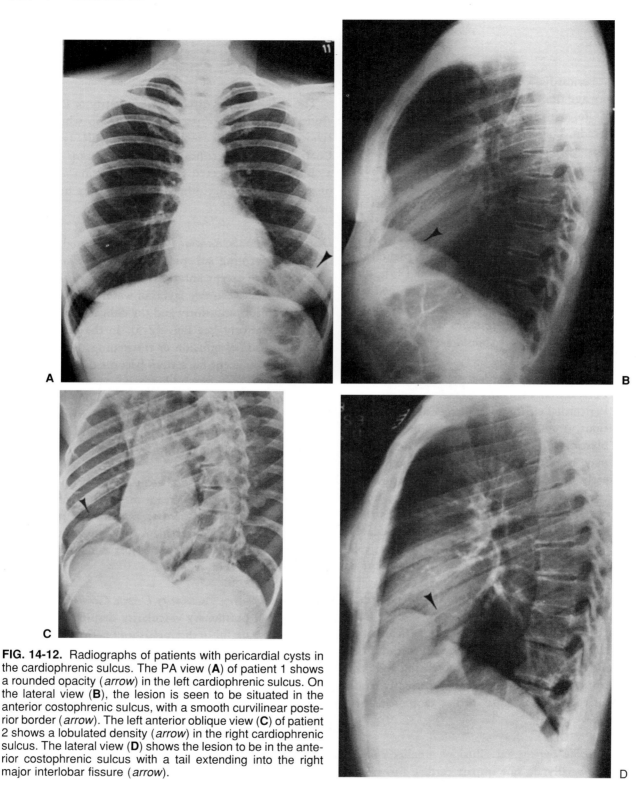

FIG. 14-12. Radiographs of patients with pericardial cysts in the cardiophrenic sulcus. The PA view (**A**) of patient 1 shows a rounded opacity (*arrow*) in the left cardiophrenic sulcus. On the lateral view (**B**), the lesion is seen to be situated in the anterior costophrenic sulcus, with a smooth curvilinear posterior border (*arrow*). The left anterior oblique view (**C**) of patient 2 shows a lobulated density (*arrow*) in the right cardiophrenic sulcus. The lateral view (**D**) shows the lesion to be in the anterior costophrenic sulcus with a tail extending into the right major interlobar fissure (*arrow*).

of the primitive lacunae to fuse may result in a pericardial cyst (27). The cyst, typically situated in the cardiophrenic sulci (Fig. 14-12A), is rarely found higher than that level (25,28). Most cysts in the cardiophrenic sulci are on the right side (Fig. 14-12C). Above this level they have a tendency to attach to the aorta, the superior vena cava, the left atrium, or the right atrium.

On radiography, the pericardial cyst usually appears as a well-defined rounded or semicircular soft-tissue density in the cardiophrenic sulcus on either side. It is attached to the pericardium and separated from the myocardium by the delicate subepicardial fat stripe. In the lateral projection it typically appears in the anterior costophrenic sulcus with a smooth posterior border (Fig. 14-12B). It is rare (2%) to find a pericardial cyst in the posterior mediastinum (25). Small cysts may assume a teardrop appearance in the lateral view, with the tail extending into the major interlobar fissure (Fig. 14-12D). Large cysts may look multilocular, but most of them (90%) are actually unilocular. The cysts range from 2 to 37 cm in diameter. They are only slightly compressible with little change in contour or size when body posture changes because they do not communicate with the pericardial cavity. When they do, they should be termed pericardial diverticulum (29). The size and shape of a pericardial diverticulum are readily affected by gravity.

Pericardial cysts and diverticula may occur at any age from infancy through the eighth decade of life, with the highest incidence in the fourth decade. There is a slight predominance among males. Most patients (75%) are asymptomatic. Symptoms include chest discomfort, dyspnea, and cough. The differential diagnosis includes pericardial lymphangioma, omental herniations through Morgagni's foramen (30,31), large pericardial fat pad, acute pericardial fat necrosis, pleural thickening, loculated pleural effusion, tumors or cysts of the thymus, and other mediastinal tumors. If there is a history of trauma, rupture of the right hemidiaphragm with herniation of a portion of the liver should be considered (30).

ACQUIRED DISEASES

Pericardial Effusion

Pericardial effusion has many causes (e.g., infectious, immunologic, traumatic, metabolic, neoplastic, and idiopathic). The pericardial fluid may be serous, exudative, or bloody. In the early stages of the disease, the nature of the effusions cannot be distinguished one from another by radiologic techniques. As the disease protracts or relapses, however, exudate and blood tend to provoke extensive fibrosis, calcification, and loculation of the pericardium with more specific radiographic signs. Transudate may undergo complete resorption with no apparent effects. Prompt recognition of acute pericardial effusion under tension (cardiac tamponade) is mandatory because of the dire consequences (i.e., hypotension and death). Immediate pericardiocentesis is usually required for the relief of acute cardiac tamponade.

Radiographic Signs

Chronic pericardial effusions <250 ml usually do not impair cardiac function and are said to be occult radiographically (32,33). The radiologist is often asked to verify or exclude the presence of pericardial effusion when echocardiography is technically difficult (see **Chapter 1**). At

other times, the radiographic signs of a clinically unsuspected pericardial effusion are unequivocal, making other diagnostic tests unnecessary.

Distinctness of Subepicardial Fat Stripes

Normally the border-forming subepicardial fat stripes are difficult to see except anteriorly, where they are sandwiched between two layers of water density: the myocardium interiorly and the delicate pericardium exteriorly (Fig. 14-5). In the presence of pericardial effusion or thickening, however, the radiolucent fat stripes become distinct on all sides against the added external opacity (34). Being farther away from the sternum, the lung, and the diaphragm for a distance proportional to the size of the effusion, the fat stripes may be interpreted as being displaced toward the center of the heart (see **Figs. 1-7, 2-18,** and **2-34**).

Rapid Change in Cardiac Size and Contour

Within days, cardiac size can increase markedly, with smoothing out of the cardiac borders. In response to proper treatment, the cardiac silhouette may return to normal just as dramatically (1,32) (Fig. 14-13).

Normal Pulmonary Vascularity Despite Cardiomegaly

Normal pulmonary vascularity despite cardiomegaly is useful in distinguishing pericardial effusion from congestive heart failure. A slowly developing pericardial effusion does not interfere with normal pulmonary blood flow. A rapidly evolving effusion, on the other hand, may compress the heart on all sides, resulting in mild cephalization of pulmonary vasculature without pulmonary edema. Normal or near-normal pulmonary vascularity is therefore characteristic of pericardial effusion despite notable enlargement of the cardiac silhouette (Fig. 14-13A; see also **Fig. 2-10**).

Obliteration of the Retrosternal Space

Probably because of a lack of pericardium over the left atrium and because of the incoming veins in the back of the heart, there is little room in the posterior compartment of the pericardium. When fluid or air enters a free pericardial sac, it has the tendency to collect first anteroinferiorly, then laterally, and last posteriorly (7,8). In fact, even with a large hydropneumopericardium, the air-fluid level hardly extends beyond the posterior border of the heart (Fig. 14-14C).

In the lateral view, when a large pericardial effusion is present, the bulk of the density appears to be situated in the retrosternal space. The cardiac silhouette bulges anteriorly and superiorly with increased vertical dimension. The heart itself is actually displaced superiorly and posteriorly by the fluid, primarily in the anteroinferior compartment of the

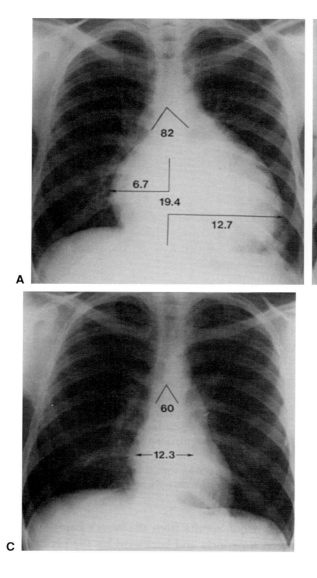

A

B

C

FIG. 14-13. The admission radiograph (**A**) of a patient with acute viral pericarditis with effusion shows gross cardiomegaly with a transverse diameter of 19.4 cm and a subcarinal angle of 82°. The pulmonary vascularity is normal. After steroid therapy for 5 days, a second film (**B**) shows marked reduction in both heart size and subcarinal angle. Follow-up 6 months later (**C**) shows further improvement. (Reproduced with permission from Chen JTT, Putman CE, Hedlund LW, et al. Widening of the subcarinal angle by pericardial effusion. *AJR Am J Roentgenol* 1982;139:883–887.)

pericardium. The left atrium then becomes the posterior border-forming structure (33). With abundant fluid in the lateral pouches, a convex and immobile border is formed behind the barium-filled esophagus, mimicking an enlarged left ventricle (32). The esophagus continues to be in contact with the left atrium and part of the left ventricle, transmitting their pulsations. It is therefore logical to think of pericardial effusion as a distinct possibility when cardiomegaly is mainly situated anteriorly in the lateral or left anterior oblique view (Fig. 14-14A).

Widening of Subcarinal Angle

Related to the previous observation is another sign of pericardial effusion, namely, the widening of the subcarinal angle in the PA view (Fig. 14-13). This phenomenon results from the heart's being displaced superiorly and backward by the pericardial effusion. It is the displaced heart that

splays the bronchi and widens the subcarinal angle. In a study of 60 patients (35), we found that the angle during pericardial effusion was significantly greater than either before or after the episode of effusion. In the group as a whole, there was also significant correlation between the subcarinal angle and the transverse diameter of the cardiopericardial silhouette, which in turn was proportional to the quantity of pericardial fluid (Fig. 14-13).

Absence of Left Atrial Enlargement

With uncomplicated pericardial effusion, there is no discrete deviation of the esophagus to suggest left atrial enlargement. Instead, a sweeping posterior displacement of the barium column (Fig. 14-15B) is usually evident as the whole heart is pushed backward by the bulk of the anterior pericardial collection. As previously mentioned, the subcarinal angle may likewise be widened (Fig. 14-15A) and thus lead to a misinterpretation of left atrial enlargement.

Differential Dampening of the Cardiac Pulsation

A small pericardial effusion may not considerably affect the cardiac pulsation (8,36,37). With an increasing quantity of pericardial fluid, however, the pulsation is progressively dampened. In the PA view, when the pericardial fluid increases, the cardiac pulsation will first be abolished over the right atrium and eventually also over the left ventricle. Without cardiac tamponade, the aortic knob, which is outside the pericardium, should pulsate normally. Decreased aortic pulsation in this context suggests cardiac tamponade with reduced stroke volume from the left ventricle. In the lateral projection, the cardiac pulsations appear to be abolished anteriorly and posterolaterally, but they are preserved posteriorly. This is explained by the tendency for more fluid to collect anterolaterally than posteriorly in a free pericardial sac.

Symmetric Enlargement of the Cardiac Silhouette

The classic picture of pericardial effusion is the "water-bottle" appearance of an enlarged cardiac silhouette (Figs. 14-13, 14-14, 14-15A). The enlargement is not always sym-metric (Fig. 14-16), however. Asymmetry of fluid distribution in the pericardium need not be accompanied by adhesions or loculations (33).

A water-bottle heart may appear relaxed or tense, depending on the intrapericardial pressure. When the pressure is normal, the cardiac contour tends to be relaxed, flabby, and triangular and has an obtuse cardiophrenic angle (Fig. 14-17). When the pressure is increased, as it is in the presence of cardiac tamponade, the cardiac contour is likely to be tense and globular and have an acute cardiophrenic angle (37) (Fig. 14-18A). Further clues to the possibility of cardiac tamponade are dilatation of systemic veins, mild pulmonary venous congestion, and dampened aortic pulsation.

Changing Cardiac Contour with Changing Posture

The cardiac contour changes when the patient changes position, with a shift of pericardial fluid to the dependent side under the influence of gravity. It is observed only when there is a large effusion in an unobstructed pericardium. As the patient moves from upright to supine, the narrow waist of the cardiac silhouette is widened by the upward shift of

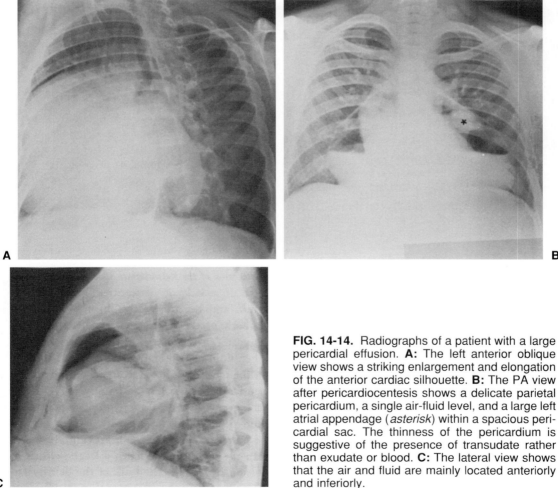

FIG. 14-14. Radiographs of a patient with a large pericardial effusion. **A:** The left anterior oblique view shows a striking enlargement and elongation of the anterior cardiac silhouette. **B:** The PA view after pericardiocentesis shows a delicate parietal pericardium, a single air-fluid level, and a large left atrial appendage (*asterisk*) within a spacious pericardial sac. The thinness of the pericardium is suggestive of the presence of transudate rather than exudate or blood. **C:** The lateral view shows that the air and fluid are mainly located anteriorly and inferiorly.

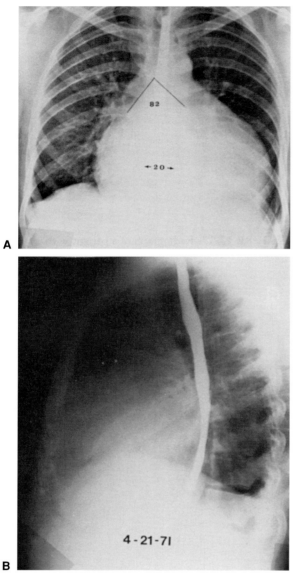

FIG. 14-15. Radiographs of a 30-year-old man with a large pericardial effusion. The PA view (**A**) shows widening of the subcarinal angle (82°) and the transverse diameter of the heart (20 cm). The lateral view (**B**) shows a mild posterior displacement of the esophagus without evidence of left atrial enlargement. (Reproduced with permission from Chen JTT, Putman CE, Hedlund LW, et al. Widening of the subcarinal angle by pericardial effusion. *AJR Am J Roentgenol* 1982; 139:883–887.)

pericardial fluid. This change is particularly pronounced along the left-upper cardiopericardial border at the level of the pulmonary trunk.

No Change in Cardiac Silhouette with Valsalva Maneuver

A dilated or normal heart usually shrinks as the intrathoracic pressure is increased (8). In the presence of pericardial

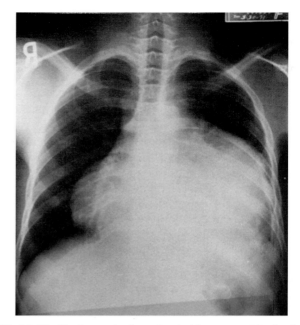

FIG. 14-16. Radiograph of a patient with asymmetric distribution of pericardial effusion.

effusion, however, no change in heart size or contour is observed with the Valsalva maneuver.

Special Diagnostic Procedures

Carbon Dioxide Atriography

Carbon dioxide atriography is briefly mentioned because of its historical value and its potential as a research tool. It is simple to perform (2,38). After intravenous injection of 100 ml of 100% carbon dioxide in the left-lateral decubitus

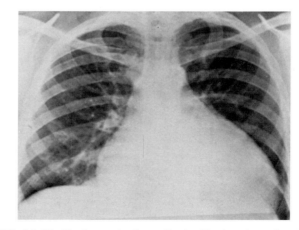

FIG. 14-17. Radiograph of a patient with chronic pericardial effusion without cardiac tamponade. Note the normal pulmonary vascularity, absence of systemic venous engorgement, and "relaxed" pericardial sac.

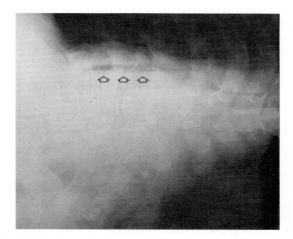

FIG. 14-19. Carbon dioxide atriogram of a patient with pericardial effusion. Arrows mark carbon dioxide inside the right atrium.

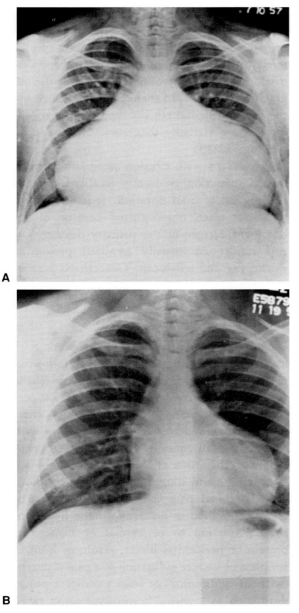

FIG. 14-18. PA radiograph (**A**) of a patient with massive pericardial effusion shows a huge cardiopericardial silhouette. Note the water-bottle configuration of the heart and the dilated superior pulmonary veins and the superior vena cava, suggestive of cardiac tamponade. Another radiograph, taken 2 years later (**B**), shows that the effusion has completely resolved. Pericardial adhesions are present, distorting the heart and creating an odd cardiac shape. Note specifically the concave right atrial border and the square left ventricular border. Despite cardiac deformity, the patient had no evidence of pericardial constriction.

of pleura. Its thickness normally ranges from 1 to 4 mm (33). A measurement >5 mm is definitely abnormal. Effusion is generally present when the extraluminal band is >1 cm (Fig. 14-19). In pericardial thickening, the extraluminal right atrial band is rigid and only mildly widened, measuring 5 to 8 mm. It tends to lose its smooth, curvilinear borders. The carbon dioxide study is misleading when there is right-sided pleural effusion, which alone may cause a thickened extraluminal band resembling pericardial effusion.

Angiocardiography

Angiocardiography is one of the most useful tests for diagnosing pericardial disease (8,33,39). A positive contrast study of the cardiac chambers in multiple projections effectively depicts the size and shape of the entire pericardium (Fig. 14-20).

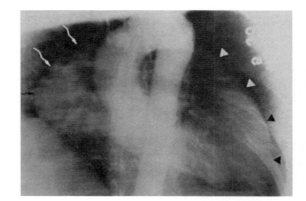

FIG. 14-20. The left ventriculogram of a patient with a large pericardial effusion. Note the markedly increased distance from the opacified chamber to the left-lateral and superior borders of the heart (*arrowheads*), which is suggestive of pericardial effusion. The bulging border of the right side of the heart (*arrows*) supports the diagnosis.

position, serial radiographs are taken in the PA projection using a horizontal x-ray beam. The extraluminal right atrial band is clearly outlined by carbon dioxide in the right atrium and by air in the right lung. The band comprises the right atrial wall, the two layers of pericardium, and the two layers

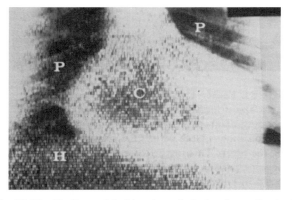

FIG. 14-21. Radionuclide blood pool study of a patient with a large pericardial effusion shows radioactivity in the heart (C), lung (P), and liver (H). The fluid-containing pericardial sac is clearly delineated by its lack of radioactivity.

Radioactive Nuclide Scanning

Comparing a radionuclide scan of the cardiac blood pool with the chest radiograph is a noninvasive procedure for the diagnosis of pericardial effusion (40) (Fig. 14-21). It can be diagnosed when the cardiac blood pool is much smaller than the radiographic image of the heart, when a zone of photon deficiency is seen between the lungs and the heart, and when the cardiac and the hepatic blood pools are separated. With technetium 99m pertechnetate as the intravenous radiopharmaceutical and the Anger camera as the image recording tool, a cardiac scan can be done in 3 minutes. An accompanying chest radiograph is not needed with this technique (41). Disadvantages of isotope scanning include a relatively poor definition of the blood pools and the necessity for the patient to cooperate. Therefore, a small pericardial effusion or pericardial thickening may be missed by this technique.

Echocardiography

Modern echocardiography has largely replaced other diagnostic procedures for assessing pericardial effusion. By virtue of its diagnostic accuracy and its noninvasive nature, ultrasonography is the method of choice in the evaluation of pericardial effusion (36) (Fig. 14-22). Unsuspected small pericardial effusions and thickening or calcification, however, may first be picked up on the chest radiograph. A small effusion in the anterior compartment of the pericardium is more readily imaged with x-ray beams than with ultrasound waves (42) (see **Chapter 1**).

Artificial Pneumopericardiography

Artificial pneumopericardiography is the most definitive way of determining the nature of pericardial disease (4). When fluid is obtained by needle aspiration, the diagnosis of pericardial effusion is made. The fluid can then be tested in

the laboratory. Second, by replacing half of the aspirated fluid with air, the pericardium can be effectively imaged in multiple projections. If the pericardium is thin, smooth, pliable, and without adhesion, the effusion may be inferred as serous (Fig. 14-14B,C). On the other hand, if thickening and adhesions of the pericardium are evident, the effusion is likely to be exudative or bloody, as is commonly found in an infectious, traumatic, or neoplastic process (Fig. 14-23).

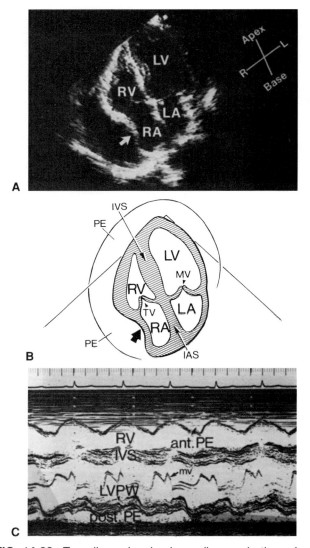

FIG. 14-22. Two-dimensional echocardiogram in the apical four-chamber view (**A**) and the corresponding diagram (**B**) of patient 1 show a large pericardial effusion (PE). Note the systolic collapse of the right atrial wall (*arrow*), which is suggestive of the presence of a hemodynamically significant PE. An M-mode echocardiogram of patient 2 (**C**) shows anterior (ant.) and posterior (post.) PE. The parietal pericardium is flattened by the effusion, whereas the visceral pericardium follows the motion of the ventricular free wall. IAS, interatrial septum; IVS, interventricular septum; L, left; LA, left atrium; LV, left ventricle; LVPW, left ventricular posterior wall; MV, mv, mitral valve leaflets; PE, pericardial effusion; R, right; RA, right atrium; RV, right ventricle; TV, tricuspid valve leaflets.

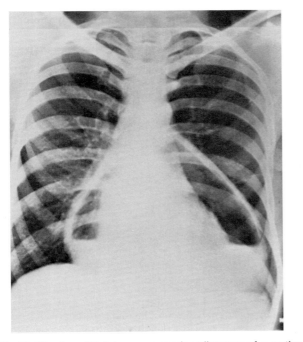

FIG. 14-23. An artificial pneumopericardiogram of a patient with constrictive pyogenic pericarditis as a complication of a stab wound. Note the markedly thickened parietal pericardium. Compare with Fig. 14-14B, in which the pericardium is thin.

Despite its apparent superiority, pericardiocentesis should not be undertaken lightly because of the rare complication of sudden death. To avoid the possibility of lacerating the myocardium, a detecting pericardial electrocardiographic lead should always be used (9). An alternative approach is to use echocardiographic guidance for accurate needle placement.

See Chapter 3 for a discussion of CT scanning in the diagnosis of pericardial diseases and Chapter 4 for assessment of MRI in the such diagnosis.

Special Forms of Pericardial Effusion

Loculated Pericardial Effusion

Loculated pericardial effusion is occasionally noted after cardiac surgery other than pericardiectomy (Fig. 14-24). A loculated pericardial effusion on the left side may mimic a left ventricular aneurysm. The simplest and most effective way to distinguish one from the other is to find the pulsating subepicardial fat stripe within the immobile zone of loculated effusion. In the patient with a left ventricular aneurysm, however, the fat stripe is stretched over the aneurysm and fluoroscopically invisible. Other helpful radiographic signs of loculated effusion include the absence of left ventricular enlargement, a peculiar cardiac contour suggestive of constrictive pericarditis, the bulging and immobile anterior cardiac border of pericardial effusion in general, and the ce-

phalic pulmonary blood flow pattern (owing to left-sided pericardial constriction) together with the absence of pulmonary edema (owing to right-sided constriction). On serial radiographs, the bulge may disappear on reabsorption of the loculated effusion. As a rule, loculated pericardial effusion either precedes or coexists with pericardial constriction (Fig. 14-25; see also **Fig. 3-15**).

Hemopericardium

Acute hemopericardium is usually caused by aneurysm of the ascending aorta dissecting into the pericardium (see **Fig. 9-18**) or rupture of the heart from myocardial infarction, trauma, or cardiac catheterization. Less common causes include blood dyscrasia (43); uncontrolled anticoagulant therapy (44); and neoplastic processes, such as metastatic carcinoma (24,44), melanoma, and lymphoma.

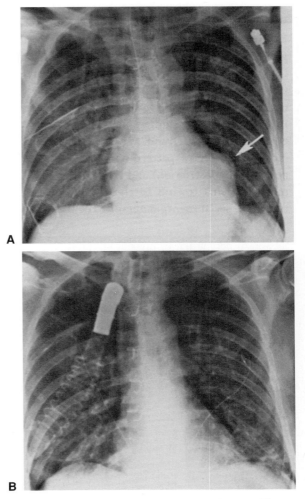

FIG. 14-24. Patient with coronary artery disease. The postoperative film (**A**) shows a bulge (*arrow*) on the left cardiac border representing a loculated pericardial effusion. A film taken 9 days later (**B**) shows that the bulge has disappeared, indicating complete resorption of the effusion.

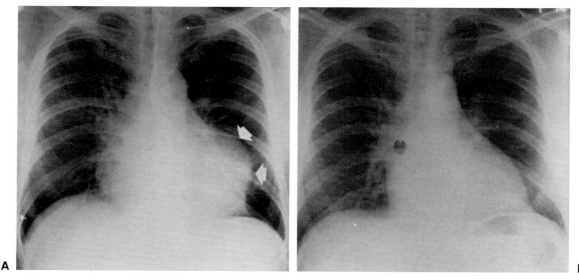

A   B

FIG. 14-25. A patient with a loculated pericardial effusion simulating a left ventricular aneurysm. His PA view (**A**) shows moderate cardiomegaly with a bulge (*arrows*) over the left ventricular border. Also note the cephalic pulmonary blood flow pattern. A film taken 2 years later (**B**), after complete resorption of the pericardial effusion, shows that the bulge has disappeared. Cephalization of pulmonary vascularity is still evident. The right heart border is flat. There are definite clinical and hemodynamic signs of constrictive pericarditis.

Postpericardiotomy Syndrome

From 1 week to 3 months, but usually 2 to 4 weeks, after pericardial or myocardial injury, an acute febrile syndrome (46) may develop in a significant percentage of patients (47). The syndrome is characterized by moderate fever, pericarditis with effusion, pleural effusion, and occasionally pneumonitis. The main clinical manifestations are fever, chest pain, cough, dyspnea, and sometimes abdominal pain and vomiting. It is generally considered an autoimmune hypersensitivity reaction to pericardial or myocardial protein or pericardial blood, resulting from as simple a procedure as ligation of a patent ductus (without cardiotomy) or from a complex procedure, such as mitral commissurotomy (with cardiotomy). Postmyocardial infarction syndrome (Dressler's syndrome) and pericarditis after chest trauma are due primarily to myocardial injuries. The similarity between these syndromes and idiopathic pericarditis suggests that they may all be due to a nonspecific immunologic response to a variety of agents capable of causing myocardial or pericardial injury (32).

A small-to-moderate pericardial effusion is seen on the radiograph, which is frequently associated with pleural effusion and now and then with patchy pneumonitis. The course of the disease may be prolonged and recurrent, with spontaneous remissions lasting from 1 to 2 weeks. The syndrome usually responds to corticosteroid therapy without surgery. But those patients who run a recurrent and chronic course in spite of temporary response to steroids may eventually develop constrictive pericarditis requiring surgical intervention.

Other Forms

Any special form of pericardial effusion has to be diagnosed according to its unique clinical, laboratory, and radiographic findings. Acute idiopathic pericarditis is characterized, for example, by acute onset of typical chest pain, the presence of fever, the exclusion of a specific infectious causation, and the very rapid and dramatic response to steroid therapy. Radiographically, the rapid change in cardiac size and the fleeting pleural effusion and pulmonary infiltrates are virtually diagnostic of this entity (Fig. 14-13).

Pericarditis with effusion stemming from myocardial infarction is usually localized, hemorrhagic, and of brief duration. It is quite common but often unrecognized because of the dominant picture of the primary disease. The end results are usually localized pericardial thickening and adhesions. Generalized pericardial effusion or hemopericardium is the exception (32).

Pericardial effusion may be a component of rheumatic pericarditis; its presence has been associated with a poor prognosis and a high incidence of severe rheumatic heart disease (48). As a rule, rheumatic pericarditis provokes localized adhesions that rarely cause pericardial constriction. Other collagen disorders are also known to cause pericarditis. Rheumatoid pericarditis tends to be focal and rarely evokes a large effusion (49). Fibrinous pericarditis with effusion in all three serous cavities is commonly seen in systemic lupus erythematosus. Pericarditis in periarteritis nodosa is less common and may be related to uremia.

Myxedema heart disease is often associated with pericardial effusion (1,50). While typical clinical manifestations of hypothyroidism may be present, pericardial effusion may be the only clue to the discovery of a silent hypothyroidism. In myxedema, the pericardial fluid has a high protein content in contrast to the low protein content in congestive heart failure. The pericardium itself is normal. Both cardiac dilatation and pericardial effusion respond to thyroid therapy, but not to anticongestive therapy.

Pericardial effusion caused by neoplastic invasion is well known. Tumors that tend to infiltrate the pericardium include bronchogenic carcinoma, breast cancer, and malignant lymphoma (see **Chapter 18**). Pericarditis with effusion may occasionally result from radiation therapy (51,52), syphilis, fungal infection, parasitic disease, infectious mononucleosis, mumps, chicken pox, viral influenza, hypersensitivity reactions, and congenital heart disease.

Pericardial Thickening

In the process of healing from a variety of injuries, the pericardium frequently becomes thickened, calcified, and adherent between its own layers (internal adhesion) or to the diaphragm, the mediastinal structures, or the large airways (external adhesion). The common causes of pericardial thickening are infection, uremia, trauma, collagen disease, cardiac surgery, and radiation therapy. Less common causes include neoplastic infiltration and metabolic disease, such as amyloidosis.

Adhesive Pericarditis

Adhesive pericarditis denotes chronic inflammation of the pericardium with adhesions of the pericardium, internally or externally or both. Since evidence of inflammation is frequently absent under such circumstances, some authors prefer to call it ''pericardial adhesion'' rather than ''adhesive pericarditis.'' Adhesions of the pericardium are likely to produce a peculiar contour of the heart and therefore can be detected radiographically. The salient features include a straight or slightly concave right atrial border, squaring off of the left cardiac border, and tenting of the pericardium (Fig. 14-18). On fluoroscopy, localized rigidity, tenting of the pericardium, or rotary movement of the heart may be seen.

Adhesive pericarditis need not imply functional disturbance of the heart (Fig. 14-25B). However, when incorporated with other measurements, radiographic signs of adhesive pericarditis are frequently the first clue to the possibility of constrictive pericarditis (see **Fig. 10-1**). Apparently pericardial adhesions without marked thickening may not cause cardiac constriction (53). Further evolution of adhesive pericarditis, however, frequently produces constrictive pericarditis (Fig. 14-26; see also **Fig. 3-14**). It is not commonly appreciated that constrictive pericarditis need not be adhesive (Fig. 14-23). Marked thickening of the pericardium (see

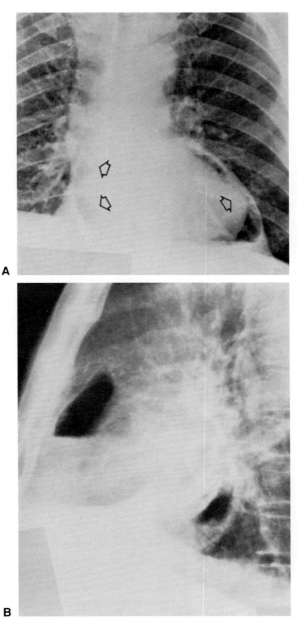

FIG. 14-26. A patient with adhesive and constrictive pericarditis. His post-pericardiocentesis PA radiograph (**A**) shows thickening and adhesions (*arrows*) of the pericardium as well as engorgement of the superior vena cava and pulmonary veins. The lateral view (**B**) shows two air-fluid levels indicative of loculated pericardial effusion.

Fig. 3-14) is the single most important determinant of constriction.

Constrictive Pericarditis

In most patients with constrictive pericarditis, the cause remains unknown, although it is likely to be viral in origin (1). Tuberculosis is the most common among the detectable

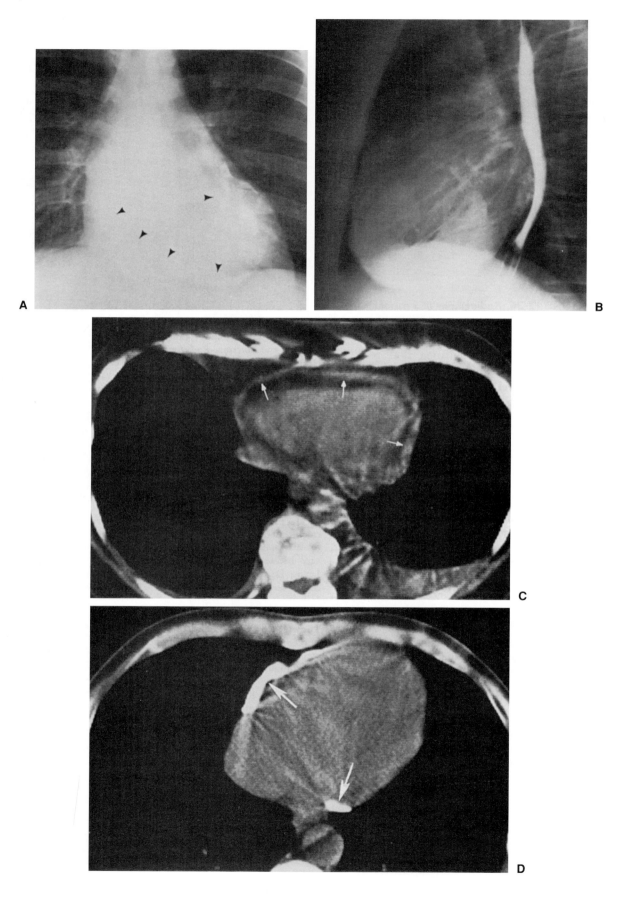

causes. More recently, trauma, cardiac surgery (54), uremia, radiation therapy, and pyogenic infection have been incriminated. The disease is usually seen in young adults, although it has been reported in all ages from 2 to 75 years (32). There is a 3:1 predominance of males. Because of the crippling effect to the patient and its high curability with modern surgery (55), early diagnosis and treatment of constrictive pericarditis are of extreme importance. Long-standing pericardial constriction is known to cause cachexia, anasarca, atrial fibrillation, liver dysfunction, and even irreversible myocardial atrophy (10,56).

Radiographic examination of the heart, aided by fluoroscopy, provides a great deal of information in the diagnosis of constrictive pericarditis. Two additional signs of constrictive pericarditis are expected, besides the appearance of adhesive pericarditis. First, abrupt termination of diastolic relaxation of the heart is usually present. This sign may or may not be associated with decreased contractility in systole. Second, heavy calcification of the pericardium is frequently accompanied by major constriction (Fig. 14-27; see also **Figs. 10–3**). Statistically, >50% of patients with pericardial calcification have constrictive pericarditis (8,37,57). In patients with constrictive pericarditis, ≤90% will show radiographic evidence of pericardial calcification. Of patients with no evidence of constrictive pericarditis, 5% to 10% may have pericardial calcification (see **Fig. 10-2**). Pericardial calcifications are more common and more extensive on the right side of the heart than they are on the left.

The heart in patients with constrictive pericarditis has been conventionally described as small and quiet (58). However, ample evidence has shown that the heart with this condition need neither be small nor quiet (1,59). Constrictive pericarditis with an enlarged heart is seen under the following conditions: compensatory hypertrophy and dilatation of the unconstricted part of the heart (e.g., left atrial enlargement is common in constrictive pericarditis) (4,57), concomitant myocardial or valvular heart disease (Fig. 14-28), associated pericardial effusion (60) (Fig. 14-23), and excessive pericardial thickening ≤2 cm (1) forming a deceptive cardiomegaly.

The cardiac pulsations usually remain normal in the absence of intense scarring of the pericardium. The distribution of scarring is often asymmetric or irregular, especially in the right and anterior aspects of the heart. Under such circumstances, areas of decreased or absent pulsation alternating with areas of normal or increased pulsation may be seen. Regional increased pulsations apparently reflect the natural compensatory mechanism.

When external pericardial adhesions are also present, the

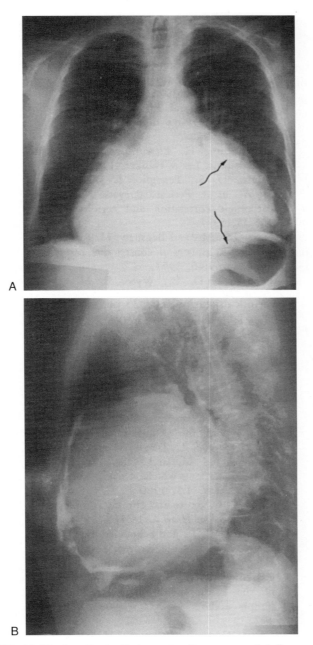

FIG. 14-28. A patient with long-standing myocardial disease complicated by calcific constrictive pericarditis. The PA view (**A**) shows gross cardiomegaly with calcification of the pericardium (*arrows*). The lateral view (**B**) shows the calcified pericardium to better advantage.

FIG. 14-27. Patients with severe constrictive pericarditis. The PA (**A**) and lateral (**B**) views of patient 1 show a cephalic pulmonary flow pattern, cardiomegaly, left atrial enlargement, and heavy pericardial calcium deposits (*arrowheads*). The CT scan of patient 2 (**C**) shows extensive irregular pericardial thickening (*arrows*). The CT scan of patient 3 (**D**) shows heavy pericardial calcification (*arrows*).

following phenomena singly or in combination may be seen (37): tugging of the left dome of the diaphragm in ventricular systole with lack of inspiratory descent, inspiratory upward and forward movement of the heart with absence of widening of the retrosternal space, lack of movement of portions of the heart with respiration, and downward movement of the trachea in ventricular systole (noted in one of our patients).

Other radiographic signs of constrictive pericarditis (57) include the following: pleural effusion in 60% of patients (34% bilateral, 26% unilateral on the right, none unilateral on the left), pulmonary venous congestion in 43% of patients, decreased cardiac pulsation in 77% of patients (23% with essentially normal cardiac pulsation, including one patient with calcification of the pericardium), dilatation of the superior vena cava in 77% of patients, dilatation of the azygos vein in 69% of patients, and left atrial enlargement in 20% of patients. Other researchers (57) have reported 76% of patients with left atrial enlargement, 33% with superior vena caval dilatation, 19% with azygos vein dilatation, 90% with pulmonary trunk dilatation, and 25% with a cardiothoracic ratio >0. 5 in constrictive pericarditis.

REFERENCES

1. Shabetai R. Diseases of the pericardium. In: Schlant RC, Alexander RW, eds. *The heart*, 8th ed. New York: McGraw–Hill, 1994: 1647–1674.
2. Scatliff JJ, Kummer AJ, Janzen AH. The diagnosis of pericardial effusion with intracardiac carbon dioxide. *Radiology* 1958;73:871–883.
3. Plum GE, Bruwer AJ, Clagett OT. Chronic constrictive pericarditis: roentgenologic findings in 35 surgically proved cases. *Proc Staff Meet Mayo Clin* 1957;32:555–566.
4. Spodick DH. *Chronic and constrictive pericarditis*. New York: Grune & Stratton, 1964.
5. Gabella G, Cardiovascular system. In: Williams PL, Bannister LH, Berry MM, et al., eds. *Gray's anatomy*, 38th ed. Edinburgh: Churchill Livingstone, 1995:1471–1479.
6. Roberts WC, Spray TL. Pericardial heart disease: a study of its causes, consequences and morphologic features. In: Spodick DH, ed. *Pericardial diseases*. Philadelphia: Davis, 1976.
7. Soulen RL, Lapayowker MS, Cortes FM. Distribution of pericardial fluid: dynamic and static influences. *Am J Roentgenol* 1968;103:583–588.
8. Steinberg I. Roentgenography of pericardial disease. *Am J Cardiol* 1961;7:33–47.
9. Ebert PA. The pericardium. In: Gibbon JH, Sabiston DC Jr, Spencer FC, eds. *Surgery of the chest*, 4th ed. Philadelphia: Saunders, 1983: 993–1010.
10. Lorell BH, Braunwald E. Pericardial disease. In: Braunwald E, ed. *Heart disease: a textbook of cardiovascular medicine*, 4th ed. Philadelphia: Saunders, 1984:1470–1527.
11. Fraser RG, Pare JAP, Pare PD, Fraser RS, Genereux GP. Pulmonary abnormalities of developmental origin. In: *Diagnosis of diseases of the chest*, vol. 2, 3rd ed. Philadelphia: Saunders, 1989:761–765.
12. Castellino RA, Blank N. Adenopathy of the cardiophrenic angle (diaphragmatic) lymph nodes. *AJR Am J Roentgenol* 1972;114:509–515.
13. Rogers CI, Seymour EQ, Brock G. Atypical pericardial cyst location: the value of computed tomography. *J Comput Assist Tomogr* 1980;4: 683–684.
14. Kelley M. Diseases of the pericardium. In: Putman CE, Ravin CE, eds. *Textbook of diagnostic imaging*, 2nd ed. Philadelphia: Saunders, 1994: 1823–1829.
15. Nath PH, Levitt RG, Gutierrez F. Heart and pericardium. In: Lee JKT, Sagel SS, Stanley RJ, eds. *Computed body tomography with MRI correlation*, 2nd ed. New York: Raven Press, 1989:387–414.
16. Ellis K, Leeds NE, Himmelstein A. Congenital deficiencies in the parietal pericardium: a review of two new cases including successful diagnosis by plain roentgenography. *Am J Roentgenol* 1959;82:125–137.
17. Larsen RL, Behar VS, Brazer SR, Chen JTT, O'Conner C. Chest pain presenting as ischemic heart disease: absence of the pericardium. *N C Med J* 1994;55:306–308.
18. Minocha GK, Falicov RE, Nijensohn E. Partial right-sided congenital pericardial defect with herniation of the right atrium and right ventricle. *Chest* 1979;76:484–487.
19. Moene RJ, Dekker A, van der Harten HJ. Congenital right-sided pericardial defect with herniation of part of the lung into the pericardial cavity. *Am J Cardiol* 1973;31:519–522.
20. Glover LB, Barcia A, Reeves TJ. Congenital absence of pericardium. *AJR Am J Roentgenol* 1969;106:542–549.
21. Pernot C, Hoeffel JC, Henry M, et al. Partial left pericardial defect with herniation of the left atrial appendage. *Thorax* 1972;27:246–250.
22. Saito R, Hotta F. Congenital pericardial defect associated with cardiac incarceration: case report. *Am Heart J* 1980;100:866–870.
23. Nasser WK, Helmen C, Tavel ME, et al. Congenital absence of the left pericardium: clinical, electrocardiographic, radiographic, hemodynamic, and angiographic findings in six cases. *Circulation* 1970;41: 469–478.
24. Chang CH, Armory HI. Congenital partial right pericardial defect associated with herniation of the right atrial appendage. *Radiology* 1965; 84:660–662.
25. Gould SE. *Pathology of the heart and blood vessels*, 3rd ed. Springfield, Ill.: Thomas, 1968:723–729.
26. Klatte EC, Yune HY. Diagnosis and treatment of pericardial cysts. *Radiology* 1972;104:541–544.
27. Lambert AV. Etiology of thin-walled thoracic cysts. *J Thorac Surg* 1940;10:1–7.
28. Feigin DS, Fenoglio JJ, McAllister HA, et al. Pericardial cysts: a radiologic-pathologic correlation and review. *Radiology* 1977;125:15–20.
29. Maier HC. Diverticulum of the pericardium with observations on mode of development. *Circulation* 1957;16:1040–1045.
30. Fraser RG, Pare JAP, Pare PD, Fraser RS, Genereux GP. Diseases of the mediastinum. In: *Diagnosis of diseases of the chest*, vol. 4, 3rd ed. Philadelphia: Saunders, 1991:2866–2877.
31. Unverferth DV, Wooley CF. The differential diagnosis of paracardiac lesions: pericardial cyst. *Cathet Cardiovasc Diagn* 1979;5:31–40.
32. Frieberg CK. Acute pericarditis. In: *Diseases of the heart*, 3rd ed. Philadelphia: Saunders, 1966:933–942.
33. Steinberg I, Von Gal HV, Finby N. Roentgen diagnosis of pericardial effusion: new angiocardiographic observations. *AJR Am J Roentgenol* 1958;79:321–332.
34. Torrance DJ. Demonstration of subepicardial fat as an aid in diagnosis of pericardial effusion or thickening. *AJR Am J Roentgenol* 1955;74: 850–854.
35. Chen JTT, Putman CE, Hedlund LW, et al. Widening of the subcarinal angle by pericardial effusion. *AJR Am J Roentgenol* 1982;139:883–887.
36. Feigenbaum H. *Echocardiography*, 5th ed. Philadelphia: Lea & Febiger, 1994.
37. Schinz HR, Baensch WE, Frommhold W, eds. *Roentgen diagnosis*, vol. 4, 2nd ed. New York: Grune & Stratton, 1970:467–491.
38. Viamonte J Jr. CO₂ angiocardiography: improved technique and results. *AJR Am J Roentgenol* 1962;88:31–37.
39. Figley MM, Bagshaw MA. Angiocardiographic aspects of constrictive pericarditis. *Radiology* 1957;69:46–52.
40. Goldenberg DB, Brogdon BG. A comparison of venous angiography and radioisotope heart scanning in the diagnosis of pericardial effusion. *AJR Am J Roentgenol* 1968;102:320–327.
41. Kriss JP. Radioisotope angiocardiography. *N Engl J Med* 1969;10:233.
42. Casarella WJ, Schneider BO. Pitfalls in the ultrasonic diagnosis of pericardial effusion. *AJR Am J Roentgenol* 1970;110:760–767.
43. Anderson GA. Spontaneous hemopericardium with cardiac tamponade and ''pericardiotomy syndrome'' complicating hemophilia. *Am J Cardiol* 1964;13:278–283.
44. Spodick DH. *Acute pericarditis*. New York: Grune & Stratton, 1959.
45. Applefeld MM, Pollock SH. Cardiac disease in patients who have malignancies. *Curr Probl Cardiol* 1980;4:5–37.
46. Engle MA, Zabriskie JB, Senterfit LB, et al. The postpericardiotomy syndrome: a new look at an old condition. *Mod Concepts Cardiovasc Dis* 1975;64:59–64.

47. Kaminsky ME, Rodan BA, Osborne DR, et al. Postpericardiotomy syndrome. *AJR Am J Roentgenol* 1982;138:503–508.

48. Thomas GT, Besterman EMM, Hollman A. Rheumatic pericarditis. *Br Heart J* 1953;15:29–36.

49. Wilkinson M. Rheumatoid pericarditis: a report of four cases. *Br Med J* 1962;2:1723–1726.

50. Kerber RE, Sherman B. Echocardiographic evaluation of pericardial effusion in myxedema. *Circulation* 1975;52:823–827.

51. Morton DL, Kagan AR, Roberts WC, et al. Pericardiectomy for radiation-induced pericarditis with effusion. *Ann Thorac Surg* 1969;8: 195–208.

52. Stewart JR, Cohn KE, Fajardo LF, et al. Radiation-induced heart disease: a study of twenty-five patients. *Radiology* 1967;89:302–310.

53. Zatuchni J, Chun RBD, Voci G. The flat right atrial border. *Am Heart J* 1961;62:603–605.

54. Cohen MV, Greenberg MA. Constrictive pericarditis: early and late complication of cardiac surgery. *Am J Cardiol* 1979;43:657–661.

55. Miller JI. Surgical management of pericardial disease. In: Schlant RC, Alexander RW, eds. *The heart*, 8th ed. New York: McGraw–Hill, 1994:1675–1680.

56. Edward JE. *An atlas of acquired diseases of the heart and great vessels.* Philadelphia: Saunders, 1961.

57. Cornell SH, Rossi NP. Roentgenographic findings in constrictive pericarditis: analysis of 21 cases. *AJR Am J Roentgenol* 1968;102:301–304.

58. Beck CS. Acute and chronic compression of the heart. *Am Heart J* 1937;14:515–525.

59. Heinz R, Abrams HL. Radiologic aspects of operable heart disease. IV. The variable appearance of constrictive pericarditis. *Radiology* 1957;69:54–61.

60. Steinberg I, Hagstrom JWC. Angiocardiography in diagnosis of effusive-restrictive pericarditis. *AJR Am J Roentgenol* 1968;102:305–319.

Essentials of Cardiac Imaging,
James T. T. Chen,
Lippincott–Raven Publishers, Philadelphia © 1998.

CHAPTER 15

Myocardial Disease

James T. T. Chen

Diseases primarily affecting the myocardium include myocarditides and the cardiomyopathies (1,2). Myocarditis is an inflammatory process of the myocardium, either infectious or noninfectious (2). Cardiomyopathy is a structural or functional disease of the myocardium unrelated to congenital, valvular, hypertensive, pericardial, or coronary abnormalities (1,2). Cardiomyopathies are classified according to their functional abnormalities into three categories: dilated, hypertrophic, and restrictive. Dilated cardiomyopathy may be the result of myocarditis (2).

MYOCARDITIS

Myocarditis may be caused by any infectious (viral, bacterial, rickettsial, mycotic, or parasitic) organism or by noninfectious agents. Among the infectious causes, coxsackievirus type B is the most common offender in the United States and western Europe (2). The noninfectious stimuli include physical agents (e.g., radiation), chemicals, and drugs (e.g., doxorubicin) (3). Depending on the virulence of the organism and the resistance of the host, infectious myocarditis may run a fulminating course with a fatal outcome or it may go unnoticed. The diagnosis may be suspected if cardiac symptoms follow on the heels of an infection. Bacteriologic investigations and endomyocardial biopsy may provide confirmatory information. Viral myocarditis tends to be serious in infants and relatively benign in adults.

The radiographic features of myocarditis are generalized cardiomegaly with a left ventricular preponderance. The ventricles contract poorly, and there is bilateral atrioventricular valve insufficiency, more severe on the left than on the right side (Fig. 15-1). Associated pericarditis with effusion is frequently seen in patients with viral myocarditis (Fig. 15-2).

Department of Radiology, Duke University School of Medicine, Durham, North Carolina 27710, U.S.A.

DILATED CARDIOMYOPATHY

Dilated cardiomyopathy is a myocardial disease characterized by four-chamber dilatation, poor ventricular contractility, bilateral atrioventricular valve insufficiency, and congestive heart failure when the left ventricular ejection fraction is <40% (the normal value exceeds 60%) (Fig. 15-3). Although a definite cause is not identifiable in most patients, many conditions appear to be closely related to dilated cardiomyopathy: myocarditides, alcoholism, pregnancy, and the puerperium (4). Mitral and tricuspid insufficiency is due to papillary muscle dysfunction as part of ventricular failure. The cardiac valves are basically normal. The regurgitant flow is small, and so is the size of the atrium because of the poor pumping ability of the markedly dilated ventricle.

Superficially, dilated cardiomyopathy may be confused with coronary heart disease; the latter can frequently be differentiated by a history of angina pectoris or myocardial infarction. Under the fluoroscope, coronary artery calcifications (5), good right ventricular contractility, and localized left ventricular asynergy all suggest the diagnosis of coronary heart disease. Both conventional and electron beam computed tomography (CT) have been found to be more sensitive than fluoroscopy in the detection of coronary artery calcifications. In dilated cardiomyopathy, the contractile abnormalities of the ventricle are more diffuse and bilateral, patients are younger than those with coronary heart disease, and coronary artery calcification is usually not present.

HYPERTROPHIC CARDIOMYOPATHY

The hallmark of hypertrophic cardiomyopathy is myocardial hypertrophy. The obstructive phase of this entity, known also as idiopathic hypertrophic subaortic stenosis (IHSS) (1,6), is discussed in **Chapter 11**. In general, the left ventricular outflow pressure gradient is quite varied in patients with IHSS. This dynamic characteristic is registered not by conventional radiologic methods, but rather by physical exami-

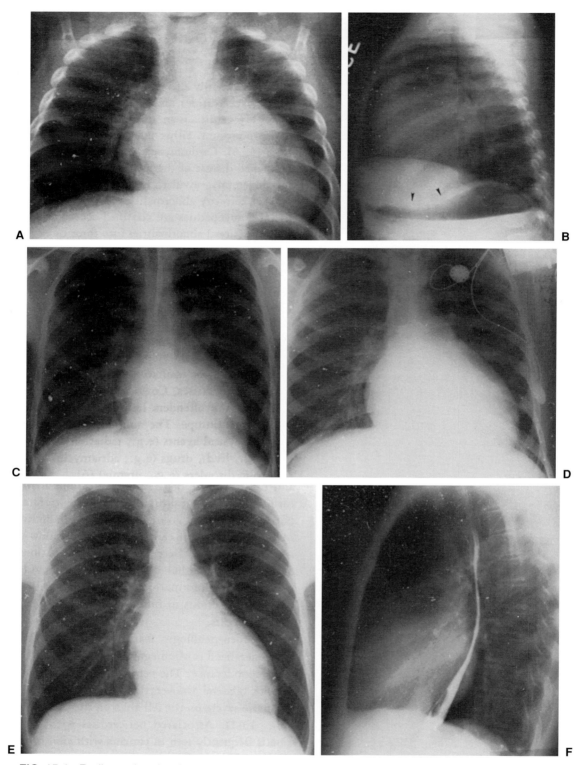

FIG. 15-1. Radiographs of patients with viral myocarditis. Posteroanterior (PA) (**A**) and lateral (**B**) views of a 2-month-old infant show gross cardiomegaly and interstitial pulmonary edema. Note that the dilated heart is impinging on the stomach; this is better appreciated on the lateral view (*arrows*). The PA view of a 15-year-old boy (**C**), taken 2 months after the onset of a tenacious viral illness, shows mild cardiomegaly with pulmonary edema. Six months later, a second radiograph (**D**) reveals gross cardiomegaly, severe pulmonary edema, and right-sided pleural effusion. The patient responded temporarily to anticongestive therapy, and the follow-up films (**E,F**) show signs of improvement. Unfortunately, the myocardium continued to deteriorate, and it failed altogether a year later.

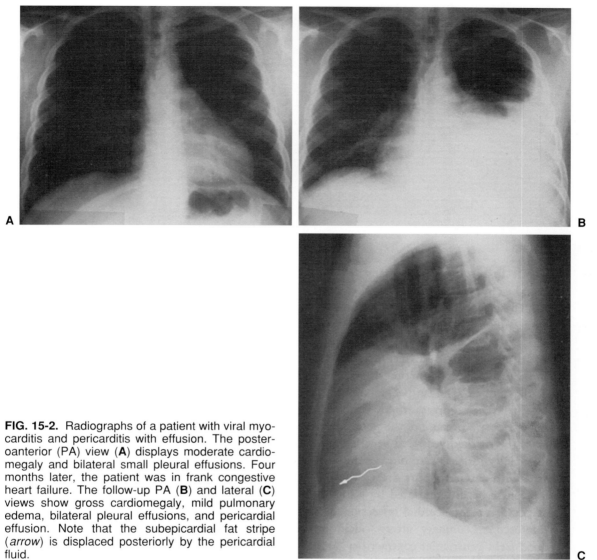

FIG. 15-2. Radiographs of a patient with viral myocarditis and pericarditis with effusion. The posteroanterior (PA) view (**A**) displays moderate cardiomegaly and bilateral small pleural effusions. Four months later, the patient was in frank congestive heart failure. The follow-up PA (**B**) and lateral (**C**) views show gross cardiomegaly, mild pulmonary edema, bilateral pleural effusions, and pericardial effusion. Note that the subepicardial fat stripe (*arrow*) is displaced posteriorly by the pericardial fluid.

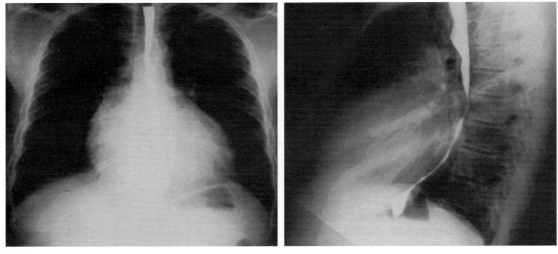

FIG. 15-3. Posteroanterior (PA) (**A**) and lateral (**B**) views of a 43-year-old man who was admitted because of a 4-year history of chronic congestive heart failure. The cardiac index was 1.4 L/minute/m^2, and the end-diastolic pressures were 22 mm Hg in the right ventricle and 34 mm Hg in the left ventricle. The radiographs show gross generalized cardiomegaly and cephalization of the pulmonary vascularity. Under the fluoroscope, the contractility of the heart was seen to be extremely poor, and there was evidence of bilateral atrioventricular valve insufficiency. The diagnosis was idiopathic dilated cardiomyopathy.

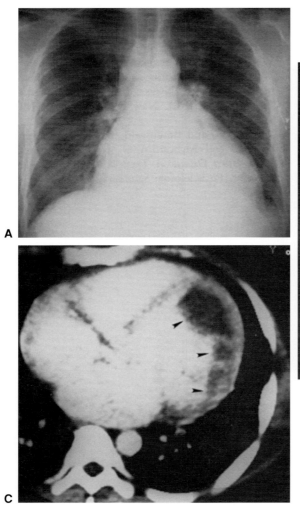

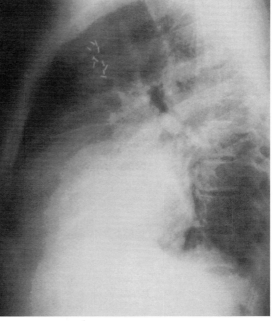

FIG. 15-4. Studies of a 32-year-old man who had had exertional dyspnea and an irregular heartbeat for 2 months. Three years before the studies, diffuse lymphadenopathy had developed, and a nodal biopsy at that time revealed sarcoidosis. Posteroanterior (**A**) and lateral (**B**) radiographs show gross cardiomegaly with pulmonary edema. A CT scan (**C**) demonstrates a mural thrombus (*arrows*) in the left ventricle.

nation, echocardiography (see **Fig. 11-8F,G**), angiocardiography (see **Fig. 11-8D**), catheterization, cine CT, and cine magnetic resonance imaging. The medical treatment of hypertrophic cardiomyopathy primarily aims at decreasing ventricular contractility by beta-adrenergic blockade or calcium channel blockers and by avoiding volume depletion. The surgical treatment consists of myotomy or myectomy (or both) of the ventricular septum (6).

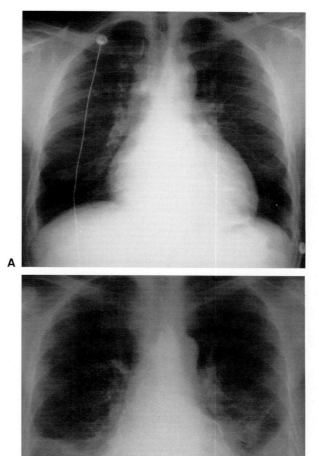

FIG. 15-6. Endomyocardial biopsy-proven amyloidosis in two patients. The posteroanterior (PA) radiograph (**A**) of the first patient, an 83-year-old man, shows mild cardiomegaly, mild interstitial pulmonary edema, and moderate bilateral pleural effusions. This is a good example of cardiac amyloidosis in its early stages. His end-diastolic pressures were 19–22 mm Hg with a left ventricular ejection fraction of 45%. The PA radiograph (**B**) of the second patient, a 53-year-old man, shows gross cardiomegaly, pulmonary vascular cephalization, dilated systemic veins, and bilateral small pleural effusions. This is a good example of cardiac amyloidosis in its late stage, simulating dilated cardiomyopathy.

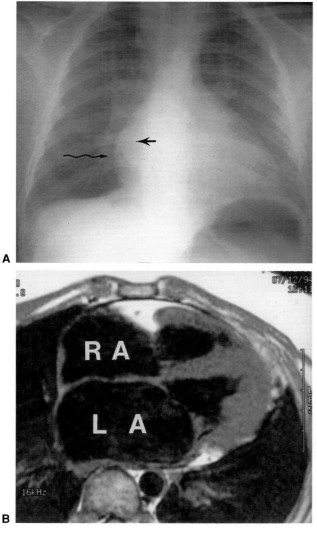

FIG. 15-5. A 7-year-old girl with restrictive cardiomyopathy had complained of fatigue and progressive shortness of breath even at rest for several months. Her cardiac catheterization showed elevated end-diastolic pressures in both sides of the heart, with normal systolic function. Endomyocardial biopsy revealed only mild patchy interstitial fibrosis. Her posteroanterior chest radiograph (**A**) shows mild cardiomegaly with significant left atrial enlargement (*short arrow*) and moderate right atrial enlargement (*long arrow*). There is cephalization of the pulmonary blood flow but no frank pulmonary edema. The spin echo (SE) magnetic resonance image (**B**) shows a huge left atrium (LA) and a moderately dilated right atrium (RA). Both ventricles are hypertrophied but not dilated.

RESTRICTIVE CARDIOMYOPATHY

The most common causes of restrictive cardiomyopathy are endomyocardial fibrosis, amyloidosis, and hemochromatosis. Sarcoidosis (Fig. 15-4) is an uncommon disease in this connection. In infants, endocardial fibroelastosis and glycogen storage disease are examples of restrictive heart disease. The characteristic sign of restrictive cardiomyopathy is stiffness of the ventricular wall, which prevents satisfactory diastolic filling of the heart. The systolic function is usually preserved in the early stages of the disease (Fig. 15-5) (1,7–9). Toward the end stage of the disease, however, both systolic and diastolic function will fail, and it becomes indistinguishable from dilated cardiomyopathy. This is exemplified by cardiac amyloidosis (Fig. 15-6) (1).

REFERENCES

1. Mason JW. Classification of cardiomyopathy. In: Schlant RC, Alexander RW, eds. *The heart*, 8th ed. New York: McGraw–Hill, 1994:1585–1590.
2. O'Connell JB, Renlund DG. Myocarditis and specific myocardial diseases. In: Schlant RC, Alexander RW, eds. *The heart*, 8th ed. New York: McGraw–Hill, 1994:1591–1608.
3. Crawley IS, Schlant RC. Effect of noncardiac drugs, electricity, poisons, and radiation on the heart. In: Schlant RC, Alexander RW, eds. *The heart*, 8th ed. New York: McGraw–Hill, 1994:1989–2006.
4. Lampert MB, Lang RM. Peripartum cardiomyopathy. *Am Heart J* 1995; 130:860–870.
5. Margolis JR, Chen JTT, Kong Y, et al. The diagnostic and prognostic significance of coronary artery calcification: a report of 800 patients. *Radiology* 1980;137:609–616.
6. Maron BJ, Roberts WC. Hypertrophic cardiomyopathy. In: Schlant RC, Alexander RW, eds. *The heart*, 8th ed. New York: McGraw–Hill, 1994.
7. Shabetai R. Restrictive cardiomyopathy. In: Schlant RC, Alexander RW, eds. *The heart*, 8th ed. New York: McGraw–Hill, 1994:1621–1636.
8. Cetta F, O'Leary PW, Seward JB, et al. Idiopathic restrictive cardiomyopathy in children: diagnostic features and clinical course. *Mayo Clin Proc* 1995;70:634–640.
9. Masui T, Finck S, Higgins CB. Constrictive pericarditis and restrictive cardiomyopathy: evaluation with MR imaging. *Radiology* 1992;182: 369–373.

Essentials of Cardiac Imaging,
James T. T. Chen,
Lippincott–Raven Publishers, Philadelphia © 1998.

CHAPTER 16

Congenital Heart Disease

James T. T. Chen

The clinical assessment of patients with congenital heart disease is greatly strengthened by the information obtained from cardiac imaging. Of the available imaging techniques, chest radiography (1–8), echocardiography (1,7–11), computed tomography (CT) (8,12,13), magnetic resonance imaging (MRI) (1,10,13–15), and radionuclide methods (1,3,7,16) are noninvasive but less precise, and contrast angiocardiography is invasive but more accurate. In conjunction with clinical and electrocardiographic data, the diagnosis can frequently be made by noninvasive techniques (see **Chapters 1–6**). When surgery is considered, cardiac catheterization (17) with angiocardiography is usually required to fully delineate the abnormal anatomy and physiology. In this chapter, congenital anomalies of the heart and great vessels are classified and discussed by the radiographic appearance of pulmonary vascularity and by the presence or absence of cyanosis. Although chest radiography is emphasized, correlations are made with information obtained from other forms of imaging.

INCREASED PULMONARY VASCULARITY WITHOUT CYANOSIS

Abnormalities that present a picture of increased pulmonary vascularity without cyanosis are left-to-right shunts and large systemic arteriovenous fistulas (see **Fig. 18-2**). Major left-to-right shunts are ventricular septal defect (VSD), atrial septal defect (ASD), atrioventricular septal defect (AVSD) or endocardial cushion defect, and patent ductus arteriosus (PDA). Minor or uncommon left-to-right shunts are aorticopulmonary septal defect (APSD) or aorticopulmonary window; coronary artery (CA) fistulas, including aberrant left coronary artery from the pulmonary artery; and aortic sinus aneurysm rupturing into the right heart (Table 16-1).

In left-to-right shunts, the pulmonary blood flow is in-

creased while the systemic flow remains normal. In systemic arteriovenous fistulas, the blood flow in both circulations is increased, and this condition should be considered one of the hyperkinetic states (see **Chapter 18**). The hemodynamic effect of a left-to-right shunt varies with the size and location of the communication between the two circulations as well as with the individual tolerance to such derangement. As a rule, a small shunt causes no functional disturbance. A moderate to large shunt under low pressure (e.g., secundum ASD) produces a high-flow, low-resistance state, which is well tolerated by most persons for years if not decades. But a large shunt under high pressure (e.g., VSD and PDA) often results in congestive heart failure or Eisenmenger syndrome. Although cyanosis is not a feature in any of these abnormalities, it may become apparent when Eisenmenger syndrome is well established and the direction of the shunt is reversed.

Ventricular Septal Defect

Ventricular septal defect is the most common congenital heart disease in children. In adults, however, it accounts for only 10% of all cardiac defects (18) because VSDs tend to close by 25% spontaneously by age 18 months, 50% by age 4 years, and 75% by age 10 years (19).

Anatomy

The anatomic classification of VSDs is important in planning surgical treatment. For example, paramembranous defects can be closed through the right atrium; a right ventriculotomy is, however, necessary for repair of supracristal defects. These defects are classified into four types (6,10,20) (Fig. 16-1), with type 2 being the most common.

Clinical Presentation

Patients with a small VSD have no symptoms but are predisposed to infective endocarditis. The typical physical

Department of Radiology, Duke University School of Medicine, Durham, North Carolina 27710, U.S.A.

TABLE 16-1. *Defects that cause increased pulmonary blood flow without cyanosis*

Left-to-right shunts
  Major defects
    Atrial septal defect
    Ventricular septal defect
    Patent ductus arteriosus
    Atrioventricular septal defect (endocardial cushion defect)
  Minor defects
    Partial anomalous pulmonary venous connection
    Aorticopulmonary septal defect (aorticopulmonary window)
    Coronary artery fistulas
    Aortic sinus aneurysm rupturing into the right heart
Systemic arteriovenous fistulas

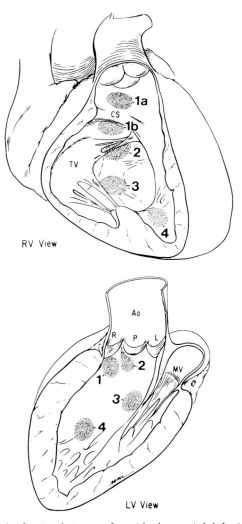

FIG. 16-1. Anatomic types of ventricular septal defects. Type 1, conal defect, subdivided into 1a (supracristal) and 1b (infracristal) defects; type 2, paramembranous defect; type 3, posterior or endocardial cushion defect; type 4, muscular defects (often multiple). Ao, aorta; CS, crista supraventricularis; L, left cusp of aortic valve; LV view, left ventricular view; MV, mitral valve; P, posterior cusp of aortic valve; R, right cusp of aortic valve; RV view, right ventricular view; TV, tricuspid valve. (Modified with permission from Kirks DR. *Practical pediatric imaging*, 2nd ed. Boston: Little, Brown, 1991.)

finding is a systolic murmur at the left sternal border. Patients with a large VSD usually suffer from recurrent congestive heart failure, respiratory infections, and poor growth. During the remission of cardiac decompensation, the physical findings include a holosystolic murmur with thrill at the left sternal border and a flow murmur (diastolic rumble) across the normal mitral valve. The electrocardiogram (ECG) usually shows biventricular hypertrophy and left atrial enlargement. With a high degree of pulmonary vascular reactivity, patients with a large VSD may follow a different course—a hyperresistant state known as Eisenmenger syndrome may develop. In such a state, the systolic murmur becomes soft or inaudible, and the ECG is right-sided in orientation (17).

Radiographic Signs

Small VSDs evidence no definite radiographic abnormalities. The typical radiographic features of VSD are usually found in patients with a medium-size defect: diffusely increased pulmonary vascularity, biventricular and left atrial enlargements, dilatation of the pulmonary trunk in proportion to the magnitude of shunt, and normal aorta and normal right atrium (Fig. 16-2).

The radiographic signs of a large VSD vary depending on a number of factors, including the patient's age and his or her individual reactivity of the pulmonary vasculature. In the neonate, the heart and lungs may look normal despite the presence of a large VSD. After about the fourth week of life, as the pulmonary vascular resistance continues to decline, a large left-to-right shunt usually becomes apparent, with the typical biventricular–left atrial enlargement. Large VSDs frequently lead to either congestive heart failure (21,22) (Fig. 16-3) or Eisenmenger syndrome (see **Figs. 8-15** and **8-16**). As Eisenmenger physiology develops, the usual features of VSD are transformed into right-sided cardiomegaly with a centralized pulmonary blood flow pattern.

Echocardiographic Signs

Echocardiographic evidence of left atrial enlargement suggests that the shunt is at the ventricular or ductal level. The two-dimensional technique (7) can actually identify the VSD.

Catheter Position and Angiography

At the time of hemodynamic evaluation, a right ventricular catheter may pass through the VSD into the aorta. Identi-

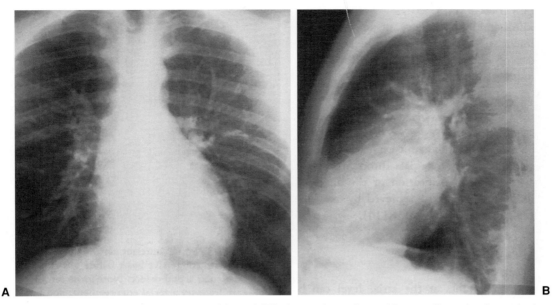

FIG. 16-2. Posteroanterior (PA) (**A**) and lateral (**B**) views of a patient with a medium-sized ventricular septal defect, showing increased pulmonary vascularity and biventricular and left atrial enlargements. The aorta and the right atrium are normal. Note that the general contour of the heart is relatively normal, suggesting a normal (nonrotatory) cardiac position. Compare with atrial septal defect with leftward cardiac rotation (see Fig. 16-10A,B,D,F) and patent ductus arteriosus with rightward rotation (see Fig. 16-21).

fication of the anatomic details of a VSD is best achieved by axial left ventricular angiocardiography (23). As with echocardiographic examination, angiographic evidence of left atrial enlargement suggests that the shunt is at the ventricular or ductal level. At the same time, an intact atrial septum can readily be verified (Fig. 16-4).

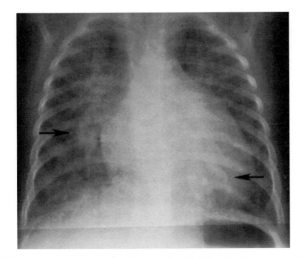

FIG. 16-3. PA view of a 6-month-old infant with congestive heart failure caused by a large ventricular septal defect. Note gross cardiomegaly, pulmonary arterial engorgement, and pulmonary venous congestion. All vessels are poorly demarcated, indicating the presence of pulmonary edema. Arrows point to the dilated pulmonary arteries, which are vertical in orientation in the lower lung zones.

Ultrafast Computed Tomography and Magnetic Resonance Imaging

Both ultrafast CT and MRI have proved quite useful in the assessment of heart disease (12,14) (see **Chapter 3** and **4**). Figure 16-5A and B provides exquisite pictures from ultrafst CT scanning of a child with a small VSD (12). Figure 16-6 is a tranaxial MR image of VSD.

Long-term Follow-up

In the adult population, one usually sees one of the three forms of congenital VSD: small VSD, surgically repaired VSD, or Eisenmenger VSD. Large VSDs (Fig. 16-7) without associated congestive heart failure or Eisenmenger physiology are exceptional. Closure of VSD is contraindicated in patients with Eisenmenger physiology when the ratio between pulmonary vascular resistance (Rp) and systemic vascular resistance (Rs) is >0.5. Patients with lower Rp/Rs ratios, however, might benefit from surgery, provided the pulmonary hypertension is due primarily to vascular spasm rather than to organic changes. Such benefits may diminish with time in some patients, and further life-saving procedures may become necessary (24) (Fig. 16-8).

Atrial Septal Defect

Anatomy

Left-to-right shunts at the atrial level can be classified as intracardiac, extracardiac, or combined. The intracardiac

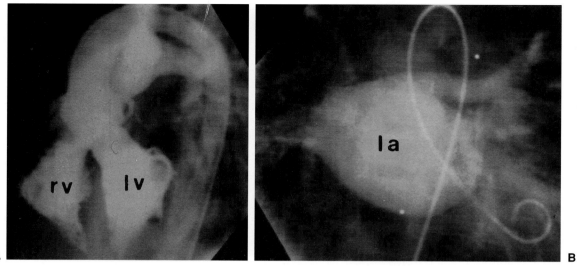

FIG. 16-4. A child with moderate VSD. A left ventriculogram in the right posterior oblique view (**A**) shows a paramembranous VSD. lv, left ventricle; rv, right ventricle. The levo phase of another left ventricular injection in the anteroposterior view (**B**) shows significant left atrium enlargement and no evidence of ASD. la, left atrium.

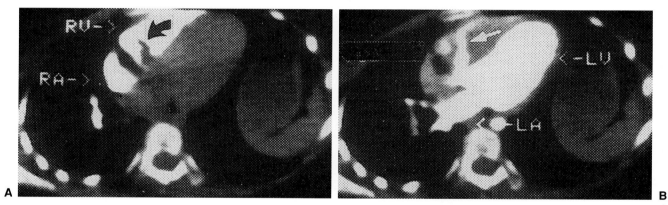

FIG. 16-5. A 4-year-old child with a small VSD. Note the negative contrast (*black arrow*) of VSD (**A**) and positive contrast (*white arrow*) of the same VSD (**B**) during right ventricular and left ventricular opacification, respectively (Reproduced with permission from Husayni TS. UFCT imaging in congenital heart disease. In: Stanford W, Rumberger JA, eds, *Ultrafast computed tomography in cardiac imaging: principles and practice.* New York: Futura, 1992.)

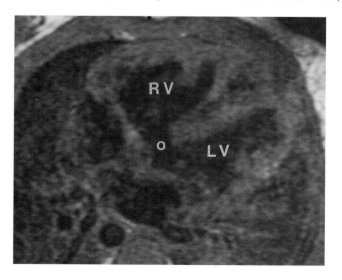

FIG. 16-6. A child with pseudotruncus arteriosus. An axial spin-echo image at the ventricular level shows right ventricular hypertrophy and a large VSD (o). RV, right ventricle; LV, left ventricle.

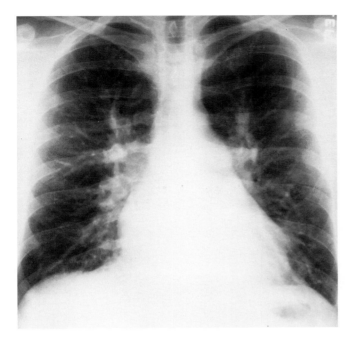

FIG. 16-7. A 28-year-old man had a 5:1 left-to-right shunt at the ventricular level with pulmonary blood flow of 26 L/minute. The PA radiograph shows a marked increase in pulmonary vascularity and left atrio-biventricular cardiomegaly.

lesions include ostium secundum, ostium primum, and sinus venosus ASDs. The extracardiac lesions comprise a variety of partial anomalous pulmonary venous connections (PAPVCs). Ostium secundum ASD, usually an isolated anomaly, is located in the middle third of the atrial septum at the level of the fossa ovalis. Ostium primum ASD is located in the lower third of the atrial septum and is frequently associated with a cleft mitral valve, representing a partial form of AVSD. Sinus venosus ASD is located in the upper third of the atrial septum, close to the entry of the superior vena cava to the right atrium (Fig. 16-9). In all three types of ASD, the incidence of coexisting PAPVC is ~15%; in sinus venosus ASD alone, however, the association is as high as 85% (17). The developmental basis of PAPVC is discussed later, in the section dealing with embryology of total anomalous pulmonary venous connection.

Clinical Presentation

Most children with ASD are asymptomatic. Mild dyspnea and easy fatigability are common among adults. The male-to-female ratio is about 3:1. On physical examination, the typical signs of uncomplicated ASD are an ejection systolic murmur along the left-upper sternal border, the fixed split-second sound, and the apical diastolic rumble of functional tricuspid stenosis due to excessive flow across a normal valve. The electrocardiographic features of uncomplicated ASDs are right axis deviation, right ventricular hypertrophy, rsR′ QRS pattern, normal sinus rhythm, and arrhythmias after the third decade of life.

Radiographic and Angiographic Signs

The radiographic features of secundum ASD right-sided cardiomegaly, increased pulmonary vascularity, a normal pulmonary blood flow pattern, and a leftward rotation of the heart and great vessels, making the aorta inappropriately small and the pulmonary trunk disproportionately large (Fig. 16-10A,B). The left atriogram or levo phase of a pulmonary arteriogram in the right posterior oblique position effectively determines the site of ASD (Fig. 16-10C). Dramatic improvement from closure of uncomplicated ASD is expected in children and young adults (25) (Fig. 16-10D,E). An incidental diagnosis of large secundum ASD in the elderly who are seen medically for reasons other than cardiovascular problems is not uncommon (Fig. 16-10F–H). Since primum ASD represents a partial form of AVSD, it is described along with AVSD.

Isolated PAPVC or PAPVC associated with ASD cannot be differentiated from uncomplicated ASD, unless the anomalous veins are clearly identified on the radiographs (Fig. 16-11A). Anomalous pulmonary veins are usually confirmed by angiocardiography (Fig. 16-11B,C). The associated sinus venosus ASD can be seen angiographically as a defect in the upper third of the septum (Fig. 16-11D).

A rare type of PAPVC is commonly seen as part of a complex congenital anomaly called scimitar syndrome (see **Fig. 8-22**). The most striking radiographic sign of this entity is the common collecting right pulmonary vein, which resembles a Turkish sword, the scimitar. It begins from the mid-lung zone, lateral and posterior to the right hilum. From there it courses downward and medially to penetrate the diaphragm and drain into the inferior vena cava. The other features of the syndrome include a hypoplastic right pulmonary artery; an aberrant arterial supply to the right-lower lobe, either from the celiac axis or the aorta; two bilobed lungs; an increased incidence of bronchiectasis or bronchial diverticulum as the source of hemoptysis; and an intact interatrial septum 95% of the time (26).

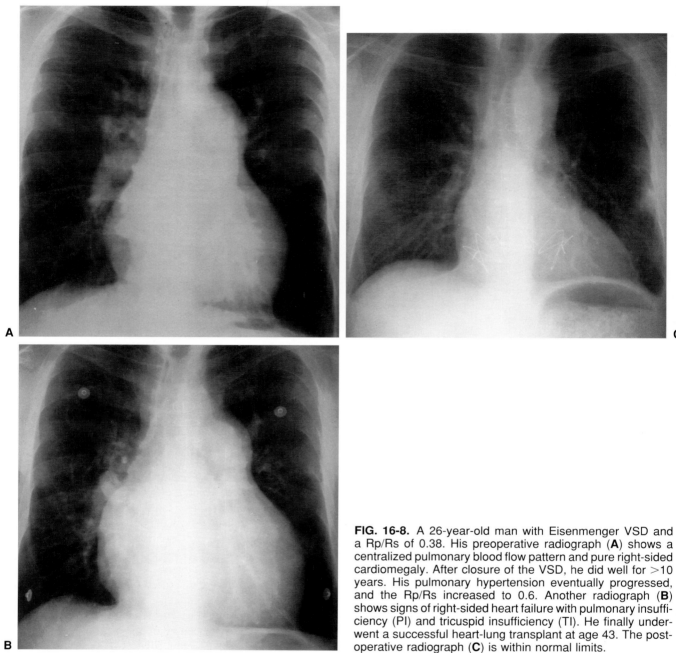

FIG. 16-8. A 26-year-old man with Eisenmenger VSD and a Rp/Rs of 0.38. His preoperative radiograph (**A**) shows a centralized pulmonary blood flow pattern and pure right-sided cardiomegaly. After closure of the VSD, he did well for >10 years. His pulmonary hypertension eventually progressed, and the Rp/Rs increased to 0.6. Another radiograph (**B**) shows signs of right-sided heart failure with pulmonary insufficiency (PI) and tricuspid insufficiency (TI). He finally underwent a successful heart-lung transplant at age 43. The postoperative radiograph (**C**) is within normal limits.

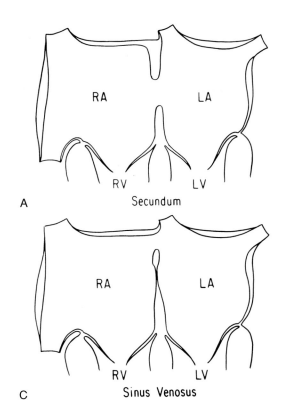

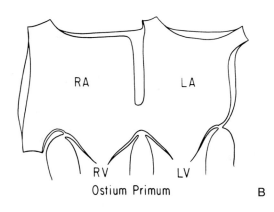

FIG. 16-9. Anatomic types of atrial septal defects. LA, left atrium; LV, left ventricle; RA, right atrium; RV, right ventricle. (Reproduced with permission from Kirks DR. *Practical pediatric imaging*, 2nd ed. Boston: Little, Brown, 1991.)

The association of ASD with mitral stenosis is known as Lutembacher's syndrome (7) (Fig. 16-12). Ostium secundum defects may be associated with skeletal abnormalities of the upper extremities as well as with conduction defects. This association is known as Holt–Oram syndrome (27) (Fig. 16-13).

Echocardiographic Signs

The echocardiographic findings of ASD are dilatation of the right ventricle, anterior systolic motion of the interventricular septum, and direct imaging of the ASD with two-dimensional or transesophageal technique. Microbubbles of air can be introduced into the bloodstream by injecting normal saline intravenously. Since such bubbles are strongly echogenic, shunting across the ASD can be readily imaged (Fig. 16-14).

Computed Tomography and Magnetic Resonance Imaging

Both CT (8,12) and MRI (14,15) have proved effective in diagnosing ASD and PAPVC.

Long-term Follow-up

Secundum ASD is the most common left-to-right shunt in the adult. The majority of patients with this condition are asymptomatic even in advanced age (Fig. 16-10F). Compared with VSD and PDA, the development of Eisenmenger physiology (Fig. 16-15) from secundum ASD is less common, particularly in the early stages of the disease. Similarly, congestive heart failure is not a feature of ASD until later in life, when arrhythmias and acquired heart disease complicate the picture. Therefore, early closure of ASD is of prime importance (17,24,25) (Fig. 16-10D,E). Large secundum ASD in adults occasionally mimics mitral stenosis in auscultatory findings (see **Fig. 2-24**). The fixed split-second sound of ASD may be confused with the opening snap of mitral stenosis; the flow murmur across the normal tricuspid valve may be mistaken for the diastolic murmur of mitral stenosis.

Atrioventricular Septal Defect

Anatomy

Atrioventricular septal defect was previously termed endocardial cushion defect. It can be classified as complete or partial. There are four component lesions for the complete form. They are low (ostium primum) ASD, cleft anterior mitral leaflet, high VSD, and cleft septal tricuspid leaflet (Fig. 16-16). As a result, a cross-shaped defect is formed in the center of the heart, which is also known as atrioventricular (AV) canal or AV communis. There are no separate AV valves in AV canal. Instead, only a common AV valve bridges the gap between atria and ventricles.

Only two component lesions exist in the most common

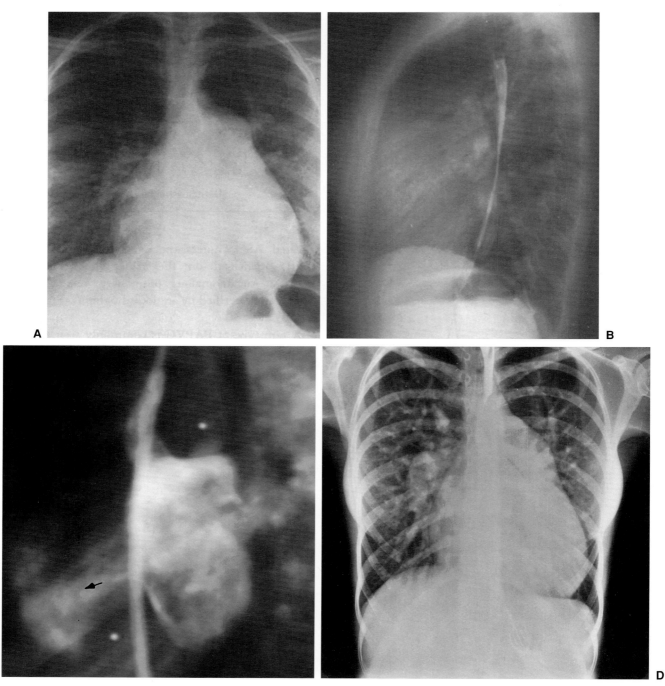

FIG. 16-10. PA (**A**) and lateral (**B**) radiographs of an 18-year-old woman with secundum ASD show increased pulmonary vascularity, right-sided cardiomegaly, a small aorta, and a big pulmonary trunk. The left-sided chambers are not enlarged. The barium-filled esophagus pursues a normal course. Angiogram (**C**) of a child with secundum ASD shows that a catheter was inserted from the inferior vena cava through the right atrium, the PFO, and the left atrium into a superior pulmonary vein. After opacification of the left atrium in the right posterior oblique position, there is a jet (*arrow*) across the middle third of the atrial septum into the right atrium. PA film (**D**) of a 23-year-old woman with a huge secundum ASD shows considerable right-sided heart enlargement and a marked increase in pulmonary blood flow.

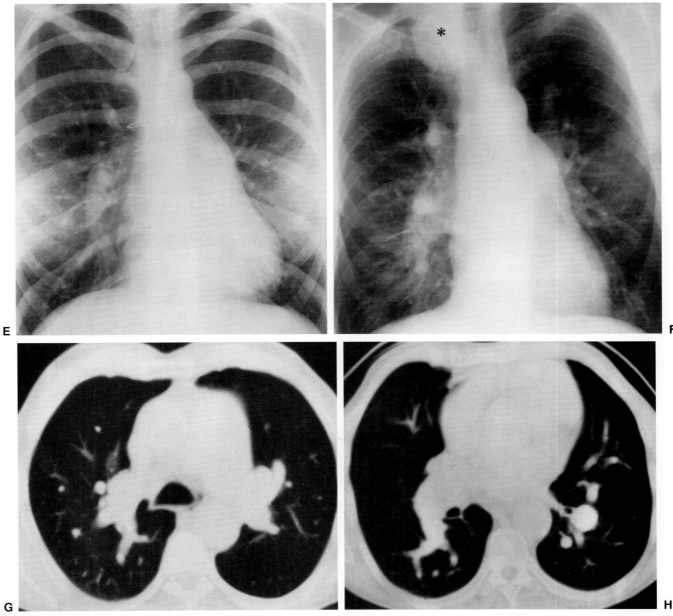

FIG. 16-10. *Continued.* The postoperative film (**E**) shows dramatic improvement. The last patient was a 62-year-old man with lung cancer. His large secundum ASD was an incidental discovery. The PA film (**F**) shows right-sided cardiomegaly, huge pulmonary arteries and veins, a normal pulmonary blood flow pattern, and a big mass (*asterisk*) in the right apex. Computed tomography at a higher level (**G**) shows huge pulmonary arteries and at a lower level (**H**) shows huge pulmonary veins. This means absence of pulmonary hypertension.

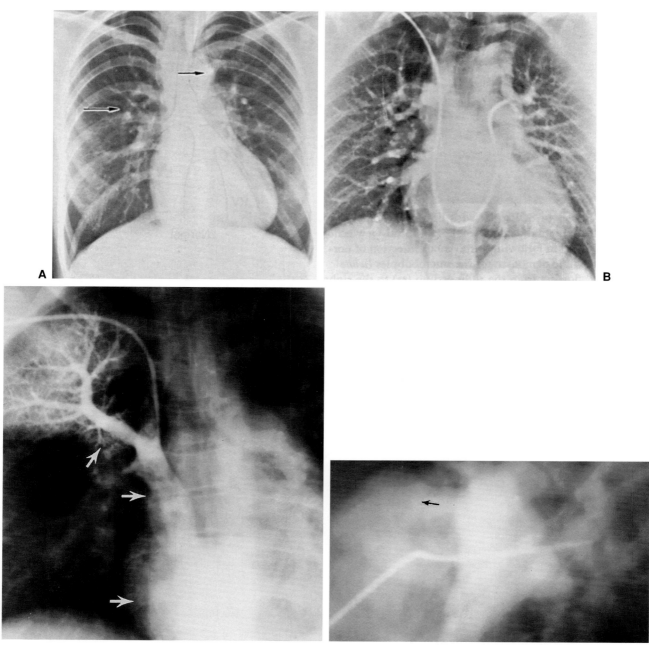

FIG. 16-11. PA radiograph (**A**) of a patient with sinus venosus ASD and bilateral upper-lobe PAPVCs shows right-sided cardiomegaly, increased pulmonary vascularity, and an anomalous vein from the right upper lobe to the superior vena cava (*lower arrow*). A bandlike density (*upper arrow*) overlapping the aortic arch suggests the presence of a left vertical vein receiving venous return from the left upper lobe. The levo phase of the pulmonary arteriogram (**B**) confirms this impression. A frontal angiogram (**C**) of another patient shows that a catheter was inserted from the superior vena cava into the right-upper-lobe anomalous vein. After injection of contrast medium there was sequential opacification of the anomalous vein (*upper arrow*), superior vena cava (*middle arrow*), and right atrium (*lower arrow*). From the third patient with sinus venosus ASD, the levo phase of the pulmonary arteriogram in the right posterior oblique position (**D**) shows good opacification of the left atrium and a jet (*arrow*) across the upper third of the atrial septum into the right atrium.

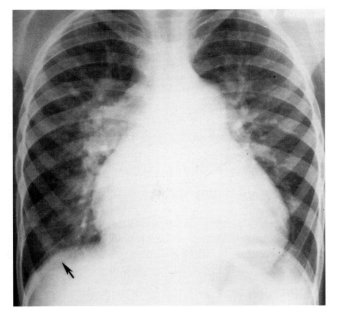

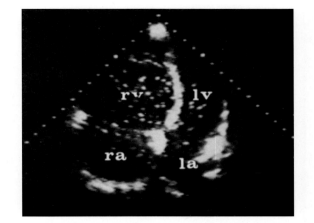

FIG. 16-12. An 8-year-old girl with Lutembacher's syndrome. PA radiograph shows increased pulmonary blood flow in cephalic distribution. The right ventricle and right atrium are markedly dilated. The left atrium is only mildly enlarged. The left ventricle is normal. Note septal lines (*arrow*) in the right costophrenic sulcus.

FIG. 16-14. Patient with Ebstein's anomaly and an ASD. The apical-view echocardiogram after intravenous injection of normal saline demonstrates the microbubbles (*white dots*) flowing from the right atrium (ra) to the right ventricle (rv) and across the ASD into the left atrium (la) and left ventricle (lv). In real time, the microbubbles were also floating to and fro across the tricuspid valve, indicating tricuspid insufficiency.

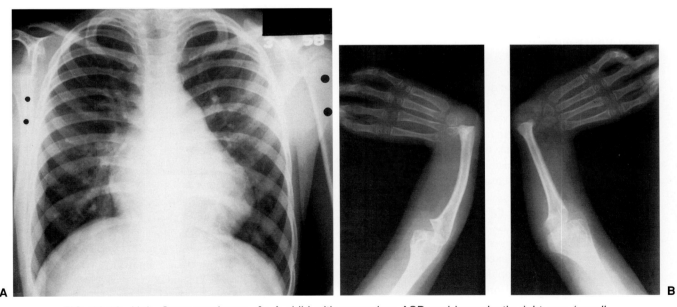

FIG. 16-13. Holt–Oram syndrome. **A:** A child with secundum ASD and hypoplastic right arm (*small dots*) compared with the normal left arm (*large dots*). Also note subluxation of the right shoulder. **B:** Another patient with tetralogy of Fallot. Note bilateral radial club hands with absent radii and thumbs.

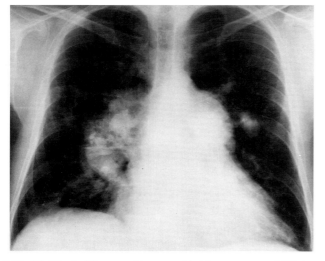

FIG. 16-15. A 42-year-old man with Eisenmenger ASD has gross right-sided cardiomegaly and striking centralization of the pulmonary blood flow. The aortic arch is quite small.

partial form of AVSD: ostium primum ASD and cleft anterior mitral leaflet. The cleft anterior mitral leaflet is attached to the upper margin of the deficient ventricular septum instead of being hung from the mitral annulus. This makes the left ventricular outflow tract more narrow and longer than normal, resulting in the so-called gooseneck deformity (6,7,28) (Fig. 16-17).

Clinical Presentation

Atrioventricular septal defect accounts for only 3% to 4% of all forms of congenital heart disease in children. The complete form usually leads quickly to death in infancy. Patients with the partial form, however, have a much better prognosis, particularly if the cleft mitral valve is functionally competent; when it is, the survival rate approaches that of ostium secundum defect. In patients with Down's syndrome, the most common heart disease is the complete form of AVSD.

On physical examination, the partial form is not distinguishable from secundum ASD unless the mitral valve is incompetent. Physical findings of the complete form are similar to those of a large VSD except for a fixed split-second sound. The electrocardiographic findings of AVSD are unique and quite helpful in distinguishing it from secundum ASD and VSD. They are a left axis deviation and a counterclockwise vector loop in the frontal plane (17).

Radiographic Signs

The radiographic signs of partial AVSD are identical to those of ostium secundum ASD unless the cleft mitral valve is functionally incompetent. In that case, mild left atrial en-

largement and a varying degree of left ventricular enlargement will be evident (Fig. 16-18). In the case of severe mitral insufficiency complicating primum ASD, the left atrium tends to be more dilated, and recurrent congestive heart failure is more frequently encountered (Fig. 16-19). The radiologic findings of complete AVSD before the development of heart failure or severe pulmonary hypertension are very similar to those found in the partial form, except for a tendency toward a more dilated right atrium and left ventricle (Fig. 16-20).

Angiographic and Magnetic Resonance Signs

On the frontal angiocardiogram or coronal MR images, narrowing and elongation of the left ventricular outflow tract (the gooseneck deformity) are characteristic of all forms of AVSD (Fig. 16-17).

Echocardiographic Signs

Two-dimensional echocardiography is capable of imaging the atrial and ventricular septa as well as the inflow and outflow tracts of both ventricles. In experienced hands, both diagnosis and classification of AVSDs can be established with this method (1,7).

Long-term Follow-up

It is not uncommon to see partial AVSD with mild mitral insufficiency in adults. Surgery is usually successful in these patients (24,29) (Fig. 16-18). On the other hand, patients with primum ASD and severe mitral insufficiency (Fig. 16-19) or those with AV canal (Fig. 16-20) typically do poorly, resulting in congestive heart failure, which is less amenable to surgery. Residual mitral and tricuspid insufficiency after closure of shunts is the most troublesome long-term problem.

Patent Ductus Arteriosus

Patency of the ductus arteriosus is essential for normal fetal circulation. Persistence of this vessel after birth, however, permits a left-to-right shunt, which may lead to congestive heart failure or Eisenmenger physiology.

Anatomy

The ductus runs from the pulmonary trunk near the origin of the left pulmonary artery to the descending aorta just distal to the left subclavian artery. In children, PDA is one of the most common congenital cardiac defects, particularly in premature infants and in those born of a mother who had rubella during the first trimester. In adults, PDA is uncom-

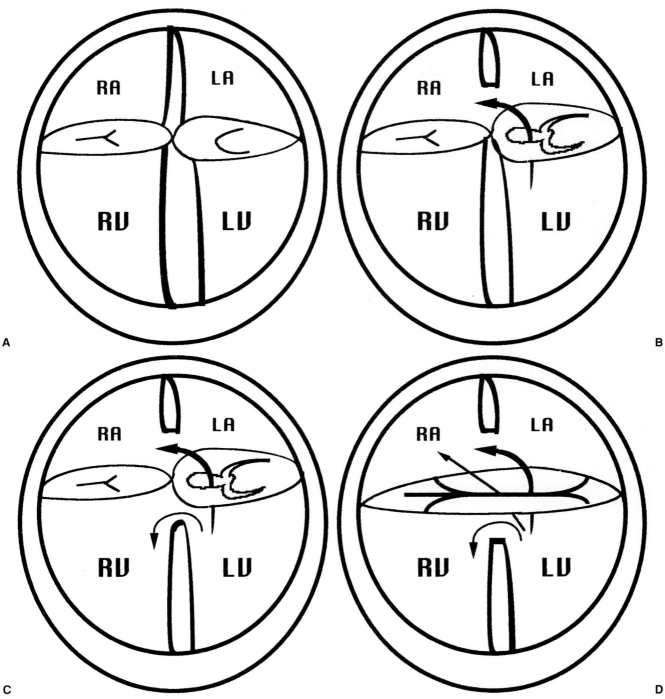

FIG. 16-16. Schematic drawings of the region of the endocardial cushions in normal subjects (**A**) and in patients with various types of atrioventricular septal defects: partial (**B**), intermediate (**C**), and complete (**D**). LA, left atrium; LV, left ventricle; RA, right atrium; RV, right ventricle.

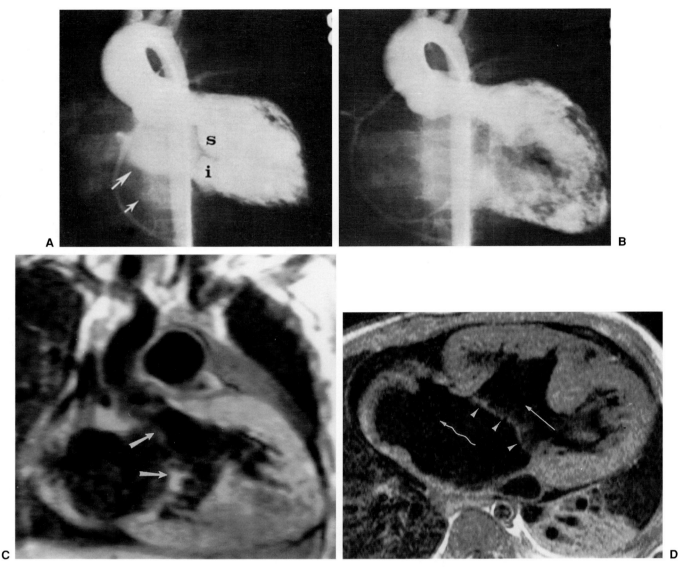

FIG. 16-17. Left ventriculogram of a patient with partial AVSD. Note that the cleft of the anterior mitral leaflet is easily seen in systole (**A**) between the superior (s) and the inferior (i) segments. The border of the cleft leaflet has the typical nodular appearance. The left atrium (*large arrow*) is opacified by the regurgitant blood from the left ventricle. The right atrium (*small arrow*) is only faintly opacified by the more diluted contrast medium from the left atrium via the ASD. In diastole (**B**) the gooseneck deformity of the left ventricle becomes more conspicuous; the scooped-out defect of the left ventricle is deepened, and the outflow tract of the left ventricle is even more narrow and elongated than it is during systole. (Modified from Kirks DR. *Practical pediatric imaging*, 2nd ed. Boston: Little, Brown, 1991.) Coronal spin-echo MR image (**C**) of another patient with AVSD shows a similar gooseneck deformity of the left ventricle (*arrows*). Axial spin-echo MR image (**D**) shows a large ASD (*spiral arrow*) and VSD (*straight arrow*) and an anterior common bridging leaflet (*arrowheads*). (MR images C and D are courtesy of Jeffrey C. Weinreb, New York University Medical Center, New York.)

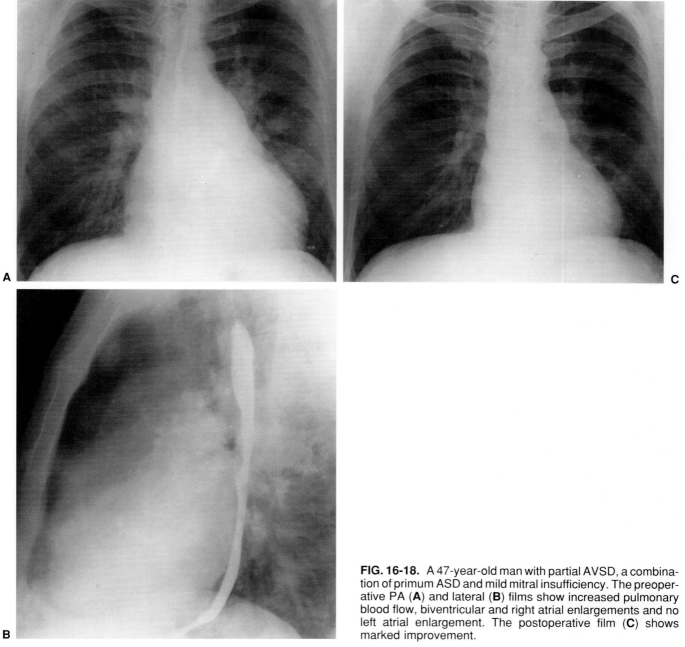

FIG. 16-18. A 47-year-old man with partial AVSD, a combination of primum ASD and mild mitral insufficiency. The preoperative PA (**A**) and lateral (**B**) films show increased pulmonary blood flow, biventricular and right atrial enlargements and no left atrial enlargement. The postoperative film (**C**) shows marked improvement.

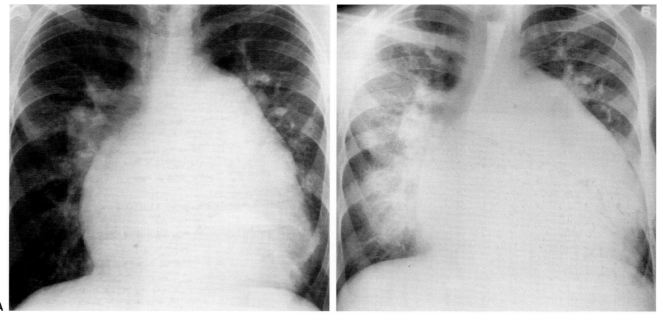

A   B

FIG. 16-19. A 16-year-old with primum ASD and severe mitral insufficiency. The initial radiograph (**A**) shows conspicuous four-chamber enlargement, a moderate increase in pulmonary blood flow, and striking cephalization. Three years later, another radiograph (**B**) shows frank congestive heart failure with gross cardiomegaly and pulmonary edema. Complete repair was attempted, but he did poorly.

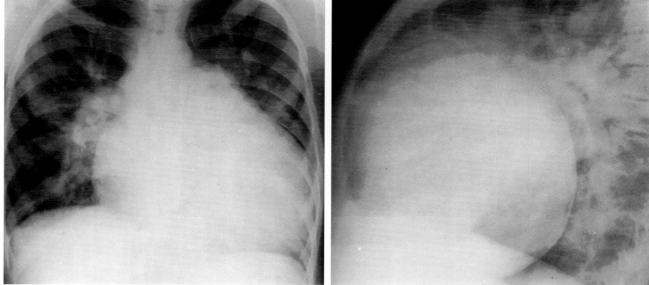

A   B

FIG. 16-20. A 14-year-old boy with complete AVSD. PA (**A**) and lateral (**B**) views show four-chamber enlargement with the left atrium being the least dilated. The pulmonary blood flow pattern is a combination of increased flow and cephalization. He developed severe congestive heart failure 9 years later, and his postoperative results were not satisfactory because of persistent mitral insufficiency and TI (not shown).

mon, mainly because of the trend toward early surgical closure of the shunt.

Clinical Presentation

Patients with a small PDA are usually asymptomatic. The clinical manifestations of a large PDA are those of congestive heart failure, which occurs either in infancy (left ventricular failure) or after the second decade of life (right ventricular failure). In preterm infants with birth asphyxia (a respiratory distress syndrome), the coexisting PDA frequently complicates their clinical course and requires prompt surgical ligation (30). Infective endocarditis is not a problem in the first 2 years of life. Thereafter it becomes increasingly prevalent with age.

On physical examination, a continuous machinery murmur with a thrill is usually found over the upper-left sternal border. The pulse pressure is widened, and the peripheral pulses are bounding. The electrocardiographic findings are typically those of left ventricular and left atrial hypertrophy. Right ventricular hypertrophy is seen only in patients with severe pulmonary hypertension.

Radiographic Signs

In patients with a small PDA, the roentgen appearance may be entirely normal. In the presence of a large PDA,

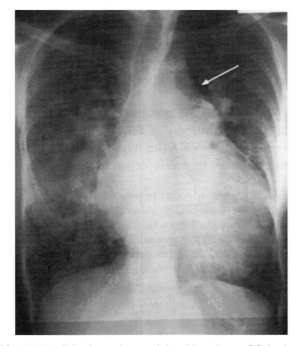

FIG. 16-21. PA view of an adult with a large PDA shows marked increase in pulmonary vascularity, left-sided cardiomegaly, and dilatation of both the pulmonary trunk and the aorta. Smooth transition from the aorta to the pulmonary trunk is evident (*arrow*).

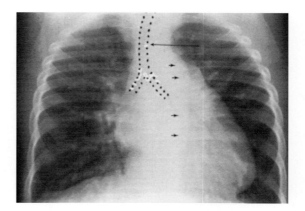

FIG. 16-22. PA view of a 13-month-old girl with a large PDA shows left-sided cardiomegaly and pulmonary plethora. The aortic arch is enlarged, causing marked deviation of the trachea to the right side (*long arrow*). The descending aorta is also enlarged (*lower arrows*). A large ductus infundibulum is clearly evident (*upper arrows*). (Modified with permission from Kirks DR. *Practical pediatric imaging*, 2nd ed. Boston: Little, Brown, 1991.

before the onset of heart failure or Eisenmenger physiology, there are two radiologic signs. First, the left-sided chambers, the aorta proximal to the ductus, and the pulmonary vasculature are all enlarged and become hyperpulsatile on fluoroscopy. Second, a smooth transition zone between the aorta and the pulmonary trunk is usually found to be the site of the PDA (6,7) (Fig. 16-21). In infants, cardiomegaly, pulmonary plethora, prominence of the aortic arch, and the presence of ductus infundibulum are all suggestive of a PDA (7) (Fig. 16-22).

Angiographic and MR Signs

An injection of contrast medium into the aortic arch or the ascending aorta is the most sensitive imaging technique in the diagnosis of PDA (Fig. 16-23). A pulmonary artery catheter frequently turns sharply downward into the descending aorta, thereby delineating the presence of a PDA (see **Fig. 7-10**). Magnetic resonance imaging is capable of differentiating PDA from APSD (see section entitled ''Aorticopulmonary Septal Defect''), allowing the surgeon to avoid the wrong surgical approach (see **Fig. 4B-5**).

Long-term Follow-up

The radiologic signs of Eisenmenger PDA may be identical to those of Eisenmenger ASD (see **Fig. 8-15**) or VSD (see **Fig. 8-16**). The possible clues to the correct diagnosis are residual aortic and left-sided heart enlargement as well as calcification of the ductus and the great arteries as a result of long-standing pressure overload (Fig. 16-24).

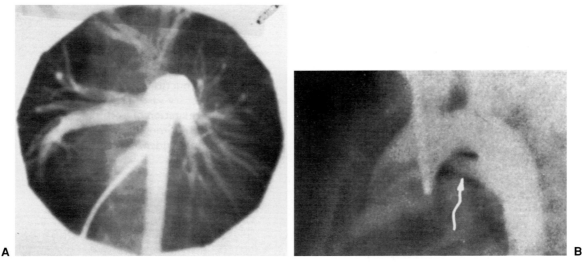

A   B

FIG. 16-23. Patients with PDA. After injection of contrast medium into the aorta of the first patient (**A**), the pulmonary arteries opacify immediately via a large PDA. A lateral aortogram of another patient (**B**) clearly shows a large PDA (*arrow*).

Aorticopulmonary Septal Defect

Aorticopulmonary septal defect is also termed aorticopulmonary window. It is a rare anomaly, representing deficient septation of the truncus arteriosus. This condition mimics a large PDA in all aspects except for its angiographic features

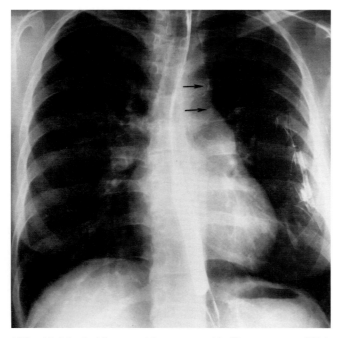

FIG. 16-24. A 41-year-old woman with Eisenmenger PDA has a centralized pulmonary blood flow pattern and right-sided cardiomegaly. The aortic arch is dilated with calcification (*upper arrow*). Immediately above the dilated pulmonary trunk and below the aortic arch, the patent ductus is also partly calcified (*lower arrow*).

(Fig. 16-25). Radiographic-hemodynamic correlation of major left-to-right shunts is shown in Table 16-2.

Coronary Artery Fistulas

Coronary artery fistulas, with decreasing incidence of myocardial ischemia, include aberrant left coronary artery from the pulmonary artery, right or anterior descending CA from the pulmonary artery, minor CA fistulas (>90% of them involve the right coronary arterial tree draining into the venous circulation) (17).

Aberrant Left Coronary Artery from the Pulmonary Artery

Aberrant (or anomalous) left CA from the pulmonary artery is an uncommon congenital abnormality. Although a left-to-right shunt exists, the magnitude of the shunt is so small that it does not manifest on radiography. Instead, a varying degree of pulmonary venous congestion is usually present, reflecting left ventricular dysfunction. In adults, the pulmonary vascularity may be within normal limits until frank left ventricular failure develops. Nevertheless, this condition is discussed here because of its similarity to PDA, APSD, CA fistula, and ruptured aortic sinus aneurysm—in all these conditions there is a continuous murmur.

Pathophysiology and Clinical Presentation

Patients with this anomaly are usually asymptomatic in the first weeks of life, despite the fact that a large mass of the myocardium is perfused with nonoxygenated blood from the pulmonary artery. As the pulmonary vascular resistance

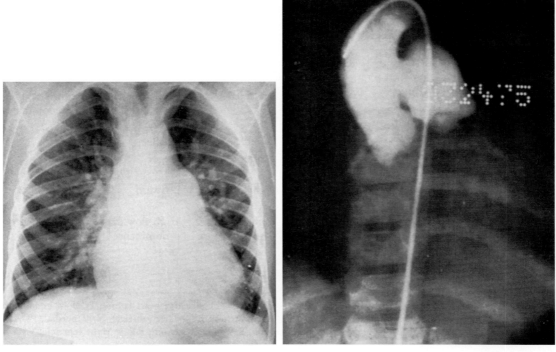

FIG. 16-25. Patients with APSD or aorticopulmonary window. Radiograph of patient 1 (**A**) shows findings indistinguishable from a large PDA. Aortogram of patient 2 (**B**) shows that the contrast medium passes from the ascending aorta through the APSD into the pulmonary trunk (Reproduced with permission from Edwards JE, Carey LS, Neufeld HN, Lester RG. *Congenital heart disease.* Philadelphia: Saunders, 1965.)

decreases, blood begins to flow in the opposite direction in the aberrant left CA. When that happens, adequate myocardial perfusion in this area depends solely on the collateral circulation from the normal right to the aberrant left CA. Since the intercoronary anastomosis takes time to develop, most patients die from myocardial infarction during the first

year of life. The survivors eventually build up abundant intercoronary collateralization and become relatively asymptomatic during childhood or in adulthood (11).

During the critical period of shunt reversing, these infants begin to have recurrent bouts of shock, possibly with profound chest pain. A typical pattern of anterolateral myocar-

TABLE 16-2. *Radiographic–hemodynamic correlation of moderate left-to-right shunts before congestive heart failure or Eisenmenger physiology*

Characteristics	2° ASD	VSD	PDA, APSD	1° ASD	AV canal
Cardiomegaly	RV, RA	RV, LV, LA	LV, LA	RV, RA, LV	RV, RA, LV, LA
Cardiac contour	Right-sided	N	Left-sided	Right-sided predom.	Right-sided predom.
Aorta	Smaller[a]	N	Larger[b]	Smaller	Smaller
PT	Larger	Proportional to flow	Smaller	Larger	Larger
Cardiac rotation	Leftward	None	Rightward	Leftward	Leftward
Hemodynamics	High flow	High flow, high press.	High flow, high press.	High flow predom.	High press., high flow
Tendency to Eisnmenger Ph or CHF	+	+ + +	+ + +	+ +	+ + + +

ASD, atrial septal defect; VSD, ventricular septal defect, PDA, patent ductus arteriosus; APSD, aorticopulmonary septal defect; AV canal, complete form of atrioventricular septal defect; RV, right ventricle; RA, right atrium; LV, left ventricle; LA, left atrium; N, normal; predom., predominant; PT, pulmonary trunk; press., pressure; Ph, physiology; CHF, congestive heart failure; 1°, primum; 2°, secundum; +, the least tendency; + + + +, the most tendency.

[a] Smaller than it actually is because of cardiac rotation.
[b] Larger than it actually is because of cardiac rotation.

dial infarction is usually evident on the ECG. On physical examination, the heart is enlarged, but no notable murmur can be heard (11). Eventually, 85% of patients die of intractable congestive heart failure.

Radiographic and Angiographic Signs

In infants, the heart is grossly enlarged, with left ventricular preponderance. The left atrium is dilated to a varying degree, depending on the severity of mitral insufficiency. The left ventricle shows poor contractility along the anterolateral wall, where an aneurysm may form. The pulmonary vessels show a pattern of venous obstruction (i.e., cephalization and pulmonary edema). A shunt vascularity is not observed (Fig. 16-26A,B). On angiography, the right CA is dilated and tortuous. The intercoronary anastomosis increases with age. The left CA fills in a retrograde fashion from the right and drains into the pulmonary artery (Fig. 16-26C,D). The left ventricle contracts abnormally along the anterolateral wall or at the apex.

Long-term Follow-up

The survivors may be entirely asymptomatic. On physical examination, a continuous murmur over the upper-left ster-

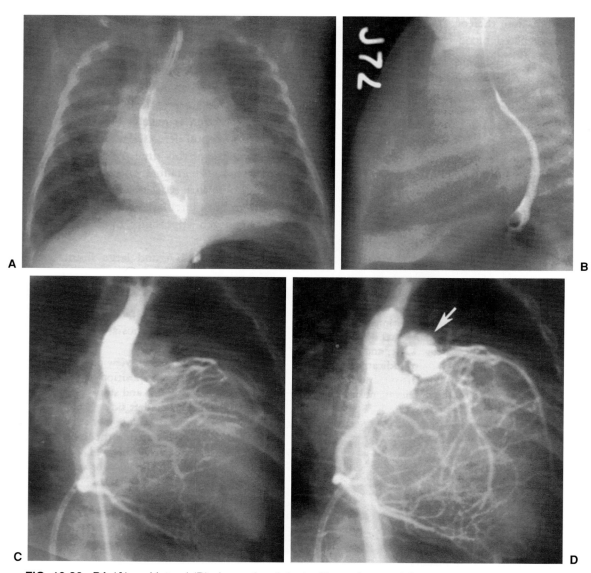

FIG. 16-26. PA (**A**) and lateral (**B**) views of an infant with an aberrant left coronary artery arising from the pulmonary trunk show gross cardiomegaly with left ventricular preponderance. The esophagus is deviated to the right and posteriorly by the enlarged left atrium. Under the fluoroscope the left ventricle contracted poorly. The early phase of the aortogram (**C**) shows that the dilated right coronary artery feeds the left coronary artery in a retrograde fashion. The later phase of the study (**D**) shows further opacification of the left coronary artery, which empties into the pulmonary trunk (*arrow*).

nal border is an outstanding clinical feature that can lead to confusion of this condition with a PDA. Other patients may be symptomatic because of myocardial ischemia, mitral insufficiency, and left ventricular aneurysm. Sudden death is a real threat even to patients who are apparently well. In adults the right CA may become aneurysmal and border-forming. When it projects to the left side, it may mimic an enlarged left atrial appendage (Fig. 16-27). Since this is a treatable disease and most patients benefit from surgery, it is mandatory that they be identified early (24).

Right Coronary Artery–Right Atrial Fistula

Isolated right CA–right atrial fistula is uncommon but may cause a significant left-to-right shunt (Fig. 16-28).

Aortic Sinus Aneurysm Rupturing into the Right Heart

This is a rare anomaly resulting from congenital weakness at the union of the aorta with the heart (11). The sinus aneu-

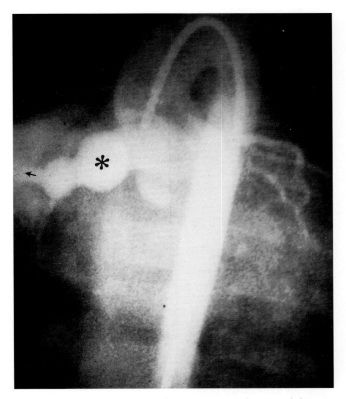

FIG. 16-28. An anteroposterior aortogram shows a right coronary artery (*asterisk*) to right atrium fistula (*arrow*), causing marked dilatation of both structures. The overall heart size is moderately enlarged. The pulmonary blood flow is increased.

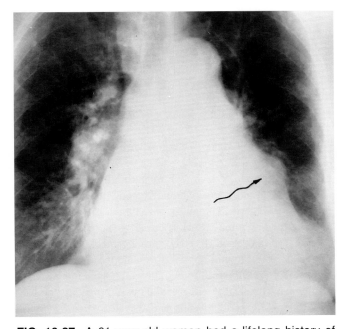

FIG. 16-27. A 61-year-old woman had a lifelong history of chest pain, dyspnea, and palpitations. She had not sought medical attention until 5 years before these tests were taken, when atrial fibrillation and congestive heart failure developed. A typical mitral insufficiency murmur and a to and fro murmur along the upper-left sternal border were heard. At catheterization, she was found to have an aberrant left coronary artery from the pulmonary artery. The right coronary artery was huge, and the giant conal branch projected to form a bulge on the left heart border (*arrow*), simulating a dilated left atrial appendage on the PA radiograph. Her other radiographic findings are those of severe ischemic heart disease in heart failure with pulmonary edema. She underwent coronary artery bypass grafting and did extremely well.

rysm forms either in the posterior noncoronary cusp or in the right coronary cusp. The former tends to be isolated and rupture into the right atrium; the latter tends to be associated with supracristal VSD and rupture into the right ventricular outflow tract (Fig. 16-29).

INCREASED PULMONARY VASCULARITY WITH CYANOSIS

Abnormalities presenting the picture of increased pulmonary vascularity in the presence of cyanosis are D-loop transposition of the great arteries (D-TGA), double-outlet right ventricle (DORV), persistent truncus arteriosus (PTA), total anomalous pulmonary venous connection (TAPVC), single ventricle (SV), and tricuspid atresia without pulmonary stenosis (Table 16-3). This group of lesions is sometimes called admixture lesions owing to the obligatory mixing of red and blue blood.

D-loop Transposition of the Great Arteries

Complete, or D-loop, transposition of the great arteries is thought to result from failure of normal spiraling of the primitive truncus arteriosus (31). In children, this anomaly

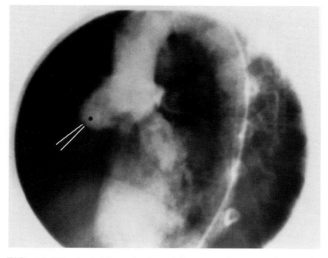

FIG. 16-29. A right posterior oblique aortogram shows the prolapsed right sinus aneurysm (*black dot*) into the right ventricle outflow tract occluding the supracristal VSD. Opacification of the left ventricle is indicative of aortic insufficiency. Note a small jet (*outlined with white lines*) from the ruptured aneurysm into the right ventricle.

accounts for ~10% of all cyanotic congenital cardiac defects (32), with a predominance among boys over girls between 2:1 and 3:1.

Pathophysiology and Clinical Presentation

With the great arteries connected to the wrong ventricles, the two circulations are separated. Oxygenated blood is delivered to the left side of the heart and from there propelled right back to the lung. On the other side of the heart, nonoxygenated blood is pumped to the body and then returned to the right ventricle. Thus, the two cycles operate indepen-

TABLE 16-3. *Abnormalities that lead to increased PBF with cyanosis (admixture lesions)*

D-TGA
Type 1 DORV
Type 2 DORV (TBC)
PTA
TAPVC
SV
TA without PS

PBF, pulmonary blood flow; D-TGA, D-loop transposition of great arteries; DORV, double-outlet right ventricle; TBC, Tassig-Bing complex; PTA, persistent truncus arteriosus; TAPVC, total anomalous pulmonary venous connection; SV, single ventricle; TA without PS, tricuspid atresia without pulmonary stenosis.

dently, and life cannot be sustained without some communication between the two.

In decreasing order of frequency, D-TGA is associated with ASD, PDA, VSD, or a combination of these conditions. Through these channels, nonoxygenated blood can mix with oxygenated blood. Bidirectional shunting is the rule; unilateral shunting will soon deplete the donor circuit. However, since the pulmonary resistance is much lower than the systemic resistance, the direction of the shunt is primarily toward the lung. When the shunts at all three levels are wide open, the lungs will be flooded, and the patient is likely to be in severe congestive heart failure with relatively mild cyanosis. Pulmonary artery banding or complete repair may have to be performed to save the patient's life. On the other hand, patients with D-TGA may have a small ASD as the only shunt to maintain life. They are usually critically ill with intense cyanosis. The treatment of choice under the circumstance is emergency balloon septostomy (Rashkind's procedure) (17) followed by complete repair.

In the neonate, when the pulmonary and systemic pressures are practically equal, shunting in either direction is meager, even in the presence of large septal defects. Patients are usually deeply cyanotic at this time. As the pulmonary vascular resistance gradually declines, mixing of blue with red blood becomes possible, the flow in both circulations increases, and the typical radiographic manifestations of D-TGA emerge (22).

Radiographic Signs

The heart and lungs of neonates with D-TGA are usually normal. Within several weeks, when the pulmonary vascular resistance gradually declines, the radiographic appearance resembles that of patients who have moderate shunts without pulmonary stenosis. The pulmonary vascularity is increased, and the heart is moderately enlarged with an "egg on the string" configuration (7). The globular shape of the heart represents the predominantly right-sided cardiomegaly resulting from pumping blood against high systemic vascular resistance. The narrow waist of the heart represents the malposition of the great arteries and the shrinkage of thymic tissue under stress (Fig. 16-30B).

Patients with D-TGA do not necessarily show all these typical radiographic features. The radiographic appearance varies according to the magnitude of the shunt and the reactivity of the pulmonary vasculature. At one end of the spectrum is a deeply cyanotic infant with a normal-sized heart with normal to diminished pulmonary vascularity, who has only a small communication between the two circulations (Fig. 16-30A). At the other end of the spectrum is a mildly cyanotic patient with gross cardiomegaly and flooded lungs. Congestive heart failure in this context results from large shunts at multiple levels (Fig. 16-30C).

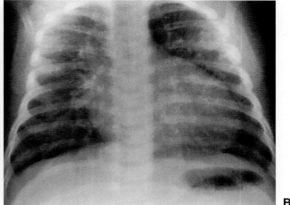

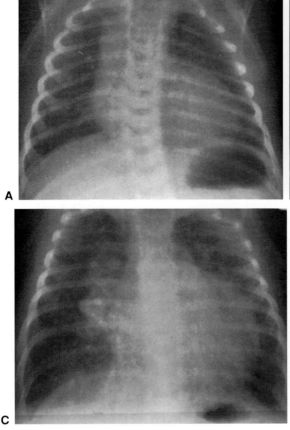

FIG. 16-30. The radiographic spectrum of D-loop transposition of the great arteries without pulmonary stenosis. **A:** There is only a small communication between the two circulations. The heart is of normal size, and the pulmonary vascularity varies from normal to decreased. The patient is deeply cyanotic. **B:** There is a medium-size systemic-to-pulmonary shunt at the atrial and ventricular levels. The patient is moderately symptomatic but not in failure. The radiograph shows increased pulmonary vascularity, moderate cardiomegaly, and an "egg on the string" configuration. **C:** There are large shunts at multiple levels. The patient is in congestive heart failure but only mildly cyanotic. Note gross cardiomegaly with an "egg on the string" contour, marked pulmonary plethora, and mild pulmonary edema.

Angiographic Signs

Selective injection of contrast medium into each ventricle provides accurate anatomic information of D-TGA and associated anomalies (Fig. 16-31). Selective angiocardiography is also crucial in the evaluation of patients who have undergone one of the definitive operations (33). A successful Mustard's operation should accomplish the following tasks: excision of the entire atrial septum, construction of a baffle using the patient's own pericardium, enclosure of all pulmonary veins inside the baffle (red atrium) so that the oxygenated blood is directed through the tricuspid valve into the right ventricle and then out to the aorta, and location of the venae cavae outside the baffle (blue atrium) so that the nonoxygenated blood is channeled through the mitral valve into the left ventricle and then out to the pulmonary artery. The common surgical complications are obstruction of flow from the vena cava to the blue atrium and abnormal communications (leaks) between the red and blue atria.

Echocardiographic Signs

The origin of the great arteries can be determined by two-dimensional echocardiography using the subxiphoid ap-

proach (7,9). The associated septal defects and pulmonary stenosis can also be imaged and assessed.

Surgical Treatment

When there is lack of communication between the two circulations, percutaneous balloon atrial septostomy (Rashkind's procedure) is the palliative treatment of choice, rather than surgical creation of an ASD, the Blalock–Hanlon operation.

Definitive surgical procedures fall into two major categories: atrial switching and arterial switching (34,35). Atrial switching or switching of the venous pathways is accomplished either by Mustard's operation (33) or by Senning's operation (17). Mustard's operation involves a few essential steps: excision of the atrial septum avoiding the sinoatrial (SA) node, construction of a baffle using pericardium or prosthetic material, enclosure of all pulmonary veins inside the baffle (red atrium) so that the oxygenated blood is directed through the tricuspid valve into the right ventricle and then out to the aorta, and location of the venae cavae outside the baffle (blue atrium) so that the nonoxygenated blood is channeled through the mitral valve into the left ventricle and then out to the pulmonary artery.

Senning's operation (36) is similar to Mustard's, except

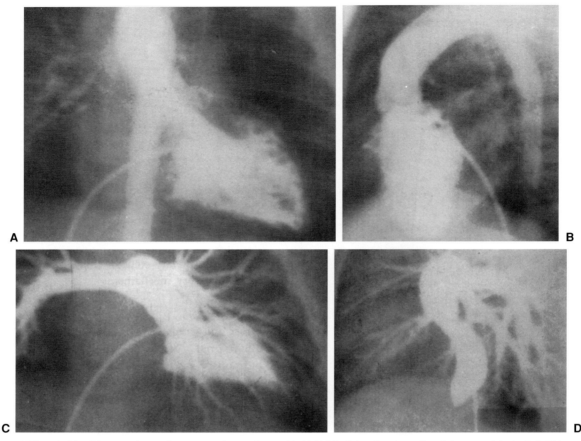

FIG. 16-31. Cine angiocardiograms of a patient with D-TGA. Injection into the right ventricle in PA (**A**) and lateral (**B**) views shows that the aorta arises from the right ventricle anteriorly and superiorly in relation to the pulmonary trunk. Faint opacification of a few branches of the pulmonary arterial system suggests some meager bronchial arterial collateralization. Injection into the left ventricle in PA (**C**) and lateral (**D**) views shows that the pulmonary trunk arises from the left ventricle posteriorly and inferiorly.

for using virtually no synthetic material to partition the atria. Surgical complications from both operations are similar, including systemic and pulmonary venous obstruction, arrhythmias, conduction defects, leaking between red and blue atria, tricuspid insufficiency, and right ventricular failure. The last complication has to do with a ventricle that is unfit to deal with the high systemic pressure load for a prolonged period of time.

Arterial switching involves switching of the distal segments of the great arteries and transfer of coronary arteries to the neo-aorta. The neo-aorta is formed by suturing the distal aorta to the proximal pulmonary artery. This operation restores the physiologic ventriculo-arterial connections and thus permits a better prognosis in the long run.

Long-term Follow-up

Both palliative and curative procedures significantly modify the usual radiographic appearance of D-TGA. Both Rashkind's procedure and the Blalock–Hanlon operation allow more flow through the lung and greater diastolic expansion of the heart. Banding of the pulmonary artery reduces the pulmonary blood flow and left-sided cardiomegaly. Successful complete repairs convert the cardiovascular image to normal (24). After atrial switching procedures, however, one may see residual right-sided cardiomegaly and a peculiar course of the transvenous pacemaker wire (Fig. 16-32).

Patients with D-TGA and large shunts rarely survive into adulthood without the benefit of surgery. If they do, a natural defense mechanism almost always exists to regulate the pulmonary blood flow so that neither congestive heart failure nor severe cyanosis develops. Increased pulmonary vascular resistance (Fig. 16-33) and coexisting pulmonary stenosis (Fig. 16-34) are such compensatory mechanisms.

Double-Outlet Right Ventricle

Double-outlet right ventricle may be considered a partial form of D-TGA. In type 1 DORV (37), both great arteries typically arise from the morphologic right ventricle. A VSD provides the only outlet from the left ventricle. In type 2 DORV (37), the aorta arises from the right ventricle, and

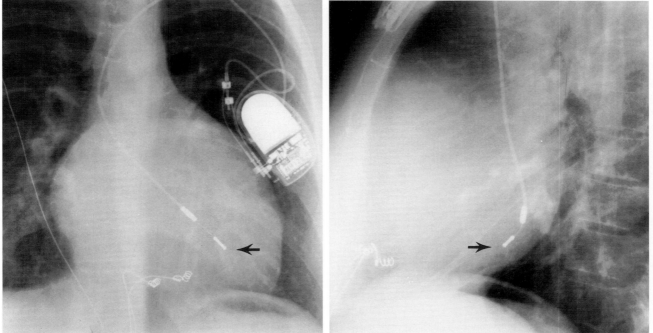

A

B

FIG. 16-32. A 26-year-old woman, after a Mustard operation for D-TGA, was seen for evaluation of her cardiac pacemaker. PA (**A**) and lateral (**B**) views show that the pacing wire is in a very peculiar position. The electrodes pass through the superior vena cava, the blue chamber (outside the baffle), the mitral valve, and the left ventricle (*arrow*).

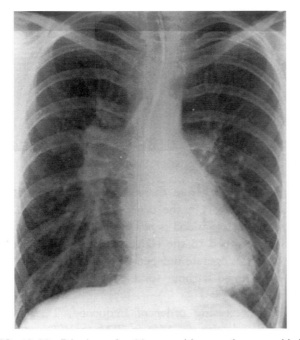

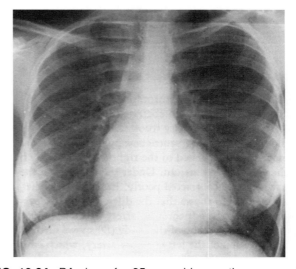

FIG. 16-34. PA view of a 35-year-old cyanotic woman with D-TGA and PS after a Blalock–Taussig shunt on the left side. Note pulmonary oligemia, which is more marked on the right side. Rib notching is noted in the upper-left thorax. The heart is moderately enlarged. The cardiac waist is narrow, though the superior vena cava is mildly dilated.

FIG. 16-33. PA view of a 23-year-old cyanotic man with D-TGA and a large VSD. Note mild cardiomegaly, a narrow waist, and a centralized pulmonary blood flow pattern indicative of pulmonary arterial hypertension. His survival into adulthood is explained by the development of protective pulmonary arterial hypertension.

the pulmonary artery straddles the VSD, receiving blood from both ventricles. Type 2 DORV is also known as Taussig-Bing complex (37). In the absence of pulmonary stenosis, type 1 tends to cause less cyanosis than either D-TGA or Taussig-Bing complex. On radiography type 1 resembles a large VSD; type 2 resembles D-TGA. Unlike D-TGA and Taussig-Bing complex, the waist of the heart is not narrowed in type 1 DORV (38). With pulmonary stenosis, DORV may mimic tetralogy of Fallot in both clinical and radiological signs. The basic angiographic findings of DORV are described later under the discussion of DORV with pulmonary stenosis (Fig. 16-48).

Persistent Truncus Arteriosus

Persistent truncus arteriosus represents a developmental failure in the division of the primitive truncus arteriosus into the aorta and pulmonary artery. As a result, the heart is drained by a single artery that supplies the coronary, systemic, and pulmonary circulations (39). The truncus arteriosus possesses somewhere between two and six cusps and straddles a large VSD. Since corrective surgery is now feasi-

ble, an early and precise diagnosis of this condition is mandatory.

Classification

The most popular classification of PTA is based on the origin of the pulmonary artery (40) (Fig. 16-35). Some patients originally classified as having type IV truncus turned out to have pseudotruncus arteriosus (the most severe form of tetralogy of Fallot) (41).

Pathophysiology and Clinical Presentation

In types I, II, and III, there is increased pulmonary blood flow owing to a predominantly left-to-right shunt. Obligatory mixing of blue and red blood occurs at the ventricular and truncal levels. Symptoms and signs in these patients depend on the magnitude of shunt and the degree of pulmonary vascular obstruction. The shunt flow is proportional to the size of the pulmonary arteries and inversely related to the pulmonary vascular resistance. Patients with large pulmonary flow are only mildly cyanotic, and most die of

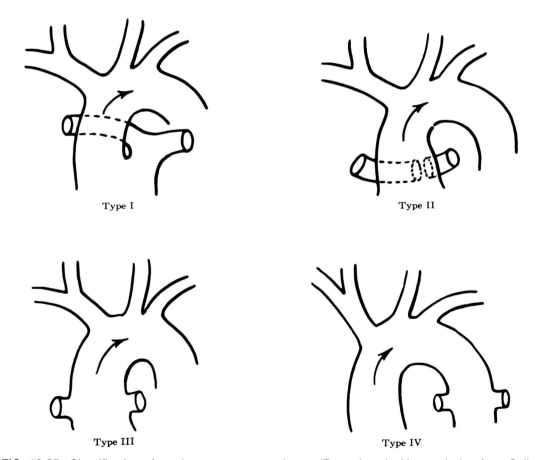

Type I

Type II

Type III

Type IV

FIG. 16-35. Classification of persistent truncus arteriosus. (Reproduced with permission from Collett RW, Edwards JE. Persistent truncus arteriosus: a classification according to anatomic types. *Surg Clin North Am* 1949;29:1245–1270.)

congestive heart failure within 1 year. Survival improves if pulmonary blood flow is restricted through either smaller pulmonary arteries or optimal increase in pulmonary vascular resistance. On physical examination, a systolic murmur along the left sternal border, a single second sound, and a diastolic murmur of truncal insufficiency are the common auscultatory findings. The pulses are bounding owing to increased pulse pressure. Biventricular hypertrophy is present on the ECG. In type IV truncus, the physiology is the same as that of pseudotruncus arteriosus, which is discussed separately.

Radiographic Signs

Patients with PTA (excluding type IV) usually have biventricular and left atrial enlargements with increased pulmonary vascularity. Pulmonary edema is expected if congestive heart failure supervenes. The pulmonary trunk segment may or may not be concave, depending on the anatomic arrangement. Concavity in this area is frequently found in types II and III. In type I truncus, the dilated pulmonary trunk may even be convex in the posteroanterior (PA) view. The truncal arch (aortic arch) is usually dilated and has increased pulsation. A right-sided arch is present in 30% to 40% of patients (39) (Fig. 16-36A). In adults, pulmonary arterial hypertension is frequently encountered (Fig. 16-37).

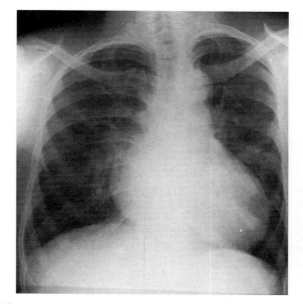

FIG. 16-37. PA view of a 20-year-old man with type I truncus arteriosus. Note bilateral cardiomegaly, prominence of the left-sided truncal arch, mild prominence of the pulmonary trunk in its usual position, and the Eisenmenger type of pulmonary vascularity.

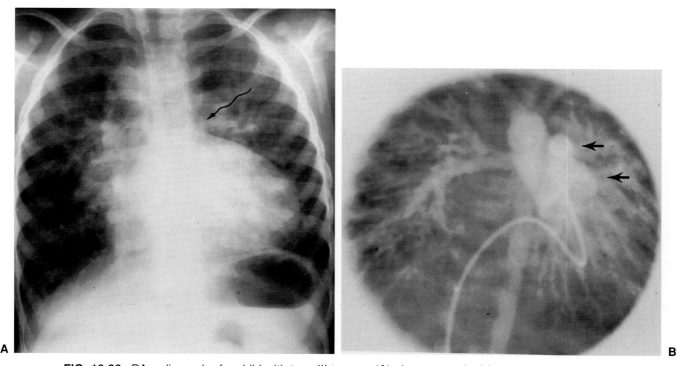

A

B

FIG. 16-36. PA radiograph of a child with type III truncus (**A**) shows a marked increase in pulmonary blood flow and left atrial–biventricular enlargement. Also note the right aortic arch and no evidence of the pulmonary trunk in its usual location (*arrow*). **B:** Another patient with type I truncus. The angiogram shows that a catheter was inserted from the inferior vena cava through the right atrium and right ventricle directly into a large truncal valve. The left sinus of Valsalva (*lower arrow*) is quite prominent. The pulmonary trunk arises from the left lateral wall of the truncus, giving rise to the left (*upper arrow*) and right pulmonary arteries. The truncal arch is left-sided.

Angiographic Signs

On angiography, the persistent truncus is connected with both ventricles on top of a large VSD. The mode of origin of the pulmonary arteries from the truncus is usually self-evident on the angiogram (39) (see Fig. 16-36B).

Long-term Follow-up

Patients without the benefit of surgery may survive into adulthood with Eisenmenger physiology (Fig. 16-37). Type I truncus is most amenable to surgery (35). Basically, the operation is performed in three steps: the pulmonary trunk is transferred from the lateral wall of the truncus to the right ventricle with a valved conduit; the VSD is closed, and the left ventricle is connected to the truncus; and the insufficient truncal valve is replaced. A successfully repaired case is shown in Fig. 16-38.

Total Anomalous Pulmonary Venous Connection

Total anomalous pulmonary venous connection comprises only 2% of all congenital cardiac defects. However, since curative surgery for TAPVC is now widely available, an early and accurate diagnosis of such lesions is imperative.

Embryology

Normally pulmonary veins derive from the venous plexus of the foregut and drain freely into the two systemic venous systems—the cardinal (forerunner of the superior vena cava, azygos vein, and coronary sinus) and the umbilicovitelline (forerunner of the portal venous system). A common pulmonary vein develops later from the primitive left atrium and connects with the pulmonary venous plexus. Further development of the lungs is accompanied by obliteration of the primitive pulmonary-systemic venous anastomotic channels. If for any reason the common pulmonary vein fails to develop or becomes obliterated secondarily, TAPVC will come about through the retention of one or more of the primitive pulmonary-systemic venous anastomoses. The development of PAPVC is due to failure of a portion of the pulmonary venous plexus to establish a connection with the common pulmonary vein; that portion drains through one of the primitive channels instead. Patients with PAPVC are not cyanotic; their pathophysiology and radiographic signs are discussed earlier in the chapter.

Anatomic Classification

Total anomalous pulmonary venous connections (42) can be classified as supradiaphragmatic or infradiaphragmatic, according to the site of connection. Pulmonary venous ob-

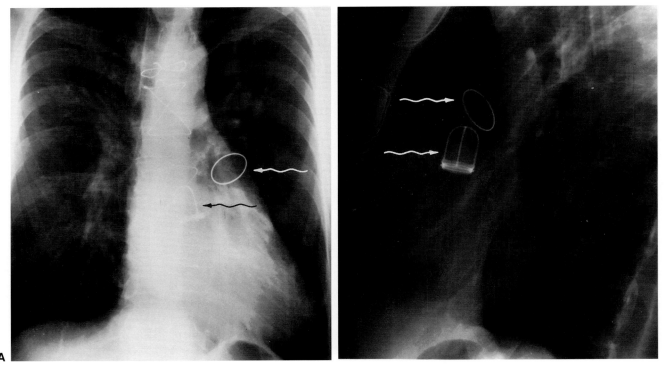

FIG. 16-38. A 24-year-old man with type I truncus. The postoperative PA (**A**) and lateral (**B**) radiographs show that the insufficient truncal valve has been replaced with a Starr-Edward valve (*lower arrow*) and that a valved (Hancock) conduit has been inserted to bridge the right ventricle and the pulmonary trunk (*upper arrow*).

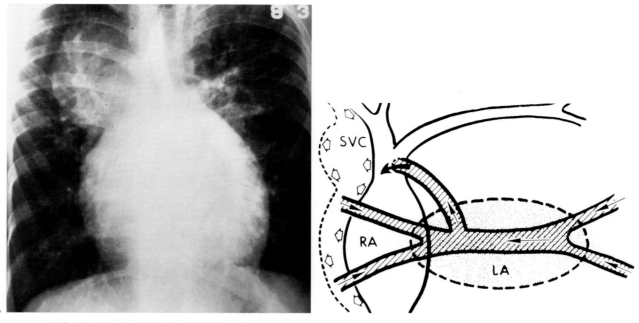

FIG. 16-39. A child with TAPVC to the superior vena cava. The PA radiograph (**A**) shows a lopsided snowman configuration. The left half of the head is absent because there is no left vertical vein. All pulmonary venous blood from both lungs drains exclusively into the right-sided superior vena cava, as shown in the schematic diagram (**B**). RA, right atrium; LA, left atrium; SVC, superior vena cava. Solid arrows show the direction of pulmonary venous blood flow; open arrows point to the dilated right atrium and superior vena cava.

struction is almost always present in infradiaphragmatic lesions but rarely in supradiaphragmatic ones. The most common supradiaphragmatic TAPVC is the so-called snowman, or figure eight, type (see **Fig. 2-13**). In this type, all pulmonary veins drain into the left brachiocephalic vein via the left vertical vein. The less common types of supradiaphragmatic TAPVC include lesions with pulmonary venous drainage to one of the following structures: superior vena cava (a lopsided snowman (Fig. 16-39) may be created), right atrium, or coronary sinus (Fig. 16-40). In the second and third conditions, no head of the snowman is formed because both lesions are at the cardiac level, not supracardiac in position.

In the infradiaphragmatic type of TAPVC, all pulmonary veins converge to a common collecting channel, which descends through the esophageal hiatus to drain into the portal venous system. From there the blood must go through the hepatic capillary bed before returning to the heart (Fig. 16-41). Because of the severe pulmonary venous obstruction and meager forward cardiac output, this anomaly would better be categorized among those with manifestations of pulmonary venous hypertension and cyanosis. Regardless of their anatomic variations, all patients with TAPVC have an ASD as the life-sustaining channel. Two thirds of these patients have no other cardiovascular abnormalities.

Radiographic and Angiographic Signs

On radiography, TAPVCs without obstruction present some features similar to uncomplicated ASDs: dilatation of

right-sided cardiac chambers, dilatation of the pulmonary trunk, and increase in pulmonary vascularity. Specific signs are related to the site of the anomalous connection. For example, TAPVC to the left vertical vein may form a snowman configuration (see **Fig. 2-13**). In patients with TAPVC directly to the right atrium or coronary sinus, however, there would not be any specific radiographic signs (Fig. 16-40), and the precise diagnosis depends on angiographic delineation. The radiographic signs for TAPVC with obstruction are a unique combination of severe pulmonary edema and a normal-sized heart (Fig. 16-41A). The angiographic features are illustrated in Fig. 16-41B.

Surgery

Surgical repair of TAPVCs is relatively simple because of a favorable anatomic arrangement between the anomalous pulmonary veins and the left atrium. There is a definite tendency for all pulmonary veins to converge into a common trunk or site, which is usually quite close to the posterior wall of the left atrium. The operative procedure (35,43) consists of ligation of the communicating vein, anastomosis of the common pulmonary vein to the posterior wall of the left atrium, and closure of ASD. For repair of TAPVC to the coronary sinus, one needs to establish a communication between the coronary sinus to the left atrium and close off the ASD.

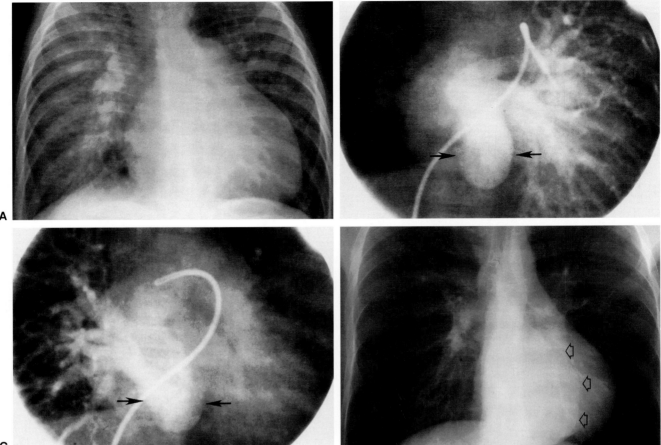

FIG. 16-40. A child with TAPVC to the coronary sinus. The PA radiograph (**A**) shows torrential pulmonary blood flow, marked right-sided cardiomegaly, a huge pulmonary trunk, and a small aortic arch. The levo phase of selective left and right PA injections (**B,C**) shows TAPVC to the coronary sinus (*arrows*). Surgical repair was quite successful. Twenty-five years later, at age 26, the patient returned for a checkup. Another PA view (**D**) shows a peculiar opacity (*open arrows*) in the middle and lower mediastinum. This opacity vividly simulates left ventricular enlargement in the lateral view (not shown). It turned out to be the residual dilatation of his coronary sinus.

Long-term Follow-up

The long-term prognosis for patients who survive hospitalization after definitive surgery is generally quite good (24). One such patient came back for routine checkup 25 years after repair. A peculiar retrocardiac opacity (Fig. 16-40D) was found on the radiographs, simulating left ventricular enlargement on the lateral view. It turned out to be a residual dilated coronary sinus following complete repair. **Figure 2-13** (D and E) shows the satisfactory surgical results in a teenager with TAPVC to the left vertical vein.

Single Ventricle

Single ventricle is also called common ventricle (44) or cor triloculare biatriatum. Only 1.5% of all congenital car-

diac defects fall into this category (45). One of the ventricles is embryologically underdeveloped. The remaining SV is usually of the left ventricular type. In the outflow tract of this ventricle, a rudimentary chamber is usually present, representing the infundibular portion of the right ventricle. The great arteries are transposed, with the aorta arising from the infundibular chamber, which is attached to the left superior aspect of the SV. The transposition of great arteries is, therefore, of the L-loop type. There are two AV valves, both connected to the SV (Fig. 16-42). Hence, this type of SV is also termed double-inlet left ventricle (17).

In spite of an SV, complete mixing of blood within the ventricle is unusual. There is a tendency for the streams from the two atria to cross so that the nonoxygenated blood from the right atrium flows preferentially to the pulmonary artery and the oxygenated blood from the left atrium flows through

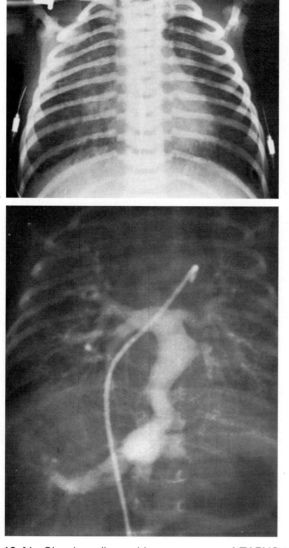

A

B

FIG. 16-41. Classic radiographic appearance of TAPVC to the portal vein. **A:** PA view shows the typical combination of severe pulmonary edema and a normal size heart. **B:** An angiocardiogram of another patient shows that all pulmonary veins converge to a common trunk and drain through the esophageal hiatus into the portal vein. (Reproduced with permission from Kirks DR. *Practical pediatric imaging*, 2nd ed. Boston: Little, Brown, 1991.)

the bulboventricular foramen into the infundibular chamber and the aorta. Therefore, before the onset of Eisenmenger physiology, there is only mild cyanosis. The clinical manifestations revolve primarily around excessive pulmonary flow and congestive heart failure. Pulmonary artery banding is usually required to keep the patient alive. After that, either of two more definitive surgical repairs can be done on an elective basis. One procedure is to separate the SV into two by putting a septation patch between; the other is to anastomose the right atrium to the pulmonary artery and leave the SV as the systemic pump (17).

Tricuspid Atresia Without Pulmonary Stenosis

Tricuspid atresia (TA) is an uncommon anomaly, accounting for only 1% of all congenital cardiac defects. The basic derangement consists of an atretic tricuspid valve, a hypoplastic right ventricle, an interatrial communication, and a VSD. Other features, related to coexisting D-TGA, pulmonary stenosis (PS), or pulmonary atresia (PA), vary.

Anatomic Classification

Tricuspid atresia has been customarily classified as follows (11). The first type is TA with normally related great arteries and with PA and an intact ventricular septum, with PS and a restrictive VSD (the most common type of TA), or with no PS and a large VSD. The second type is TA with TGA and with PA and a large VSD, with PS and a large VSD, or with no PS and a large VSD. Under the heading of increased pulmonary vascularity with cyanosis we are concerned only with TA with normally related great arteries with no PS and a large VSD and TA with TGA with no PS and a large VSD.

Pathophysiology and Clinical Presentation

In both of the afore-mentioned lesions of concern, there is no restriction to blood flow in either direction. Most patients have large communications between the two sides of the heart, allowing free right-to-left shunting at the atrial level and left-to-right shunting at the ventricular level. Since pulmonary vascular resistance is much lower than systemic vascular resistance, there is a tendency for patients to suffer from excessive pulmonary flow, congestive heart failure, and mild cyanosis. As the pulmonary vascular resistance rises, symptoms of heart failure may ease off at the price of increasing cyanosis. Since the right ventricle is hypoplastic, the left ventricle is the only pumping chamber, and the right atrium is markedly enlarged, the electrocardiographic findings are unique: left axis deviation, left ventricular hypertrophy, and peaking of P waves. These signs help distinguish TA from other forms of cyanotic heart disease, which are usually associated with right axis deviation.

In the circumstance of intractable congestive heart failure, emergency pulmonary artery banding may be a life-saving measure. A more definitive and physiologic procedure (Fontan operation) consists of closure of shunts, right atrium–pulmonary artery anastomosis, and superior vena cava–right pulmonary artery anastomosis (Glenn procedure) (17).

Radiographic and Angiographic Signs

In patients with TA with normally related great arteries with no PS and a large VSD, the radiographic findings are

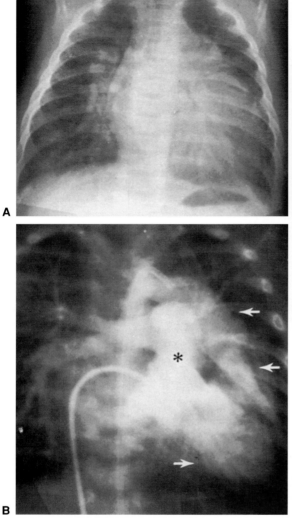

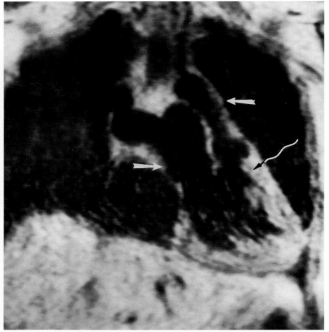

FIG. 16-42. PA radiograph (**A**) of a patient with a single ventricle shows gross cardiomegaly, torrential pulmonary blood flow, and pulmonary edema. Note the bulge along the left-upper cardiac border typical of L-TGA. The angiocardiogram (**B**) shows that the catheter is inserted from the right atrium through the tricuspid valve directly into the single ventricle. After contrast opacification, the single ventricle (*lower arrow*) appears to be smooth and of the left ventricular type. The infundibular chamber (*middle arrow*) is typically connected to the left superior aspect of the single ventricle (SV). The aorta (*upper arrow*) originates from the infundibular chamber, forming the left-lateral convexity. The pulmonary trunk (*asterisk*) arises medially from the ventricle. The coronal spin-echo MR image (**C**) of another patient, an adult, shows that the larger pulmonary artery (*lower arrow*) arises from the medio-inferior aspect of the single ventricle and that the smaller aorta (*upper arrow*) arises from the infundibular chamber (*spiral thin arrow*).

similar to those of a VSD. However, the nature of TA may be revealed by a heart border flattened on the right side and bulging on the left. Since both the left atrium and the left ventricle receive blood from the right atrium and the pulmonary veins, their enlargement is expected. Pulmonary vascularity increases (Fig. 16-43) before the onset of heart failure or Eisenmenger syndrome. The radiographic features of TA with TGA with no PS and a large VSD are similar, except for the narrow waist peculiar to the associated D-TGA.

With the first type of lesion, the basic angiographic findings include dilatation of the right atrium, right-to-left shunt at the atrial level, enlargement of the left atrium and ventricle, left-to-right shunt at the ventricular level, and free flow through the small right ventricle and pulmonary valve to the pulmonary circulation. In the second type of lesion, the great arteries are transposed. Both the right atrium and right ventricle are hypoplastic and therefore have flat borders on radiography. A levoposed right atrial appendage immediately above the left atrial appendage (46) is a common feature for all types of TA (Fig. 16-44C).

DECREASED PULMONARY VASCULARITY WITH CYANOSIS

Abnormalities causing decreased pulmonary vascularity and cyanosis include tetralogy of Fallot (TOF), PA, TA with PS, D-TGA with PS, DORV with PS, SV with PS, Ebstein's anomaly, and Uhl's disease (Table 16-4). Uhl's disease is extremely rare, usually appearing as severe right-sided heart failure and tricuspid insufficiency simulating Ebstein's anomaly. The pathologic basis of Uhl's disease is severe dysplasia of the right ventricle with paper-thin walls (4).

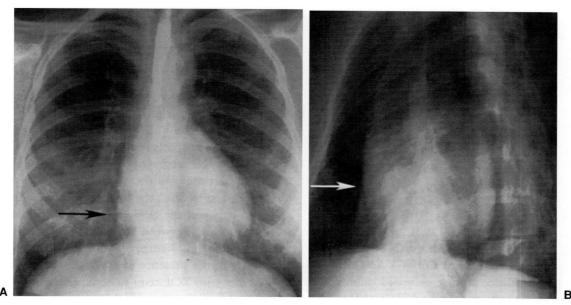

FIG. 16-43. PA (**A**) and left anterior oblique (**B**) views of a 22-year-old cyanotic woman with tricuspid atresia without pulmonary stenosis show mild cardiomegaly of the left atrium and left ventricle. The pulmonary blood flow is mildly increased. Both the right atrial border (*black arrow*) and the right ventricular border (*white arrow*) are flat.

Tetralogy of Fallot

Most patients with TOF are not overtly symptomatic until late in infancy, childhood, or even adulthood. For this reason, TOF is the most common cyanotic congenital heart disease of older children and adults. In contrast, patients with other cyanotic conditions usually die quickly unless treated surgically.

Anatomy

The four basic component lesions of TOF are infundibular PS, VSD, overriding aorta, and right ventricular hypertrophy. Of these lesions, only the first two are hemodynamically important. Although the infundibulum is the usual site of PS, obstruction may also be found at the pulmonary valve.

Pathophysiology and Clinical Presentation

The combination of PS and VSD encompasses a broad spectrum of hemodynamic and clinical expressions. At one end is the so-called pink tetralogy, when the shunt is predominantly left-to-right, the pulmonary obstruction mild, the VSD large, and the clinical presentation essentially that of a VSD. At the other end is ''end-stage'' tetralogy—pseudotruncus arteriosus—when the pulmonary obstruction is complete, the flow unidirectionally right to left, and the clinical expression that of severe cyanosis. Between the two extremes, all degrees of right ventricular outflow obstruction exist in the context of VSD.

Patients with TOF tend to be acyanotic until they are 3 to 6 months old. After age 4, tetralogy is the most common cyanotic congenital cardiac disease (6). The classic auscultatory findings are a systolic murmur and a single second sound. The electrocardiographic findings include right axis deviation and right ventricular hypertrophy. Squatting for relief of exertional dyspnea in childhood is well known (47). Hypoxemic spells with loss of consciousness generally suggest the presence of severe PS or PA. Endocarditis and brain abscess are serious complications.

Radiographic and Angiographic Signs

On radiography, most patients show signs of pulmonary oligemia (see **Figs. 8-13** and **8-23**). Occasionally, normal pulmonary vascularity may be found in patients with marked PS (Fig. 16-45). When in doubt, the size of the hilum in the lateral view can be a helpful marker (Fig. 16-46B). A small hilar image always indicates decreased pulmonary blood flow. In addition, marked oligemia is commonly accompanied by bronchial arterial collateralization. These systemic collaterals are small and tortuous, best seen in the upper-medial lung zones near their origin (see **Fig. 8-23**).

The overall cardiac size is usually normal (Fig. 16-46) because there is no volume overload in the presence of a large VSD. The contour of the heart is, however, distinctly abnormal, and has been likened to a wooden shoe (coeur en sabot) (Fig. 16-46; see also **Fig. 8-23**). It is formed by a dilated and hyperpulsatile aorta due to a large right-to-left shunt at the ventricular level, a concave pulmonary artery segment stemming from infundibular PS and hypoplasia of

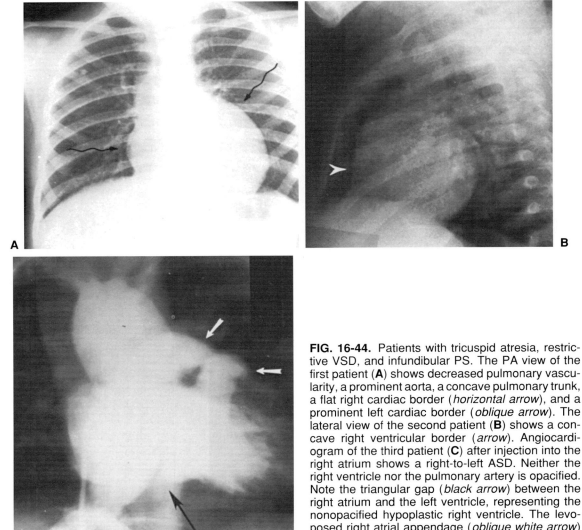

FIG. 16-44. Patients with tricuspid atresia, restrictive VSD, and infundibular PS. The PA view of the first patient (**A**) shows decreased pulmonary vascularity, a prominent aorta, a concave pulmonary trunk, a flat right cardiac border (*horizontal arrow*), and a prominent left cardiac border (*oblique arrow*). The lateral view of the second patient (**B**) shows a concave right ventricular border (*arrow*). Angiocardiogram of the third patient (**C**) after injection into the right atrium shows a right-to-left ASD. Neither the right ventricle nor the pulmonary artery is opacified. Note the triangular gap (*black arrow*) between the right atrium and the left ventricle, representing the nonopacified hypoplastic right ventricle. The levoposed right atrial appendage (*oblique white arrow*) is seen immediately above the dilated left atrial appendage (*horizontal white arrow*).

pulmonary arteries, and an upturned cardiac apex representing the left ventricle posterosuperiorly displaced by the hypertrophied right ventricle.

The angiocardiogram reveals a heavily trabeculated right ventricle pumping blood through a stenotic infundibulum to a small pulmonary artery. The pulmonary valve may also be stenotic and sometimes bicuspid. The wider outlet for the right ventricular output is the infracristal VSD, through which a large right-to-left shunt is visible. A right-sided aortic arch is present in 20% to 25% of patients (Fig. 16-47). The incidence of right aortic arch increases proportionately with the severity of PS. For instance, patients with pseudotruncus arteriosus have a much higher incidence (50% to 60%) of right aortic arch than those with TOF. In the presence of a right aortic arch, the PDA almost always inserts

between the left subclavian and the left pulmonary arteries. An aortogram or a selective coronary arteriogram is used to rule out the 5% possibility of an aberrant anterior descending coronary artery from the right coronary artery (35). Such an aberrant vessel lies in front of the right ventricle and can be inadvertently severed during right ventriculotomy for complete repair of TOF.

In diagnosing pseudotruncus arteriosus, selective bronchial arteriography or wedging pulmonary venography is needed preoperatively to answer two questions: whether a true pulmonary arterial tree is present (see **Fig. 8-24A**), and, if it is, whether the left and right pulmonary arteries converge to form the pulmonary trunk (see **Fig. 8-24B**). Fibrous continuity between the anterior mitral leaflet and the posterior aortic cusp is an important angiographic feature seen in nor-

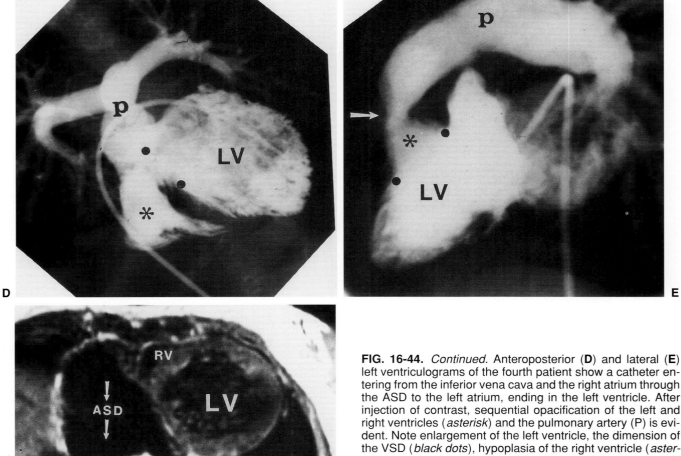

FIG. 16-44. *Continued.* Anteroposterior (**D**) and lateral (**E**) left ventriculograms of the fourth patient show a catheter entering from the inferior vena cava and the right atrium through the ASD to the left atrium, ending in the left ventricle. After injection of contrast, sequential opacification of the left and right ventricles (*asterisk*) and the pulmonary artery (P) is evident. Note enlargement of the left ventricle, the dimension of the VSD (*black dots*), hypoplasia of the right ventricle (*asterisk*), persistent opacification of the right ventricle without influx of nonopacified blood from right atrium (diagnostic of TA), and infundibular PS (*arrow*) on the lateral view (**E**). The axial spin-echo MR image (**F**) of the last patient shows a right-to-left ASD (*arrows*), an enlarged left ventricle, and a hypoplastic right ventricle filled only through a restrictive VSD.

mal persons and in patients with TOF. Discontinuity of the two structures suggests the possibility of DORV (Fig. 16-48A,B).

Echocardiographic Signs

The echocardiogram may evidence certain features of TOF: an overriding aorta with a malaligned VSD or a septal-aortic discontinuity (7,11,17), a normal left atrium, and fibrous continuity between the mitral and aortic valves.

Surgery and Follow-up

Palliative procedures for the treatment of TOF are some of the surgical systemic-pulmonary shunts designed to improve pulmonary blood flow only (17,35). All procedures are reviewed here for the sake of convenience, although not all are suitable for TOF. These procedures are the Blalock–Taussig

shunt (subclavian artery to ipsilateral pulmonary artery anastomosis) (Fig. 16-49), a modified Blalock–Taussig procedure (performed by using a synthetic conduit between the two arteries), the Potts' shunt (descending aorta to left pulmonary artery anastomosis), the Waterston shunt (ascending aorta to

TABLE 16-4. *Abnormalities that cause decreased PBF with cyanosis*

TOF
PA
Ebstein's anomaly
TA with PS
Uhl's disease
Admixture lesions + PS

TOF, tetralogy of Fallot; PA, pulmonary atresia; TA with PS, tricuspid atresia with pulmonary stenosis; PS, pulmonary stenosis.

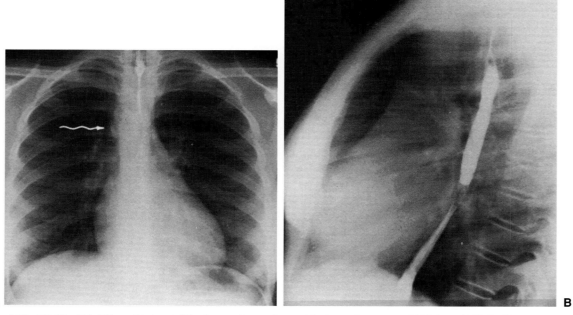

FIG. 16-45. PA (**A**) and lateral (**B**) views of a patient with the avian type of RAA and TOF. The aorta is right-sided (*arrow*), displacing the trachea and esophagus to the left. The esophagus and trachea are normal in position on the lateral view. There are no obvious radiographic signs of TOF.

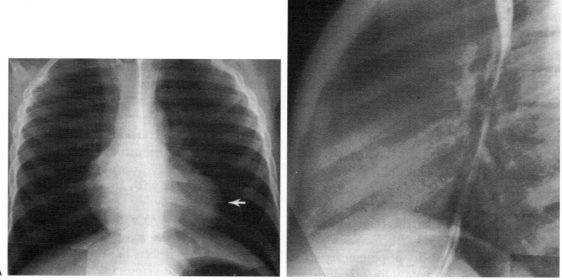

FIG. 16-46. Radiographs of a child with tetralogy of Fallot. The PA view (**A**) shows pulmonary oligemia and a boot-shaped cardiovascular configuration. The arrow points to the upturned left ventricular apex. The overall cardiac size is within normal limits. The lateral view (**B**) shows right ventricular enlargement, small hila, and a flat posterior cardiac border.

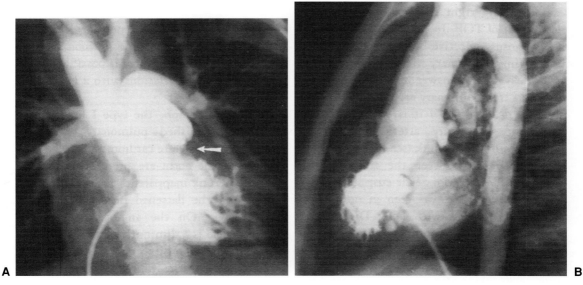

FIG. 16-47. Right ventriculograms of patients with TOF. The frontal view of patient 1 (**A**) shows RAA and severe infundibular PS (*arrow*). The lateral right ventriculogram of another patient (**B**) shows infundibular PS, right-to-left VSD, and overriding of the aorta.

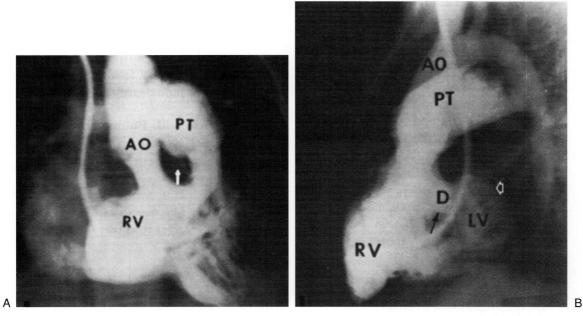

FIG. 16-48. A patient with DORV and PS. Frontal right ventriculogram (**A**) shows that both great arteries arise side by side from the right ventricle. The aortic and pulmonary valves are at the same horizontal level, with the crista supraventricularis (*arrow*) positioned between. In the lateral angiocardiogram (**B**), there is a lack of continuity between the aortic and mitral valves. The site of the mitral valve is marked by an open arrow. AO, aorta; D, ventricular septal defect; LV, left ventricle; PT, pulmonary trunk; RV, right ventricle. (Reproduced with permission from Hallermann FJ, Kincaid OW, Ritter DG, Ongley PA, Titus JL. Angiocardiographic and anatomic findings in origin of both great arteries from the right ventricle. *AJR Am J Roentgenol* 1970;109:51–66.)

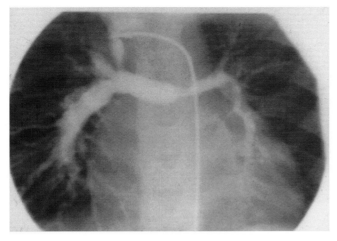

FIG. 16-49. A child with tricuspid atresia, after a Blalock–Taussig shunt. The retrograde aortic catheter was used to inject contrast medium into the right subclavian artery, which was anastomosed to the side wall of the right pulmonary artery.

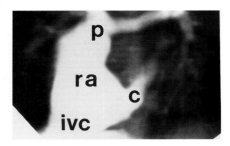

FIG. 16-51. Modified Fontan procedure. Injection into the right atrium shows the dilated right atrium (ra), inferior vena cava (ivc), and coronary sinus (c). Note the functioning right atrium (ra)–pulmonary artery (p) anastomosis.

right pulmonary artery shunt), a central shunt (ascending aorta to pulmonary trunk shunt using synthetic conduit), the Glenn shunt (superior vena cava to right pulmonary artery end-to-end anastomosis) (Fig. 16-50A), a modified Glenn shunt (superior vena cava to right pulmonary artery end-to-side anastomosis), a bidirectional cavopulmonary connection (Fig. 16-50B), the Fontan operation (Glenn shunt plus inferior vena cava–pulmonary artery anastomosis with valved conduits), and modified Fontan procedures (including right atrio-pulmonary artery anastomosis) (Fig. 16-51).

The most frequently used surgical shunts for TOF are the

first two. The third and fourth procedures are seldom used because of significant postoperative complications. The fifth procedure is commonly used for infants. The last four procedures were originally designed for treatment of TA and later also for PA, SV, and other lesions with only one functioning ventricle.

Complete surgical repair of TOF consists of two major steps: infundibulectomy for treatment of PS and closure of VSD. For patients with severe PS and hypoplastic pulmonary annulus, Dacron or a pericardial patch (transannular patch) may have to be used to widen the outflow tract all the way through the pulmonary trunk. Sometimes a valved conduit (most commonly containing a Hancock porcine valve) is used for this purpose. Finally, the VSD is closed with a Dacron patch (17,35). Homografts have also been used with success for right ventricular outflow tract reconstruction (35,48,49).

Postoperative changes are frequently seen on the follow-

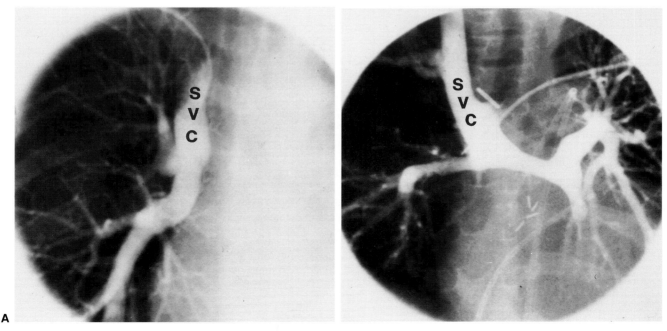

FIG. 16-50. Glenn shunts: classic Glenn (A), modified Glenn (B). SVC, superior vena cava.

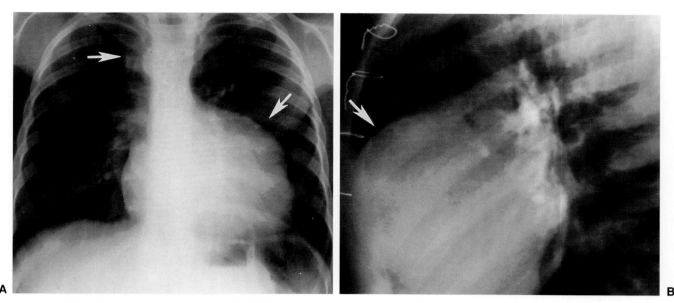

FIG. 16-52. A 4-year-old boy with TOF after complete repair. PA (**A**) and lateral (**B**) views show RAA (*horizontal arrow in A*), clear lungs, and a huge right ventricle with aneurysmal dilatation of the outflow tract (*oblique arrows*). On both clinical examination and catheterization he had severe PI.

up chest radiographs. Unilateral upper-rib notching (see **Fig. 2-5**) on the side of a Blalock–Taussig shunt is well known. Closure or severe stenosis of a shunt may manifest as worsened oligemia; too wide a shunt may lead to congestive left-sided heart failure. After complete repair, one sees (a) a median sternotomy; (b) dilatation of the right ventricular outflow tract (if isolated and stable it has no clinical significance, but an enlarging aneurysm needs surgical intervention) (Fig. 16-52); (c) significant right-sided cardiomegaly, which means right-sided heart failure with PI (Fig. 16-52) or PI and TI; (d) increased pulmonary blood flow, which may signal a leaking of the interventricular patch in the absence of PS; and (e) calcification of the outflow tract patch (11), which suggests PS with or without PI and right-sided heart failure (Fig. 16-53).

Pulmonary Atresia with an Intact Ventricular Septum

Pulmonary atresia with an intact ventricular septum is one of the most common cyanotic congenital cardiac defects in neonates (11,50). Most infants die as the ductus closes in the first weeks of life if the natural downhill course is not interrupted. This condition can be classified into two types according to the size of the right ventricle. In type I, the right ventricle is small and the tricuspid valve competent; in type II, the right ventricle is either normal or dilated with tricuspid valve insufficiency. A patent foramen ovale is usually present, permitting right-to-left shunting at the atrial level. A left-to-right shunt at the ductal level is crucial for survival. When the ductus undergoes spontaneous closure, death will ensue.

Medical management is aimed at maintaining the patency

of the ductus by prostaglandin infusion until surgery can be done. Surgical shunts may be used to improve the pulmonary blood flow. More definitive surgery is possible only for patients with type II lesions with a larger right ventricle.

On the radiograph, the type I lesion shows markedly diminished pulmonary vascularity with mild-to-moderate cardiomegaly. The right atrium and the aorta are prominent, and the pulmonary trunk inapparent. The right ventricular arc may be flattened in the left anterior oblique view. On the angiocardiogram, the right ventricle is a diminutive and thick-walled chamber in which a blind pouch is found at the site of the atretic pulmonary valve. The tricuspid valve is small but competent. The enlarged myocardial sinusoids provide the only outlet for the right ventricle to drain in a retrograde fashion into the CA and aorta (Fig. 16-54).

The type II lesion displays severe tricuspid insufficiency with markedly dilated right atrium and ventricle. Owing to right-to-left shunting at the atrial level, pronounced pulmonary oligemia is the rule. This entity mimics severe valvular PS with intact ventricular septum (Fig. 7-4) as well as Ebstein's anomaly.

Tricuspid Atresia with Pulmonary Stenosis

The most common type of TA is associated with PS and a restrictive VSD. In contradistinction to TA without PS, there is cyanosis at birth; the lungs are markedly oligemic. Clues to the diagnosis of TA are electrocardiographic evidence of left axis deviation and left ventricular hypertrophy, radiographic evidence of left-sided cardiomegaly, a flat or concave right ventricular border, bulging along the mid-left

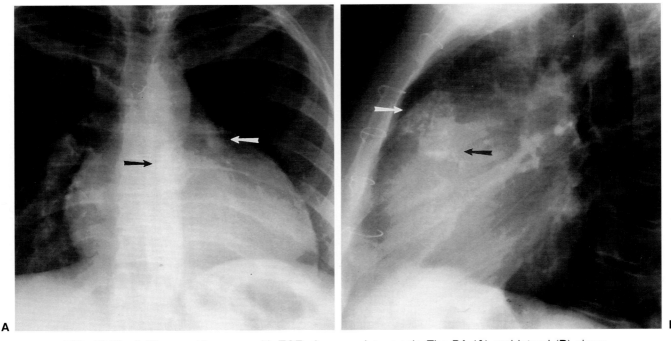

FIG. 16-53. A 25-year-old woman with TOF after complete repair. The PA (**A**) and lateral (**B**) views show clear lungs, moderate right-sided heart enlargement, and calcification of both the outflow tract (*white arrow*) patch and the ventricular septal (*black arrow*) patch. The patient had clinical evidence of significant PI, mild PS and TI.

cardiac border, concavity of the pulmonary trunk, and an enlarged aorta (Fig. 16-44).

On angiography, the only exit seen from the right atrium is an ASD. The systemic and pulmonary venous blood mixes in the left atrium. The mixed blood is propelled primarily through the enlarged aorta to the systemic circulation. Very little blood enters the pulmonary circulation through the restrictive VSD and the stenotic right ventricular outflow tract. The inferior vena cava is dilated, as are the right and left atria, the left ventricle, and the aorta. The great arteries are almost always normally related. Juxtaposition of the atrial appendages is a common feature (Fig. 16-44C). A PDA may be present; if so, the clinical course is more mild and the lungs less oligemic.

A palliative systemic-to-pulmonary artery shunt is indicated for severely cyanotic infants. Otherwise, a Fontan-type procedure (51) is usually performed (see previous discussion on palliative surgical procedures to improve pulmonary blood flow under the heading Tetralogy of Fallot).

D-loop Transposition of Great Arteries with Pulmonary Stenosis

Patients with D-TGA, VSD, and PS tend to have more mild cyanosis and better survival than those without PS. A moderate degree of obstruction to the pulmonary blood flow decreases the threat of congestive heart failure and increases

the flow of oxygenated blood from the left ventricle through the VSD into the aorta (see Fig. 16-34).

Double-Outlet Right Ventricle with Pulmonary Stenosis

Double-outlet right ventricle with pulmonary stenosis (38) closely resembles TOF both clinically and radiographically. On angiocardiography, both great arteries are seen to originate from the right ventricle. The semilunar valves are situated at the same horizontal level, with the crista supraventricularis placed between. There is discontinuity between the aortic and the mitral valves. This feature distinguishes DORV from TOF. The PS is usually in the subpulmonary area (Fig. 16-48).

Single Ventricle with Pulmonary Stenosis

Single ventricle is rarely associated with normally related great arteries. When it is, PS is generally present. This is another lesion that closely resembles TOF in both clinical and radiographic features. The overall cardiac size, however, tends to be larger than that found in TOF.

Ebstein's Anomaly

Ebstein's anomaly is an uncommon congenital heart disease; it is important because most patients live into childhood

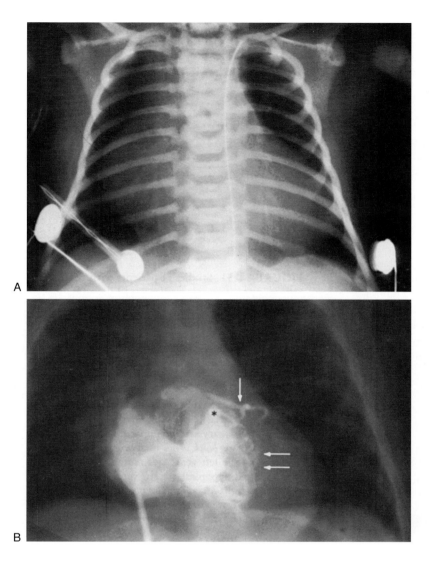

FIG. 16-54. Studies of a neonate with marked cyanosis caused by type 1 pulmonary atresia with an intact ventricular septum. **A:** A chest film taken in the supine position shows severe right-sided cardiomegaly and pulmonary oligemia. **B:** A frontal right ventriculogram shows a small right ventricle with a blind pouch (*asterisk*) at the site of the atretic pulmonary valve. There is reflux of contrast medium across the tricuspid valve into the markedly dilated right atrium. The myocardial sinusoids (*transverse arrows*) are visible, and the coronary arteries are filled in a retrograde fashion. The vertical arrow marks the distal segment of the left main coronary artery. (Modified with permission from Kirks DR. *Practical pediatric imaging*, 2nd ed. Boston: Little, Brown, 1991.)

or beyond. The basic abnormality consists of downward displacement of the tricuspid valve, severe tricuspid insufficiency, and some arrhythmias, usually in the form of supraventricular tachycardia. Ebstein's anomaly is thought to represent an incomplete undermining process of the wall of the right ventricle (52). When the process is complete, much of the redundant valvular sheets over the inner layer of the ventricular muscle is resorbed from the apex to the tricuspid annulus, leaving behind only the normal tricuspid apparatus. In Ebstein's anomaly, two of the three leaflets of the tricuspid valve remain attached to, and therefore appear to arise from, the right ventricular wall. Only the anterior leaflet originates normally from the annulus.

The consequences of such a developmental abnormality are that a large functionless atrialized right ventricle is created, the remaining right ventricle is small and ineffective, the inflow to the right ventricle at the atrialized chamber is obstructed, the tricuspid valve is severely insufficient, a right-to-left shunt across the patent foramen ovale is created, and pulmonary oligemia and clinical cyanosis develop.

The clinical manifestations of Ebstein's anomaly vary widely, in keeping with the broad spectrum of the underlying disease. As a rule, the larger the atrialized right ventricle, the smaller the normally functioning portion of the chamber and the greater the physiologic derangement of the heart. Patients with mild defects may be entirely asymptomatic. In severe disease, symptoms may begin shortly after birth. Cyanosis, dyspnea, and feeding difficulties may lead to death within weeks. The neonatal course of the disease may swing rapidly for two reasons. Improvement usually coincides with the decline of pulmonary vascular resistance, and worsening coincides with spontaneous closure of the PDA. Most patients, however, survive into childhood, adolescence, or even adulthood. The major symptoms of older patients are cyanosis, dyspnea, and palpitations. The electrocardiographic findings include right axis deviation, peaked P waves, right bundle branch block, and a 25% incidence of Wolff-Parkinson-White syndrome (53). Medical treatment primarily involves management of congestive heart failure and arrhythmias. Surgical intervention consists of replacement of the tricuspid valve and plication of the atrialized portion of the right ventricle and closure of ASD.

Radiographic and Angiographic Signs

On radiography, the picture varies widely, depending on the severity of the anomaly. In extreme cases, the right side of the heart is massively dilated with the right ventricle forming the left cardiac border on the PA view. The left-sided cardiac chambers are displaced posteriorly and compressed by the dilated right heart. The pulmonary vascularity is diminished. The hilar shadows are small (see **Fig. 2-6**).

Superficially the radiographic appearance of Ebstein's anomaly resembles that of pericardial effusion. However, some features of Ebstein's anomaly militate against such a diagnosis. First, the subepicardial fat stripe is not displaced, and the pericardium is not thickened. Second, the cardiac borders are pulsatile instead of dampened. Third, the pulmonary vascularity is diminished rather than normal.

On angiocardiography, the markedly dilated right atrium is clearly outlined, with the tricuspid annulus displaced to the left side. The atrialized right ventricle forms a sharply demarcated inferior border between the right atrium and the remaining portion of the right ventricle (Fig. 16-55).

Echocardiographic Signs

Right ventricular diastolic overload and paradoxical septal motion are usually visible on the echocardiogram. More specifically, the tricuspid valve may show exaggerated motion

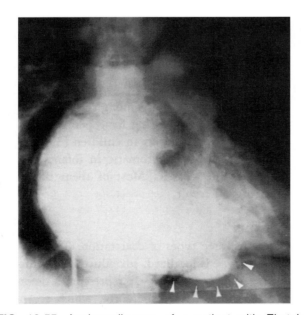

FIG. 16-55. Angiocardiogram of a patient with Ebstein's anomaly. Both the right atrium and the right ventricle are enormous. The right ventricle is actually border-forming on the left side. Note a third compartment (*arrows*) between the right atrium and the right ventricle. This is the so-called atrialized right ventricle between the tricuspid annulus and the malpositioned tricuspid leaflets.

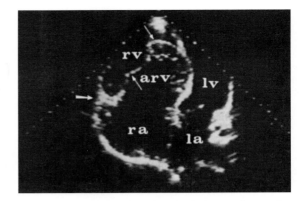

FIG. 16-56. Two-dimensional apical-view echocardiogram shows downward displacement of the posterior and septal leaflets of the tricuspid valve (*thin arrows*) and marked dilatation of the right atrium (ra) and the atrialized right ventricle (arv). The remaining right ventricle (rv), left atrium (la), and left ventricle (lv) are small. The thick arrow marks the level of the tricuspid annulus. The atrial septum appears to be defective.

and delayed closure. The two-dimensional technique is capable of recording both the anatomic and physiologic abnormalities of the anomaly (7,17) (Figs. 16-14 and 16-56).

NORMAL PULMONARY VASCULARITY WITHOUT CYANOSIS

In the noncyanotic group of patients, congenital cardiac lesions that manifest normal pulmonary vascularity are the distal left-sided obstructive lesions before congestive heart failure, such as aortic stenosis, aortic insufficiency, Marfan syndrome, and coarctation or pseudocoarctation of the aorta. Lesions with aortic insufficiency are considered to have pathophysiologic rather than anatomical obstructions. Also considered in the differential diagnosis are uncomplicated L-loop transposition of the great arteries, most aortic arch anomalies, some cardiac malpositions, and all hemodynamically insignificant congenital anomalies (Table 16-5). How-

TABLE 16-5. *Abnormalities that manifest normal PBF without cyanosis*

Distal left-sided obstructions[a]
AS
AI
CoA
PsCoA
L-TGA[b]
Most arch anomalies
Some cardiac malpositions
(+) CHD

As, aortic stenosis; AI, aortic insufficiency; CoA, coarctation of aorta; PsCoA, pseudocoarctation of aorta; L-TGA, L-loop transposition of great arteries; (+) CHD, all hemodynamically insignificant congenital heart disease.

[a] Status before congestive heart failure.
[b] Without associated lesions.

ever, only three of the conditions are discussed here. Others are considered later in this chapter or in **Chapter 11**.

Coarctation of the Aorta

Coarctation of the aorta is among the most common anomalies, accounting for 8% of all congenital cardiac defects in children (54). Patients tend to be symptomatic in infancy and after the third decade. Most of them benefit from surgical repair.

Anatomy

There are three types of coarctation. The most common type is termed localized, juxtaductal, postductal, or adult coarctation. It represents a deformity of the media of the aorta, which eccentrically narrows the lumen by a curtainlike infolding of the wall. The second type is called diffuse, pre-

ductal, or infantile coarctation. It is characterized by a tubular hypoplasia of the aortic isthmus (between the left subclavian artery and the ductus arteriosus) with or without a localized coarctation. The third type is known as pseudocoarctation, mild coarctation, or nonobstructive coarctation.

All types of coarctation are prone to manifest a bicuspid aortic valve (55); the incidence is estimated to be as high as 85% (56). Ventricular septal defects occasionally accompany the localized form of coarctation and precipitate congestive heart failure in early infancy. This is known as the coarctation syndrome (50). The diffuse form of coarctation is often associated with complex intracardiac defects and a poor prognosis (22).

Pathophysiology

Coarctation of the aorta becomes hemodynamically important when the aortic lumen is reduced by 50%, or when its cross-sectional area is reduced by 75%. The characteristic

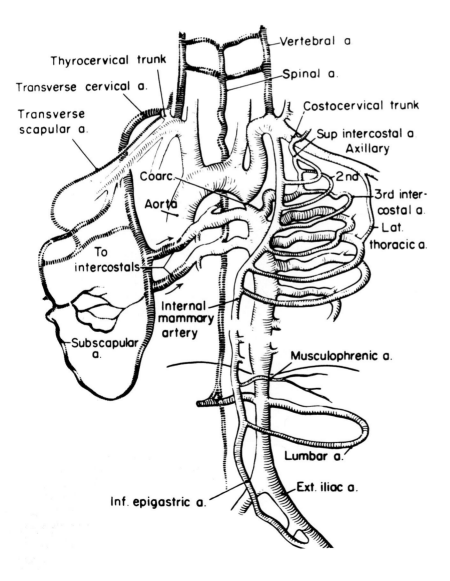

FIG. 16-57. Collateral circulation in the presence of coarctation of the aorta (see text). (Reproduced with permission from Roberts WC, ed. *Congenital heart disease.* Philadelphia: Davis, 1979.)

hemodynamic alterations include hypertension proximal and hypotension distal to the site of obstruction, as well as subsequent development of collateral channels between the two compartments. Starting from the subclavian artery, the collaterals are formed both anteriorly and posteriorly on both sides (Fig. 16-57). The anterior system delivers blood primarily from the internal mammary artery through the epigastric to the ileofemoral arteries. Part of the flow is channeled through the intercostal arteries to the descending aorta. The posterior system is concerned mainly with delivering blood through the thyrocervical trunk, the transverse cervical, the scapular, and the intercostal arteries to the descending and abdominal aortas.

Clinical Presentation

The clinical presentation of coarctation depends on the site and severity of the obstruction as well as on the presence of associated anomalies. Congestive heart failure occurs either in infancy or after the third decade of life. Most children and young adults with uncomplicated coarctation are asymptomatic. The diagnosis is usually suggested by hypotension in the lower and hypertension in the upper extremities. On auscultation, a systolic or continuous murmur is usually present over the sternal borders, the back, and the spinous process. In the presence of a bicuspid aortic valve, a diastolic murmur of aortic insufficiency may also be audible. The ECG usually shows left ventricular hypertrophy in patients with an isolated coarctation and biventricular or predominantly right ventricular hypertrophy in those with a complicated lesion.

The treatment for isolated aortic coarctation is surgical resection with end-to-end anastomosis or placement of a graft. Late development of calcific aortic stenosis from a bicuspid valve is common. Other complications (57) include infective endocarditis, aneurysm at the site of coarctation, and congestive heart failure. Rupture of an aneurysm of the circle of Willis, although rare, is a well-documented complication of coarctation (58).

Radiographic Signs

In isolated coarctation, the pulmonary vascularity is normal before congestive heart failure. The left ventricle may appear hypertrophied. Calcium should always be sought in the aortic valve in patients who are >30 years old (Fig. 16-58). The incidence of rib notching increases with the patient's age; it is rare in infants, uncommon in children, but present in 75% of adults (59). The notches are typically found along the lower margin of the third through the eighth ribs posterolaterally. They represent pressure erosion of the ribs inflicted by dilated, tortuous, and hyperpulsatile intercostal arteries in the costal grooves (Figs. 2-2, 16-59). The anterior ribs are spared because they are outside the costal grooves; the first and second ribs are also spared because their intercostal arteries originate from the costocervical trunk rather than the descending aorta.

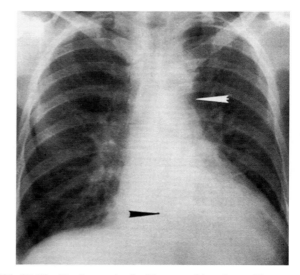

FIG. 16-58. Radiograph of a 60-year-old patient with coarctation of the aorta and calcific aortic stenosis. The black arrow points to the heavily calcified aortic valve. Congestive heart failure is evident by cardiomegaly and pulmonary edema. Note the figure-three sign of coarctation of the aorta (white arrow).

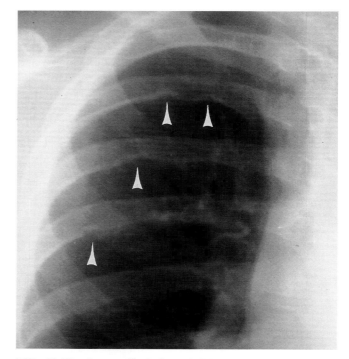

FIG. 16-59. A magnified view of right-upper chest of a 17-year-old boy with coarctation of the aorta shows multiple notched ribs (arrows). The sclerotic margin of each notch represents the reparative process of laying down new bones. In fact, all the involved ribs show a sclerotic lower margin even before the typical notching forms.

Since the pressure erosion is constantly being repaired with new bone deposition, genuine notches are always outlined by a sclerotic margin. Rib notching is usually present bilaterally. Unilaterality of the sign suggests an uncommon location of the coarctation. When the obstruction is proximal to the left subclavian artery, rib notching is absent on the left side, because that artery, being in the low-pressure compartment, does not participate in the development of collateral flow. Unilateral right-sided rib notching also occurs when the origin of the left subclavian artery is encroached on by the coarctation. Unilateral left-sided rib notching develops when the coarctation is situated between the left subclavian and the aberrant right subclavian arteries.

The site of coarctation can frequently be identified on the standard PA radiograph as a figure-three sign. The upper arc of the figure three represents either the dilated aortic arch or the dilated left subclavian artery proximal to the obstruction; the lower arc is the poststenotic dilatation of the descending aorta (60). When the esophagus is opacified, a reversed figure-three, or E, sign will be noted on the barium column, marking the other side of the deformed aorta (Fig. 16-60A,B). The figure-three sign is usually absent when the coarctation is located way down in the lower thoracic or abdominal aorta (see **Fig. 2-2**).

In the lateral view, left ventricular enlargement and ascending aortic dilatation are usually evident. Occasionally

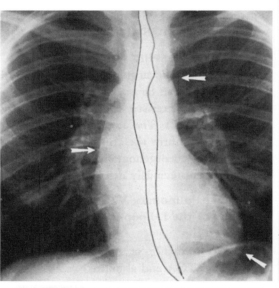

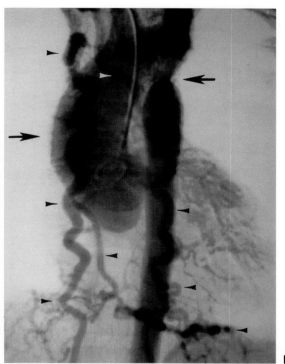

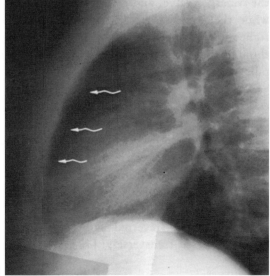

FIG. 16-60. Patients with coarctation of the aorta. **A:** PA view of patient 1 shows dilatation of the ascending aorta (*lower horizontal arrow*), a figure-three sign (*upper horizontal arrow*), and an *E* sign on the barium-filled esophagus (*outlined with black lines*). The hypertrophied left ventricle (*oblique arrow*) has a more convex contour and extends more inferiorly and to the left than normal. **B:** A frontal aortogram of patient 2 shows a striking coarctation of the aorta in the usual location (*upper arrow*), forming a figure-three deformity. Also note the dilated ascending aorta (*lower arrow*) and multiple collaterals (*arrowheads*) from the high-pressure compartment to the low-pressure compartment. **C:** The lateral view of patient 3 shows a serpentine density in the retrosternal region (*arrows*), representing the tortuous internal mammary arteries. The aortic arch is not visible.

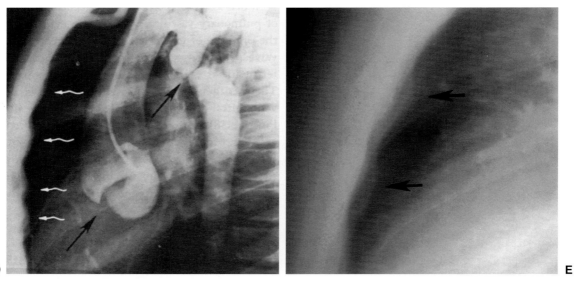

FIG. 16-60. *Continued.* **D:** Lateral aortogram of patient 4 shows rich collateral circulation and the serpentine internal mammary arteries (*horizontal arrows*). The aortic arch is deformed, and all the brachiocephalic branches are markedly dilated. These are the main reasons why the aortic arch is frequently invisible on the lateral radiograph. The upper oblique arrow marks the site of coarctation. The lower oblique arrow points to the bicuspid aortic valve. **E:** A magnified lateral view of patient 3 shows the serpentine density (*arrows*) to better advantage.

a serpentine density is seen in fragments behind the sternum, representing the dilated and tortuous internal mammary arteries (Fig. 16-60C,D). The absence of the aortic arch in this view is another sign of coarctation, which can sometimes be the only clue to the diagnosis (14) (Fig. 16-60C,D).

Pseudocoarctation of the aorta (1) causes little or no obstruction to the flow of blood. It is also associated with a high incidence of bicuspid aortic valve. The unique features of the condition are elongation and buckling of the aorta (Fig. 16-61). The two bumps of the aorta form two aortic knobs in the PA view, one being too high and the other too low for a normal aortic arch (Fig. 16-61A). A webbing of the neck of Turner's syndrome can sometimes manifest in the chest radiograph. This should prompt the observer to look for evidence of coarctation.

Angiographic Signs

A selective injection of contrast medium in the ascending aorta usually depicts all component lesions of coarctation as well as the extent of collateral flow around the obstruction (Fig. 16-60B,D). The unique features of pseudocoarctation are readily confirmed on the aortogram (Fig. 16-61C,D).

L-Loop Transposition of the Great Arteries

Transposition of the great arteries is thought to result from failure of the primitive truncus arteriosus to spiral normally. The anteroposterior relationship between the two arteries is consequently reversed—each arises from the wrong ventricle. There are two types of TGA (1,7,17). One is called the "complete" TGA, or D-TGA, and the other is "congenitally corrected" TGA, or L-TGA (Fig. 16-62).

The term complete refers to a physiologically uncorrected transposition in which systemic venous blood is delivered to the aorta and pulmonary venous blood is delivered to the pulmonary artery (Fig. 16-62A). The term corrected implies that despite the transposed great arteries, oxygenated blood is directed to the aorta and nonoxygenated blood to the pulmonary artery, thereby creating a physiologically corrected TGA. This is effected by inversion of ventricles with their corresponding AV valves, so that the morphologic right ventricle is situated on the left side, connected to the left atrium through the tricuspid valve and giving rise to the aorta, while the morphologic left ventricle is on the right side, connected to the right atrium through the mitral valve and giving rise to the pulmonary artery (Fig. 16-62B).

The term D-loop (Fig. 16-62A) means that the TGA is associated with embryologic right (dextro) looping of the cardiac tube, so that the right ventricle is situated on the right side; L-loop (Fig. 16-62B) indicates that the TGA is associated with embryologic left (levo) looping of the cardiac tube, so that the morphologic right ventricle is situated on the left side. In L-TGA, the great arteries are both transposed (reversed sagittally) and inverted (reversed transversely) (32,61).

Clinical Presentation

Patients with isolated L-loop TGA are usually asymptomatic and may live a normal life span. One reported patient was alive at age 73 (36). This longevity is exceptional, how-

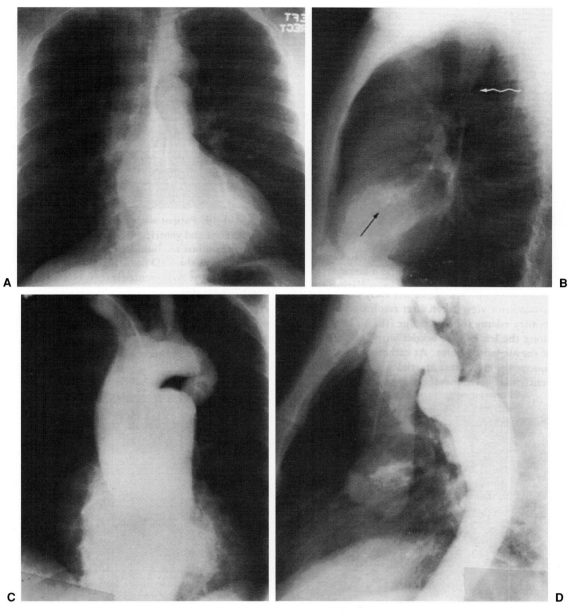

FIG. 16-61. The PA view (**A**) of an adult with pseudocoarctation of the aorta shows two aortic knobs, one being too high and the other too low for the normal aortic arch. The ascending aorta and the left ventricle are enlarged. The pulmonary vascularity is normal. Note that there is no rib notching. A lateral view (**B**) shows elongation and buckling (*white arrow*) of the thoracic aorta. Heavy calcification is noted in the aortic valve (*black arrow*). At catheterization, notable stenosis of a bicuspid aortic valve was found to coexist with pseudocoarctation. PA (**C**) and lateral (**D**) aortograms from another asymptomatic adult patient show characteristic angiographic findings of pseudocoarctation.

ever, for most such patients usually develop one of two problems. First, heart block may occur and progress after the second decade. Second, the left-sided AV valve may become incompetent. The unique electrocardiographic findings are orientation of the initial ventricular depolarization to the left, rather than to the right, anteriorly; large upright T waves in the precordial leads; and AV conduction delay of varying degrees. Beside heart block and tricuspid insufficiency, VSD may coexist with L-TGA. Even in patients with isolated L-TGA, late development of right ventricular failure remains a problem because the right ventricle is not designed to pump blood against systemic resistance.

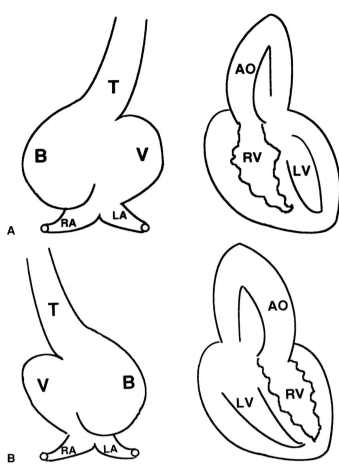

FIG. 16-62. Schematic drawing of D-loop VS L-loop TGA. **A:** D-loop. **B:** L-loop. T, truncus arteriosus; B, bulbus cordis; V, ventricular portion of the primitive cardiac tube; LA, left atrium; LV, left ventricle; RA, right atrium; RV, right ventricle.

Radiographic Signs

On the PA radiographic view, there are several features of isolated L-TGA. Rightward convexity of a normal ascending aorta is absent; instead, a leftward convexity of the transposed ascending aorta is present. The pulmonary trunk, on the other hand, is medially placed and may impinge on the left border of the barium-filled esophagus. A second bulge along the left cardiac border may be seen immediately below the convexity of the left-sided ascending aorta, representing the protruding border of the morphologic right ventricle (Figs. 16-63 and 16-64).

Angiographic Signs

Even before angiocardiography, the diagnosis of L-TGA can be made with confidence by noting the characteristic catheter positions (see **Figs. 7-11** and **7-12**). Angiocardiograms (Fig. 16-64) help confirm the clinical, electrocardiographic, and radiographic suggestions of this condition, as previously described.

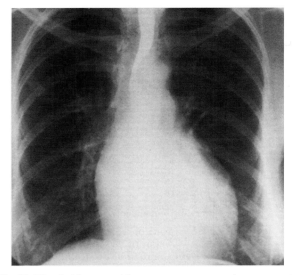

FIG. 16-63. A 45-year-old woman was seen for congestive heart failure and a mitral insufficiency murmur that she had experienced since early childhood. The PA view taken after resolution of pulmonary edema shows a bulging left-lower cardiac border; the ascending aorta is not visible in its usual location. At catheterization, L-TGA with a left-sided atrioventricular valve (tricuspid) insufficiency was diagnosed.

Abnormal Pulmonary Vascularity in the Presence of L-TGA

For the convenience of presentation, patients with L-TGA and abnormal vascularity are also discussed here. When associated with a VSD, the shunt type of pulmonary vascular-

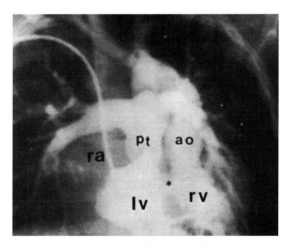
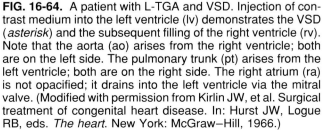

FIG. 16-64. A patient with L-TGA and VSD. Injection of contrast medium into the left ventricle (lv) demonstrates the VSD (*asterisk*) and the subsequent filling of the right ventricle (rv). Note that the aorta (ao) arises from the right ventricle; both are on the left side. The pulmonary trunk (pt) arises from the left ventricle; both are on the right side. The right atrium (ra) is not opacified; it drains into the left ventricle via the mitral valve. (Modified with permission from Kirlin JW, et al. Surgical treatment of congenital heart disease. In: Hurst JW, Logue RB, eds. *The heart.* New York: McGraw–Hill, 1966.)

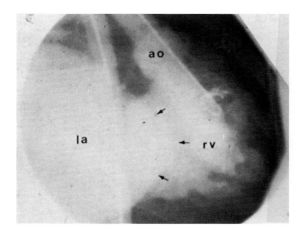

FIG. 16-65. Angiocardiogram of a patient with L-TGA and tricuspid insufficiency. Injection of contrast medium into the left-sided right ventricle (rv) demonstrates retrograde filling of the markedly dilated left atrium (la) through the insufficient tricuspid valve (*arrows*). Also note the ascending aorta (ao), which arises from the right ventricle and courses superiorly and to the midline of the chest.

ity is usually evident. In the context of severe left-sided AV valve (tricuspid) insufficiency, a cephalic pulmonary blood flow pattern with or without pulmonary edema is usually observed. The radiographic appearance resembles that of severe mitral insufficiency (Figs. 16-63 and 16-65). Pulmonary stenosis, generally coexistent with a VSD, may also complicate the picture of L-TGA. In this situation, the pulmonary vascularity may be decreased, and the cardiovascular contour may mimic that of TOF.

PULMONARY VENOUS HYPERTENSION WITHOUT CYANOSIS

When congestive heart failure develops, all the above-mentioned lesions manifest signs of pulmonary venous hy-

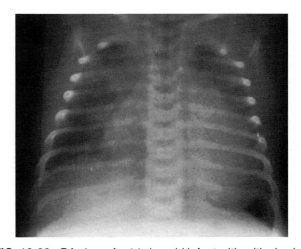

FIG. 16-66. PA view of a 14-day-old infant with critical valvular aortic stenosis. Note gross cardiomegaly and pulmonary edema.

pertension, such as severe aortic stenosis with left ventricular failure. In the neonate, common anomalies causing pulmonary venous hypertension are critical aortic stenosis (Fig. 16-66), cor triatriatum (Fig. 16-67), atresia of the common pulmonary vein, systemic arteriovenous fistula, and intrauterine myocarditis. The most frequently encountered conditions in the first 2 months of life are coarctation of the aorta, aortic stenosis, endocardial fibroelastosis, glycogen storage disease, hypertrophic cardiomyopathy, cor triatriatum, mitral stenosis, systemic arteriovenous fistula, viral myocarditis, and aberrant left CA from the pulmonary artery (see Fig. 16-26) (Table 16-6).

Endocardial fibroelastosis, glycogen storage disease, viral myocarditis, and aberrant left CA from the pulmonary artery all have similar clinical and radiographic features (see Fig. 16-26A,B): bilateral but predominantly left-sided cardiomegaly, bilateral but predominantly left-sided congestive heart failure, bilateral but predominantly left-sided AV valve insufficiency, and signs of pulmonary venous hypertension with or without frank pulmonary edema.

PULMONARY VENOUS HYPERTENSION WITH CYANOSIS

Cyanotic heart diseases with pulmonary venous hypertension commonly seen in the neonate are hypoplastic left heart syndrome and TAPVC with obstruction (Table 16-7). Hypoplastic left heart syndrome consists of three major component lesions: aortic atresia, mitral atresia, and interruption of the aortic arch. These three may be present alone or in combination. The left atrium and ventricle are hypoplastic. The shunting of blood is usually bidirectional—left to right

TABLE 16-6. *Abnormalities causing PVH without cyanosis*

Any age
    All lesions listed in Table 16-5 + CHF
In the neonate
    Aortic stenosis
    Pulmonary vein atresia
    Intrauterine myocarditis
    Cor triatriatum
    Systemic AV fistula
In the first 2 months of life
    Coarctation of aorta
    Endocardial fibroelastosis
    Glycogen storage disease
    Systemic AV fistula
    Hypertrophic cardiomyopathy
    Aortic stenosis
    Cor triatriatum
    Mitral stenosis
    Viral myocarditis
    ALCA from PA

PVH, pulmonary venous hypertension; CHF, congestive heart failure; AV, arteriovenous, ALCA from PA, aberrant left coronary artery from pulmonary artery.

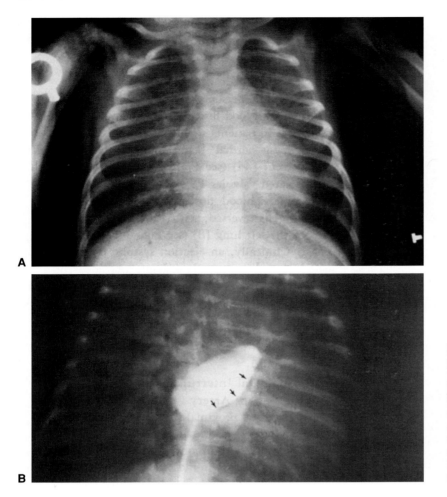

FIG. 16-67. Two-month-old boy with cor tria-triatum. PA view (**A**) shows moderate cardio-megaly with severe pulmonary edema. An in-jection into the left atrium (**B**) shows a linear filling defect (*arrows*) representing the parti-tion between the accessory left atrial chamber above (larger and more dense area) and the true left atrium below (smaller and less dense area). (Modified with permission from Kirks DR. *Practical pediatric imaging*, 2nd ed. Bos-ton: Little, Brown, 1991.)

at the atrial level and right to left at the ductal level. The right ventricle usually is the only pumping chamber of the heart (Fig. 16-68). The pulmonary venous blood in TAPVC with obstruction almost invariably drains infradiaphragmati-cally into the portal vein (Fig. 16-41).

LATERALIZED FLOW PATTERN WITHOUT CYANOSIS

A lateralized pulmonary blood flow pattern is observed in two acyanotic congenital anomalies, namely, valvular PS

TABLE 16-7. *Diseases leading to PVH with cyanosis in the neonate*

TAPVC with obstruction
  Severe pulmonary edema
  Normal heart size
Hypoplastic left heart syndrome
  Severe pulmonary edema
  Moderated cardiomegaly

  TAPVC, total anomalous pulmonary ve-nous connection.

and proximal interruption of one pulmonary artery (Table 16-8).

Valvular Pulmonary Stenosis

In normal persons, the right-to-left ratio of pulmonary blood flow is ~52% to 48%. In patients with secundum ASD, this ratio remains normal at ~53% to 47% (16) (Fig. 16-10). In those with isolated valvular PS, however, the normal pulmonary blood flow pattern between the two lungs is re-versed, with a markedly greater flow to the left lung (3,62) (see **Fig. 8-17**). On clinical examination an ejection systolic murmur is heard in the pulmonic area, both in valvular PS and in secundum ASD—hence the frequent misdiagnosis of one for the other. On radiography, however, the two condi-tions are easily differentiated by their unique pulmonary blood flow pattern, as previously described.

Congenital Interruption of One Pulmonary Artery

Congenital proximal interruption of one pulmonary artery was previously called congenital absence of one pulmonary

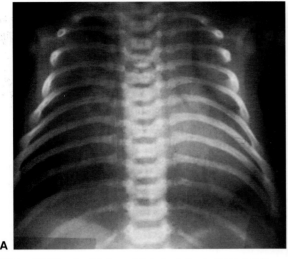

A

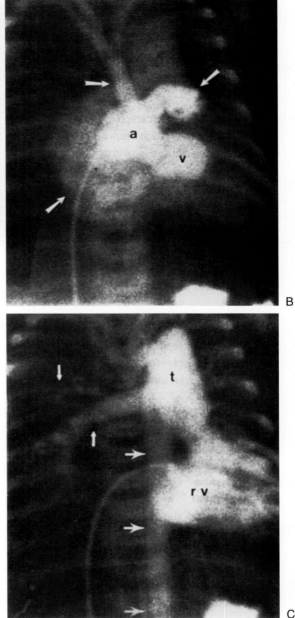

B

C

FIG. 16-68. A 17-day-old infant had intractable congestive heart failure and cyanosis. PA view (**A**) shows moderate cardiomegaly and severe pulmonary edema. Frontal angiocardiogram (**B**) after injection into the small left atrium (a) shows sequential filling of the hypoplastic left ventricle (v), ascending aorta (*horizontal arrow*), and brachiocephalic vessels. The right atrium (*lower oblique arrow*) is just beginning to be opacified via an ASD. The upper oblique arrow points to the left atrial appendage. The aortic arch and descending aorta are not visible, indicating interruption of the aorta. Another frontal angiocardiogram (**C**) after injection into the dilated right ventricle (rv) demonstrates sequential filling of the dilated pulmonary trunk (t), the pulmonary arteries (*vertical arrows*), and the descending aorta (*horizontal arrows*). The right-to-left shunt is at the ductal level.

artery. This is a misnomer, because in most patients there is only an interruption between the pulmonary trunk and one of the pulmonary arteries. All the branches distal to the interruption are usually present and fed by bronchial arterial collaterals.

TABLE 16-8. *Anomalies accompanied by lateralized flow pattern without cyanosis*

Valvular pulmonary stenosis with left lateralization
Proximal interruption of RPA with right lateralization

RPA, right pulmonary artery.

Although a pulmonary artery can be interrupted on either side, it is usually on the right side, opposite the aortic arch. When that is the case, the lesion is typically isolated. When the interruption occurs on the side of the aortic arch, associated intracardiac defects are frequently encountered, most commonly in the form of a VSD or TOF. Eighty percent of the patients with isolated interruption of a pulmonary artery are asymptomatic (see **Fig. 8-18**). In the remaining 20%, pulmonary arterial hypertension develops early in life, and the patients do poorly. Patients with associated intracardiac defects have a grave prognosis; they may die of unilateral pulmonary edema in infancy. Two acquired diseases are considered in the differential diagnosis of this anomaly: Swyer-James syndrome (see **Fig. 8-19**) and Westermark's sign of massive pulmonary embolism (see **Fig. 8-20**).

LOCALIZED FLOW PATTERN WITHOUT CYANOSIS

A localized flow pattern without cyanosis is seen in pulmonary artery branch stenosis (62), pulmonary vein varix, and partial anomalous pulmonary venous connection (Table 16-9).

Pulmonary Artery Branch Stenosis

Pulmonary artery branch stenosis (62) may be single, but more commonly it is multiple and bilateral. It is also called distal pulmonary artery stenosis. Associated intracardiac lesions are, in descending order of frequency, valvular PS, VSD, and ASD. On clinical and hemodynamic examination, patients with isolated pulmonary artery branch stenoses usually have severe pulmonary arterial hypertension and right ventricular strain. Pulmonary artery branch stenosis may be confused with primary pulmonary artery hypertension or valvular PS. Pulmonary arteriography (see **Fig. 8-21B**) and careful pressure measurements during cardiac catheterization are definitive diagnostic procedures. Surgical treatment of bilateral multiple pulmonary artery stenoses is difficult. Recent advances in balloon dilation and stenting of hypoplastic pulmonary arteries has led to a better prognosis for these patients (63).

Pulmonary Vein Varix

Pulmonary vein varix is a rare congenital anomaly that seldom causes symptoms, though hemoptysis has been re-

ported. It usually affects the right-lower-lobe pulmonary vein near its entrance into the left atrium. The varix may become more conspicuous in the presence of pulmonary venous hypertension, such as that stemming from severe mitral insufficiency.

On radiography, a varicose pulmonary vein appears as a rounded or lobulated opacity in the lower-medial lung zone. Its connection with the incoming venous branches and the left atrium can be better appreciated on conventional or CT scanning. Under the fluoroscope, the compressibility of the lesion can be seen with a Valsalva maneuver and a rebound pulsation on the release of the breath. The diagnosis of a pulmonary vein varix can be confirmed by an enhanced CT scan (see **Fig. 8-22D,E,F**) or MRI.

Partial Anomalous Pulmonary Venous Connection

The abnormal course of anomalous veins may be clearly visible on the radiograph. The best example is the so-called scimitar syndrome, in which a swordlike vessel is seen to descend from the right perihilar region to the diaphragm (see **Fig. 8-22**) (see discussion on scimitar syndrome in the section of left-to-right shunts). Other types of PAPVC are less commonly visible on the chest radiograph but more frequently diagnosed on CT or MRI or angiography (7,12,15) (Fig. 16-11B,C).

LOCALIZED FLOW PATTERN WITH CYANOSIS

Pulmonary arteriovenous fistula is the only congenital anomaly with a localized flow pattern and cyanosis (Table 16-9). It is a developmental defect in the terminal capillary loops, leading to the formation of a thin-walled aneurysm, which is fed by a pulmonary artery and drained by a pulmonary vein (64). In approximately one third of patients, there are several lesions, most commonly found in the lower lobes. In 40% to 65% of patients with pulmonary arteriovenous fistulas, similar vascular lesions are also present in the skin, mucous membrane, and other organs. This condition has been known as Rendu–Osler–Weber disease or hereditary hemorrhagic telangiectasia.

Although they are congenital, these lesions tend to remain clinically silent until the patient reaches adulthood, after the vessels have been stretched under pressure for a long time. When pulmonary arteriovenous fistulas are large or numerous, the patient usually has hemoptysis and dyspnea. Cyanosis, finger clubbing, and a continuous murmur over the lesion are the common objective signs of the disease. Besides recurrent hemoptysis, rupture of the arteriovenous aneurysm into the nearby pleural cavity is another life-threatening complication. Unlike its systemic counterparts, pulmonary arteriovenous fistulas seldom cause congestive heart failure. Per-

TABLE 16-9. *Anomalies causing localized flow pattern*

Without cyanosis
  PA branch stenosis
    Nodular poststenotic opacities
    Dilated pulmonary trunk
    Right-sided cardiomegaly
  PV varix
    Rounded mass at RLCB
    Frequently with MI
  Partial APVC
    Abnormal course of vessel(s)
    Frequently with ASD
With cyanosis
  Pulmonary AV fistula(s)
    Feeding PA → aneurysm → draining PV → LA

PA, pulmonary artery; PV, pulmonary vein; RLCB, right-lower cardiac border, MI, mitral insufficiency; APVC, anomalous pulmonary venous connection; ASD, atrial septal defect, AV, arteriovenous; LA, left atrium.

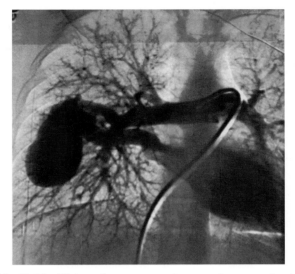

FIG. 16-69. Right pulmonary arteriogram of a cyanotic child with pulsatile masses in both lungs. Note a large pulmonary arteriovenous fistula. Smaller fistulas were evident on the left pulmonary arteriogram (not shown).

haps this finding is related to the low-pressure, low-resistance characteristics of the pulmonary circulation in which fistulas rarely provoke a notable increase in cardiac output.

On radiography, the fistulas are typically rounded or oval-shaped opacities, more commonly found in the lower than the middle and upper lobes. By the aid of fluoroscopy in multiple views, the dilated afferent pulmonary artery can be distinguished from the hilum, and the dilated efferent pulmonary vein can be seen coursing toward the left atrium. Usually, intrinsic pulsations of the vascular complex can also be observed under the fluoroscope. The vessels, too, tend to shrink with a Valsalva maneuver and to rebound with more vigorous pulsations when the breath is released. Other diagnostic imaging methods, such as enhanced CT scanning and MRI, may be used when necessary. The ultimate preoperative evaluation depends on high-quality selective right and left pulmonary angiograms (Fig. 16-69). The treatment of choice for larger fistulas is surgical resection. For the smaller ones, transcatheter embolization of the pulmonary artery with suitable materials is preferred (65).

AORTIC ARCH ANOMALIES

Aortic arch anomalies are important for three major reasons: they are common (with an incidence between 0.5% and 3%) (13), they may cause compression symptoms, and certain anomalies are associated with a high incidence of congenital heart disease. Almost all arch anomalies can be explained by the double-arch model proposed by Stewart et al. (66) (Fig. 16-70). Normally the right aortic arch gradually disappears, leaving a normal left arch. On the contrary, the

left arch may regress, forming a right aortic arch. If both arches should persist, then a double aortic arch will result. For practical reasons, only four relatively common anomalies are discussed.

Right Aortic Arch

Of the five types of right aortic arch (RAA) (67), only two are of practical importance. Fortunately, they are easily recognized radiographically, with or without barium in the esophagus. Computed tomography and MRI have become increasingly important in the diagnosis of arch anomalies (13,14).

Avian Type (Type 1)

The avian type of RAA is normal for birds but devastating for mankind. It results from breakage of the double aortic ring between the left ductus and the descending aorta (Fig. 16-70). In the experience of Stewart and co-workers (68), 98% of patients with this anomaly had congenital heart dis-

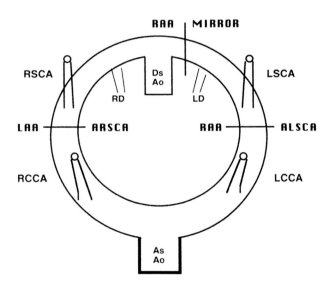

FIG. 16-70. Drawing of Edwards' double aortic arch model. Depending on the site of breakage of the ring, the following anomalies are formed: between the right common carotid artery and the right subclavian artery: left aortic arch with aberrant right subclavian artery; between the left ductus and the descending aorta: right aortic arch with mirror image branching; between the left common carotid artery and left subclavian artery: right aortic arch with aberrant left subclavian artery. As Ao, ascending aorta; RCCA, right common carotid artery; LAA-ARSCA, left aortic arch with aberrant right subclavian artery; RSCA, right subclavian artery; RD, right ductus; Ds Ao, descending aorta; RAA-MIRROR, right aortic arch with mirror image branching; LD, left ductus; LSCA, left subclavian artery; RAA-ALSCA, right aortic arch with aberrant left subclavian artery; LCCA, left common carotid artery.

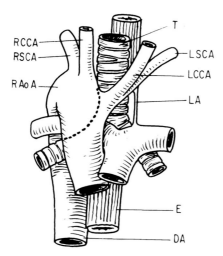

FIG. 16-71. Drawing of type 1 (avian type, anterior type) RAA shows mirror-image branching of the arch. The aortic arch is anterior to the trachea and esophagus, as is usual. DA, descending aorta; E, esophagus; LA, ligamentum arteriosum; LCCA, left common carotid artery; LSCA, left subclavian artery; RAoA, right aortic arch; RCCA, right common carotid artery; RSCA, right subclavian artery; T, trachea. Compare with Fig. 16-70.

ease. Approximately 90% of the cardiac defects were TOF. Other lesions, with much lower incidences, in their study were PTA, transposition of the great arteries, left-to-right shunts, and coarctation of the aorta. The aorta branches as a mirror image of the normal arrangement. The first branch is the left innominate (brachiocephalic) artery, followed by the right common carotid and then the right subclavian (Fig. 16-71). In this type of RAA, there is no posterior component of the arch to push either the esophagus or the trachea forward (Fig. 16-45). Therefore, in the lateral radiograph the trachea and esophagus are entirely normal (Fig. 16-45B). On the PA view, the superior mediastinum is completely empty to the left of midline owing to the absence of a big aortic diverticulum (Fig. 16-45A).

Patients with this anomaly usually, but not always, show the telltale radiographic signs of TOF. They are decreased pulmonary vascularity owing to right-to-left shunting across a VSD and the coeur en sabot (boot-shaped) cardiovascular contour due to right ventricular enlargement, hypoplasia of the pulmonary artery, and enlargement of the aortic arch. The right-sided position of the aortic arch by itself says nothing about the underlying pathophysiology, however.

Common Type (Type 3)

Type 3 RAA is more common in the general population than the avian type (68). However, it is infrequently seen in hospitalized patients because most patients with this anomaly are healthy. In one study (68), only 12% of patients with this condition had congenital heart disease. The prevailing

lesion was TOF (71%). Other lesions included left-to-right shunts (21%) and coarctation of the aorta (7%).

This arch anomaly results from breakage of the double aortic ring between the left subclavian artery and the left common carotid artery (Fig. 16-70). In this context, the aberrant left subclavian artery arises from the aortic diverticulum in the proximal descending aorta (Fig. 16-72). The aortic diverticulum is usually quite large, representing the remnant of the left arch; it is typically clearly visible in the superior mediastinum to the left of midline at the same horizontal level as the RAA on the PA view (Fig. 16-73A) and pushing the esophagus and the trachea forward on the lateral view (Fig. 16-73B).

Four separate arteries arise from the arch in the following order: the left common carotid, the right common carotid, the right subclavian, and the aberrant left subclavian. The aberrant artery courses leftward and superiorly toward the left arm, occasionally causing a shallow, oblique indentation on the barium-filled esophagus. More frequently, though, the esophagus is markedly displaced from behind by the huge diverticulum, and there is no trace of the crossing left subclavian, which is much smaller (Fig. 16-73). When the esophagus is not visible with barium, the air-filled trachea (tracheogram) can be used to diagnose the type of right arch. Again, it is the lateral view that clearly distinguishes one type of RAA from the other.

To recapitulate the importance of distinguishing one type of RAA from the other, see Table 16-10. The major radiographic differences between the two types are seen on the

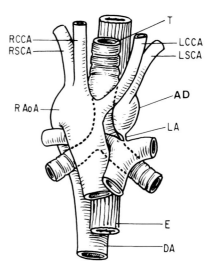

FIG. 16-72. Drawing of type 3 (common type, posterior type) right-sided aortic arch. There is an aberrant left subclavian artery arising from an aortic diverticulum. The aortic diverticulum represents a remnant of the left aortic arch. The diverticulum is usually quite large, displacing the esophagus and trachea anteriorly. It also bulges toward the left of the midline. AD, aortic diverticulum. Other abbreviations are the same as those in Fig. 16-71 (compare with Fig. 16-70).

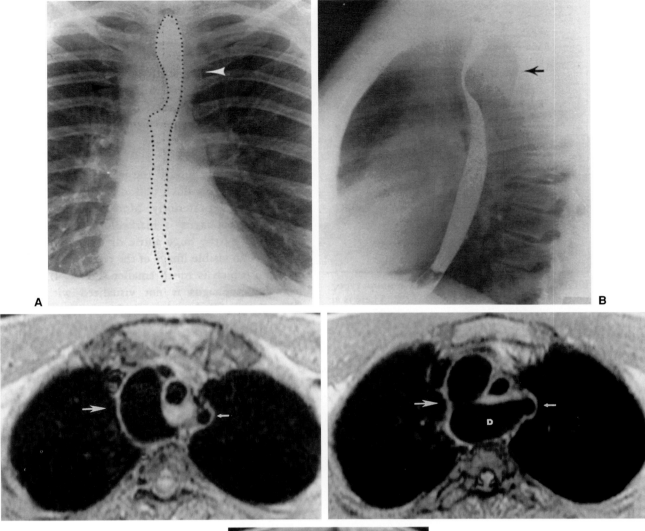

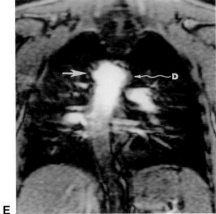

FIG. 16-73. PA (**A**) and lateral (**B**) views of a patient who was referred for evaluation of a right superior mediastinal mass. A: The RAA is marked by the black arrow. The barium-filled esophagus (*marked by dotted lines*) is deviated to the left side. The huge aortic diverticulum protrudes to the left of the midline (*white arrow*). B: The diverticulum (*arrow*) displaces the esophagus and the trachea anteriorly. The patient was otherwise well, and the radiographs showed normal results. Unnecessary surgery was avoided by the typical radiographic signs of type 3 RAA. Axial spin-echo MR images of another patient with the same conditions (**C,D**) show the RAA (*large arrow*) with huge retroesophageal diverticulum (D) giving rise to an aberrant left subclavian artery (ALSA) (*small arrow*). The coronal gradient-echo MR image (**E**) shows the RAA (*large arrow*) with the diverticulum (D) *spiral arrow*) extending to the left of the midline (compare with PA radiograph in A).

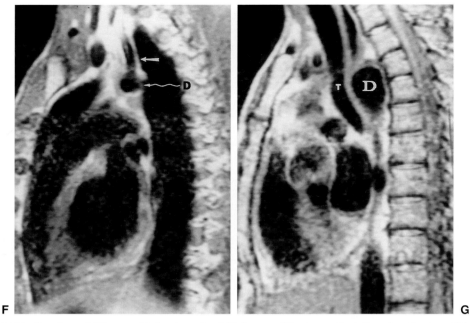

F   G

FIG. 16-73. *Continued.* The sagittal spin-echo MR image (**F**) shows that the diverticulum (D) (*spiral arrow*) gives rise to the aberrant left subclavian vein (*arrow*). Another, more medial sagittal spin-echo MR image (**G**) shows the huge diverticulum (D) displacing the trachea (T) forward (compare with lateral radiograph in B).

lateral view, and the following paradox may prove helpful. A normal lateral view is bad news; an abnormal lateral view is good news (or at least much better news).

Double Aortic Arch

A double aortic arch represents the persistence of Edwards' hypothetical aortic arch system (66). The right arch is typically higher, posterior, and larger than the left (Fig. 16-74). Both arches are usually functioning. As a rule, the aorta descends on the left side. On radiography, indentations are seen on both sides of the esophagus on the PA view

(Fig. 16-75A). On the lateral view the esophagus is displaced anteriorly by the larger right arch from behind; the trachea is displaced posteriorly by the smaller left arch from the front (Fig. 16-75B,C). The clinical importance of double aortic arch is twofold. First, it frequently causes compression symptoms in infants, but rarely creates any problem in adults until they are >60 years old. Second, this anomaly is not

TABLE 16-10. *Incidence of ICD in RAAs*

MIRROR (98%)
  TOF (90%)
  Truncus (2.5%)
  TGA (1.5%)
  L→R (0.5%)
ALSCA (<12%)
  TOF (71%)
  L→R (21%)
  CoA (7%)

ICD, intracardiac defects; RAAs, right aortic arch anomalies; TOF, tetralogy of Fallot; TGA, transposition of great arteries; L→R, left-to-right shunts; CoA, coarctation of aorta.

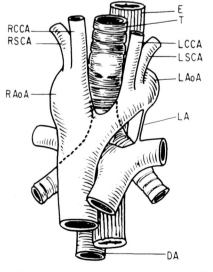

FIG. 16-74. Drawing of a double aortic arch. The brachiocephalic branches are symmetric, each arch giving rise to two separate arteries. LAoA, left aortic arch. Other abbreviations are the same as in Fig. 16-71.

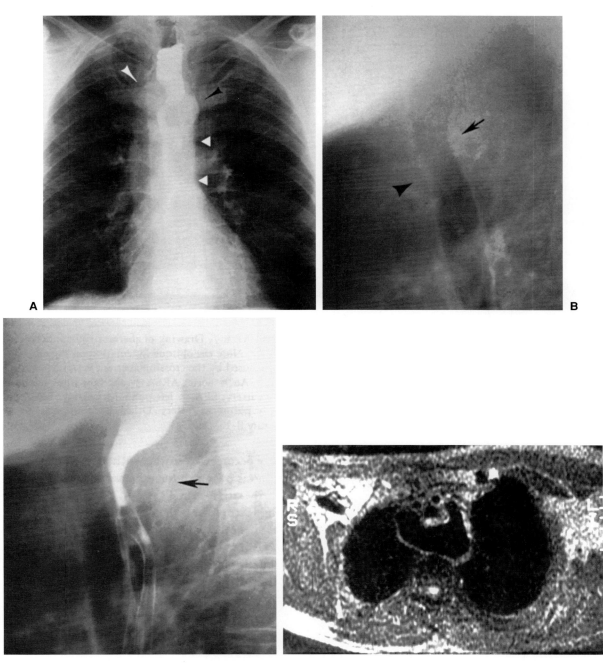

FIG. 16-75. A 52-year-old man was seen for evaluation of indigestion. A loose double aortic arch (DAA) was incidentally diagnosed with a barium swallow. On the PA view (**A**), the esophagus is indented bilaterally, by the right arch (*white long arrow*) superiorly and by the left arch (*black long arrow*) inferiorly. The common descending aorta (*short arrows*) is typically on the left side. On the lateral view (**B**), both the anterior wall (*arrowhead*) and the posterior wall (*arrow*) of the trachea are indented. On the lateral view with barium (**C**), the esophagus is indented and displaced forward by the right aortic arch (*arrow*). The same patient became symptomatic with dysphagia at age 64, when severe atherosclerotic changes caused the vascular ring to tighten. Taken for preoperative evaluation, the spin-echo MR image 3 cm below the sternal notch (**D**) shows a larger right-sided and posterior component and a smaller left-sided and anterior component of the double aortic arch. Both the esophagus and the trachea are compressed.

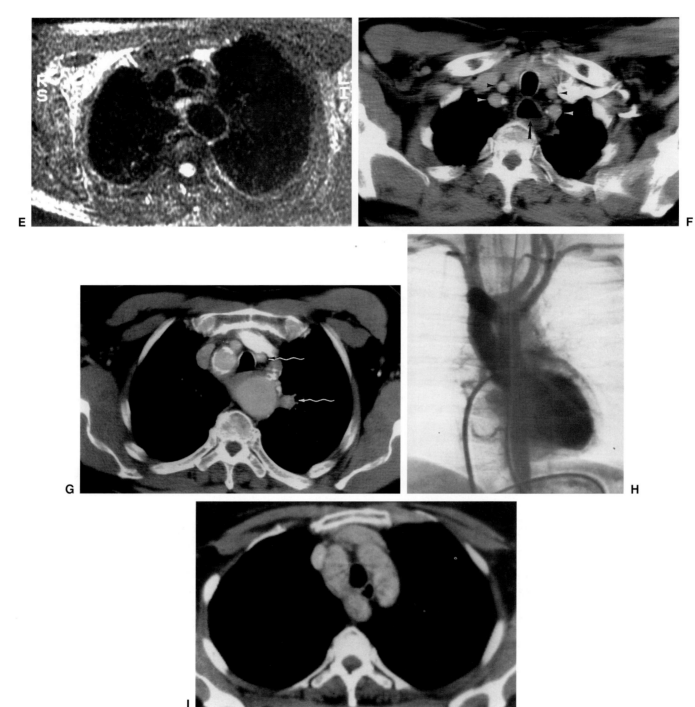

FIG. 16-75. *Continued.* The second MR image, ~1.5 cm lower (**E**), shows both arches beginning to converge to form their common ascending and descending aortae. Following ligation and division of his left arch between the left common carotid artery (LCCA) and the left subclavian artery (LSCA), his dysphagia improved but did not disappear. A postoperative CT scan above the sternal notch (**F**) shows two symmetrical pairs of brachiocephalic vessels (*arrowheads*), typical of double aortic arch. Also note the air-fluid level in the dilated esophagus (*arrow*). Another CT scan, 4 cm lower (**G**), shows that the esophagus is still somewhat compressed by the dilated and calcified double aortic arch. Note that the left common carotid artery (*upper arrow*) and left subclavian artery (*lower arrow*) are now far apart as a result of surgical division. The second patient was a child with compression symptoms. The subtraction aortogram (**H**) shows a rather typical double aortic arch, both arches functioning. Nasogastric and endotracheal tubes are enclosed in the vascular ring. The third patient, an asymptomatic adult (**I**), has the classic CT appearance of double aortic arch.

associated with an increased incidence of congenital heart disease (67).

Aberrant Right Subclavian Artery

Left aortic arch with aberrant right subclavian artery is a common anomaly, occurring in about one in 200 persons (67) (Figs. 16-76 and 16-77A,B). It results from breakage of the double aortic ring between the right common carotid artery and the right subclavian artery (Fig. 16-70). It is remarkable for its lack of clinical importance except in the following conditions.

When the aberrant right subclavian artery arises distal to a coarctation of the aorta in infants, it may be confused with severe aortic stenosis owing to the decreased or absent pulses in the right arm (17). In older children, the right arm blood pressures may be deceptively normal even when the coarctation is severe. Rib notching is seen only on the left side in this circumstance. The right subclavian artery serves as a large communicating channel between the arch and the descending aorta, eliminating the need for the usual collateral pathways on the right side.

Knowledge of this anomaly is important when using Sones' technique for coronary arteriography (69). If the right brachial artery is chosen for catheterizing the coronary arterial system, reaching the ascending aorta may be very difficult when aberrant right subclavian artery is present. Similarly, the pediatric cardiologist may encounter difficulties

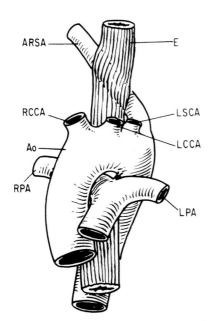

FIG. 16-76. Drawing of a left aortic arch with aberrant right subclavian artery. Note the oblique indentation on the esophagus caused by the aberrant vessel crossing from behind. Ao, aorta; ARSA, aberrant right subclavian artery; LPA, left pulmonary artery; RPA, right pulmonary artery. Other abbreviations are the same as in Fig. 16-71 (compare with Fig. 16-70).

catheterizing the ascending aorta via the right brachial artery. One of the reasons for obtaining radiographs with barium in the esophagus (Fig. 16-77A,B) before cardiac catheterization is to exclude the possibility of this anomaly. The diagnosis of this condition is readily made with CT or MRI (12–14).

In the elderly, an aneurysmal dilatation of the origin of the aberrant right subcvlavian artery, termed diverticulum of Kommerell, may cause compression symptoms (13) (Fig. 16-77C–G). Similar difficulties can sometimes appear in infants or young children; the condition is known as dysphagia lusoria (70).

Late Problems of Asymptomatic Arch Anomalies

Adult patients with double aortic arch, type 3 RAA, or left aortic arch with aberrant right subclavian artery usually show no signs of tracheal or esophageal compression as long as their arteries are young and pliable. However, as they age (when they reach the seventh decade) the once loose aortic ring begins to tighten up coincident with the development of severe atherosclerosis (13,71,72) (Figs. 16-75D–G and 16-77C–G).

CARDIAC MALPOSITIONS

According to Elliott and Schiebler, a cardiac malposition is present when the heart, the stomach, or both are out of the normal left-sided position (6). This definition helps clarify the possible confusion between RAA and cardiac malposition. In patients with a RAA, both the heart and the stomach are in the normal position. Before considering the possibility of cardiac malposition, hearts displaced by pulmonary, skeletal, or diaphragmatic disease should also be ruled out. And they should be termed dextroposition or levoposition of the heart instead. From the standpoint of statistical diagnosis, certain radiologic landmarks are important. They indicate, with a remarkable degree of accuracy, the position and the interrelationships of the cardiac chambers, the great arteries, and the abdominal viscera. These landmarks are the descending aorta (the aortic arch), the stomach, the venae cavae, the bronchi, and the liver.

With rare exceptions, there is visceroatrial concordance (17,73,74). The morphologic right atrium is found on the same side as the liver, inferior vena cava, eparterial bronchus, and trilobed lung; the left atrium is found on the side of the stomach, descending aorta, spleen, hyparterial bronchus, and bilobed lung (6,17,73). In other words, the position of the atria can be determined by the position of the abdominal viscera—hence the term visceroatrial situs (17,73–75).

Situs Solitus

Situs solitus means normal position of the heart and the abdominal and thoracic viscera. The PA radiograph shows

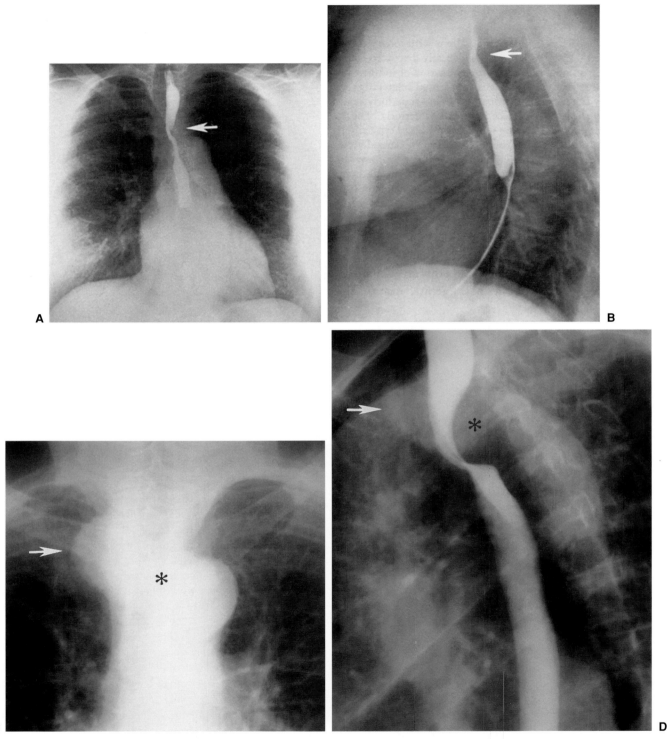

FIG. 16-77. PA (**A**) and lateral (**B**) views of an asymptomatic 55-year-old woman show evidence of an aberrant right subclavian artery. Note the oblique indentation on the esophagus posteriorly (*arrows*). Another patient, a 68-year-old woman, was examined because of dysphagia. Her PA (**C**) and left anterior oblique (**D**) radiographs, anteroposterior subtraction aortogram (**E**), and two CT scans (**F,G**) show a large diverticulum of Kommerell (*asterisk*) (D) displacing and compressing the esophagus forward. In addition, there is aneurysmal dilatation of the more distal segment of the vessel (*arrow*) more superiorly and to the right side.

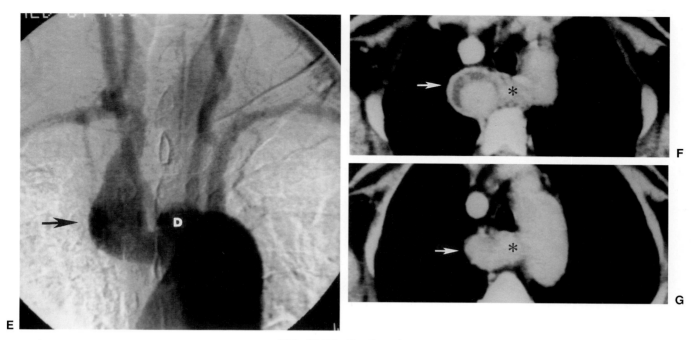

FIG. 16-77. *Continued.*

an aortic arch–gastric bubble concordance on the left side (5).

Situs Inversus

Situs inversus is the mirror image of situs solitus. The PA radiograph shows an aortic arch–gastric bubble concordance on the right side (5) (Fig. 16-78).

Situs Ambiguus

Situs ambiguus is the pattern of abnormal visceroatrial relationships in patients with a splenic malformation, a circumstance in which the laterality characteristics of the atria and other viscera are lost, making it impossible to identify the situs as being solitus or inversus by the usual radiologic landmarks (as described in the preceding paragraphs). Such patients tend to have a common atrium with bilateral left-sidedness or bilateral right-sidedness, depending on the type of splenic anomaly present (6,17,75) (Fig. 16-79) (Table 16-11).

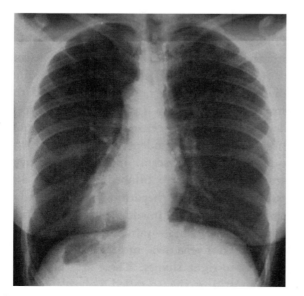

FIG. 16-78. PA view of an asymptomatic person with situs inversus and dextrocardia.

TABLE 16-11. *Asplenia vs. polysplenia syndrome*

Asplenia	Polysplenia
Bilateral right-sidedness	Bilateral left-sidedness
No spleen	Multiple small spleens
Heinz bodies in blood smear	No Heinz bodies in blood smear
Frequent hepatic symmetry	Less frequent
Frequent midline stomach	Less frequent
Frequent dextrocardia	Less frequent
Usually bilateral SVC	Frequently bilateral SVC
AO & IVC on same side	Normal
No	Enlarged AV or HAV
No	Interruption of IVC
Presents in early infancy	Often seen in adults
Severe cyanotic disease	Mild acyanotic disease
High mortality	Low mortality
Oligemia or PVH	Plethora or normal PBF

SVC, superior vena cava; AO, aorta; IVC, inferior vena cava; AV, azygous vein; HAV, hemiazygous vein; PVH, pulmonary venous hypertension; PBF, pulmonary blood flow.

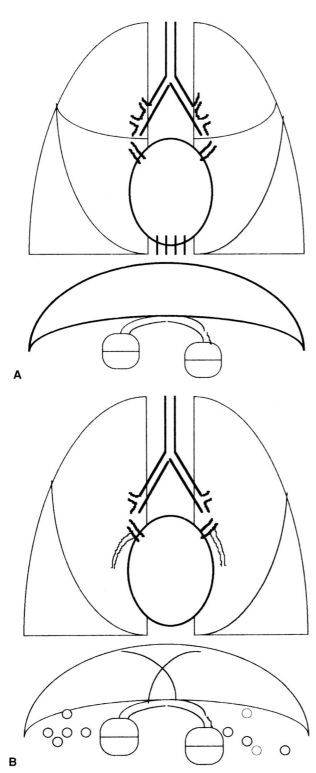

FIG. 16-79. Diagrams of anatomic features of thoracic and abdominal organs in patients with asplenia syndrome (**A**) and polysplenia syndrome (**B**). (Modified from Stanger P, Rudolph AM, Edwards JE. Cardiac malpositions: an overview based on study of 65 necropsy specimens. *Circulation* 1977; 56:159–172, and Kelley MJ, Jaffe CC, Kleinman CS. *Cardiac imaging in infants and children.* Philadelphia: Saunders, 1982.)

Levocardia

Levocardia simply means that the heart is on the left side. Levocardia can be associated with either situs solitus or inversus.

Levocardia with Situs Solitus

This is the normal arrangement, and the incidence of congenital heart disease is ~0.75%.

Levocardia with Situs Inversus

This is drastically abnormal and almost always associated with serious intracardiac defects (6,11,75,76), namely, L-TGA, VSD, and PS. This condition was previously termed levoversion, implying that the ventricular apex failed to swing to the right side to match all other right-sided structures (Fig. 16-80). This may be considered a mirror image of dextrocardia with situs solitus (discussed later).

Dextrocardia

Dextrocardia simply means that the heart is on the right side. It can be associated with situs solitus or inversus.

Dextrocardia with Situs Solitus

This combination is also drastically abnormal (75) and is associated with a 98% incidence of intracardiac defects. Of these defects, 85% are cyanotic anomalies (5,76). The most

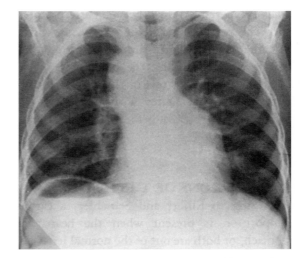

FIG. 16-80. PA radiograph of a patient with situs inversus with levocardia. Associated cardiac defects were VSD, PS, and L-TGA. Note that both the aorta and the stomach are right-sided, whereas the heart is left-sided.

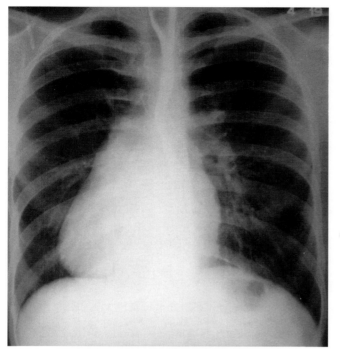

FIG. 16-81. A young adult with mild cyanotic heart disease (L-TGA + VSD + PS). His aorta and stomach are left-sided, whereas his heart is right-sided (situs solitus + dextrocardia).

common lesion is L-TGA. The next is a combination of VSD and PS (5,76). More frequently than not, all three are present simultaneously (Fig. 16-81; see also **Fig. 2-19**). This anomaly was previously termed dextroversion, implying a failure of the ventricular apex to swing to the left side as the last stage of cardiac development toward maturity in utero (5). In other words, the situs is normal, but the ventricles alone remain on the wrong side. The ventricles are likely to be twisted against all other normally positioned structures and, hence, the extremely high incidence of congenital heart disease (compare with levocardia with situs inversus).

Dextrocardia with Situs Inversus

This is a mirror image of normal (see Fig. 16-78). Because all structures are still normally related, except for a left-to-right reversal, there is only a threefold increase of congenital heart disease over the general population, from 0.75% to 2.5% (6). The so-called Kartagener's syndrome, or immotile cilia syndrome, represents a triad of dextrocardia, sinusitis, and bronchiectasis (77,78).

Asplenia Syndrome

Asplenia syndrome was first described by Ivemark (79) in 1955. There is agenesis of the spleen with Howell–Jolly

bodies in the erythrocytes. On radiology, situs ambiguus is seen, with a common atrium and bilateral right-sidedness of the viscera, including two eparterial bronchi, two trilobed lungs, two right pulmonary arteries, two superior venae cavae, absent or midline gallbladder, and hepatic symmetry (80). A specific angiographic finding is the presence of the inferior vena cava and abdominal aorta together on the same side of the spine (81). In contrast to polysplenia, patients with asplenia usually have cyanotic heart disease with decreased pulmonary vascularity (Figs. 16-79A, 16-82) and die in infancy (Table 16-11).

Polysplenia Syndrome

Polysplenia syndrome (80) is the most common anomaly associated with situs ambiguus in adults. Usually there is a combination of interruption of the hepatic segment of the inferior vena cave with azygos continuation, multiple small spleens, and left-to-right shunts (5). Patients with this syndrome are usually seen for treatment in childhood or adulthood, and they are acyanotic. Other unique features are a discordant aortic arch–gastric bubble relationship, and a tendency for bilateral left-sidedness of the viscera, including two hyparterial bronchi, two bilobed lungs, two left pulmonary arteries, hepatic symmetry, and a common atrium (Fig. 16-83) (Table 16-11) (6). The radiographic findings of interruption of the inferior vena cava with azygos continuation are a huge azygos arch and an absent image of the inferior vena cava in the lateral view (Figs. 16-79B and 16-83B).

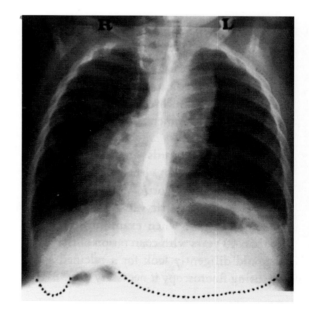

FIG. 16-82. Radiograph of an infant with asplenia syndrome. Note the hepatic symmetry (lower margin of the liver enhanced with dots). The pulmonary vascularity is decreased owing to TA with a restricted VSD. L, left side; R, right side.

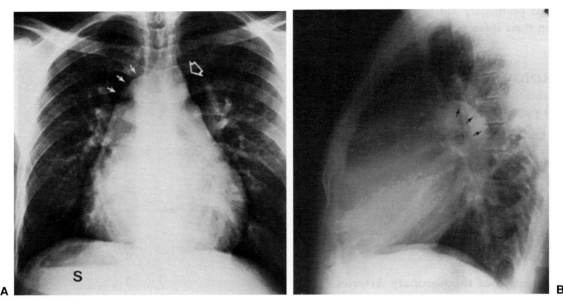

FIG. 16-83. PA (**A**) and lateral (**B**) radiographs of a patient with polysplenia syndrome. The hepatic segment of the inferior vena cava is interrupted with azygos continuation. Note the large azygos vein (*small arrows*) on both views, the left-sided aortic arch (*open arrow*), and the right-sided stomach (S). On the lateral view (**B**), the inferior vena cava image is not seen. Increased pulmonary vascularity is due to an atrial septal defect.

REFERENCES

1. Burrows PE, Smallhorn JF, Moes CAF. Congenital cardiovascular disease. In: Putman CE, Ravin CE, ed. *Textbook of diagnostic imaging*, 2nd ed. Philadelphia: Saunders, 1994:1739–1740.
2. Chen JTT, Khoury M, Kirks DR, et al. Obscured aortic arch on lateral radiographs in coarctation of aorta. *Radiology* 1984;153:595–596.
3. Chen JTT, Robinson AE, Goodrich FK, et al. Uneven distribution of pulmonary blood flow between left and right lungs in isolated pulmonary stenosis. *AJR Am J Roentgenol* 1969;107:343–350.
4. Edwards JE, Carey LS, Neufeld HN, Lester RG. *Congenital heart disease*. Philadelphia: Saunders, 1965.
5. Elliott LP, Jue KL, Amplatz K. A roentgen classification of cardiac malpositions. *Invest Radiol* 1966;1:17–28.
6. Elliott LP, Schiebler GL. *The x-ray diagnosis of congenital heart disease in infants, children, and adults*, 2nd ed. Springfield, Ill.: Thomas, 1979.
7. Kelley MJ, Jaffe CC, Kleinman CS. *Cardiac imaging in infants and children*. Philadelphia: Saunders, 1982.
8. Steiner RM, Gross GW, Flicker S, et al. Congenital heart disease in the adult patient: the value of plain film chest radiology. *J Thorac Imaging* 1995;10:1–25.
9. Bierman FZ, Williams RG. Prospective diagnosis of D-transposition of the great arteries in neonates by subxiphoid two-dimensional echocardiography. *Circulation* 1979;60:1496–1502.
10. Kirks DR. *Practical pediatric imaging*, 2nd ed. Boston: Little, Brown, 1991.
11. Perloff JK. *The clinical recognition of congenital heart disease*, 4th ed. Philadelphia: Saunders, 1994.
12. Husayni TS. UFCT imaging in congenital heart disease. In: Stanford W, Rumberger JA, eds. *Ultrafast computed tomography in cardiac imaging: principles and practice*. New York: Futura, 1992.
13. Vandyke CW, White RD. Congenital abnormalities of the thoracic aorta presenting in the adult. *J Thorac Imaging* 1994;9:230–245.
14. Bisset GS. Magnetic resonance imaging of congenital heart disease in the pediatric patient. *Radiol Clin North Am* 1991;29:279–291.
15. Vesely TM, Julsrud PR, Brown JJ. MR imaging of partial anomalous pulmonary venous connections. *J Comput Assist Tomogr* 1991;15:752–756.
16. Perloff JK, LeBauer EJ, Miall A, et al. Differential quantification of pulmonary arterial flow in left-to-right shunt atrial septal defect using ^{131}I macroaggregated albumin [Abstract]. *Am J Cardiol* 1969;23:132.
17. Nugent EW, Plauth WH, Edwards JE, et al. Congenital heart disease. In: Schlant RC, Alexander RW, ed. *The heart*, 8th ed. New York: McGraw–Hill, 1994:580–728.
18. Krovetz LJ, Gessner IH, Schiebler GL. *Handbook of pediatric cardiology*. New York: Hoeber–Harper, 1981.
19. Alpert BS, Cook DH, Varghese PJ, et al. Spontaneous closure of small ventricular septal defects: 10-year follow-up. *Pediatrics* 1979;63:204–206.
20. Kirklin JW, Harshbarger HG, Donald DE. Surgical correlation of ventricular septal defect: anatomy and technical considerations. *J Thorac Surg* 1957;33:45–59.
21. Blackstone EH, Kirklin JW, Bradley EL, et al. Optional age and results in repair of large ventricular defects. *J. Thorac. Cardiovasc. Surg* 1976;72:661–679.
22. Rudolph AM. *Congenital diseases of the heart*. Chicago: Year Book, 1974.
23. Elliott LP, Bargeron LM, Bream PR, et al. Axial cineangiography in congenital heart disease. *Circulation* 1977;56:1084–1093.
24. Moller JH, Anderson RC. 1,000 consecutive children with a cardiac malformation with 26- to 37-year follow-up. *Am J Cardiol* 1992;70:661–667.
25. Speechly-Dick ME, John R, Pugsley WB, et al. Secundum atrial septal defect repair: long-term surgical outcome and the problem of late mitral regurgitation. *Postgrad Med* 1993;69:912–915.
26. Kiely B, Filler J, Stone S. Syndrome of anomalous venous drainage of the right lung to the inferior vena cava: a review of 67 reported cases and three new cases in children. *Am J Cardiol* 1967;20:102–116.
27. Holt M, Oram S. Familial heart disease with skeletal malformations. *Br Heart J* 1960;22:236–242.
28. Gedgaudas E, Moller JH, Castabeda-Zuniga WR, et al. *Cardiovascular radiology*. Philadelphia: Saunders, 1985.
29. Bergin ML, Warnes CA, Tajik MA, et al. Partial atrioventricular canal defect: long-term follow-up after initial repair in patients ≥40 years old. *J Am Coll Cardiol* 1995;25:1189–1194.
30. Higgins CB, Rausch J, Friedman WF, et al. Patent ductus arteriosus in preterm infants with idiopathic respiratory distress syndrome: radiographic and echocardiographic evaluation. *Radiology* 1977;124:189–195.

31. Swischuk LE. *Plain film interpretation in congenital heart disease*, 2nd ed. Baltimore: Williams & Wilkins, 1979.

32. Fisher E, Paul MH. Transposition of the great arteries: recognition and management. *Cardiovasc Clin* 1970;2:211–230.

33. Mustard WT. Successful two-staged correction of transposition of the great vessels. *Surgery* 1964;55:469–472.

34. Dunn JM. Jatene's arterial repair for transposition of the great vessels. *Ann Thorac Surg* 1991;51:511–514.

35. Sabiston DC, ed. *Textbook of surgery*, 4th ed. Philadelphia: Saunders, 1991.

36. Roberts WC, ed. *Congenital heart disease in adults*, Philadelphia: Davis, 1979.

37. Neufeld HN, Lucas RV Jr, Lester RG, et al. Origin of both great vessels from right ventricle without pulmonary stenosis. *Br Heart J* 1962;24:393–408.

38. Van Praagh R, Perez-Trevino C, Reynolds JL, et al. Double outlet right ventricle with subaortic ventricular septal defect and pulmonary stenosis. *Am J Cardiol* 1975;35:42–53.

39. Hallermann FJ, Kincaid OW, Tsakiris AG, et al. Persistent truncus arteriosus: a radiographic and angiographic study. *AJR Am J Roentgenol* 1969;107:827–834.

40. Collett RW, Edwards JE. Persistent truncus arteriosus: a classification according to anatomic types. *Surg Clin North Am* 1949;29:1245–1270.

41. Sotomora RF, Edwards JE. Anatomic identification of so-called absent pulmonary artery. *Circulation* 1978;57:624–633.

42. Gatham GE, Nadas AS. Total anomalous pulmonary venous connection: clinical and physiologic observations of 75 pediatric patients. *Circulation* 1970;42:143–154.

43. Rodriguez-Collado JR, Attie F, Zabal C, et al. Total anomalous pulmonary venous connection in adults: long-term follow-up. *J Thorac Cardiovasc Surg* 1992;103:877–880.

44. Elliott LP, Anderson RC, Edwards JE. The common cardiac ventricle with transposition of the great vessels. *Br Heart J* 1964;26:289–301.

45. Keith JD, Rowe RD, Vlad P. *Heart disease in infancy and childhood*, 3rd ed. New York: Macmillan, 1978.

46. Charuzi Y, Spanos PK, Amplatz K, et al. Juxtaposition of the atrial appendages. *Circulation* 1973;47:620–627.

47. Hurst JW, Morris DC. The history: symptoms and past events related to cardiovascular disease. In: Schlant RC, Alexander RW, eds. *The heart*, 8th ed. New York: McGraw–Hill, 1994:205–216.

48. Bando K, Danielson GK, Schaff HV, et al. Outcome of pulmonary and aortic homografts for right ventricular outflow tract reconstruction. *J Thorac Cardiovasc Surg* 1995;109:509–518.

49. Murphy JG, Gersh BJ, Mair DD, et al. Long-term outcome in patients undergoing surgical repair of tetralogy of Fallot. *N Engl J Med* 1993;329:593–599.

50. Gyepes MT, Vincent WR. *Cardiac catheterization and angiocardiography in severe neonatal heart disease*. Springfield, Ill.: Thomas, 1974.

51. Reul GJ, Gregoric ID. Recent modifications of the Fontan procedure for complex congenital heart disease. *Tex Heart Inst J* 1992;19:223–231.

52. Netter FH. *Heart: the Ciba collection of medical illustrations*, vol. 5 Summit, N.J.: Ciba, 1969:133–164.

53. Bialostozky D, Horwitz S, Espino-Vela J. Ebstein's malformation of the tricuspid valve. *Am J Cardiol* 1972;29:826–836.

54. Nadas AS. *Pediatric cardiology*, 3rd ed. Philadelphia: Saunders, 1972.

55. Maron BJ. Coarctation of the aorta in the adult. In: Roberts WC, ed. *Congenital heart disease in adults*. Philadelphia: Davis, 1979.

56. Edwards JE. The congenital bicuspid aortic valve. *Circulation* 1961; 23:485–488.

57. Nanton MA, Olley PM. Residual hypertension after coarctectomy in children. *Am J Cardiol* 1976;37:769–772.

58. Campbell M, Baylis JH. Course and prognosis of coarctation of aorta. *Br Heart J* 1956;18:475–495.

59. Figley M. Accessory roentgen signs of coarctation of the aorta. *Radiology* 1954;62:671–686.

60. Holman E. On circumscribed dilatation of an artery immediately distal to a partially occluding band: poststenotic dilatation. *Surgery* 1954;36:3–24.

61. Angelini P. Embryology and congenital heart disease. *Tex Heart Inst J* 1995;22:1–12.

62. Castaneada-Zuniga WR, Formanek A, Amplatz K. Radiologic diagnosis of different types of pulmonary stenoses. *Cardiovasc Radiol* 1977;1:2–14.

63. O'Laughlin MP, Mullins CE. Balloon dilation and stenting of hypoplastic pulmonary arteries. *Tex Heart Inst J* 1992;19:185–189.

64. Fraser RG, Pare JA. *Diagnosis of diseases of the chest*, 2nd ed. Philadelphia: Saunders, 1977:640–645.

65. Gomes AS, Mali WP, Oppenheimer WL. Embolization therapy in the management of congenital arteriovenous malformations. *Radiology* 1982;144:41–49.

66. Stewart JR, Kincaid OW, Edwards JE. *An atlas of vascular rings and related malformations of the aortic arch system*. Springfield, Ill.: Thomas, 1964.

67. Shuford WH, Sybers RG. *The aortic arch and its malformations*. Springfield, Ill.: Thomas, 1974.

68. Stewart JR, Kincaid OW, Titus JL. Right aortic arch: plain film diagnosis and significance. *Am J Roentgenol* 1966;97:377–889.

69. Sones FM, Shirey EK. Cine coronary arteriography. *Mod Concepts Cardiovasc Dis* 1962;31:735–738.

70. Gross RE. Surgical treatment for dysphagia lusoria. *Ann Surg* 1946; 124:532–534.

71. Copleman B. Anomalous right subclavian artery. *AJR Am J Roentgenol* 1945;54:270–275.

72. Harrison LH, Batson RC, Hunter DR. Aberrant right subclavian artery aneurysm: an analysis of surgical options. *Ann Surg* 1994;57:1012–1014.

73. Bream PR. Case 27: questions 94 through 97. In: Cooley RN, Capp MP, Lester RG, et al. *Plain film diagnosis of cardiovascular disease syllabus*. Chicago: American College of Radiology, 1979:293–303.

74. Keith J, Rees S. *Clinical cardiac radiology*. London: Butterworth, 1973:139–240.

75. Winer-Muram HT. Adult presentation of heterotaxic syndromes and related complexes. *J Thorac Imaging* 1995;10:43–57.

76. Schad N. Congenital anomalies of the heart and great vessels. In: Schinz HR, ed. *Roentgen diagnosis*. New York: Grune & Stratton, 1970:30–331.

77. Gershoni-Baruch R, Gottfried E, Pery M, et al. Immotile cilia syndrome. *Am J Med Genet* 1989;33:390–393.

78. Katz M, Benzier EE, Nangeroni L, et al. Kartagener's syndrome. *N Engl J Med* 1953;248:730–731.

79. Ivemark BL. Implications of agenesis of the spleen on the pathogenesis of cono-truncus anomalies in childhood. *Acta Paediatr* 1955;44(suppl. 104):590–592.

80. Stanger P, Rudolph AM, Edwards JE. Cardiac malpositions: an overview based on study of 65 necropsy specimens. *Circulation* 1977;56:159–172.

81. Elliott LP, Cramer GG, Amplatz K. The anomalous relationships of the inferior vena cava and abdominal aorta as a specific angiographic sign in asplenia. *Radiology* 1966;87:859–863.

Essentials of Cardiac Imaging,
James T. T. Chen,
Lippincott–Raven Publishers, Philadelphia © 1998.

CHAPTER 17

Cardiac Pacemakers and Prosthetic Valves

James T. T. Chen

Artificial cardiac pacing and valve replacement are now commonplace (1–4). Radiologic examinations play an important role in ensuring the proper placement and function of various pacemakers and valve prostheses. All parts of pacemakers and most elements of prosthetic valves are readily identified on the chest radiograph. Fluoroscopic observations (5) and cine radiographic examinations (6) of these devices help detect obscure causes of their malfunctions.

CARDIAC PACEMAKERS

The first clinical trial of cardiac pacing was reported in 1952, when a patient in ventricular asystole was successfully resuscitated by external electric stimulation (1,7). In the past three decades, considerable advances in pacemaker systems have been made. At the present time, in the United States alone, at least 500,000 patients have implanted pacemakers (2). The purposes of cardiac pacing are to correct bradycardias and tachycardias and to diagnose arrhythmias by pace-mapping various atrial and ventricular sites.

The essential parts of a pacemaker are the pulse generator as the power source, the conducting wires, and the electrodes by which the electric stimuli are delivered to the myocardium or the endocardium. The electrodes and the wires are collectively called the pacing lead. Pacemakers may be used either temporarily or permanently. To deliver the stimuli to the myocardium, the electrodes are implanted transmediastinally to the atrial or ventricular wall or both (1,8). When the stimuli are directed to the endocardium, the electrodes are introduced transvenously into the right atrium or ventricle or both.

The pacemakers are capable of performing two functions: stimulating (pacing) the heart and recognizing (sensing) the intrinsic cardiac impulses. The information obtained by sensing is used to modulate the timing of the succeeding stimulus to ensure its responsiveness to and coordination with the spontaneous cardiac electrical events. Two kinds of pacing electrodes are the bipolar and the unipolar systems. In bipolar systems, both the anode and cathode electrodes are placed in the heart. In unipolar systems, the cathode alone is placed in the heart with the anode located away from the heart, as is the metallic housing of the pulse generator.

Right Ventricular Pacing

The most commonly implanted pacemaker is the demand ventricular pacemaker (2). It recognizes ventricular activity and stimulates the ventricle only when needed. The proper position of the electrodes of such a pacer is shown by line b in Fig. 17-1 and by the ventricular lead b in Fig. 17-2.

In the posteroanterior (PA) radiograph, the tip of the pacing lead should be at, but medial to, the right ventricular apex, which is located at about the midpoint between the midline of the thorax and the apex of the heart, in the absence of marked right ventricular enlargement. The electrodes in this position are usually entrapped by the trabeculae and move synchronously with and at the same amplitude as the right ventricular wall. Any excessive movement within the cardiac chamber denotes dislodgment of the electrodes. When the tip of the pacing lead moves beyond the confines of the right ventricular apex, myocardial perforation should be suspected; the more lateral the displacement of the electrodes, the more likely it is that such a complication has occurred.

Since the interventricular septum near the cardiac apex is much thicker than the right ventricular wall, the electrodes usually enter the pericardium (Fig. 17-1A, line c; Fig. 17-3A) rather than the left ventricle. Under the fluoroscope, excessive or erratic movements of the electrodes are observed. Such movements are asynchronous with those of the ventricle. The electric stimuli may be delivered to the diaphragm instead of the ventricle; the pacemaker may continue to work, work intermittently, or fail altogether. The

Department of Radiology, Duke University School of Medicine, Durham, North Carolina 27710, U.S.A.

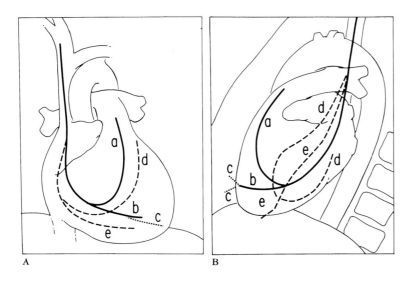

FIG. 17-1. PA (**A**) and lateral (**B**) representation of catheter positions in ventricular and atrial pacing (see text for discussion). (Reproduced with permission from Hewitt MJ, Chen JTT, Ravin CE, Gallagher JJ. Coronary sinus atrial pacing: radiographic considerations. *Am J Roentgenol* 1981;136:323–328.)

position of the electrodes in the pulmonary artery is readily determined with the lead sitting in either the pulmonary trunk or one of its branches (see Fig. 17-1A, line a). Such malpositions are accompanied by failure to pace.

In the lateral projection, the tip of the pacing lead normally appears behind the sternum, immediately above the anterior costophrenic sulcus, interior and posterior to the subepicardial fat stripe, which is the divider between the pericardium and the myocardium (Fig. 17-1B, line b; and Fig. 17-2B,

lead b). Once the tip gets beyond the fat plane, it has penetrated the myocardium and intruded into the pericardium (9) (Fig. 17-3B). Further protrusion from the chamber may cause the lead to deflect upward or downward (Fig. 17-1B, dotted line c; and Fig. 17-3B). The position of the lead in the pulmonary artery is indicated by line a in Fig. 17-1.

Most right ventricular perforations are not accompanied by notable bleeding, and no specific treatment is indicated other than withdrawal of the lead and proper repositioning

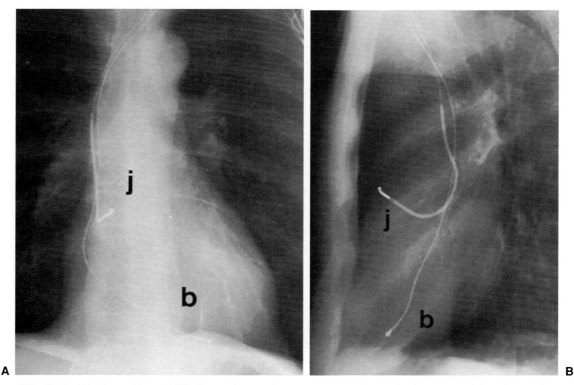

FIG. 17-2. PA (**A**) and lateral (**B**) views of normal transvenous atrioventricular sequential pacing catheters. j, atrial lead; b, ventricular lead.

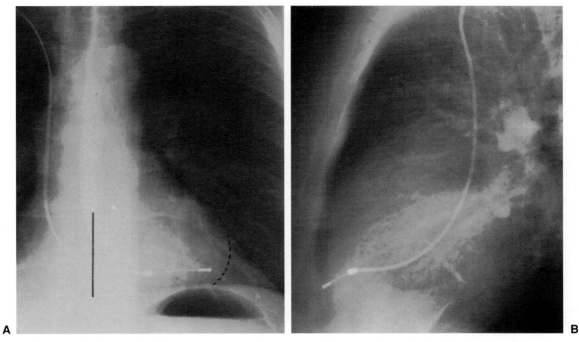

FIG. 17-3. Patients with right ventricular perforation. **A:** PA view of a patient with pacemaker failure. The pacing catheter is situated beyond the confines of the right ventricle. The tip of the pacing lead is too far left from the midline (*solid line*), approaching the left ventricular apex (*broken line*). **B:** Lateral view of another patient with pacing failure. The tip of the electrode is obviously outside the myocardium, going through the subepicardial fat stripe into the pericardium.

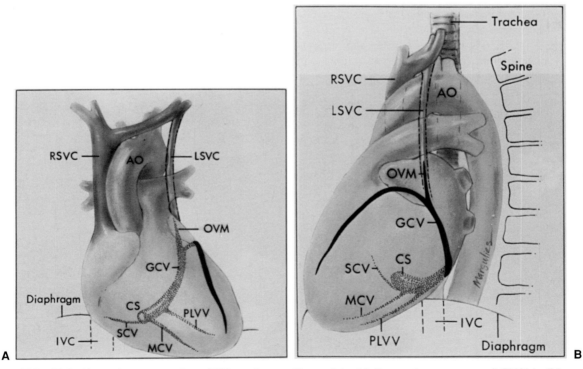

FIG. 17-4. Normal coronary sinus (CS) anatomy with persistent left superior vena cava (LSVC) in PA (**A**) and lateral (**B**) projections. The aorta (AO), great cardiac vein (GCV), inferior vena cava (IVC), middle cardiac vein (MCV), oblique vein of Marshall (OVM), posterior left ventricular vein (PLVV), right superior vena cava (RSVC), and small cardiac vein (SCV) are visible. (Reproduced with permission from Hewitt MJ, Chen JTT, Ravin CE, Gallagher JJ. Coronary sinus atrial pacing: radiographic considerations. *AJR Am J Roentgenol* 1981;136:323–328.)

(10). In rare instances, however, such myocardial penetrations may result in cardiac tamponade requiring emergency treatment.

Coronary Sinus Atrial Pacing

Transvenous atrial pacing through the coronary sinus has become popular for both diagnosis and therapy of cardiac arrhythmias. Atrial and atrioventricular sequential pacing has the advantage of restoring natural cardiac function and output by preserving atrioventricular synchrony (1).

The coronary sinus is the persistent left horn of the sinus venosus (11). It enters the atrioventricular groove posteriorly from the right atrium and continues to run in the groove for a distance of ~23 mm before becoming the great cardiac vein. In addition to the great cardiac vein, the tributaries of the coronary sinus are small cardiac, middle cardiac, posterior left ventricular, and anterior interventricular veins. In patients with persistent left superior vena cava, the oblique vein of Marshall is open, channeling blood downward from the junction of the left jugular and left brachiocephalic veins to the coronary sinus (Fig. 17-4).

The electrodes in coronary sinus pacing may be seen in any of the tributaries of the coronary sinus, but most commonly in either the great cardiac vein (Fig. 17-5) or the middle cardiac vein (Fig. 17-6). Since all cardiac veins, including the coronary sinus, are embedded in the subepicardial fat stripes (12), the electrodes within the veins are actually outside the myocardium when viewed in tangent on the radiograph (Figs. 17-5B, and 17-6B). This appearance should not be misinterpreted as myocardial penetration.

As the pacing lead passes from the right atrium through the coronary sinus into the great cardiac vein, it runs in the left atrioventricular groove, forming a smooth curve leftward, posteriorly, and superiorly (Fig. 17-5). Such a typical radiographic appearance helps prevent echocardiographic misdiagnosis of the coronary sinus pacer lead as a left atrial mass (13).

As the lead extends from the coronary sinus into the middle cardiac vein, it pursues a route lower than the tricuspid valve, extending more laterally and inferiorly from the right ventricular apex in the PA view and more inferiorly and posteriorly in the lateral view. In either view, the electrodes are more peripheral in position, lying between the myocardium and the pericardium within the fat stripe in the posterior interventricular groove (Fig. 17-6). The middle cardiac vein pacer lead may seem as though it is in a right ventricular position on the PA view (compare Fig. 17-2A with Fig. 17-6A). For that reason, the lateral view in this situation is more helpful than the PA view.

Right Atrial Pacing

Another site of atrial pacing is the right atrial appendage. The J-shaped lead can be easily manipulated into the appendage under the fluoroscope in the lateral projection. The tip of the lead should be pointing anteriorly and upward in this view. As soon as this is accomplished, the position of the lead should be double-checked in the PA view, where the tip should be pointing upward and medially (14) (Fig. 17-2, lead j).

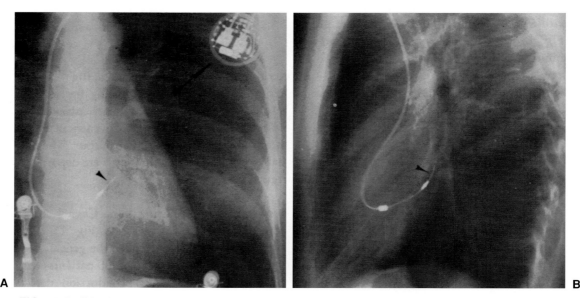

A   **B**

FIG. 17-5. PA (**A**) and lateral (**B**) views of the normal position of the coronary sinus catheter with its tip in the great cardiac vein. The flexible tip (*short arrow*) extends beyond the electrode to prevent dislodgment and to avoid ventricular pacing. Attached to the chest wall is the radiofrequency pacemaker control (*long arrow*). In the lateral view (B), the wire appears to be quite peripheral (*short arrow*) in position, lying in the subepicardial fat along the left atrioventricular groove.

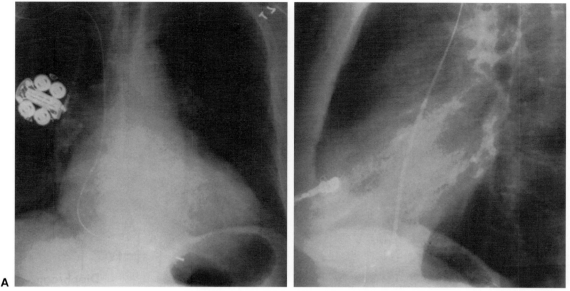

FIG. 17-6. PA (**A**) and lateral (**B**) views of a pacing catheter in the middle cardiac vein. Note the position of the pacing lead lower than the tricuspid valve, with its tip in the subepicardial fat outside the myocardium on both views; note also the straight course of the pacing lead and its anterior turn at the termination on the lateral view. (Reproduced with permission from Hewitt MJ, Chen JTT, Ravin CE, Gallagher JJ. Coronary sinus atrial pacing: radiographic considerations. *AJR Am J Roentgenol* 1981; 136:323–328.)

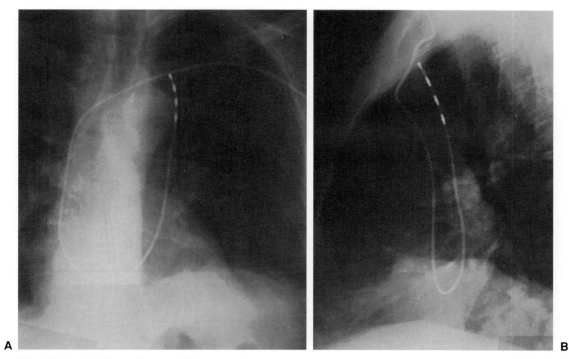

FIG. 17-7. PA (**A**) and lateral (**B**) views of a pacing catheter in a patient with persistent left superior vena cava. Note that the catheter is inserted from the left basilic vein. After passing through the left brachiocephalic vein, the right superior vena cava, the right atrium, the coronary sinus, and the persistent left superior vena cava, the catheter tip goes back to the junction between the persistent left superior vena cava and the left brachiocephalic vein. (Reproduced with permission from Hewitt MJ, Chen JTT, Ravin CE, Gallagher JJ. Coronary sinus atrial pacing: radiographic considerations. *AJR Am J Roentgenol* 1981;136:323–328.)

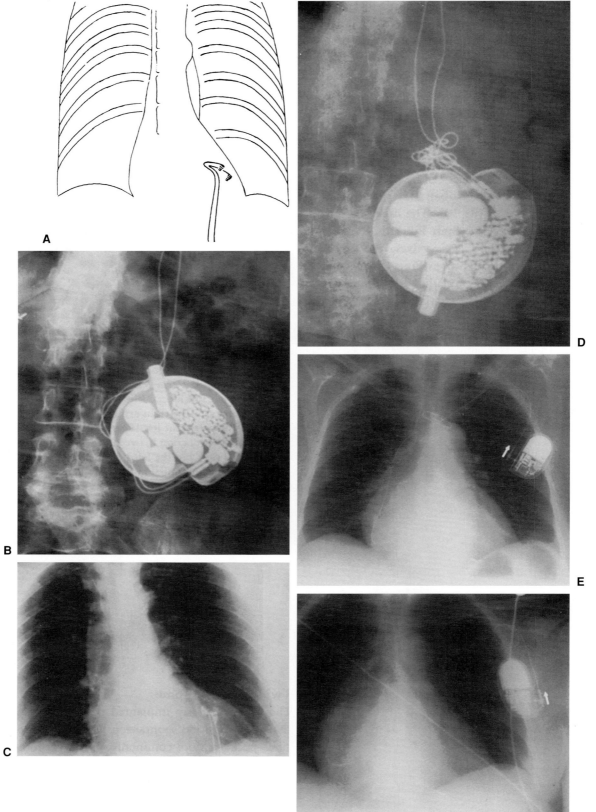

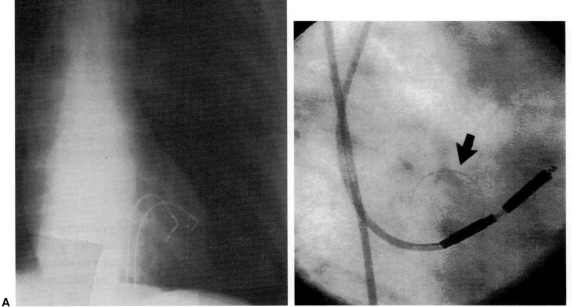

FIG. 17-9. Patients with fractured pacing leads. **A:** PA view of the first patient shows fractured electrodes of a transmediastinal pacemaker. **B:** Digital fluoroscopic image in the right anterior oblique view from the second patient with fractured retention wire (*arrow*) almost totally extruded through insulation. (Reproduced with permission from Lloyd MA, Hayes DL, Stanson AW, et al. Snare removal of a Telectronics Accufix atrial J retention wire. *Mayo Clin Proc* 1995;70:376–379.)

Atrioventricular Sequential Pacing

Atrioventricular sequential pacing has recently become preferred to right ventricular pacing for preserving normal atrioventricular synchrony and raising cardiac output (1). The normal positions of the pacing leads are depicted in Fig. 17-2. Persistent left superior vena cava (Fig. 17-7) occurs in 0.28% to 0.50% of the general population and in 4.50% of patients with congenital atrioventricular conduction defects (11).

Transmediastinal Pacing

In addition to the transvenous pacing techniques already discussed, the transmediastinal approach can be used by placing the electrodes directly into the left ventricular myo-cardium (Figs. 17-8 and 17-9). This is accomplished either by open thoracotomy or via the percutaneous approach through the chest wall (1,8).

Twiddler's Syndrome

The subcutaneously implanted pacemaker may change its position spontaneously within a spacious pocket. More commonly, however, rotation of the pulse generator results from the patient's habit of twiddling the pacemaker, which causes displacement or breakage of the electrodes and failure to pace (15) (Fig. 17-8A–D). When the pulse generator is implanted in the pectoral region, a twiddling-induced 180° flip (Fig. 17-8E,F) may cause stimulation of the pectoralis muscle, demand pacemaker myopotential inhibition, and failed or aberrant programming and interrogation. Radiographic

FIG. 17-8. Patients with twiddler's syndrome. **A:** Line drawing of the PA view of the first patient shortly after implantation of a transmediastinal pacemaker. Note the normal curve of the pacing wires and electrodes. **B:** Abdominal film taken 1 year after initial implant shows a normal relationship between the wires and the impulse generator. **C:** Four years later, after the patient manifested symptoms of pacemaker malfunction. Note the stretched wires, absence of previous curve, and closer electrodes. **D:** Film taken 2 years later shows a 180° rotation of the impulse generator. Wires close to the generator are twisted. (Reproduced with permission from Rodan BA, Lowe JE, Chen JTT. Abdominal twiddler's syndrome. *AJR Am J Roentgenol* 1978;131:1084–1085.) **E:** PA radiograph of the second patient immediately after insertion of a pacemaker shows clockwise exit of pacing leads (*parallel to arrow*). **F:** A second radiograph after pulse-generator flip shows counterclockwise exit of pacing leads (*parallel to arrow*). (Reproduced with permission from Karis JP, Ravin CE. Counterclockwise exit of cardiac pacemaker leads: sign of pulse–generator flip. *Radiology* 1990;174:711–712.)

evidence of such a flip is a counterclockwise, instead of the normal clockwise, exit of the pacemaker leads (16).

Fracture of the Lead

Breakage of a pacing wire or electrode is uncommon with the newer models of pacemakers. It usually occurs at a fixation point: near the generator, across the intercostal space, or at the point of insertion (Fig. 17-9A). Breakage of a wire within an intact cover of insulating material frequently escapes radiographic examination, which mostly encompasses diastolic images. In systole under the fluoroscope, however, such subtle fractures may become conspicuous when the fractured fragments form an angulation at the point of breakage (10). A recall of the Telectronics Accufix atrial J leads (models 330-801 and 329-701) has been issued because of reports of fracture and extrusion of the J-shaped retention wire (5) (Fig. 17-9B). More than 42,000 of these leads have been implanted worldwide. Detection and prompt treatment of such fractures are mandatory if serious, even fatal, consequences are to be avoided. Because of its small size, the retention wire is not visible on chest radiography, echocardiography, computed tomography, or cardiac catheterization. Digital fluoroscopy turned out to be the diagnostic tool of choice. The best treatment has been snare removal of the wire alone, leaving the atrial lead intact (5).

Implantable Cardioverter–Defibrillator

For nearly a decade, the implantable cardioverter–defibrillator (ICD) has been used for the prevention of sudden death in ambulatory patients with malignant ventricular arrhythmias. Newer and more simple devices with diagnostic and therapeutic capabilities continue to be made (17). One of the nonthoracotomy lead systems in use at present is the Endotak system. It consists of a transvenous endocardial electrode and a subcutaneous rectangular patch electrode. In some patients, however, the defibrillation thresholds may be achieved using the endocardial electrode alone (Fig. 17-10). The radiographic aspects of most ICDs have been reviewed and illustrated in the literature (6,18). Most recently, a single transvenous lead system with consistently low defibrillation thresholds has been described (19). With that system a subcutaneous patch is no longer needed. The new ICD pulse generator is small enough to be implanted in the subpectoral area (20). This approach is better than the cumbersome abdominal placement.

PROSTHETIC VALVES

Since the advent of open heart surgery more than three decades ago, an increasing number of patients have benefited from cardiac valve replacement. Despite continued improvements in the design and engineering of prosthetic valves,

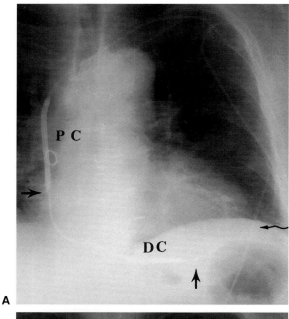

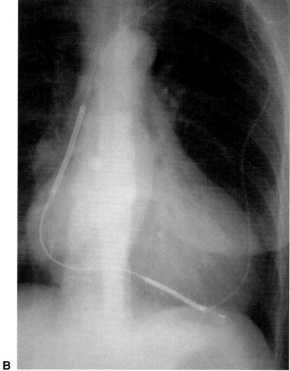

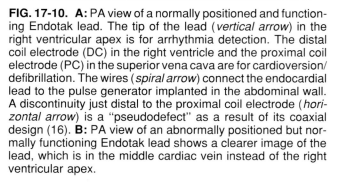

FIG. 17-10. A: PA view of a normally positioned and functioning Endotak lead. The tip of the lead (*vertical arrow*) in the right ventricular apex is for arrhythmia detection. The distal coil electrode (DC) in the right ventricle and the proximal coil electrode (PC) in the superior vena cava are for cardioversion/defibrillation. The wires (*spiral arrow*) connect the endocardial lead to the pulse generator implanted in the abdominal wall. A discontinuity just distal to the proximal coil electrode (*horizontal arrow*) is a "pseudodefect" as a result of its coaxial design (16). **B:** PA view of an abnormally positioned but normally functioning Endotak lead shows a clearer image of the lead, which is in the middle cardiac vein instead of the right ventricular apex.

none of the currently used prostheses is considered ideal. Radiology is important in identifying an artificial valve and detecting its malfunctions (3,4,21–26).

Classification

At present two basic types of cardiac valve prostheses are in use: mechanical and tissue. Mechanical valves, though more durable than tissue valves (3,4,27,28) have the disadvantage of requiring permanent anticoagulation (27). Tissue valves, on the other hand, have a much lower associated

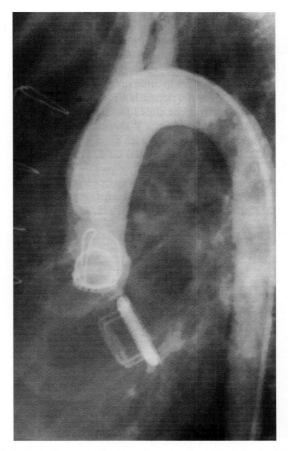

FIG. 17-12. Normal lateral aortogram showing a Beall caged-disk valve in the mitral position and a Starr–Edwards caged-ball valve in the aortic position.

rate of thrombogenicity, eliminating the need for long-term anticoagulants (27). The main drawback of tissue valves is their tendency to early breakdown, necessitating surgical replacement within a few years (28). This problem is most serious in children and patients on ongoing hemodialysis, in whom calcific valvular stenosis develops often and rapidly (3,4,28–30).

Identification

Mechanical prostheses can be divided into three categories (3,4,29,31): caged ball, caged disk, and tilting disk. The caged-ball type is represented by the Starr–Edwards (Fig. 17-11) and the Smellof–Cutter valves, the caged-disk type by the Beall valve (Fig. 17-12), and the tilting-disk type by the Bjork–Shiley (Fig. 17-13) and the St. Jude (Fig. 17-14) valves. The Bjork–Shiley valves have been discontinued because of significant complications (26).

The commonly used tissue valves are the porcine and the bovine pericardial valves. Porcine valves include the Hancock (Fig. 17-13) and the Carpentier–Edwards (Fig. 17-15) valves. The bovine valve is called the Ionescu–Shiley valve

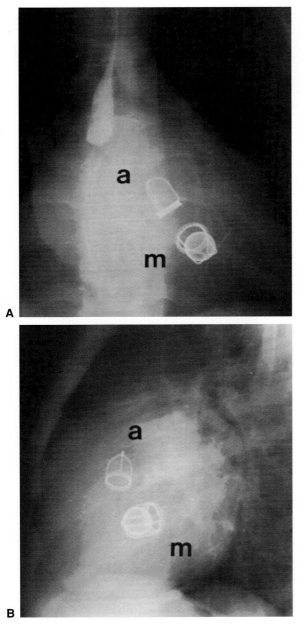

FIG. 17-11. Two Starr–Edwards prostheses. One is in the mitral (m) and the other in the aortic (a) position. **A:** PA view. **B:** Lateral view.

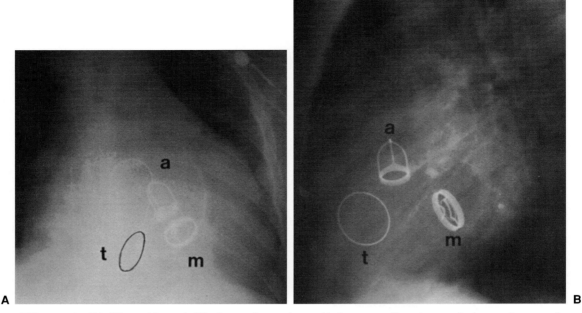

FIG. 17-13. PA (A) and lateral (B) views of a patient with long-standing rheumatic heart disease. A Starr–Edwards valve is in the aortic (a) position, a Bjork–Shiley valve is in the mitral (m) position, and a Hancock porcine valve is in the tricuspid (t) position.

(4,29) (Fig. 17-16). Unfortunately, Ionescu–Shiley valves have shown evidence of rapid structural deterioration after 10 years of use and have been discontinued (28).

At present the commonly used cardiac prostheses are the St. Jude and the Carpentier–Edwards. In general, the selection of mechanical versus tissue prostheses is based on the patient's age, childbearing potential, lifestyle, increased risk of anticoagulation, and other individual factors (28,29). Valves in patients with pure mitral or tricuspid insufficiency may be surgically repaired rather than replaced (8,32). Repair involves a plastic reconstruction of the annulus and the leaflets, using multiple-point fixation to a semiflexible ring, for example, the Carpentier annuloplasty ring (Fig. 17-17).

Detection of Malfunctions

Some malfunctions of prosthetic valves are diagnosed by radiologic techniques alone, others by correlating radiologic (3,4,29,32) with clinical and echocardiographic findings (3,4,22,24–26,29,31).

Prosthetic Instability

A normally functioning prosthetic valve moves to and fro in the direction of blood flow with only a negligible tilt between systole and diastole. A phasic tilt of >12° or an apparently rocking prosthesis indicates instability related to

sutures pulling loose (see **Fig. 2-35**). An unstable prosthesis is almost always associated with radiographic signs of significant valvular insufficiency (Fig. 17-18). The causes of such a complication include faulty surgical technique, infective endocarditis, and tissue deterioration at the site of valve implantation, as is often found in patients with mitral valve prolapse or Marfan's syndrome.

Paravalvular Leak

Leaking around the prosthetic valve may or may not coexist with prosthetic instability, depending on the site and extent of tissue damage and the number of sutures pulling loose from the annulus. In the absence of prosthetic instability, paravalvular leak cannot be differentiated from valvular insufficiency of other origins.

Valvular Insufficiency

Incompetence of a prosthetic valve in the absence of valvular instability usually results from cuspal tears and perforations of the tissue valves and from thrombosis, degeneration, or wear of the mechanical valves. In patients with double valve replacement, the stent or ring of the mitral prosthesis may prevent the aortic poppet from seating in diastole, thereby causing aortic insufficiency (4).

Outlet strut fractures involving the Bjork–Shiley valve

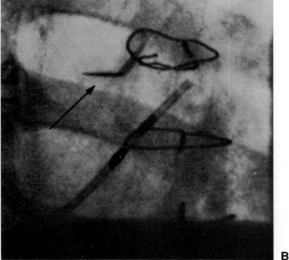

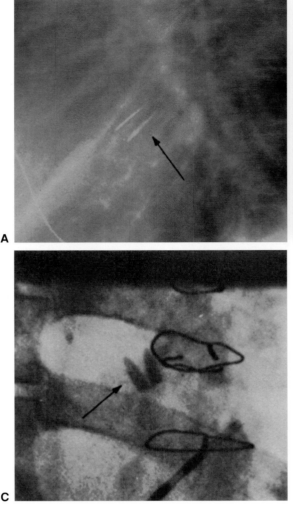

FIG. 17-14. A: A normally functioning St. Jude mitral valve is caught in diastole when the two radiopaque leaflets are open and viewed from the top as two parallel linear densities (*arrow*). When the valve is closed in systole, the leaflets are viewed face on and therefore become invisible (not shown). **B:** A side view of a normally functioning St. Jude aortic valve in the closed position. Note that the two leaflets form a V-shaped configuration (*arrow*). **C:** The same valve caught in an open position (*arrow*). (Both B and C views were reproduced with permission from Kotler MN, Panidis J, Mintz GS, et al. The role of noninvasive technique in the evaluation of the St. Jude cardiac prosthesis. In: DeBakey ME, ed. *Advances in cardiac valves: clinical perspectives*. New York: Yorke, 1983:213–228.)

have been reported (26). A sudden onset of profound heart failure usually develops coincident to the loss of the auscultatory clicks of the prosthesis. In the preparation for lifesaving surgery, prompt radiographic identification of the defective strut and the disk embolus is preferred to time-consuming cardiac catheterization.

With the increasing use of the bileaflet St. Jude prosthesis for cardiac valve replacement, some rare but life-threatening complications have been reported (24,25). A 12-year-old boy suddenly lost one of the two leaflets from his St. Jude valve, causing severe mitral insufficiency. The valve was repaired by emergency operation (25). Two other patients died from obstruction of one of the two leaflets in an aortic St. Jude prosthesis (24). These complications can be promptly detected by fluoroscopy with videotape recording, cine radiography (22), or echocardiogaphy (31). Radiographic signs of insufficient cardiac valves are presented elsewhere in this book, particularly in **Chapters 2** and **11**.

Valvular Stenosis

Prosthetic valve stenosis primarily results from calcification of a tissue valve or thrombotic obstruction of a mechanical valve. In either case, the decreased or absent excursion of a ball or disk poppet can be observed fluoroscopically or on cine radiography (22) or echocardiography (31). A calcified prosthetic valve is diagnosed more easily by fluoroscopy or cine radiography (6,22,24) than by conventional radiography.

Another cause of obstruction to a prosthetic valve is the size disproportion between the prosthesis and the ventricle or the ascending aorta. If the mitral prosthesis is too big, it can cause obstruction of left atrial emptying and, less commonly, obstruction of the outflow tract of the left ventricle. When an oversized prosthesis is implanted in the aortic position, proper emptying of the left ventricle may be disrupted. Radiologic findings of stenotic cardiac valves are discussed elsewhere, particularly in **Chapters 2** and **11**.

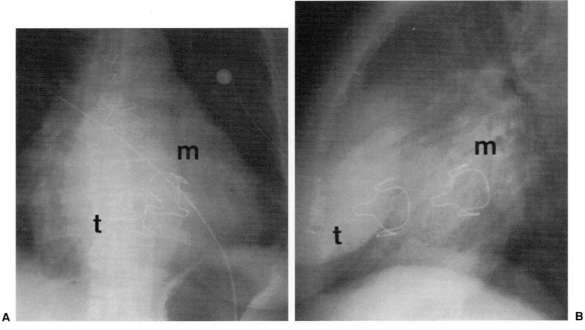

A   B

FIG. 17-15. PA (**A**) and lateral (**B**) views of a patient with rheumatic mitral stenosis and tricuspid insufficiency. Both valves were replaced. A Carpentier–Edwards porcine valve is seen in each position. m, mitral; t, tricuspid.

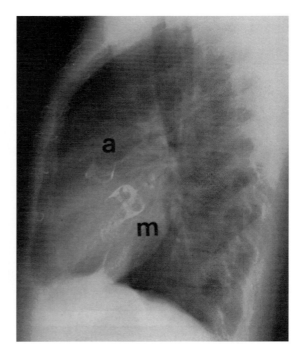

FIG. 17-16. Two Ionescu–Shiley valves are seen, one in the mitral (m) and the other in the aortic (a) position.

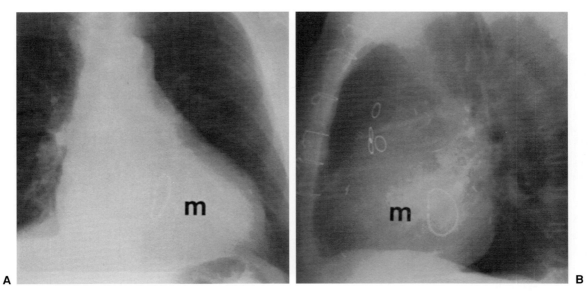

FIG. 17-17. PA (**A**) and lateral (**B**) views of a patient with mitral insufficiency after myocardial infarction. A Carpentier annuloplasty ring is implanted in the mitral position (m) with good results.

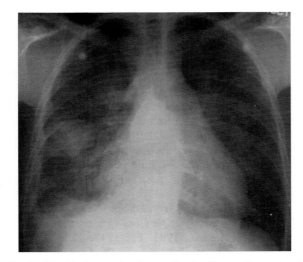

FIG. 17-18. Radiograph of a patient with aortic and mitral valve prostheses. The artificial mitral valve was unstable and leaking, causing congestive heart failure.

REFERENCES

1. Mond HG. Permanent cardiac pacemakers: techniques of implantation, testing, and surveillance. In: Schlant RC, Alexander RW, eds. *The heart*, 8th ed. New York: McGraw–Hill, 1994:815–842.
2. Barold SS, Zipes DP. Cardiac pacemakers and antiarrhythmic devices. In: Braunwald E, ed. *Heart disease: a textbook of cardiovascular medicine*, 4th ed. Philadelphia: Saunders, 1992:726–755.
3. Mehlman DJ. A pictorial and radiographic guide for identification of prosthetic heart valve devices. *Prog Cardiovasc Dis* 1988;30:441–464.
4. Hancock EW. Artificial valve disease. In: Schlant RC, Alexander RW, eds. *The heart*, 8th ed. New York: McGraw–Hill, 1994:1539–1546.
5. Lloyd MA, Hayes DL, Stanson AW, et al. Snare removal of a Telectronics Accufix atrial J retention wire. *Mayo Clin Proc* 1995;70:376–379.
6. Takasugi JE, Godwin JD, Bardy GH. The implantable pacemaker-cardioverter-defibrillator: radiographic aspects. *RadioGraphics* 1994;14:1275–1290.
7. Zoll P. Resuscitation of the heart in ventricular standstill by external electric stimulation. *N Engl J Med* 1952;247:768–771.
8. Sabiston DC Jr, Spencer FC. *Surgery of the chest*, 5th ed. Philadelphia: Saunders, 1990:1532–1535.
9. Hanabergh E, Rahim A, Agatston A, et al. Coronary sinus pacer lead simulating left atrial mass. *J Ultrasound Med* 1982;1:83–85.
10. Sorkin RP, Schaurmann BJ, Simon AB. Radiographic aspects of permanent cardiac pacemakers. *Radiology* 1976;119:281–286.
11. Hewitt MJ, Chen JTT, Ravin CE, Gallagher JJ. Coronary sinus atrial pacing: radiographic considerations. *AJR Am J Roentgenol* 1981;136:323–328.
12. McAlpine WA. *The heart and coronary arteries: an anatomic atlas for clinical diagnosis, radiologic investigation and surgical treatment.* New York: Springer, 1976.
13. Ormond RS, Rubenfire M, Anbe DT, et al. Radiographic demonstration of myocardial penetration by permanent endocardial pacemakers. *Radiology* 1971;98:35–37.
14. Bognolo DA, Vijayanagar R, Eckstein PF, et al. Implantation of permanent transvenous atrial J lead using lateral view fluoroscopy. *Ann Thorac Surg* 1981;31:574–576.
15. Rodan BA, Lowe JE, Chen JTT. Abdominal twiddler's syndrome. *AJR Am J Roentgenol* 1978;131:1084.
16. Karis JP, Ravin CE. Counterclockwise exit of cardiac pacemaker leads: sign of pulse-generator flip. *Radiology* 1990;174:711–712.
17. Brooks R, Ruskin JN. The implantable cardioverter-defibrillator. In: Schlant RC, Alexander RW, eds. *The heart*, 8th ed. New York: McGraw–Hill, 1994:847–858.
18. Drucker EA, Brooks R, Garan H, et al. Malfunction of implantable cardioverter defibrillators placed by a nonthoracotomy approach: frequency of malfunction and value of chest radiography in determining cause. *AJR Am J Roentgenol* 1995;165:275–279.
19. Strickberger SA, Do KCM, Daoud E, et al. Effect of first-phase polarity of biphasic shocks on defibrillation threshold with a single transvenous lead system. *J Am Coll Cardiol* 1995;25:1605–1608.
20. Hammel D, Block M, Geiger A, et al. Single-incision implantation of cardioverter defibrillators using nonthoracotomy lead systems. *Ann Thorac Surg* 1994;58:1614–1616.
21. Morse D, Steiner RM. *The pacemaker and valve identification guide.* Garden City, N.Y.: Medical Examination, 1978.

22. Aoyagi S, Higa Y, Matsuzoe S, et al. Obstruction of the St. Jude medical valve: diagnostic and therapeutic values of cineradiography. *Thorac Cardiovasc Surg* 1993;41:357–363.

23. Tomazic BB, Edwards WD, Schoen FJ. Physicochemical characterization of natural and bioprosthetic heart valve calcific deposits: implications for prevention. *Ann Thorac Surg* 1995;60:S322–327.

24. Kotler MN, Panidis J, Mintz GS, et al. The role of noninvasive technique in the evaluation of the St. Jude cardiac prosthesis. In: DeBakey ME, ed. *Advances in cardiac valves: clinical perspectives.* New York: Yorke, 1983:213–228.

25. Ross EM, Roberts WC. A precaution when using the St. Jude medical prosthesis in the aortic valve position. *Am J Cardiol* 1984;54:231.

26. Wills J, ed. Complications of convexoconcave heart valves. *FDA Drug Bull* 1984;14:22.

27. Koppensteiner R, Moritz A, Schlick W, et al. Blood rheology after cardiac valve replacement with mechanical or bioprostheses. *Am J Cardiol* 1991;67:79–83.

28. Tyers GFO, Jamieson WRE, Munro AI, et al. Reoperation in biological and mechanical valve populations: fate of the reoperative patient. *Ann Thorac Surg* 1995;60:S464–469.

29. Jamieson WRE, David TE. Introduction: the Sixth International Symposium for Cardiac Bioprostheses. *Ann Thorac Surg* 1995;60:S61–64.

30. Braunwald E. Valvular heart disease. In: Braunwald E, ed. *Heart disease: a textbook of cardiovascular medicine*, 3rd ed. Philadelphia: Saunders, 1992:1007–1077.

31. Nanda NC, Cooper JW, Mahan EF. Echocardiographic assessment of prosthetic valves. *Circulation* 1991;84(suppl 1):I-228–I-239.

32. Craver JM. Surgical reconstruction for regurgitant lesions of the mitral valve. In: Schlant RC, Alexander RW, eds. *The heart*, 8th ed. New York: McGraw–Hill, 1994:1557–1566.

Essentials of Cardiac Imaging,
James T. T. Chen,
Lippincott–Raven Publishers, Philadelphia © 1998.

CHAPTER 18

Miscellaneous Heart Diseases

James T. T. Chen

HYPERDYNAMIC STATES

An adult is said to be in a hyperdynamic or high cardiac output state when his or her cardiac output exceeds the upper limit of 3.9 L/min/m² at rest (1). A hyperdynamic circulation such as that encountered in athletes (Fig. 18-1) and pregnant women (see **Fig. 8-4A**) is a normal variant. A high cardiac output is typically found in patients with systemic arteriovenous fistula, renal failure, anemia, hyperthyroidism, and Paget's disease.

Systemic Arteriovenous Fistula

Systemic arteriovenous fistulas may be congenital or acquired. Congenital lesions are exemplified by cerebral, hepatic, and peripheral arteriovenous fistulas; acquired fistulas are caused by trauma and surgically related shunts. In neonates or infants, arteriovenous fistulas that cause congestive heart failure are commonly situated in the brain or the liver. Cerebral arteriovenous shunts tend to involve the posterior cerebral arteries and Galen's vein, which is usually the site of an aneurysm (2).

In older children, congenital arteriovenous fistulas may be found in an extremity in the form of numerous subcutaneous arteriovenous shunts. Since these lesions develop during the period of bone growth, the involved extremity may become longer and bigger than its contralateral mate (3) (Fig. 18-2). In adults, systemic arteriovenous fistulas are most commonly found in patients with gunshot wounds (Fig. 18-3). Less often, they may be iatrogenic in origin or surgically constructed for the purpose of hemodialysis. Rarely, an abdominal aortic aneurysm may rupture spontaneously into the inferior vena cava, causing congestive heart failure (4).

Department of Radiology, Duke University School of Medicine, Durham, North Carolina 27710, U.S.A.

Pathophysiology and Clinical Presentation

The decreased peripheral vascular resistance in the context of systemic arteriovenous fistulas must be compensated for by increased cardiac output to maintain adequate blood pressure and blood supply to the tissues (1). The mean systemic arterial pressure is kept within normal limits by raising the systolic pressure to compensate for the unusually low diastolic pressure. The pulse pressure, as a result, is widened, and the peripheral pulses become brisk. A continuous murmur with systolic accentuation is typically heard over the site of the fistula.

The high level of cardiac output is maintained by augmenting the stroke volume and by increasing the heart rate. These adjustments are manifested by tachycardia, hypertro-

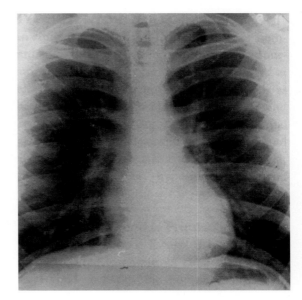

FIG. 18-1. Posteroanterior view of a trained athlete whose resting cardiac output was 10.5 L per minute. Note the mild engorgement of the heart and all vessels. The pulmonary blood flow pattern remains within normal limits.

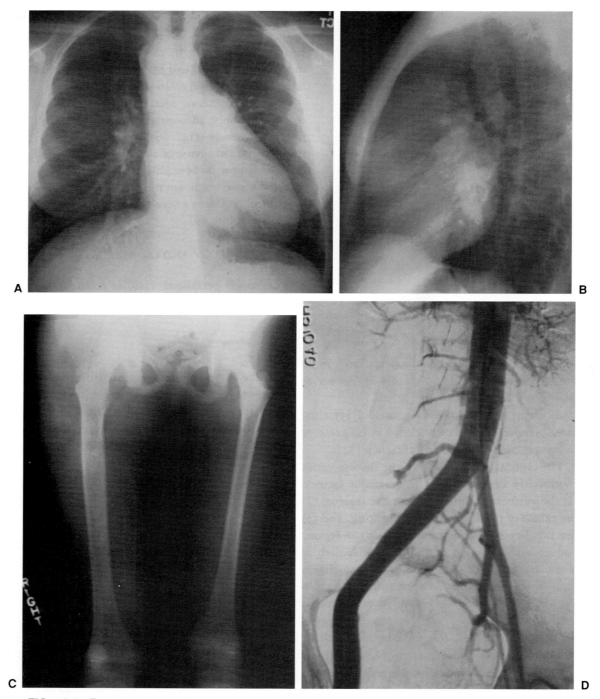

FIG. 18-2. Posteroanterior (**A**) and lateral (**B**) views of a patient with large systemic arteriovenous fistulas show a right-sided aortic arch with aberrant left subclavian artery, moderate cardiomegaly, and increased pulmonary vascularity. The radiograph of her lower limbs (**C**) shows a larger and longer right leg. The abdominal aortogram (**D**) reveals a much larger right iliac artery.

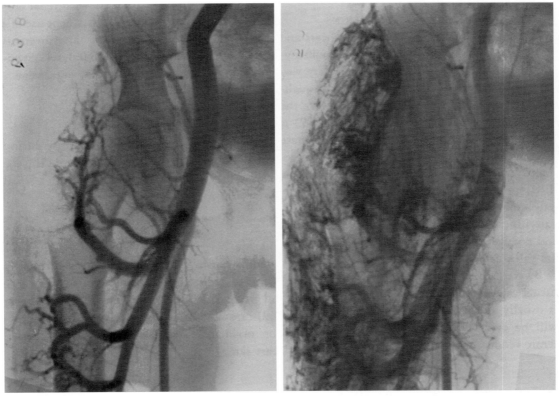

E   F

FIG. 18-2. *Continued.* Arterial (**E**) and early venous (**F**) phases of the right iliac arteriogram show numerous arteriovenous fistulas in the swollen right thigh.

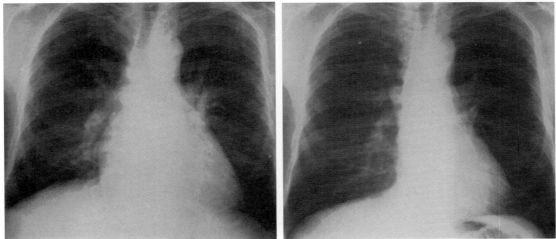

A   B

FIG. 18-3. A: A patient with a large traumatic arteriovenous fistula in the left leg that led to congestive heart failure. **B:** Following closure of the fistula, improvement is dramatic.

phy, and dilatation of the heart and vessels. By manual compression of the fistula, the heart rate can be brought down notably, and this is known as Branham's sign. A useful clue to the diagnosis of systemic arteriovenous fistula is a widened pulse pressure in the absence of aortic insufficiency (1).

The clinical presentation of the disease varies enormously depending on three major factors: the vastness of individual cardiac reserve, the extent of the arteriovenous shunting, and the rapidity of the development of the lesion. Sudden establishment of a large fistula, such as would happen with a gunshot wound, almost always leads to congestive heart failure (Fig. 18-3). On the other hand, slow development of numerous arteriovenous fistulas, such as is seen in Paget's disease, may be well tolerated by the patient. People who have preexisting cardiac conditions adapt poorly to the additional burden imposed by a newly formed fistula.

Radiographic and Angiographic Signs

Before congestive heart failure, the heart and vessels are diffusely enlarged with accompanying heightened pulsations. The pulmonary vascularity is increased. A varying degree of equalization of the pulmonary blood flow between the upper and lower lung zones (Fig. 18-2) is typically seen when there is a moderate arteriovenous shunt. Gravity, however, remains the main controlling force of the flow distribution—the lower lobes still receive markedly more blood than the upper (see **Chapter 8**). Curvilinear calcifications of the dilated vessels and nodular calcifications of multiple phleboliths are valuable radiographic signs of such fistulas.

By the time a chronic systemic arteriovenous fistula causes congestive heart failure, the heart is usually already massively enlarged, and there will be evidence of both pul-monary and systemic venous hypertension (Fig. 18-3). On the angiocardiogram, the fistulas are clearly evident, and their location and extent can be accurately determined (Fig. 18-2D–F). The heart is usually both dilated and hypertrophied, with increased contractility before and decreased contractility after failure.

Renal Failure

Hypervolemia in patients with renal disease is due partly to abnormal salt and water retention and partly to an increased metabolic rate (4). Since the myocardium is generally normal in patients with renal failure, the stroke volume and the contractility of the heart are usually increased. In spite of pulmonary edema, the pulmonary blood flow distribution remains relatively normal. There is a diffuse vascular engorgement but no cephalization of the pulmonary vascularity to suggest left ventricular failure (Fig. 18-4). The blood volume in patients with renal failure is further augmented by the frequent use of a surgically constructed systemic arteriovenous fistula for the purpose of hemodialysis. Eventually, congestive heart failure may supervene.

Pregnancy

The cardiac output continues to increase during normal pregnancy. By the seventh month, the increase may reach 50% above normal (4) (see **Fig. 8-4**).

Anemia

Anemia causes high cardiac output primarily owing to reduced peripheral vascular resistance and decreased blood

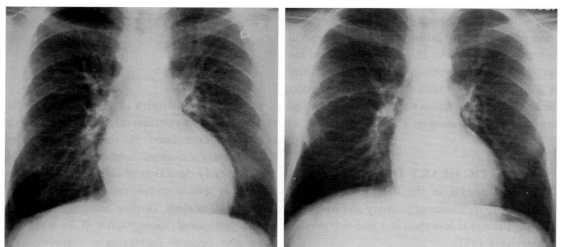

FIG. 18-4. A: Radiographs of a patient with renal failure show cardiomegaly and increased pulmonary vascularity with minimal interstitial pulmonary edema. **B:** After successful renal transplantation, the cardiovascular status improved.

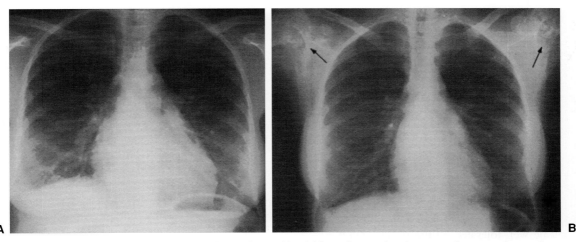

FIG. 18-5. A: Posteroanterior view of a patient with sickle cell anemia shows an increase in cardiac size and pulmonary vascularity. Pleural and pulmonary scars are seen in the right costophrenic sulcus. **B:** Another film taken 2 months later shows that the patient's condition in general has improved. Findings of bone infarction are now evident in both humeral heads (*arrows*).

viscosity (1). As in other conditions causing high cardiac output, there is a combination of increased stroke volume and increased heart rate. Although the radiographic signs of an anemic heart are nonspecific, there are other findings that may favor and even confirm the diagnosis. First, there may be telltale bony changes to suggest sickle cell or other kinds of severe anemia (Fig. 18-5). Second, there may be pulmo-

nary opacities from recurrent pneumonias or pulmonary thromboembolic disease (Figs. 18-5A and 18-6A), which could lead to pulmonary hypertension (Fig. 18-6B). Third, a gallstone may be seen in a teenager or young adult (Fig. 18-7), again suggesting the possibility of sickle cell anemia. In the case of radiolucent gallstones, an ultrasound study helps make the diagnosis.

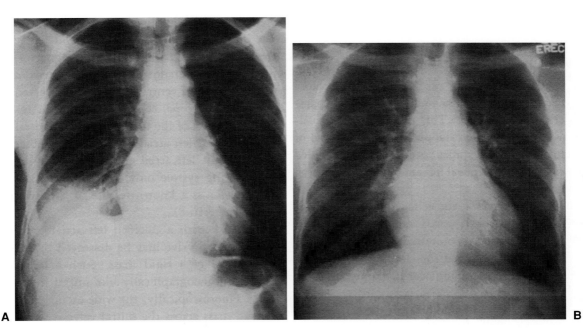

FIG. 18-6. A: Posteroanterior view of a patient with sickle cell anemia and recurrent pulmonary thromboembolic disease leading to pulmonary hypertension. Note the mild cardiomegaly and increased pulmonary blood flow. An opacity in the right costophrenic sulcus probably represents another episode of pulmonary embolism. **B:** Three years later, the cardiac contour has changed, suggesting predominantly right-sided cardiomegaly. The pulmonary trunk is dilated, and there is a centralized pulmonary blood flow pattern suggestive of pulmonary arterial hypertension.

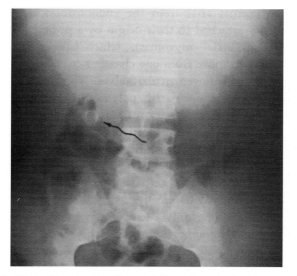

FIG. 18-7. The chest radiograph (not shown) of a 22-year-old man with a 9-year history of recurrent severe stomachache demonstrates cardiomegaly with increased pulmonary vascularity. The abdominal film shows hepatosplenomegaly and a gallstone (*arrow*).

NEOPLASTIC HEART DISEASE

Neoplastic disease of the heart is uncommon. The autopsy incidence of primary and metastatic cardiac tumors is <0.1% and 6.0%, respectively (5). Cardiac tumors may mimic common heart diseases and remain misdiagnosed and mismanaged until tumor fragments embolize to arteries in the brain or aortic bifurcation. A left atrial myxoma, for instance, may be treated as rheumatic mitral stenosis until tumor cells are discovered from the embolic material lodged in the abdominal aortic bifurcation.

Fortunately, our awareness of cardiac tumors has been considerably heightened by the experience accumulated in the past three decades. Concurrently, modern noninvasive diagnostic tools for early detection of cardiac tumors, most noticeably echocardiography, gated radionuclide cardiac imaging, dynamic computed tomography (CT) scanning, and cine magnetic resonance imaging, have also become increasingly available. The role of radiography and fluoroscopy is still important, for it occasionally provides the first clue to the unsuspected disease.

Primary Cardiac Tumors

By far the most common primary tumors of the heart are myxomas. Others, in descending order of frequency, include lipoma, papillary fibroelastoma, angiosarcoma, rhabdomyoma, rhabdomyosarcoma, fibroma, hemangioma, fibrosarcoma, teratoma, malignant lymphoma, and thymoma (6). More than 75% of primary cardiac tumors are benign.

Myxomas

Myxomas are benign tumors of the mesenchyme. Local recurrence after resection and growth at the site of tumor embolization, however, may occur. About 75% of cardiac myxomas are located in the left atrium, 18% in the right atrium, and 4% equally in either the right or the left ventricle (6). Myxomas arise from the endocardium, frequently attached by a pedicle (as seen in atrial myxomas), which allows the tumors to move from one chamber to the other across the atrioventricular valve. They usually appear as pedunculated, polypoid, gelatinous, and friable intracavitary masses ranging from 1 to 15 cm. Areas of hemorrhage and thrombosis are usually found inside the myxoma (7).

Left Atrial Myxomas

Left atrial myxomas mimic mitral stenosis in clinical signs and radiologic appearance, providing only a few subtle clues for the experienced diagnostician. First, cardiac myxomas tend to provoke constitutional manifestations, such as fever, fatigue, anemia, weight loss, elevated erythrocyte sedimentation rate, and increased serum immunoglobulin. These are supposedly immunologic symptoms, as a result of host reaction to the tumor antigens.

Second, the severity of pulmonary venous obstruction and the quality of heart murmurs tend to change drastically when the patient's posture changes. Dyspnea, for example, may be relieved with the patient's assuming a recumbent position. Such peculiar phenomena can be explained by the movability of the tumor within the heart under the influence of gravity. Third, systemic embolization frequently occurs in patients with left atrial myxoma, owing to the friable nature of the tumor and its tendency to break up within a dynamic organ and embolize distally.

On physical examination, the opening snap of mitral stenosis is often unusually late and low pitched, and this is known as a "tumor plop." In addition, there may be other auscultatory signs of associated mitral insufficiency. On the radiograph, noncalcified left atrial myxomas typically mimic mitral valve stenosis, causing a combination of pulmonary venous hypertension and left atrial–right ventricular enlargement. There are, however, some deviations from the classic picture of mitral stenosis. First, the left ventricle is mildly enlarged, owing partly to the diastolic intracavitary tumor and partly to the tumor-provoked, minor mitral regurgitation. Second, a paradoxic movement between the left atrium and ventricle is usually observed under the fluoroscope, corresponding to the to-and-fro excursion of the tumor across the mitral valve. When the left atrial wall remains pliable, an intermittent left atrial enlargement may be present during systole only. Intermittent pulmonary edema is a known feature of left atrial myxoma (Fig. 18-8).

In patients with a calcified left atrial myxoma, the mitral valve may be destroyed by the bombardment of a rigid mass.

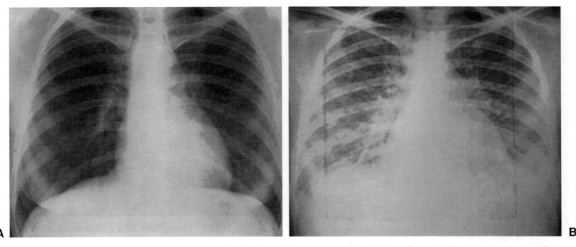

FIG. 18-8. Radiographs of a patient with a left atrial myxoma show intermittent pulmonary edema. On the posteroanterior view (**A**) there is prominence of the left atrium and normal pulmonary vascularity. Within 1 year before surgery, repeated episodes of pulmonary edema occurred (**B**).

On radiography, this lesion has features similar to mitral insufficiency. On fluoroscopy, the wide excursion of a calcified mass across the mitral valve is virtually diagnostic of such a tumor (see **Fig. 10-16**). The frequency of calcification of this tumor is ~10%.

Two-dimensional echocardiography (see **Fig. 6-5**) is superior to the M-mode technique (Fig. 18-9) in evaluating cardiac myxomas because of its capability to image all four cardiac chambers simultaneously. This procedure is particularly valuable when the possibility of biatrial or multicentric myxomas needs to be excluded before the removal of an obvious left atrial myxoma. Transesophageal echocardiography has become popular for its capability of imaging within the thorax and gaining better pictures (Fig. 18-10).

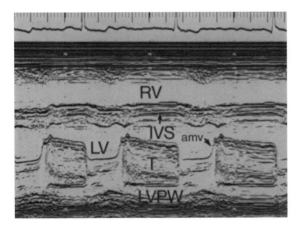

FIG. 18-9. An M-mode echocardiogram shows the left atrial myxoma (T) prolapsing into the left ventricle (LV) during diastole. A clear space between the anterior mitral valve leaflet (amv) and the tumor is typically present, representing the delay between the time the mitral valve opens and the tumor settles in the left ventricle. IVS, interventricular septum; LVPW, left ventricular posterior wall; RV, right ventricle.

If, for any reason, the echocardiographic diagnosis is equivocal, enhanced CT, electron beam CT (Fig. 3-13), or cine magnetic resonance imaging (see **Fig. 4-9A**) may be undertaken for clarification. Cardiac catheterization and angiocardiography are indicated only when other associated cardiac diseases are suspected and hemodynamic data are needed in the preparation for surgery.

In catheterization, catheters should not be introduced into the left side of the heart for fear that the friable myxoma may break up and its fragments embolize the systemic arteries. The angiocardiogram should be obtained by injecting contrast medium into the pulmonary trunk to image the levophase of the study, namely, the opacified left atrium and ventricle (Fig. 18-11). If associated right atrial myxoma is also suspected, rather than intubating the right side of the heart, contrast medium should be injected into the superior or inferior vena cava. This precaution is imperative to avoid disturbing a right-sided myxoma and risking pulmonary embolism.

Right Atrial Myxomas

Right atrial myxomas are much less common than their left atrial counterparts, accounting for only one fifth of all cardiac myxomas. These tumors, before calcification, typically mimic tricuspid stenosis. Calcified right atrial myxomas, on the other hand, tend to destroy the tricuspid leaflets and cause valvular insufficiency in addition to obstruction. Since isolated tricuspid valve disease of a rheumatic nature never exists alone, the differential diagnosis of right atrial myxoma is not as difficult as that of left atrial myxoma. Again, the combination of constitutional, cardiac, and embolic manifestations suggests the correct diagnosis. If a patent foramen ovale is present, a right-to-left shunt may develop in the face of right atrial pressure and volume overload.

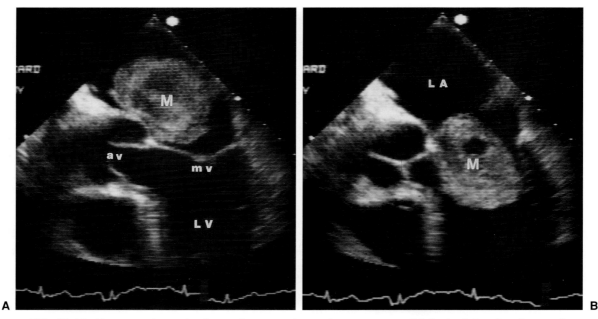

FIG. 18-10. Transesophageal echocardiograms show a large myxoma (M) in the left atrium in systole (**A**) and in the left ventricle in diastole (**B**). av, aortic valve; mv, mitral valve; LV, left ventricle; LA, left atrium.

Consequently, certain patients may become cyanotic or may sustain a paradoxic embolism or both.

On the radiograph, signs of right-sided heart failure are apparent in most patients (Fig. 18-12; see also **Fig. 9-11**). They are decreased pulmonary vascularity reflecting low cardiac output and low pulmonary blood flow with or without a right-to-left shunt; right atrial and ventricular enlargements; and fluoroscopic evidence of tricuspid stenosis and insufficiency. The principles and applications of other imaging methods for the diagnosis of right atrial

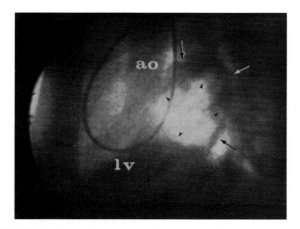

FIG. 18-11. Levophase of a pulmonary arteriogram in systole shows a large lobulated filling defect (*arrowheads*) representing the myxoma inside the opacified left atrium (*arrows*). The left ventricle (lv) and the aorta (ao) are also faintly opacified. In diastole (not shown), the tumor is inside the left ventricle.

myxomas (Fig. 18-12B) are similar to those for left-sided lesions.

Rhabdomyomas

Rhabdomyomas are probably hamartomas of the myocardium rather than true neoplasms. They are most commonly encountered in children. About one third of the patients with rhabdomyoma also evidence the signs of tuberous sclerosis. Symptoms are produced by arrhythmias and intracavitary obstructions (5,7,8).

Primary Pericardial Tumors

Although some authors classify pericardial cysts in the category of neoplasms, the vast majority of these lesions represent a congenital malformation from persistence of the ventral recess of the coelom (see **Chapter 14**). Primary pericardial tumors include malignant and benign teratomas and mesotheliomas as well as malignant fibrosarcoma and angiosarcoma.

Teratomas

Most thoracic teratomas are located outside the heart in the anterior mediastinum. Intrapericardial teratomas are most commonly found in infants and children (6). They are bulky tumors, displacing and compressing the heart and

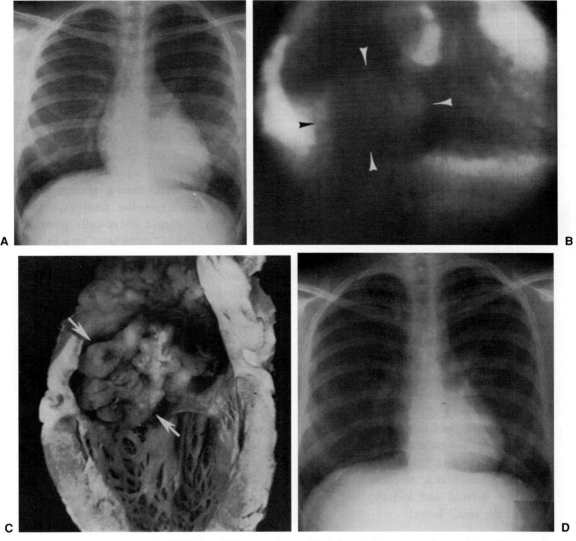

FIG. 18-12. Posteroanterior (PA) view (**A**) of a patient with right atrial myxoma shows right-sided cardiomegaly with decreased pulmonary vascularity. This patient's right anterior oblique view is seen in **Fig. 9-11**, which demonstrates dilatation of the superior vena cava (SVC), inferior vena cava, and azygos vein. An injection into the superior vena cava (**B**) shows a large lobulated filling defect (*arrows*) in the right atrium, causing obstruction of flow to the right ventricle. The specimen (**C**) evidences a huge, lobulated, and gelatinous tumor (*arrows*) inside the right atrium. The postoperative posteroanterior view (**D**) shows a return to the normal state.

great vessels and at times provoking pericardial effusion. Since they are usually benign, surgical cure is expected.

Mesotheliomas

Mesotheliomas from the pericardium are usually malignant, although benign lesions have been encountered and removed successfully (9).

Thymomas

Intrapericardial thymomas have been reported (8). A thymic cyst may arise from or adhere to the pericardium, causing marginal calcification.

Metastatic Tumors

Metastatic neoplasms of the pericardium and heart are 20 to 40 times more common than their primary counterparts. The mode of spread to the heart is through the bloodstream, via the lymphatic channels, by direct extension, or a combination of these methods (8). Renal cell carcinoma is known to spread along the inferior vena cava into the right atrium. Cardiac metastases usually originate from carcinoma of the bronchi, lungs, and breast. Other malignancies that tend to invade the heart include melanoma, lymphoma, sarcoma (10), carcinoma of the thyroid and kidney, and carcinoid tumor of the small bowel.

Clinical Presentation

Metastatic lesions of the heart and pericardium tend to remain clinically silent until cardiac function is severely jeopardized. It is not too surprising to find acute cardiac tamponade, atrial fibrillation, complete heart block, rapid onset of congestive heart failure, or superior vena cava syndrome as the first sign of cardiac metastasis. The more insidious forms of the disease include persistent pericarditis with effusion and constrictive pericarditis.

The cardiac lesions from a malignant carcinoid are typi-

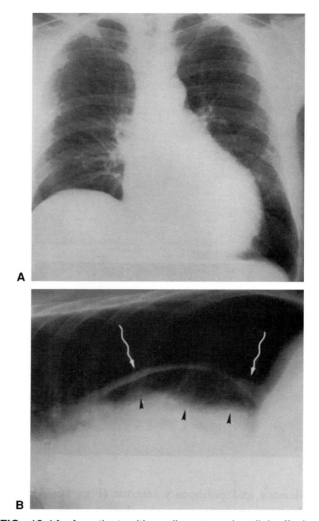

FIG. 18-14. A patient with malignant pericardial effusion caused by recurrent bronchogenic carcinoma. The posteroanterior radiograph (**A**) shows cardiomegaly and evidence of right thoracotomy. A post-pericardiocentesis radiograph (**B**) was taken in the right lateral decubitus position. Note the irregular thickening of both parietal (*arrows*) and visceral (*arrowheads*) layers of the pericardium due to tumor infiltration.

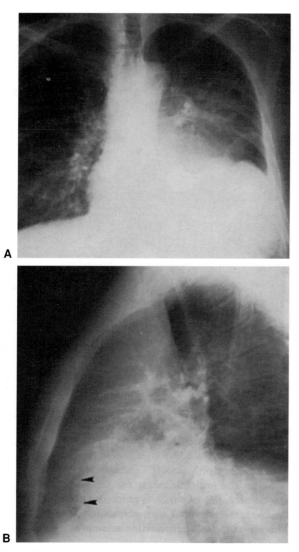

FIG. 18-13. A patient with oat-cell carcinoma, which invades the heart and causes pericardial effusion and tamponade. The posteroanterior view (**A**) shows gross cardiomegaly, engorgement of the azygos vein, cephalization of pulmonary vascularity, left-sided pleural effusion, and opacities in the left lung. The lateral view (**B**) shows posterior displacement of the subepicardial fat stripe (*arrows*) by the opaque pericardial effusion.

cally a combination of tricuspid insufficiency and pulmonary stenosis. The carcinoid tumor secretes large circulating quantities of serotonin, which is normally inactivated by the liver, lungs, and brain. In the presence of hepatic metastasis, however, serotonin may pass through the liver unaltered, reach the right side of the heart, and provoke the formation of fibrous plaques over the tricuspid and pulmonary valves. The left-sided cardiac valves are protected by the detoxifying ability of the lungs. In addition to cardiac findings, metastasizing carcinoid tumor is typically portrayed by cutaneous flushing, asthmatic attacks, and diarrhea. Tricuspid valve replacement and pulmonary valvulotomy are usually indicated in the treatment of patients with carcinoid heart disease. Surgery should not be denied even if there is hepatic metastasis, for these patients usually survive >10 years after the onset of metastases.

Radiographic Signs

The most common radiologic sign of cardiac metastasis is pericardial effusion with or without evidence of cardiac tamponade. In this situation, the displaced subepicardial fat stripe in the retrosternal space may be the first clue to the diagnosis (Fig. 18-13). The pericardial tap is frequently bloody, and tumor cells may be discovered. On the radiograph taken after pericardiocentesis and intrapericardial air injection, tumor infiltrates may be visible on either layer of the pericardium (Fig. 18-14).

In patients with bronchogenic carcinoma or malignant melanoma, the clinical suspicion of superior vena cava syndrome may be strengthened by the presence of a large soft-tissue mass in the right superior mediastinum. Furthermore, associated air trapping may be present to suggest its bronchogenic origin. The radiographic manifestations of carcinoid heart disease are the same as tricuspid insufficiency and pulmonary stenosis (Fig. 18-15). In contrast to congenital valvular pulmonary stenosis, however, no poststenotic dilatation of the pulmonary trunk and left pulmonary artery is observed in carcinoid pulmonary stenosis (Fig. 18-15).

TRAUMATIC HEART DISEASE

With the increasing incidence of automobile accidents, physical violence, and invasive medical procedures, traumatic cardiovascular disease has become commonplace. Serious cardiac trauma can be overlooked unless medical professionals remain actively alert to the signs (11). The immediate complications of cardiac trauma are exsanguination and cardiac tamponade. In patients who survive the acute phase of trauma, complications such as myocardial infarction, aneurysm, pseudoaneurysm, ventricular septal defect, valvular injury, pericarditis, and pericardial constriction may develop later (11).

Patients who are hemorrhaging usually undergo emer-

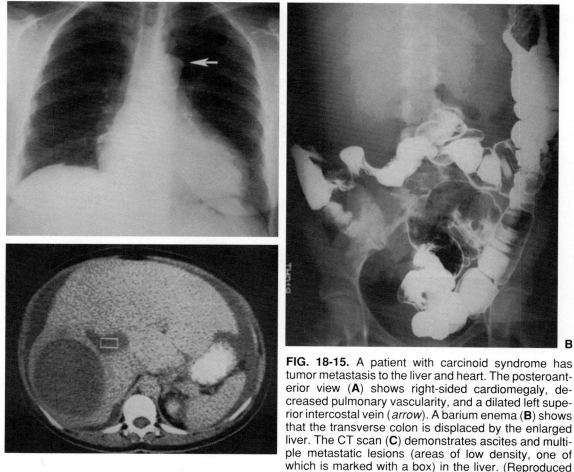

FIG. 18-15. A patient with carcinoid syndrome has tumor metastasis to the liver and heart. The posteroanterior view (**A**) shows right-sided cardiomegaly, decreased pulmonary vascularity, and a dilated left superior intercostal vein (*arrow*). A barium enema (**B**) shows that the transverse colon is displaced by the enlarged liver. The CT scan (**C**) demonstrates ascites and multiple metastatic lesions (areas of low density, one of which is marked with a box) in the liver. (Reproduced with permission from Thompson WM. Film interpretation session/case 6. *Radiology* 1983;149:8.)

gency thoracotomy without the benefit of imaging procedures. Rarely is there time enough for even a portable chest radiograph. Patients with cardiac tamponade, however, may be sustained long enough for radiography or echocardiography to be done before therapeutic pericardiocentesis is performed.

Acute Radiographic Manifestations

The following are changes noted during the acute stage of trauma:

1. Signs of pericardial effusion with or without cardiac tamponade, resulting from injury to the pericardium (12) (Fig. 18-16)
2. Signs of congestive heart failure with pulmonary edema resulting from injury to the myocardium, coronary artery, or cardiac valves (11–14) (Fig. 18-17 and 18-18A)
3. Widening of the mediastinum, apical capping, and pleural effusion, resulting from injury to the heart and great vessels with active bleeding (11,14,15), which is particularly likely in patients with transection of the aorta (see **Fig. 19-12**) and penetrating injury to the thin-walled structures, such as the atria and pulmonary artery. Unlike the ventricles, thin-walled structures seldom seal spontaneously (11)
4. Foreign body retention, resulting from penetrating injury to the heart (Fig. 18-18; see also **Fig. 2-36**)

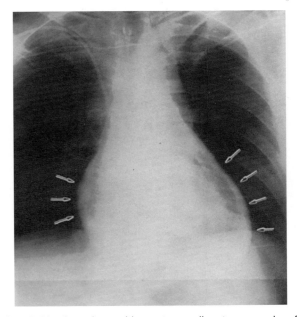

FIG. 18-16. A patient with acute cardiac tamponade after catheter perforation of the left ventricle during angiocardiography. About 40 ml of 75% Hypaque was injected into the pericardium. A radiograph taken immediately after the accident shows a small amount of opacified fluid in the pericardium (*arrows*). The mean pressure in the superior vena cava was 11 mm Hg.

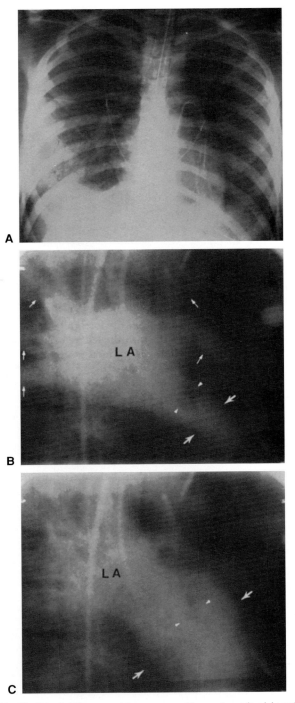

FIG. 18-17. A 20-year-old woman with acute mitral insufficiency from blunt chest trauma. A portal film (**A**) shows severe pulmonary edema and a normal-sized heart. A left ventriculogram in systole (**B**) demonstrates a filling defect (*arrowheads*), representing the amputated stump of a papillary muscle. The left ventricle (*arrows*) is well contracted. The left atrium (LA) is markedly dilated, as are the pulmonary veins (*small arrows*). In diastole (**C**), the left ventricle (*arrows*) is dilated and the left atrium (LA) is well contracted. The filling defect (*arrowheads*) has persisted.

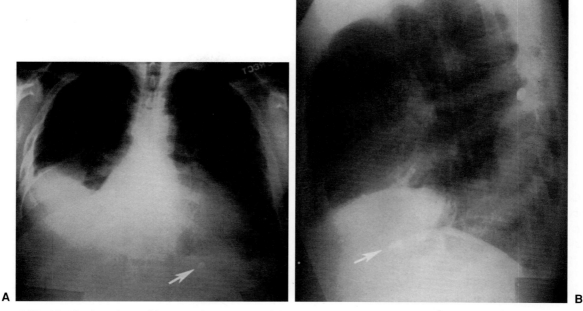

FIG. 18-18. A patient with a gunshot wound of the chest. The posteroanterior view (**A**) shows pleural and pericardial effusions and a bullet (*arrow*) in the inferior left ventricular wall. The lateral view (**B**) confirms the location of the bullet (*arrow*). Under the fluoroscope, the foreign body was moving synchronously with the left ventricular wall, indicative of its stable intramural position. The bullet was successfully removed.

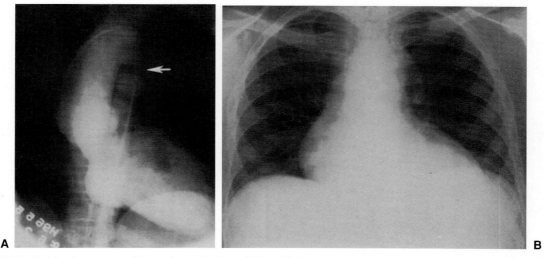

FIG. 18-19. A patient with aortic and tricuspid insufficiency stemming from blunt chest trauma. An aortogram (**A**) shows severe aortic insufficiency due to rupture of the aortic valve. Also noted is a transection of the aorta (*arrow*). Six months after replacement of the aortic valve and repair of the dissection, the radiograph (**B**) demonstrates a deformed aortic arch, moderate cardiomegaly, and decreased pulmonary vascularity.

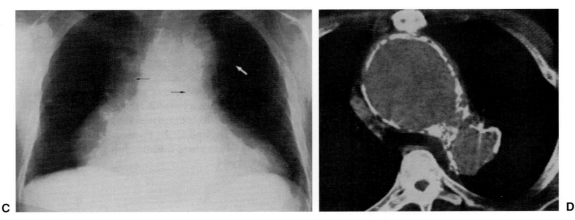

C

D

FIG. 18-19. *Continued.* In retrospect, the prominence of the right cardiac border (right atrial enlargement) and decreased pulmonary flow are suggestive of traumatic tricuspid insufficiency. The patient returned 12 years later (**C**) with gross cardiomegaly, evidence of severe tricuspid insufficiency, a leaky aortic prosthesis, a markedly deformed and calcified aortic arch (*oblique arrow*), and a calcified ascending aortic aneurysm (*transverse arrows*). A CT scan (**D**) shows a huge calcific aneurysm extending from the ascending aorta to the proximal descending aorta.

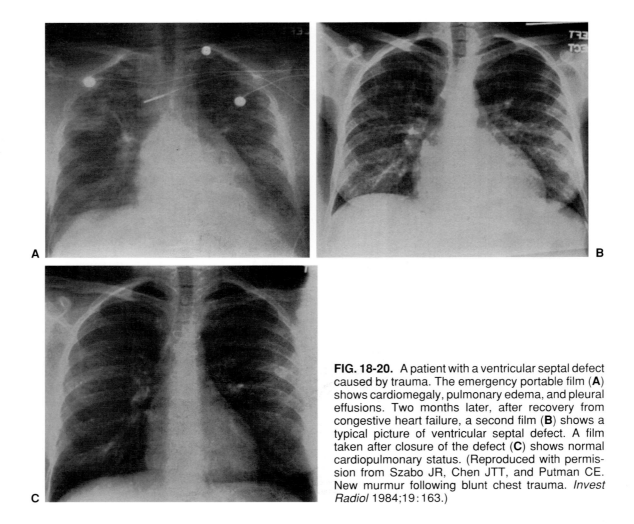

A

B

C

FIG. 18-20. A patient with a ventricular septal defect caused by trauma. The emergency portable film (**A**) shows cardiomegaly, pulmonary edema, and pleural effusions. Two months later, after recovery from congestive heart failure, a second film (**B**) shows a typical picture of ventricular septal defect. A film taken after closure of the defect (**C**) shows normal cardiopulmonary status. (Reproduced with permission from Szabo JR, Chen JTT, and Putman CE. New murmur following blunt chest trauma. *Invest Radiol* 1984;19:163.)

Chronic Radiographic Manifestations

The following long-term changes may be noted:

1. Postpericardiotomy syndrome with late development of pericardial and pleural effusions, resulting from injury to the pericardium, the myocardium, or both (16)
2. Signs of constrictive or constrictive-effusive pericarditis, resulting from hemorrhage or infection of the pericardium (14,15) (see **Fig. 14-22**)
3. Signs of cardiac herniation through a traumatic pericardial defect with or without strangulation (11) (see **Fig. 14-11**)
4. Signs of ventricular aneurysm or pseudoaneurysm, resulting from injury to the myocardium (14)
5. Aortic pseudoaneurysm (17) with or without wall calcification (Fig. 18-19)
6. Foreign body retention (Fig. 18-19; see also **Fig. 2-36**)
7. Traumatic ventricular septal defect (11–13). The increased pulmonary vascularity and the dynamic changes of a ventricular septal defect (Fig. 18-20B) do not manifest until the myocardium has regained its strength in response to anticongestive measures. At first, only a nonspecific pattern of congestive heart failure is evident (Fig. 18-20A).
8. Valvular insufficiency resulting from injury to the cardiac valves or the papillary muscles (11,12,14) (Figs. 18-17 and 18-18)
9. Posttraumatic myocardial calcification or ossification (18)

REFERENCES

1. Fowler NO. High-cardiac-output states. In: Schlant RC, Alexander RW, eds. *The heart*, 8th ed. New York: McGraw–Hill, 1994:503–514.
2. Kelley MJ, Jaffe CC, Kleinman CS. *Cardiac imaging in infants and children*. Philadelphia: Saunders, 1982:200–202.
3. Young JR. Diseases of the peripheral arteries. In: Hurst JW, ed. *The heart*, 6th ed. New York: McGraw–Hill, 1985:1339–1363.
4. Grossman W, Braunwald E. High-cardiac-output states. In: Braunwald E, ed. *Heart disease: a textbook of cardiovascular medicine*, 2nd ed. Philadelphia: Saunders, 1984:807–822.
5. Rosenthal DS, Handin RI, Braunwald E. Hematologic-oncologic disorders and heart disease. In: Braunwald E, ed. *Heart disease: a textbook of cardiovascular medicine*, 4th ed. Philadelphia: Saunders, 1992: 1742–1766.
6. McAllister HA, Fenoglio JJ. Tumors of the cardiovascular system. In: Firminger HI, ed. *Atlas of tumor pathology*. Washington, D.C.: Armed Forces Institute of Pathology, 1978.
7. Hall RJ, Cooley DA, McAllister HA, Frazier OH. Neoplastic heart disease. In: Schlant RC, Alexander RW, eds. *The heart*, 8th ed. New York: McGraw–Hill, 1994:2007–2030.
8. Gould SE. *Pathology of the heart and blood vessels*, 3rd ed. Springfield, Ill.: Thomas, 1968:870–872.
9. Davis RD, Oldham HN, Sabiston DC. The mediastinum. In: Sabiston DC, Spencer FC, eds. *Surgery of the chest*, 6th ed. Philadelphia: Saunders, 1995:676–712.
10. Seibert KA, Rettenmier CW, Waller BF, et al. Osteogenic sarcoma metastatic to the heart. *Am J Med* 1982;73:136–141.
11. Cohn PF, Braunwald E. Traumatic heart disease. In: Braunwald E, ed. *Heart disease: a textbook of cardiovascular medicine*, 4th ed. Philadelphia: Saunders, 1992:1517–1526.
12. Parmley LF, Manion WC, Mattingly TW. Nonpenetrating traumatic injury to the heart. *Circulation* 1958;18:371–396.
13. Danzil DF, Thomas DM, Miller JW. Ventricular septal defect following blunt chest trauma. *Ann Emerg Med* 1980;9:150–154.
14. Gay W. Blunt trauma to the heart and great vessels. *Surgery* 1982;91: 507–509.
15. Fallahnejad M, Kutty ACK, Wallace HW. Secondary lesions of penetrating cardiac injuries. *Ann Surg* 1980;191:228–233.
16. Kaminsky ME, Rodan BA, Osborne DR, et al. Postpericardiotomy syndrome. *Am J Roentgenol* 1982;138:503–508.
17. Ayella RJ, Hankins JR, Turney SZ, et al. Ruptured thoracic aorta due to blunt trauma. *J Trauma* 1977;17:199–205.
18. Grossman CM. Posttraumatic ossification of the myocardium. *J Trauma* 1974;14:85–89.

Essentials of Cardiac Imaging,
James T. T. Chen,
Lippincott–Raven Publishers, Philadelphia © 1998.

CHAPTER 19

Diseases of the Aorta

James T. T. Chen

Most of the thoracic aorta is surrounded by air-filled lungs, and its outline is clearly visible on chest radiographs (1). The mediastinal portions of the aorta can be imaged with computed tomography (CT) because of its ability to discriminate fat from water density (2) (see **Chapters 3** and **20**). Echocardiography (3) (see **Chapter 6**) and magnetic resonance imaging (MRI) (3) (see **Chapter 4**) have the further advantage of making visible the cardiovascular lumens without the use of contrast medium. The dynamic nature of the aorta can be appreciated by fluoroscopy, echocardiography, cine CT (ultrafast CT or electron beam tomography) (2), and cine MRI (gradient-echo MRI) in multiple planes (3). Changes of the aorta often reflect the status of the left ventricle centrally and that of the systemic circulation peripherally.

RADIOGRAPHIC ANATOMY OF THE AORTA

The aorta is the main trunk of the systemic arterial tree. It arises from the left ventricle at about the midline of the thorax, courses superoanteriorly and rightward for about 5 cm (ascending aorta), then bends to the left and posteriorly (the aortic arch) to descend on the left side of the trachea and the spine (descending aorta). It measures ~3 cm at its origin and tapers distally. The abdominal aorta at the level of the fourth lumbar vertebra measures only 1.75 cm in diameter (4).

On the posteroanterior (PA) view on chest radiography, the ascending aorta is not border-forming in children and young adults. In older persons, it emerges as a smooth and slightly rightward convexity (5,6). The aortic arch is not evident, except where it contributes to the visibility of the aortic knob immediately distal to the origin of the left subclavian artery. The descending aorta is outlined by the left lung, sometimes all the way to the diaphragm and at other times only to the midpoint of the thorax, where it courses medially

to disappear in the mediastinum. The brachiocephalic branches of the aortic arch are not discernible except in a lordotic view, where the lateral margin of the innominate and that of the left subclavian arteries are brought into relief. The anteromedial border of the distal aortic arch and the descending aorta can be outlined by the barium-filled esophagus. The medial and posterior borders of the ascending aorta are not seen unless they are calcified.

In the lateral view, the proximal, intrapericardial segment of the ascending aorta is sometimes outlined by the subepicardial fat stripe, particularly under the fluoroscope. This landmark points to the site of the aortic valve immediately posterior to the lower end of the fat stripe (Fig. 19-1). The rest of the ascending aorta, up to the origin of the innominate artery, can also be seen against the right lung. The aortic arch begins to be seen after the takeoff of the left subclavian artery. Only the proximal descending aorta is visible in children and young adults. The remainder of its course is well within the mediastinum, away from the lung, and therefore invisible. Again, the anteromedial border of the distal aortic arch and the descending aorta can be outlined by the barium column in the esophagus (Fig. 19-2A,B; see also **Fig. 9-22**). The posterior wall of the ascending aorta and most of the inferior wall of the aortic arch are not evident unless they are calcified. The left anterior oblique view is the best view for evaluating the thoracic aorta on radiography or by aortography because it effectively uncoils the aorta into a profile (Fig. 19-3D; see also **Fig. 9-22**).

FUNCTION OF THE AORTA

The aorta is composed of three layers: the intima, the media, and the adventitia. The intima is lined by the endothelium. The vasa vasorum, lymphatics, and nerves enter the aortic wall through the adventitia. The strength of the aorta lies in the media, which consists of large amounts of elastic tissue and relatively little smooth muscle. Over the life span of an average person, the aorta is able to absorb the impact

---

Department of Radiology, Duke University School of Medicine, Durham, North Carolina 27710, U.S.A.

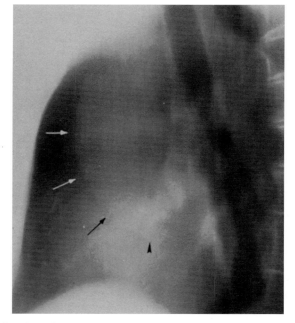

FIG. 19-1. A lateral tomogram of a patient with calcific aortic stenosis shows the subepicardial fat stripe (*arrows*) outlining the anterior border of the ascending aorta. The lower end of the fat stripe marks the anterior aspect of the aortic valve, which is calcified (*arrowhead*).

of three billion heartbeats and effectively deliver 200 million liters of blood to all parts of the body. Experimentally, the aorta can successfully resist the pressure of thousands of millimeters of mercury (1).

In systole, the aorta is distended by the blood ejected into its lumen. At the same time, part of the force imparted by the left ventricle is transformed into potential energy stored in the stretched wall of the aorta. During diastole, as the aorta relaxes, the potential energy is converted into kinetic energy to milk the blood further distally against the closed aortic valve and the narrowed aorta (1).

DISEASES OF THE AORTA

Diseases of the aorta can be classified as congenital or acquired. Important congenital abnormalities of the aorta are described in **Chapter 16**. Acquired diseases of the aorta include atherosclerosis, cystic medial degeneration, various types of aortitis, and trauma. They are discussed in this chapter and **Chapter 20**.

Atherosclerosis

The pathology of atherosclerosis is detailed in **Chapter 13** in the discussion of coronary heart disease. Generally, the initial yellow streaks represent the intimal depositions of lipid. Next comes the formation of fibrous plaques con-

taining fibrous tissue in addition to large amounts of lipid and cellular elements. Eventually, hemorrhage, ulceration, calcification, and thrombosis occur in these plaques, forming the typical advanced lesion of atherosclerosis.

The aorta, or its major branches, may become occluded by the bulky plaques with superimposed thrombus. Although atherosclerosis begins in the intima, the underlying media may be notably weakened, leading to the formation of an aneurysm (3). Aortic dissection only occasionally results from perforation through an atherosclerotic plaque (1).

Cystic Medial Degeneration

Mild cystic medial degeneration takes place as part of the aging process and is associated with dilatation, elongation, and rigidity of the aorta. Whether this predisposes the patient to aortic dissection is debatable (1). Patients with Marfan's syndrome typically show massive degeneration of elastic fibers of the media. They usually have long extremities (long hands and feet), a high-arched palate, kyphoscoliosis, lax ligaments, and dislocated lens. Frequently, an identical form of cystic medial degeneration occurs in patients who have no other signs of Marfan's syndrome. The end result of severe, medial degeneration is a combination of ascending aortic aneurysm and proximal aortic dissection (see **Fig. 11-11**).

Aortitis

Aortitis is inflammation of the aorta with or without a known cause. Examples of aortitis with a known cause are syphilitic aortitis (see **Fig. 10-18**), tuberculous aortitis, and mycotic aneurysms (7) (Fig. 19-4); those without known cause include Takayasu's disease, giant-cell arteritis (see **Fig. 20-5**), aortitis due to ankylosing spondylitis, and Reiter's syndrome.

Trauma

Injuries to the heart and great vessels in general are discussed in **Chapter 18**. In this chapter trauma to the aorta is covered only in the section False Aneurysm of the Aorta (8).

DIFFUSE ABNORMALITIES OF THE AORTA

Small Aorta

The smallness of the aorta in the PA view may sometimes be more apparent than real. This is exemplified in patients with atrial septal defect, where the aorta rotates with the heart to the left side and folds in on itself (see **Chapter 2**). The actual smallness of a portion of the thoracic aorta is seen in supravalvular aortic stenosis with hypoplasia of the

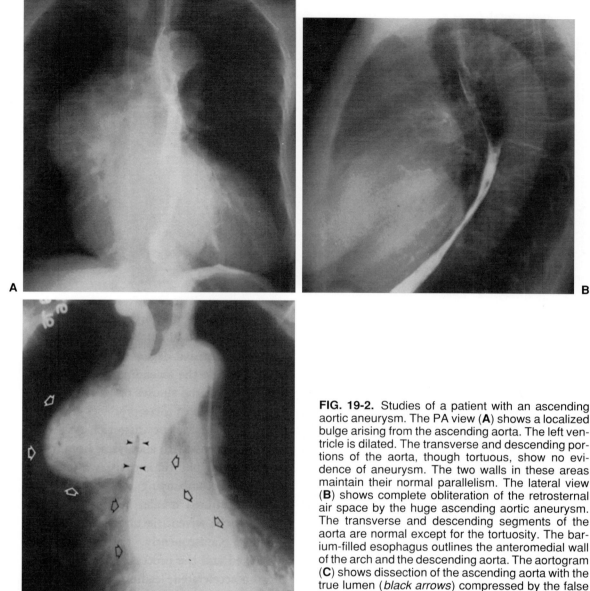

FIG. 19-2. Studies of a patient with an ascending aortic aneurysm. The PA view (**A**) shows a localized bulge arising from the ascending aorta. The left ventricle is dilated. The transverse and descending portions of the aorta, though tortuous, show no evidence of aneurysm. The two walls in these areas maintain their normal parallelism. The lateral view (**B**) shows complete obliteration of the retrosternal air space by the huge ascending aortic aneurysm. The transverse and descending segments of the aorta are normal except for the tortuosity. The barium-filled esophagus outlines the anteromedial wall of the arch and the descending aorta. The aortogram (**C**) shows dissection of the ascending aorta with the true lumen (*black arrows*) compressed by the false lumen (*white arrows*). Arrowheads mark the intimal flap.

ascending aorta and in some cases of coarctation with diffuse hypoplasia of the aorta in addition to discrete constriction.

Diffuse Dilatation and Tortuosity

The size or the degree of tortuosity of the aorta can be assessed by measuring the transverse diameter of the frontal aortic arch and by comparing the result with the predicted value on the tomogram (9) (Fig. 19-5). Values exceeding 10% of the predicted diameter are abnormal. Another method of gauging the size of the aorta is to measure the distance between the outermost border of the aortic knob and the lateral margin of the indented trachea or the barium-filled esophagus. The normal value is 2.5 to 3.0 cm. The upper limit of normal in older individuals is 4.0 cm (10) (Fig. 19-6). According to Ungerleider and Gubner (9), the diameter of the frontal aortic arch increases with age. A gradual increase in prominence of the aortic image is considered normal, coincidental with the progressive loss of elastic tissue in the media.

As a rule of thumb, tortuosity of the aorta in patients <40 years old is more important than it is in persons >40 years

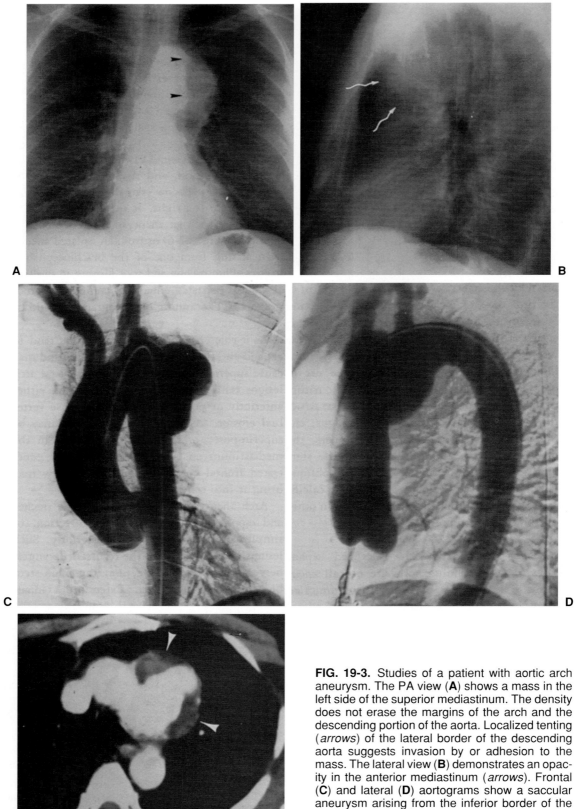

FIG. 19-3. Studies of a patient with aortic arch aneurysm. The PA view (**A**) shows a mass in the left side of the superior mediastinum. The density does not erase the margins of the arch and the descending portion of the aorta. Localized tenting (*arrows*) of the lateral border of the descending aorta suggests invasion by or adhesion to the mass. The lateral view (**B**) demonstrates an opacity in the anterior mediastinum (*arrows*). Frontal (**C**) and lateral (**D**) aortograms show a saccular aneurysm arising from the inferior border of the arch and protruding leftward, anteriorly, and cranially. A CT scan (**E**) shows an arch aneurysm springing leftward and anteriorly. Mural thrombi are evident (*arrows*).

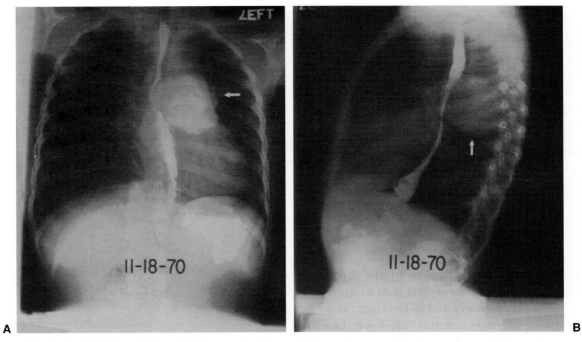

FIG. 19-4. PA (**A**) and lateral (**B**) views of a 5-year-old boy with a mycotic descending aortic aneurysm simulating a nonvascular mediastinal mass. The aneurysm (*arrow*) is at the site of the coarctation of the aorta. Both lesions were confirmed on angiography and surgery.

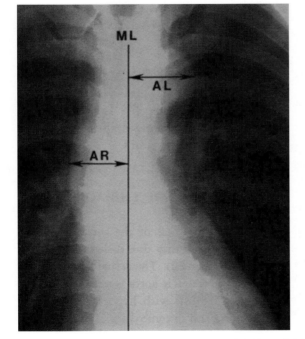

FIG. 19-5. Measurement of the aorta using the Ungerleider method (13). AL, maximum extension of the aorta to the left of midline; AR, maximum extension of the aorta to the right of midline; AR + AL, transverse diameter of the aorta; ML, midline of the spine.

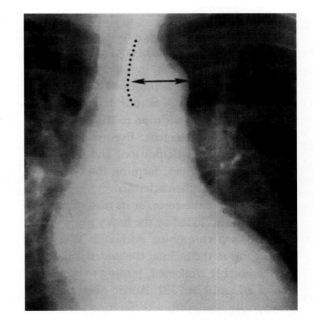

FIG. 19-6. Aortic measurements using the trachea or the esophagus as a reference. The dimension of the aortic knob is measured from the lateral margin of the trachea or the barium-filled esophagus to the outermost border of the aortic arch.

old (11). In younger people, it suggests the presence of systemic hypertension or aortic insufficiency, or both, depending on the size of the left ventricle and the status of the pulmonary vasculature (**Chapter 11**). Tortuosity with calcification of the aorta in younger persons is even more worrisome, since it suggests the presence of risk factors such as hypercholesterolemia and hypertension, with the implication of a shorter life span (12).

Radiographic Signs

The radiographic signs of diffuse dilatation and tortuosity of the aorta are as follows:

1. The transverse diameter of the frontal aorta exceeds the predictive value by 10% (9).
2. The aorta becomes uncoiled and buckles laterad and craniad against the air-filled lung, thereby widening the aortic window.
3. The descending aorta becomes visible in its entirety in both PA and lateral views.
4. The barium-filled esophagus is pulled to the left and posteriorly in conformity with the tortuous course of the aorta (Fig. 19-2A,B), with the two structures crossing each other distally, causing a marked indentation on the esophagus, even to the point of inducing dysphagia.
5. In extreme cases, the descending aorta may buckle to the contralateral side and form the right border of the cardiovascular silhouette (Fig. 19-7).
6. The borders of the tortuous aorta remain smooth and parallel without localized dilatation or narrowing.

Thoracic Aortic Aneurysm

Regardless of cause, aortic aneurysms form at the sites of damage to the media. Perhaps systemic hypertension is the single most important contributing factor in the development of such lesions, as it exposes weakness and accelerates degeneration of the elastic fibers of the media (3). Once the aorta begins to dilate, tension in its wall rises by the law of Laplace. Higher wall tension leads to further dilatation of the aneurysm. A vicious cycle may become established, eventually ending in rupture (1,3). Unlike generalized dilatation and tortuosity, aortic aneurysms are localized expansions of the aorta.

Cause and Pathology

Atherosclerosis is the leading cause of aortic aneurysm. Aneurysms of this nature tend to be fusiform and located in the aortic arch and distally. Extension into the abdomen is common (3). Both cystic medial degeneration and syphilis primarily invade the ascending segment of the aorta, including the sinuses of Valsalva. Aneurysms attributable to these processes tend to be saccular. Proximal aortic dissection occurs frequently in patients with aneurysms from medial degeneration. Syphilitic aortitis is a disease of the media. Accompanying the reparative process of the injured media, however, both the intima and the adventitia undergo fibrosis

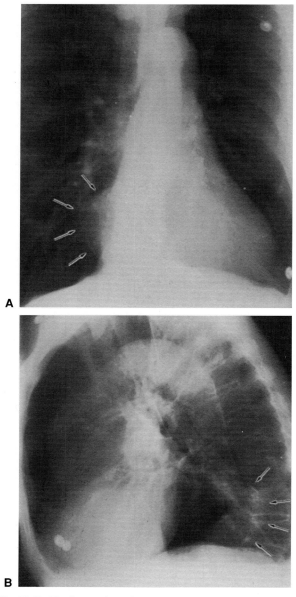

FIG. 19-7. Radiographs of a patient with a tortuous aorta. PA (**A**) and lateral (**B**) views show a very tortuous aorta with the lower descending segment (*arrows*) forming the right cardiac border. There is, however, no evidence of aneurysm or dissection.

and thickening. Consequently, the coronary ostia are involved, and the process of intimal atherosclerosis is accelerated, leading to selective calcification of the ascending aorta. Other rare forms of the disease include mycotic aneurysms (Fig. 19-4), aneurysms at the site of coarctation repair (see **Fig. 4-28**), and aneurysms resulting from Takayasu's disease and giant-cell aortitis.

Clinical Presentation

Patients with aortic aneurysm may be entirely asymptomatic. Under this circumstance, the diagnosis is usually made by the evidence of radiographic abnormalities or by the discovery of a murmur of aortic insufficiency. The most common symptom is chest pain. Compression symptoms from an arch aneurysm include cough, dyspnea, dysphagia, hoarseness, or superior vena cava syndrome. Unfortunately, exsanguination can occur without warning. At other times, hemoptysis, hematemesis, or widening of the mediastinum may precede a fatal hemorrhage into the airways, the esopha-

gus, the mediastinum, and the pleural and extrapleural spaces. Rupture into the pericardium causes cardiac tamponade. Rupture into the systemic venous system establishes an arteriovenous fistula. The risk of rupture increases with the size of the aneurysm (3,13). An aneurysm 6 cm or larger, particularly in a symptomatic patient, should be resected on an emergency basis. Congestive heart failure may occasionally become the predominant clinical manifestation of an

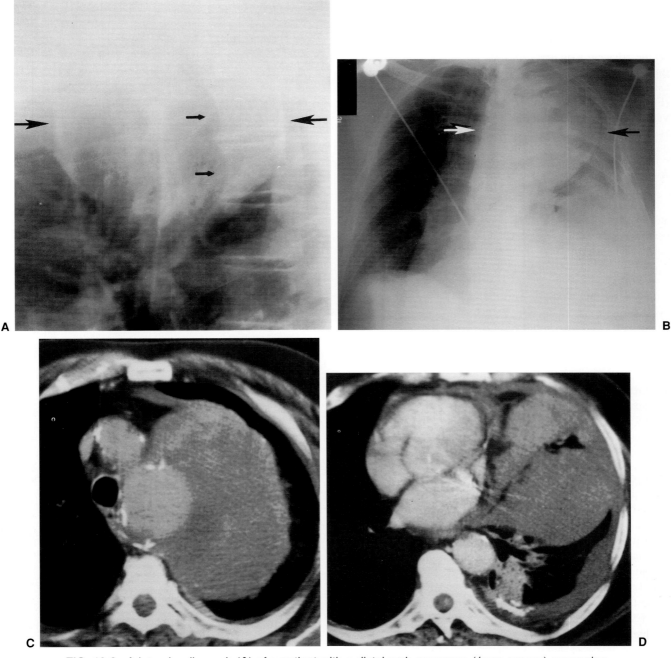

FIG. 19-8. A lateral radiograph (**A**) of a patient with a distal arch aneurysm (*large arrows*) measuring 8 × 9 cm. Note compression bone erosion of T5 and T6 (*small arrows*). A second radiograph in the PA view (**B**), taken 7 years later, shows interval growing of the aneurysm to 13.5 × 14.5 cm (*arrows*); it has begun to leak into the left lung and left pleural space. Computed tomography scans at the levels of the arch (**C**) and the left atrium (**D**) confirm the radiographic evidence.

ascending aortic aneurysm, owing to the associated severe aortic insufficiency. The therapy of choice or by necessity is surgical repair.

Radiographic Signs

Routine chest films should be carefully scrutinized for the detection of aortic diseases. Most of the time the size, shape, location, and direction of expansion of a thoracic aortic aneurysm is clearly delineated by the lung. The medial extent of the lesion can be outlined by the barium-filled esophagus. Fluoroscopy and the use of oblique views can help in the evaluation of the dynamic nature of the lesion and its effect on the adjacent structures, such as the airways, the esophagus, the pulmonary arteries, the cardiac chambers, the mediastinum, the lung, the pleura, the sternum, and the spine (Fig. 19-8). Fluoroscopy and oblique radiographs are also valuable in detecting calcifications in the wall of an aneurysm and in other cardiovascular structures.

Ascending Aortic Aneurysms

Localized expansions of the ascending aorta are not all aneurysms. The most notable condition that mimics an ascending aneurysm is the poststenotic dilatation of valvular aortic stenosis. In general, aortic aneurysms remain connected to the aorta in all views of the chest (11). The most outstanding examples of ascending aortic aneurysm are those caused by syphilitic aortitis and Marfan's syndrome or its forme fruste (11) (Fig. 19-2; see also **Figs. 4-22, 10-18**, and **11-11**). The complications of ascending aortic aneurysm are aortic insufficiency (see **Figs. 10-18 and 11-11**), pressure erosion of the sternum and adjacent ribs, compression of the right mainstem bronchus and right phrenic nerve, and rupture into the pericardium (see **Fig. 11-11**) with resultant cardiac tamponade.

Aortic Arch Aneurysms

Depending on its exact location, extension, and shape, an arch aneurysm can cast a shadow cranially or caudally, to the left or to the right. It may be difficult to differentiate such a lesion from a mediastinal tumor or an isolated aneurysm from one of the brachiocephalic arteries (Fig. 19-3). Arch aneurysms tend to displace the trachea and esophagus laterad in either direction or simply compress them anteroposteriorly. They may also compress the recurrent laryngeal nerve, the phrenic nerve, and the mainstem bronchus on either side. Extending craniad, arch aneurysms may affect the brachiocephalic arteries, causing cerebral symptoms and differential blood pressures and pulses between the two arms (11).

As a rule, proximal arch aneurysms tend to expand anteriorly and to the right side and may cause superior vena cava syndrome. Distal arch lesions tend to extend to the left side,

superiorly and posteriorly, and may cause vertebral erosion (Fig. 19-8). The central type of arch aneurysm arising from its inferior border deserves special mention because of its unique radiographic manifestations (Fig. 19-3). It typically extends to the left side and anteriorly, making it difficult to understand why an apparent descending aortic lesion on the PA view projects anteriorly into the ascending territory on the lateral view. This paradox, however, turns out to be a useful clue to the correct diagnosis (see Fig. 20-1).

Descending Aortic Aneurysms

Aneurysms arising from the proximal descending aorta extend leftward and posteriorly (Fig. 19-9). Lower descend-

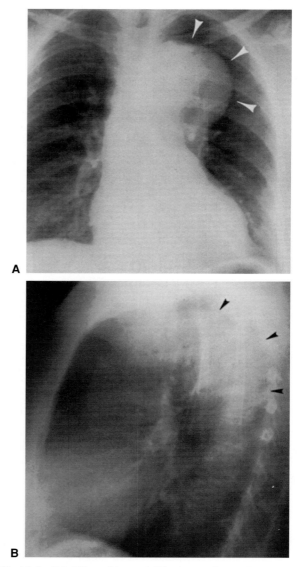

FIG. 19-9. PA (**A**) and lateral (**B**) views of a patient show a large proximal descending aortic aneurysm (*arrows*). The rest of the aorta remains normal. The diagnosis was verified by aortography and at surgery.

ing aortic aneurysms displace the esophagus (or nasogastric tube) and the left stem bronchus to the right and anteriorly (Fig. 19-4) and may cause left lung collapse (Fig. 19-10). In the posterior mediastinum, an aneurysm should be distinguished from a lung mass, a paraspinal abscess, and a neurogenic tumor (Fig. 19-9). The most serious complication of an aneurysm is rupture. This can happen swiftly, without warning. Sometimes a temporarily contained hematoma may be evident before the fatal exsanguination. This occurs more commonly in the left hemithorax (Fig. 19-8) than in the right (Fig. 19-11).

Aortography, Computed Tomography and Magnetic Resonance Imaging

If the diagnosis of aortic aneurysm remains in doubt, aortography (Figs. 19-2C; 19-3C,D; 19-12B; and 19-13C) may be required for clarification. Recently, CT scanning with enhancement (2,3) (see **Chapter 20**) and MRI (see **Chapter 4**) have been used effectively in selected cases (Fig 19-3E; see also Figs. **4-22, 4-28, 4-29** and **20-1**) to confirm the diagnosis. Both technologies have the following advantages over aortography: they do not require catheterization; they are superior in distinguishing aneurysm from other mediastinal masses; they better delineate the thrombus contained in the aneurysm; they can assess the thickness of the aortic wall and more accurately measure the diameter and length of the aneurysm; and they are more effective in detecting associated abnormalities, such as hematoma, pleural effusion, collapsed lung, and bony erosion.

Magnetic resonance imaging has the further advantage of multiplanary display of findings and of distinguishing slow blood flow from clots (see **Fig. 4-20**). However, CT is suffi-

cient for diagnosis in most cases and is less expensive than MRI. Aortography, on the other hand, may be indispensable when hemodynamic information and detailed branch vascular anatomy are needed in the preparation for surgery (2).

Aortic Dissection

Acute aortic dissection is also known as dissecting hematoma or dissecting aneurysm. The incidence of this disease is about 2,000 patients per year in the United States. Aortic dissection usually begins with a tear in the intima, allowing the blood to enter the aortic wall under high pressure. The dissecting hematoma may extend into the aortic root, causing aortic insufficiency (see **Fig. 11-11**). It may eventually rupture through the adventitia into the pericardium, the left pleural space, or anywhere along the course of the aorta (1). An intramural hematoma (the false lumen) may cause a second intimal rupture distally at its reentry to the aorta (the true lumen). Occasionally, a dissection begins as an intramural hematoma from hemorrhage of the vasa vasorum. Under such circumstance, an intimal tear is not present initially (11,14) and therefore may be impossible to differentiate from an aneurysm with large thrombus (Fig. 19-14D).

Aortic dissection has been classified by DeBakey and colleagues (14) into three types: type I involves all segments of the aorta (Fig. 19-15B), type II is limited to the ascending aorta (Fig. 19-2C), and type III begins in the descending aorta (Figs. 19-14, 19-15A, and 19-16) and extends distally. Daily and associates (15) proposed reclassifying aortic dissection form into two types, with type A including all dissections affecting the ascending aorta and type B encompassing those confined to the descending aorta.

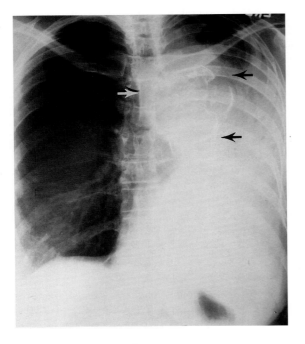

FIG. 19-10. A PA radiograph of a patient with a huge calcified descending aortic aneurysm (*arrows*) compressing the left stem bronchus and causing subtotal collapse of the left lung.

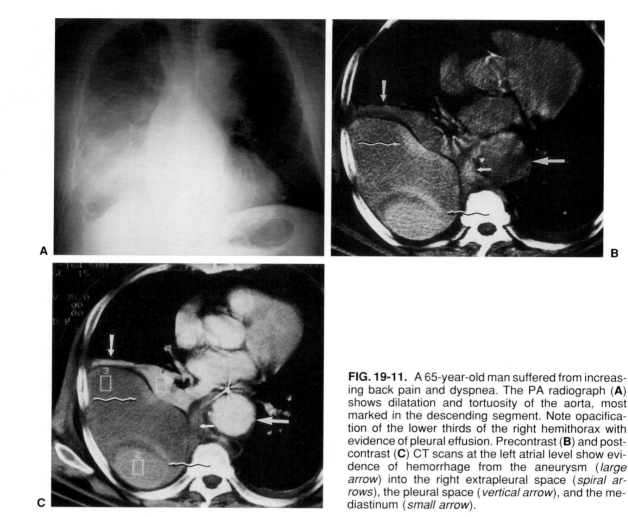

FIG. 19-11. A 65-year-old man suffered from increasing back pain and dyspnea. The PA radiograph (**A**) shows dilatation and tortuosity of the aorta, most marked in the descending segment. Note opacification of the lower thirds of the right hemithorax with evidence of pleural effusion. Precontrast (**B**) and postcontrast (**C**) CT scans at the left atrial level show evidence of hemorrhage from the aneurysm (*large arrow*) into the right extrapleural space (*spiral arrows*), the pleural space (*vertical arrow*), and the mediastinum (*small arrow*).

Clinical Presentation

Severe chest pain is the most common symptom of aortic dissection. It is commonly associated with sweating, nausea, vomiting, fainting, and apprehension. Anterior chest pain suggests proximal dissection, and interscapular pain indicates distal dissection. Congestive heart failure usually results from aortic insufficiency as a complication of proximal dissection. Syncope without focal neurologic deficits suggests the presence of cardiac tamponade resulting from dissection into the pericardium. On physical examination, pulse deficits, neurologic signs, and aortic insufficiency are commonly evident in the patient with proximal dissection (16).

Radiographic Signs

On radiography, most patients show evidence of long-standing severe systemic hypertension in the form of diffuse dilatation and tortuosity of the aorta and left ventricular hypertrophy. In addition to this background of hypertensive cardiovascular changes, more localized expansion of the aorta is usually present (Fig. 19-16). The involved segments tend to be elongated with lobulated borders. Under the fluoroscope, pulsations are absent or markedly diminished, in contrast to the adjacent normally pulsating aorta.

There are three radiographic signs highly suggestive of aortic dissection: progressive enlargement of the same segment or segments on serial films (Fig. 19-16); double density of the aortic image, or the "aorta within aorta" sign, which represents the composite shadow of two lumina of the aorta (Fig. 19-14); and the displaced calcium sign, which becomes positive when the calcium depicted in the intima is >6 mm within the outer border of the dilated aorta. With regard to the last sign, the superimposition of two segments of the aorta in the region of the aortic knob in the PA view must not be mistaken as a positive displaced calcium sign. To avoid such error, a steep left anterior oblique view should be obtained.

Angiographic Signs

On aortography both the true and false lumina can be opacified, with the intimal flap appearing as a linear lucency

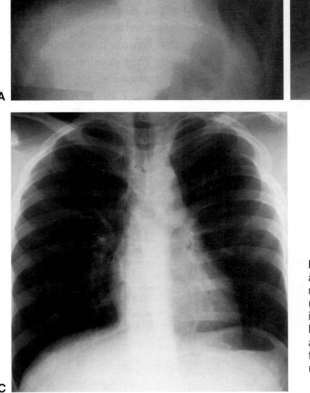

FIG. 19-12. Studies of a child with transection of the aorta. The PA view (**A**) shows a markedly widened mediastinum and left apical capping. An aortogram (**B**) demonstrates the site of transection to be the isthmus of the aorta (*arrow*). The opacified blood leaks into the mediastinum (*arrowhead*). The left apical cap has widened (*open arrow*). A postoperative radiograph taken 3 months later (**C**) shows remarkable improvement.

between them (Fig. 19-15). In this manner the site of origin and the extent of the dissection, as well as the distal circulation of the vital organs, can all be determined (16). Sometimes, the degree of narrowing of the true lumen by the false lumen and the point of reentry of the false lumen can also be documented. Delayed filling and emptying may be observed in either the true or the false lumen. The information on associated aortic insufficiency and left ventricular function may be obtained in the same sitting.

Other Imaging Methods

In the diagnosis of aortic dissection, imaging techniques other than aortography have also been used. They include CT (3,18) (see **Chapter 20**), transesophageal echocardiography (3,17,18) (see **Chapter 6**), and MRI (3) (see **Chapter 4**). Although transesophageal echocardiography has the benefits of speed, convenience, accuracy, and reasonable cost (see **Fig. 6-9**), it is somewhat invasive, with an incidence of complications of 2.8% (17). Computed tomography can accurately identify the intimal flap, the true and false lumina, and calcifications (see **Figs. 20-2 and 20-4**). However, if only one lumen is filled with contrast agent and no calcium is visible, it can be difficult to differentiate between a thrombosed dissection and a fusiform aneurysm by CT alone (3,18). Other disadvantages of CT include pulsation artifacts, the need to perform dynamic scans with contrast medium, and the inability of the technique to assess aortic valve and branch vessels. Aortography, although invasive, remains the

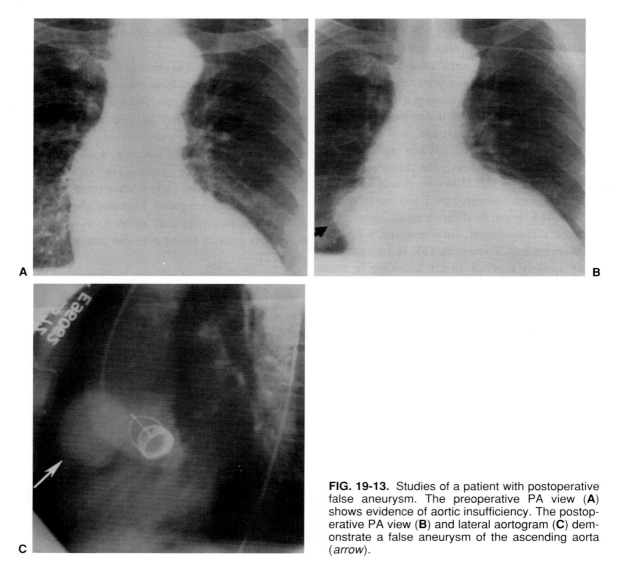

FIG. 19-13. Studies of a patient with postoperative false aneurysm. The preoperative PA view (**A**) shows evidence of aortic insufficiency. The postoperative PA view (**B**) and lateral aortogram (**C**) demonstrate a false aneurysm of the ascending aorta (*arrow*).

procedure of choice when dissection is strongly suspected and emergency operation is seriously considered. Computed tomography is indicated when the diagnosis of dissection is not so strongly entertained, in patients with chronic dissections and in those who need postoperative follow-ups (2,18).

Magnetic resonance imaging has advantages in assessing suspected aortic dissection: no contrast medium is required; a multiplanary display of information is possible; the cine technique can assess the function of the aortic valve and left ventricle; and, like CT, the method can detect mediastinal hematoma, hemothorax, and hemopericardium. The disadvantages of MRI are that some patients are excluded for safety reasons, it is more time-consuming than CT, artifacts are seen more often than with CT, and greater experience is required to interpret MR images accurately. Taking all these considerations into account, under favorable conditions, MRI is probably the most versatile and accurate single

test for the detection of aortic dissection (3,18) (see **Figs. 4-1, 4-12, 4-13, 4-21,** and **20-3** and **Chapter 4**).

False Aneurysm of the Aorta

False aneurysms of the aorta most commonly result from blunt chest trauma from automobile accidents (8,19,20). Occasionally they develop postoperatively as a surgical complication.

Transection of the Aorta

A false aneurysm accompanying transection of the aorta most frequently results from injuries associated with blunt chest trauma (8,19,20). Sudden deceleration of the body in automobile accidents or as a result of falls from a height

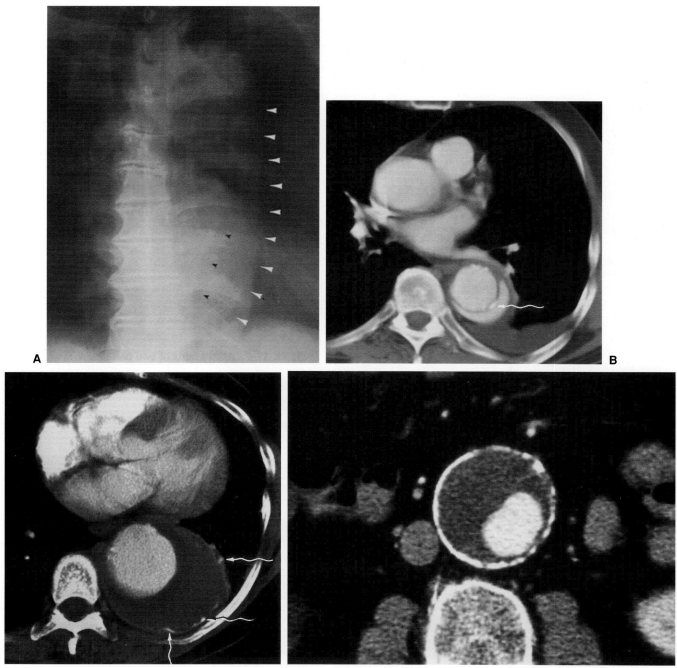

FIG. 19-14. Bucky film (**A**) of a patient with dissection of the descending aorta. Note the double density (*black arrows*) in the descending aorta (*white arrows*). Another, similar patient whose enhanced CT image (**B**) shows two equally opacified lumens with an intimal flap between. Note the calcific deposits within the intimal flap (*arrow*). In comparison, the CT scan (**C**) of patient 3 shows an aneurysm with a large thrombus and peripheral calcified intima (*arrows*). An enhanced CT scan (**D**) of patient 4 shows a compressed aortic lumen, large nonopacified thrombus, and peripheral calcification. Whether this represents an aneurysm with a thrombus or an intramural hematoma is very difficult to tell.

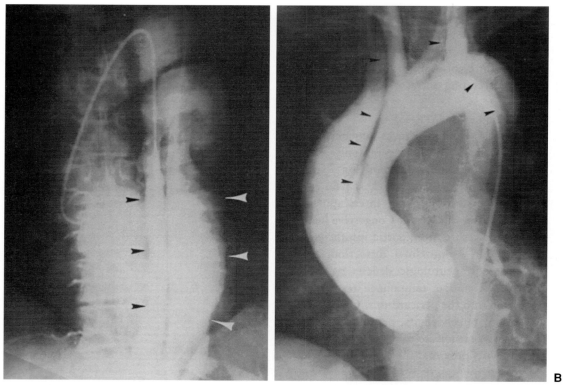

FIG. 19-15. Aortograms of two patients with aortic dissection. The aortogram (**A**) obtained from patient 1 demonstrates the the true (*black arrows*) and false (*white arrows*) lumina of the descending aorta with the intimal flap in between. The aortogram (**B**) of patient 2 reveals extensive aortic dissection involving all segments of the thoracic aorta. Arrows point to the intimal flap between the true and false lumina.

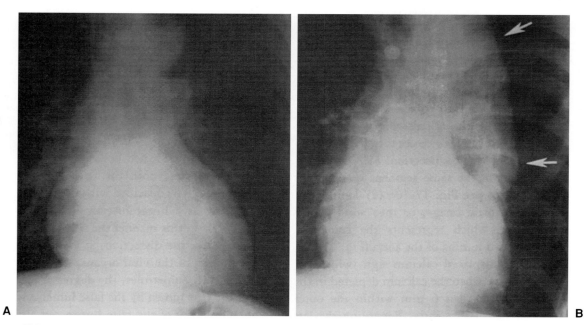

FIG. 19-16. Radiographs (**A,B**), made 2 years apart, of a patient with evolving dissection of the descending aorta show the increasing prominence of the proximal descending aorta (*arrows*).

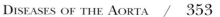

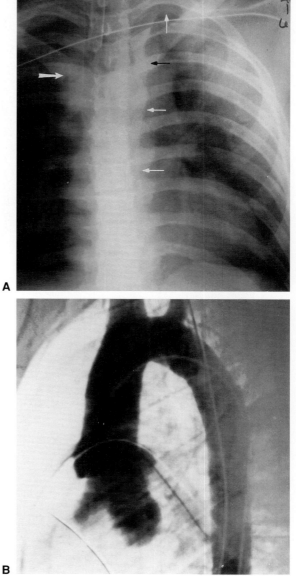

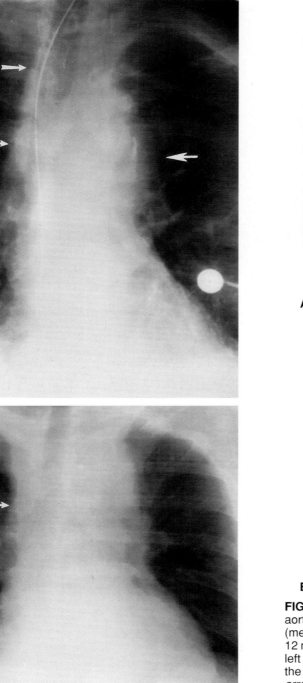

FIG. 19-17. Two adults with transection of the aorta at the isthmus. The PA radiograph (**A**) of patient 1, an 82-year-old woman, shows widening of the mediastinum (measuring 9.8 cm) and of the right paratracheal stripe (measuring 12 mm) (*small arrows*). Also note a mass (*large arrow*) in the antero-posterior window (measuring 18 mm lateral to the calcified intima of the descending aorta). Both the trachea and the esophagus are displaced to the right side. The anteroposter-ior view (**B**) of patient 2, a 37-year-old man, shows marked widening of the mediastinum (measuring 11 cm) and of the right paratracheal stripe (*arrows*) (measuring 30 mm). Left apical capping is visible. The trachea is deviated to the right side.

FIG. 19-18. A 21-year-old man with deceleration injury of the aorta. The radiograph (**A**) shows widening of the mediastinum (measuring 9.5 cm) and right paratracheal stripe (measuring 12 mm) (*arrow*). The trachea is deviated to the right side. The left paraspinal line (*small arrows*) is deformed, extending to the left and superiorly to form the left apical cap (*vertical arrow*). Also note a contusion of the left-upper lung. The aorto-gram (**B**) shows an unusual site of transection, just above the aortic valve.

have a violent shearing effect on the aorta where a mobile portion is connected to a fixed segment. In 90% of patients the site of rupture is in the aortic isthmus, where the vessel is fixed by the ligamentum arteriosum (1). The uncommon sites of transection are in the ascending segment and the arch of the aorta.

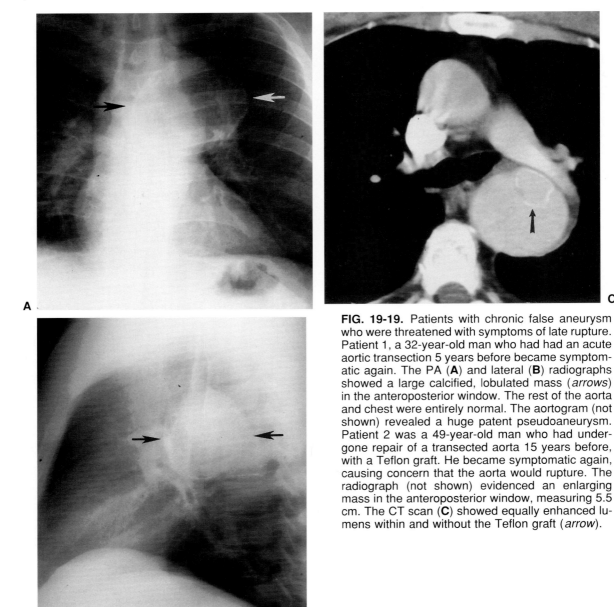

FIG. 19-19. Patients with chronic false aneurysm who were threatened with symptoms of late rupture. Patient 1, a 32-year-old man who had had an acute aortic transection 5 years before became symptomatic again. The PA (**A**) and lateral (**B**) radiographs showed a large calcified, lobulated mass (*arrows*) in the anteroposterior window. The rest of the aorta and chest were entirely normal. The aortogram (not shown) revealed a huge patent pseudoaneurysm. Patient 2 was a 49-year-old man who had undergone repair of a transected aorta 15 years before, with a Teflon graft. He became symptomatic again, causing concern that the aorta would rupture. The radiograph (not shown) evidenced an enlarging mass in the anteroposterior window, measuring 5.5 cm. The CT scan (**C**) showed equally enhanced lumens within and without the Teflon graft (*arrow*).

Clinical Presentation

Two thirds of patients with transection of the aorta have obvious evidence of other chest trauma. Aortic rupture itself may be relatively asymptomatic (8). Compression symptoms may arise in the form of dyspnea, stridor, dysphagia, and superior vena cava syndrome. Rarely, but typically, acute coarctation with blood pressure discrepancy between the upper and lower extremities may develop. A systolic murmur is usually heard over the interscapular area (1). About 80% of patients with transection of the aorta die immediately. Death frequently occurs among the survivors within the first week.

Without the benefit of surgery, only 2% to 5% live long enough to develop a chronic pseudoaneurysm at the site of the aortic rupture. Old traumatic aneurysms may become infected, and even calcified ones may rupture; for this reason, they should always be repaired surgically (1).

Radiographic Signs

The radiographic signs of aortic transection are nonspecific but important to keep in mind, since a decision must be made promptly as to the need for aortography (8). Widening of the mediastinum over 8 cm is suggestive of aortic transection (Figs. 19-12, 19-17, and 19-18), and progressive widening over a short period of time, in particular, is a probable sign of aortic rupture with active bleeding. As the blood accumulates in the mediastinum, widening near the aortic isthmus becomes most marked; this widening is followed by deviation of the trachea and esophagus (as often outlined by a nasogastric tube) to the right side. Eventually, the blood is spilled over into the extrapleural space and assumes the form of an apical cap, which is most commonly seen on the left side but may be found bilaterally. Other suggestive signs are widening of the right paratracheal stripe exceeding 5 mm., rib and spinal fractures, lung contusion, and pleural effusion (Figs. 19-12, 19-17, 19-18).

Angiographic Signs

Aortography is the procedure used to confirm the diagnosis before thoracotomy. The injected contrast medium promptly outlines the lumen of the aorta and depicts the site of rupture and extravasation into the false aneurysm and the mediastinum (18) (Figs. 19-12B and 19-18B).

Computed Tomography and Magnetic Resonance Imaging

The literature suggests that CT may play a role in the assessment of suspected traumatic aortic rupture (19,20). If the portal chest radiograph gives equivocal results, CT may help determine whether mediastinal hematoma is present. If it is not present, no further study is needed. If it is (see Fig. 20-8 and 20-9), aortography should be undertaken. When confronting the problems of monitoring and sustaining the trauma patient, MRI is less practical. In the evaluation of patients with chronic false aneurysm, either CT or MRI would be appropriate (Fig. 19-19C; see also **4-14** and **4-25**) (see **Chapters 4** and **20**).

Postoperative Pseudoaneurysm

Postoperative rupture of the aorta, forming a false aneurysm, is rare. Such cases are only occasionally seen following aortic valve replacement (Fig. 19-13) and aortonomy for cardiopulmonary bypass or coronary artery bypass grafting (see **Figs. 20-6** and **20-7**).

REFERENCES

1. Eagle KA, De Sanctis RW. Diseases of the aorta. In: Braunwald E, ed. *Heart disease: a textbook of cardiovascular medicine*, 4th ed. Philadelphia: Saunders, 1992:1528–1557.
2. Rooholamini SA, Stanford W. Ultrafast computed tomography in the diagnosis of aortic aneurysms and dissections. In: Stanford W, Rumberger J, eds. *Ultrafast computed tomography in cardiac imaging: principles and practice*. Mount Kisco, N.Y.: Futura, 1992:287–310.
3. Lindsay J, DeBakey ME, Beall AC. Diagnosis and treatment of diseases of the aorta. In: Schlant RC, Alexander RW, eds. *The heart*, 8th ed. New York: McGraw–Hill, 1994:2163–2180.
4. Gabella G. Cardiovascular system. In: Williams PL, Bannister LH, Berry MM, et al., eds. *Gray's anatomy*, 38th ed. Edinburgh: Churchill Livingstone, 1995:1505–1574.
5. Meszaros WT. *Cardiac roentgenology*. Springfield, Ill.: Thomas, 1969: 146–199.
6. Baron MG. Anatomy of the heart. In: Taveras JM, Ferrucci JT, eds. *Radiology: diagnosis—imaging—intervention*. Philadelphia: Lippincott, 1987:1–13.
7. Oldham HN Jr, Phillips JF, Jewett PH, et al. Surgical treatment of mycotic aneurysm associated with coarctation of the aorta. *Ann Thorac Surg* 1973;15:411–418.
8. Woodring JH. The normal mediastinum in blunt traumatic rupture of the thoracic aorta and brachiocephalic arteries. *J Emerg Med* 1990;8: 467–476.
9. Ungerleider HE, Gubner R. Evaluation of heart size measurements. *Am Heart J* 1942;24:494–510.
10. Kreuzfuchs S. Die Brustaorta im Röntgenbilt. *Wien Klin Wochenschr* 1916;29:701–705.
11. Thurn P. Heart diseases. In: Schinz HR, Baensch WE, Frommhold W, et al., eds. *Roentgen diagnosis*, 2nd ed. New York: Grune & Stratton, 1970:527–557.
12. Bell MF, Schaaf RS, Jernigan TP. The prognostic import of calcification of the aortic knob. *Trans Assoc Life Insur Med Dir Am* 1963;47: 33.
13. Fomon JJ, Kurzweg FT, Broadway RK. Aneurysms of aorta: a review. *Ann Surg* 1967;165:557–563.
14. DeBakey ME, Henly WS, Cooley DA, et al. Surgical management of dissecting aneurysms of the aorta. *J Thorac Cardiovasc Surg* 1965;49: 130–149.
15. Daily PO, Trueblood HW, Stinson EB, et al. Management of acute aortic dissection. *Ann Thorac Surg* 1970;10:237–247.
16. Tonkin IL. Diseases of the thoracic aorta. In: Putman CE, Ravin CE, eds. *Textbook of diagnostic imaging*, 2nd ed. Philadelphia: Saunders, 1994:1843–1859.
17. Khandheria BK, Seward JB, Tajik AJ. Transesophageal echocardiography. *Mayo Clin Proc* 1994;69:856–863.
18. Fann JI, Miller DC. Management of ascending aortic dissection. *American College of Cardiology Current Journal Review* May/June 1995: 39–41.
19. Morgan PWE, Goodman LR, Aprahamian C, at el. Evaluation of traumatic aortic injury: Does dynamic contrast-enhanced CT play a role? *Radiology* 1992;182:661–666.
20. Raptopoulos V, Sheiman RG, Phillips DA, et al. Traumatic aortic tear: screening with chest CT. *Radiology* 1992;182:667–673.

Essentials of Cardiac Imaging,
James T. T. Chen,
Lippincott–Raven Publishers, Philadelphia © 1998.

CHAPTER **20**

Computed Tomography and Magnetic Resonance Imaging of the Thoracic Aorta

Edward F. Patz, Jr.

Chest radiographs remain the most common radiologic study performed. The thoracic aorta is imaged on each study, and although plain films provide a tremendous amount of information, additional studies are often necessary in making the correct diagnosis. Aortography, computed tomography (CT), and magnetic resonance imaging (MRI) are the most commonly used examinations, depending on the clinical question, the chest radiographic findings, and the patient's condition (1–5). Aortic diseases can be divided into congenital and acquired abnormalities, although this review will focus on advanced imaging techniques of acquired diseases of the thoracic aorta. There are four major acquired abnormalities of the thoracic aorta: aneurysm, dissection, aortitis, and trauma (see **Chapter 19**).

AORTIC ANEURYSM

Aortic aneurysms are predominantly atherosclerotic in nature, representing one of the two major complications of atherosclerosis, the other being aortic dissection (4,6–12). Therefore, in the presence of aortic aneurysm, milder atherosclerotic lesions are usually evident elsewhere in the aorta. They are typically found in older individuals, particularly patients with hypertension, diabetes, and a history of smoking. Contrast-enhanced CT or MR manifestations of atherosclerotic disease are focal luminal irregularity, ectasia, tortuosity, and variable amounts of thrombus and plaque formation. Thick localized calcification is a typical finding in older individuals. It is usually present within the wall and occasionally within intraluminal plaque formation.

True aortic aneurysms represent a focal ballooning of the aorta with preservation of the vessel wall. They are usually described as saccular or fusiform, depending on the configu-

ration, and are typically found distal to the transverse aortic arch. The plain film appearances are variable and may be confused with those of other mediastinal abnormalities. Contrast-enhanced CT or MRI generally clarifies the abnormality and defines its exact location, origin, and relationship to other mediastinal structures and the extent of intraluminal thrombus (Fig. 20-1). Computed tomographic findings have been well described and include an area of focal aortic enlargement with luminal enhancement and variable amounts of thrombus and calcification (1,6,7,10,13,14). Similar information, with the exception of wall calcification, can be gained by MRI. These features are useful not only for making the diagnosis but also for therapeutic decisions (9,15–17). A progressively enlarging aneurysm, particularly when it is >5 to 6 cm in diameter, has a tendency to rupture (see **Figs. 19-7** and **19-11**), and surgical repair is often suggested.

AORTIC DISSECTION

Aortic dissection is ordinarily seen in hypertensive patients, although it may complicate a number of aortic disorders, such as Marfan's syndrome. It begins as an intimal tear that creates a false channel into the wall of the aorta. Aortic dissections often originate either at the level of the aortic valve or at the isthmus (just below the takeoff of the left subclavian artery). It is essential to differentiate the types of dissection, because those dissections involving the ascending aorta are considered surgical candidates and those involving only the descending aorta are treated more conservatively with medical therapy (aiming at controlling the patient's hypertension). Two different classifications describe aortic dissections. The DeBakey classification has three types: type 1 encompasses the entire aorta, type 2 involves just the ascending aorta, and type 3 involves only the descending aorta. The Stanford classification is somewhat

Department of Radiology, Duke University Medical Center, Durham, North Carolina 27710, U.S.A.

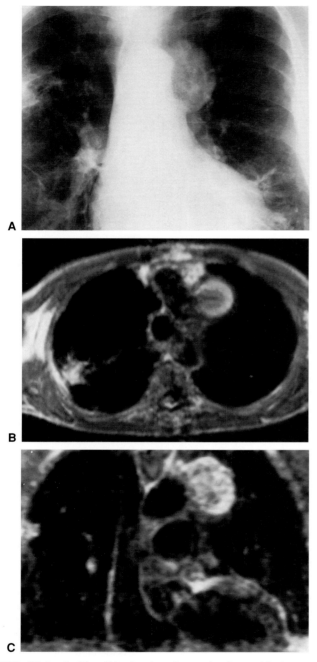

FIG. 20-1. A: The PA chest radiograph of an elderly man with a long history of hypertension and diabetes demonstrates a smoothly marginated mediastinal mass projecting over the region of the anteroposterior window. **B:** Axial T2-weighted MRI at the level of the aortic arch shows a predominantly high-signal-intensity abnormality suggestive of a thrombosed aortic arch aneurysm. **C:** Coronal MRI confirms the presence of a thrombosed saccular aneurysm.

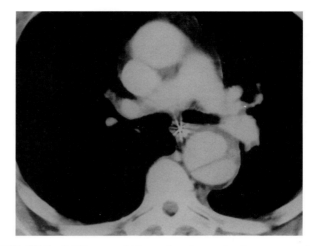

FIG. 20-2. A 52-year-old hypertensive patient was seen for assessment of back pain. An axial CT image with contrast demonstrates an intraluminal flap with flow in both the true and false lumens in the descending aorta. This finding was suggested a type B dissection.

simpler: type A affects the ascending aorta, while type B only affects the descending aorta.

Patients are usually symptomatic, and although the diagnosis may be suggested on plain films, additional studies are almost always performed. The next study depends on the patient's stability and other relevant information (i.e., status of the aortic valve and coronary arteries). In the vast majority of cases, transesophageal echocardiography, MRI, or CT provides diagnostic information, and aortography is not necessary (7,16,18–22). The absolute evidence of an aortic dissection in all of these studies is an intraluminal intimal flap. In most cases (70%), there will be flow in both the true and false lumens, which confirms the diagnosis (Figs. 20-2 and 20-3) (18,23–25). Limitations of transesophageal echocardiography includes its operator dependence and the fact that subtle abnormalities may not be clearly defined (26,27). Magnetic resonance imaging can be limited by the patient's clinical status and by technical difficulties.

Both of these studies, however, do not require intravenous contrast administration; this is a significant advantage over CT in patients with renal failure. In patients with normal renal function, CT is the study of choice at our institution, since helical CT studies can be performed with a uniformly optimal bolus of intravenous contrast in a short period of time. In cases in which the false lumen is thrombosed, other signs should suggest the diagnosis (7,28): a hyperdense soft-tissue rind due to clot surrounding the lumen on noncontrast studies (Fig 20-4) (29), displacement of intimal calcification, a pleural (usually left-sided) effusion, or a pericardial effusion.

AORTITIS

Inflammatory lesions of the aorta are uncommon. They may be caused by an infectious process, including syphilis,

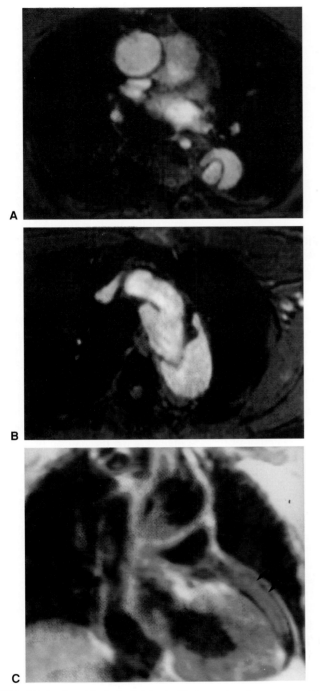

FIG. 20-3. An elderly individual with hypertension was seen for assessment of mild back pain. **A:** Gradient-refocused axial MR images show flow in the ascending and descending aorta with an intraluminal flap dividing the true and false lumen, suggestive of a dissection. **B:** An axial image of a similar patient demonstrates an intraluminal flap in the aortic arch. **C:** Coronal MRI of the same patient evidences increased signal (*long arrows*) within the pericardium, suggesting the presence of fluid and an intraluminal flap (*short arrows*) in the aortic arch. This constellation of findings is diagnostic of aortic dissection rupturing into the pericardium.

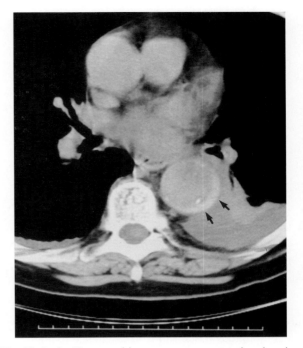

FIG. 20-4. A 68-year-old women was experiencing back pain. The CT image shows an asymmetric hyperdense soft-tissue rind surrounding the descending aorta (*arrows*), indicating intramural thrombus from a type B aortic dissection.

tuberculosis, or other bacterial diseases. As a result of infection, mycotic aneurysms may be produced. The typical findings of aortitis, on contrast-enhanced CT or MRI, are asymmetric focal enlargement of the aortic lumen and thickening of the aortic wall (30). There may be atelectasis of the adjacent lung and a pleural effusion.

Noninfectious causes of aortitis include Takayasu's arteritis, giant-cell arteritis, and, rarely, some of the spondyloarthropathies, such as Reiter's syndrome or ankylosing spondylitis. These inflammatory processes usually have systemic manifestations. While plain chest radiographs often give nonspecific results, findings on CT or MRI may suggest the correct diagnosis. These features include aortic luminal narrowing, annulo-aortic ectasia, and varying degrees of aortic wall thickening (Fig 20-5) (31). Associated findings may also include similar findings in other thoracic vessels. In Takayasus aortitis, a thin rim of aortic wall calcification may be seen in association with other findings, for example, stenosis and/or dilation of the brachiocephalic vessels.

TRAUMA

A number of studies have addressed the problem of diagnosing and treating patients with potential aortic trauma, although there still does not exist a unified approach. Trauma of the aorta can be divided into two general categories: penetrating and nonpenetrating injuries. These injuries create a perforation or tear of the aortic wall and produce a pseudoan-

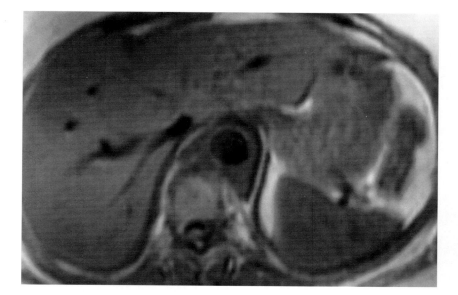

FIG. 20-5. A 47-year-old woman had an elevated sedimentation rate and multiple systemic complaints. The axial T2-weighted MR scan shows marked thickening of the descending aorta, which suggested the patient's eventual diagnosis of vasculitis, presumed to be giant-cell aortitis.

eurysm. Pulsatile blood flow into the abnormality is contained by fibrous tissue and clot. Computed tomography or MRI usually demonstrates a narrow channel of blood arising from the aorta and flowing into a heterogeneous soft-tissue abnormality representing the thrombus (32). In the acute stage, there is no calcification, although chronic (>6 months) pseudoaneurysms often show fine curvilinear calcification surrounding the abnormality.

A penetrating wound due to sharp or projectile objects or to surgical procedures, such as aortotomy for cardiopulmonary bypass, can cause focal aortic lacerations (Figs. 20-6, and 20-7) (32,33). Plain film findings that are suggestive of

aortic injury necessitate further evaluation. Direct visualization of the vessels with angiography remains the study of choice, since the site and extent of injury can be identified.

Nonpenetrating injuries, most commonly due to motor vehicle accidents, cause a shear or compression injury to the aorta. These injuries vary in degree, from small intimal tears to complete transection (34–37). The diagnostic workup of these patients is still a subject of controversy and depends on a number of factors, including the mechanism of injury, plain film findings, the patient's stability, and the institution (38–40). Some studies have suggested screening low-risk patients with equivocal findings on portable chest radio-

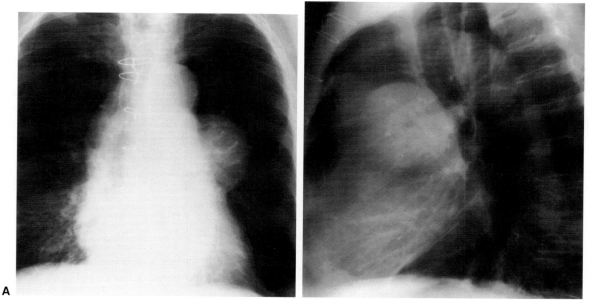

A

B

FIG. 20-6. A 67-year-old man was seen for follow-up after sternotomy and coronary artery bypass. A: The PA chest radiograph shows a smoothly marginated mass projecting over the left hilum. B: The lateral radiograph confirms the presence of a mediastinal mass anterior to the left hilum.

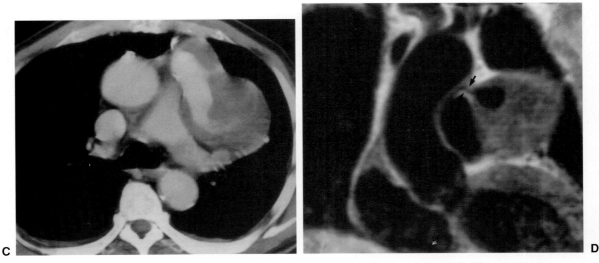

C

D

FIG. 20-6. *Continued.* **C:** The axial CT image demonstrates swirling contrast within this partially thrombosed pseudoaneurysm, which was thought to arise from the ascending aorta at the level of the previous aortotomy. **D:** Coronal MRI reveals a narrow neck (*arrows*) into this partially thrombosed pseudoaneurysm.

graphs using contrast-enhanced CT (38,41). Completely normal CT findings in these patients obviate the need for aortography, since there have been very few, if any, false-negative CT cases reported (i.e., aortic injury and normal CT findings) (42,43).

If the CT demonstrates an abnormal mediastinum, including infiltration of the mediastinal fat due to hemorrhage, particularly around the ligamentum arteriosum (the most common site of aortic injury in patients who survive the initial insult), or irregularity of the aortic lumen, patients should go directly to aortography. In some series, only 10% of those patients with abnormal CT findings have been found to have an aortic transection, and the remaining patients most likely had findings due to shearing of small mediastinal vessels (37,38,41). Occasionally, a direct tear of the aorta with pseudoaneurysm formation can be diagnosed on CT, particularly with helical studies using thin sections (3 to 5 mm) (Figs. 20-8 and 20-9). These patients need no further evaluation. It is suggested at most institutions that if this injury is detected in the acute stage, patients proceed directly to sur-

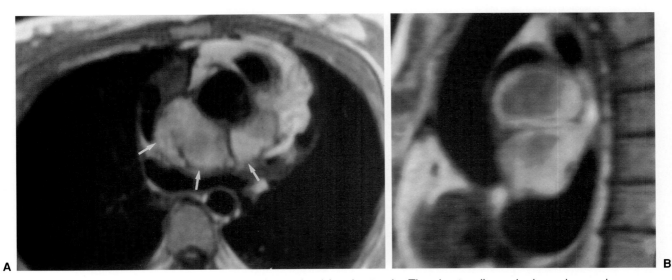

A

B

FIG. 20-7. A 42-year-old woman was examined for chest pain. The chest radiograph showed normal findings. **A:** An axial T2-weighted MR scan demonstrates a heterogeneous mass (*arrows*) posterior to the ascending aorta, which displaces the right atrium laterally and the left atrium posteriorly. **B:** A sagittal oblique MR scan confirms the heterogeneous signal intensity mass displacing both the pulmonary artery and the left atrium.

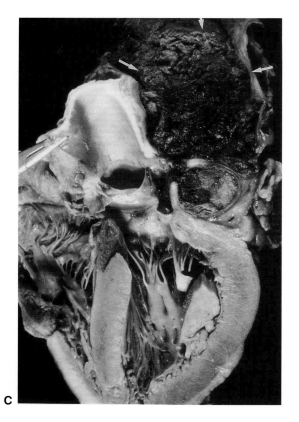

C

FIG. 20-7. *Continued.* **C:** The patient died several days later, and at autopsy this abnormality was shown to be a partially thrombosed sinus of Valsalva aneurysm (*arrows*).

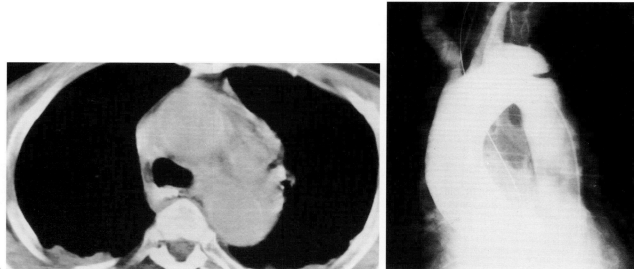

A

B

FIG. 20-8. A 57-year-old man had mediastinal widening following a motor vehicle accident. **A:** An axial CT image at the level of the anteroposterior window shows marked soft-tissue infiltration of the mediastinum, suggestive of mediastinal hematoma. There was concern about a possible aortic rupture. **B:** Aortography confirms the intimal tear from the patient's MVA. The patient was taken to surgery for repair.

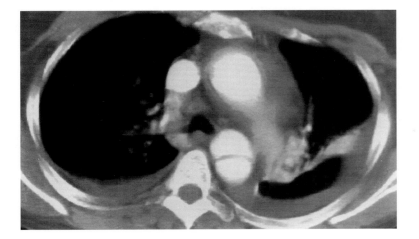

FIG. 20-9. A 51-year-old woman with persistently abnormal chest radiography findings 12 days after a motor vehicle accident. Contrast-enhanced CT at the level of the anteroposterior window shows a tear through the descending aorta with infiltration of the mediastinal fat and a left pleural effusion. The patient went directly to thoracotomy for repair of an aortic transection.

gery for definitive repair, since they are at high risk of rupture and exsanguination.

In high-risk patients with abnormal chest radiography findings, most institutions still proceed directly to aortography, which has a 10% true-positive rate in most series (38,41–43). Even though this rate is low, delayed diagnosis has a significant impact on the patient's outcome. As the technology continues to improve, noninvasive imaging with CT may prove to be a more expeditious means to diagnose this devastating disorder in patients who often have no other underlying medical problem.

REFERENCES

1. Godwin JD. Conventional CT of the aorta. *J Thorac Imaging* 1990;5:18–31.
2. Costello P, Ecker CP, Tello R, Hartnell GG. Assessment of the thoracic aorta by spiral CT. *AJR Am J Roentgenol* 1992;158:1127–1130.
3. Hartnell GG, Finn JP, Zenni M, et al. MR imaging of the thoracic aorta: comparison of spin-echo, angiographic, and breath-hold techniques. *Radiology* 1994;191:697–704.
4. Webb WR, Sostman HD. MR imaging of thoracic disease: clinical uses. *Radiology* 1992;182:621–630.
5. Link KM, Lesko NM. Role of MR imaging in the evaluation of acquired diseases of the thoracic aorta. *AJR Am J Roentgenol* 1992;158:1115–1125.
6. Stanford W, Rooholamini SA, Galvin JR. Ultrafast computed tomography in the diagnosis of aortic aneurysms and dissections. *J Thorac Imaging* 1990;5:32–39.
7. Kazerooni EA, Bree RL, Williams DM. Penetrating atherosclerotic ulcers of the descending thoracic aorta: evaluation with CT and distinction from aortic dissection. *Radiology* 1992;183:759–765.
8. Welch TJ, Stanson AW, Sheedy PFII, Johnson CM, McKusick MA. Radiologic evaluation of penetrating aortic atherosclerotic ulcer. *RadioGraphics* 1990;10:675–685.
9. Hirose Y, Hamada S, Takamiya M, Imakita S, Naito H, Nishimura T. Aortic aneurysms: growth rates measured with CT. *Radiology* 1992;185:249–252.
10. Posniak HV, Olson MC, Demos TC, Benjoya RA, Marsan RE. CT of thoracic aortic aneurysms. *RadioGraphics* 1990;10:839–855.
11. Stanford W, Rooholamini SA, Galvin JR. Ultrafast computed tomography in the diagnosis of aortic aneurysms and dissections. *J Thorac Imag* 1990;5–4:32–39.
12. Yucel EK, Steinberg FL, Egglin TK, Geller SC, Waltman AC, Athanasoulis CA. Penetrating aortic ulcers: diagnosis with MR imaging. *Radiology* 1990;177:779–781.
13. Posniak HV, Demos TC, Marsan RE. Computed tomography of the normal aorta and thoracic aneurysms. *Semin Roentgenol* 1989;24:7–21.
14. Torres WE, Maurer DE, Steinberg HV, et al. CT of aortic aneurysms: the distinction between mural and thrombus calcification. *AJR Am J Roentgenol* 1988;150:1317–1319.
15. Hirose Y, Hamada S, Takamiya M, et al. Aortic aneurysms: growth rates measured with CT. *Radiology* 1992;185:249–252.
16. Demos TC, Posniak HV, Marsan RE. CT of aortic dissection. *Semin Roentgenol* 1989;24:22–37.
17. Gonda RL Jr, Gutierrez OH, Azodo MVU. Mycotic aneurysms of the aorta: radiologic features. *Radiology* 1988;168:343–346.
18. Tottle AJ, Wilde P, Hartnell GG, et al. Diagnosis of acute thoracic aortic dissection using combined echocardiography and computed tomography. *Clin Radiol* 1992;45:104–108.
19. Luker GD, Glazer HS, Eagar GM, Gutierrez FR, Sagel SS. Aortic dissection: effect of prospective chest radiographic diagnosis on delay to definitive diagnosis. *Radiology* 1994;193:813–819.
20. Hamada S, Takamiya M, Kimura K, Imakita S, Nakajima N, Naito H. Type A aortic dissection: evaluation with ultrafast CT. *Radiology* 1992;183:155–158.
21. Wolff KA, Herold CJ, Tempany CM, Parravano JG, Zerhouni EA. Aortic dissection: atypical patterns seen at MR imaging. *Radiology* 1991;181:489–495.
22. Yamada T, Tada S, Harada J. Aortic dissection without intimal rupture: diagnosis with MR imaging and CT. *Radiology* 1988;168:347–352.
23. Spittell PC, Spittell JA Jr, Joyce JW, et al. Clinical features and differential diagnosis of aortic dissection: experience with 236 cases (1980 through 1990). *Radiology* 1994;191:879.
24. Cigarroa JE, Isselbacher EM, DeSanctis RW, et al. Medical progress: diagnostic imaging in the evaluation of suspected aortic dissection. Old standards and new directions. *AJR Am J Roentgenol* 1993;161:485–493.
25. Petasnick JP. Radiologic evaluation of aortic dissection. *Radiology* 1991;180:297–305.
26. Shively BK. Transesophageal echocardiography in the assessment of aortic pathology. *J Thorac Imaging* 1990;5:40–47.
27. Shively BK. Transesophageal echocardiography in the diagnosis of aortic disease. *Semin Ultrasound CT MR* 1993;14:106–116.
28. Fisher ER, Stern EJ, Goodwin II JD, Otto CM, Johnson JA. Acute aortic dissection: typical and atypical imaging features. *RadioGraphics* 1994;14:1263–1271.
29. Landay MJ, Virolainen H. "Hyperdense" aortic wall: potential pitfall in CT screening for aortic dissection. *J Comput Assist Tomogr* 1991;15:561–564.
30. Mantello MT, Panaccione JL, Moriarty PE, et al. Impending rupture of nonaneurysmal bacterial aortitis: CT diagnosis. *J Comput Assist Tomogr* 1990;14:950–953.
31. Yamada I, Numano F, Suzuki S. Takayasu arteritis: evaluation with MR imaging. *Radiology* 1993;188:89–94.
32. Woodard PK, Patz EF, Sostman HD. Pseudoaneurysms at aortic cannulation site after coronary artery bypass graft: MR findings. *J Comput Assist Tomogr* 1992;16:883–887.

33. Sherry CS, Harms SE. MR imaging of pseudoaneurysms in aortocoronary bypass graft. *J Comput Assist Tomogr* 1989;13:426–429.

34. Fisher RG, Chasen MH, Lamki N. Diagnosis of injuries of the aorta and brachiocephalic arteries caused by blunt chest trauma: CT vs aortography. *AJR Am J Roentgenol* 1994;162:1047–1052.

35. Cohen AM, Crass JR, Thomas HA, et al. CT evidence for the ''osseous pinch'' mechanism of traumatic aortic injury. *AJR Am J Roentgenol* 1992;159:271–274.

36. Groskin SA. Selected topics in chest trauma. *Radiology* 1992;183:605–617.

37. Cohen AM, Crass JR. Traumatic lacerations of the aorta and great vessels with a normal mediastinum at radiography. *J Vasc Interv Radiol* 1992;3:541–544.

38. Morgan PW, Goodman LR, Aprahamian C, et al. Evaluation of traumatic aortic injury: Does dynamic contrast-enhanced CT play a role? *Radiology* 1992;182:661–666.

39. Madayag MA, Kirshenbaum KJ, Nadimpalli SR, et al. Thoracic aortic trauma: role of dynamic CT. *Radiology* 1991;179:853–855.

40. Crass JR, Cohen AM, Motta AO, et al. Proposed new mechanism of traumatic aortic rupture: the osseous pinch. *Radiology* 1990;176:645–649.

41. Raptopoulos V, Sheiman RG, Phillips DA, et al. Traumatic aortic tear: screening with chest CT. *Radiology* 1992;182:667–673.

42. Brooks AP, Olson LK, Shackford SR. Computed tomography in the diagnosis of traumatic rupture of the thoracic aorta. *Clin Radiol* 1989;40:133–138.

43. Ishikawa T, Nakajima Y, Kaji T. Role of CT in traumatic rupture of the thoracic aorta and its proximal branches. *Semin Roentgenol* 1989;24:38–46.

Subject Index

Subject Index

Note: Page numbers in italics indicate figures. Page numbers followed by "t" indicate tables.